A Guide to Management of Urological Cancers

Prabhjot Singh
Brusabhanu Nayak
Sridhar Panaiyadiyan
Editors

A Guide to Management of Urological Cancers

Springer

Editors
Prabhjot Singh
Department of Urology
All India Institute of Medical Sciences
New Delhi, Delhi, India

Brusabhanu Nayak
Department of Urology
All India Institute of Medical Sciences
New Delhi, Delhi, India

Sridhar Panaiyadiyan
Department of Urology
All India Institute of Medical Sciences
New Delhi, Delhi, India

ISBN 978-981-99-2340-3 ISBN 978-981-99-2341-0 (eBook)
https://doi.org/10.1007/978-981-99-2341-0

This Springer imprint is published by the registered company Springer Nature Singapore Pte Ltd.
The registered company address is: 152 Beach Road, #21-01/04 Gateway East, Singapore 189721, Singapore

Foreword

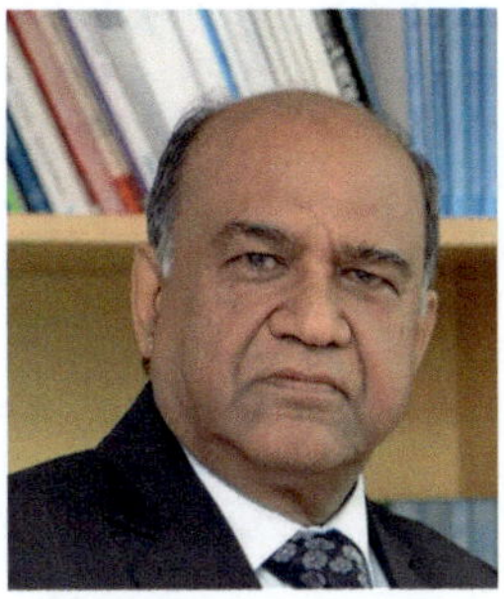

During the period of my career in urology, over the last 50 years, we have come full circle in the arena of management of urogenital cancers. We remain mindful that cancer continues to be a deadly disease if left undetected and untreated in time whereas if detected early when the disease is localized and properly treated, patients can have a normal lifespan as given by God. We have to also remember that one size fits all is unacceptable and proper evaluation by biomarkers, imaging, and genetic assessment is important for personalized care of a urogenital cancer patient.

With the increase in aging population, better imaging, tumor markers, and awareness in doctors and public, the number of cases of genitourinary cancers is increasing worldwide. Science is evolving and every day new research is published in cancer management. Voluminous literature is published in various textbooks and monographs on urogenital cancer. One may get lost how to utilize this literature in clinical management of a patient.

In this book, the authors have divided urogenital cancer into different sections organized by organs. Each section is further subdivided into clinically important topics. Each topic nicely summarizes the existing knowledge available to guide the clinical management of cases. The language is simple and lucid and has relevant bibliography.

I strongly believe that this material will run into a great reference book in urogenital cancer. This will be useful for practicing uro-oncologists, urologists, and postgraduates of urology to understand the subject and use it as a guide for treating patients with urogenital cancers.

I compliment the authors and editors for choosing such an important subject of clinical importance and converting it into a reference book.

N.P. Gupta
Professor Emeritus, Medanta, Medicity Hospital
Gurugram, India

Formerly Professor and Head of Urology,
All India Institute of Medical Sciences
New Delhi, India

Foreword

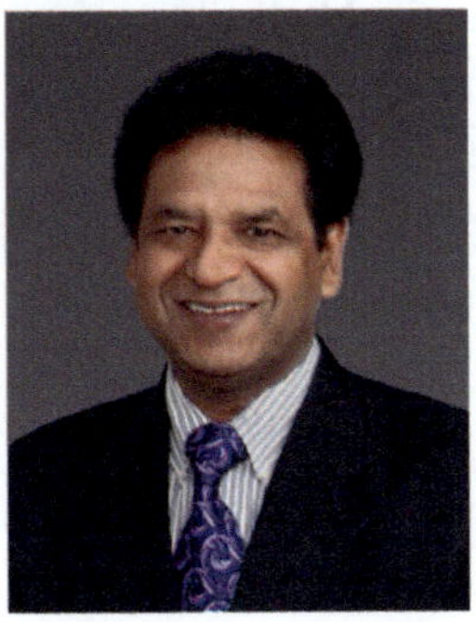

It has been a great privilege and honor for me to write a foreword for this book. The practice of uro-oncology is constantly changing given newer developments, techniques, and research. The editors have done an amazing job inviting devoted and celebrated authors to contribute to this book following evidence-based medicine and guidelines in areas of early detection and cancer prevention, technological innovations, and data sciences with input of precision immunotherapies, chemo-immunotherapy along with personalized medicine. After going through it, I can say this textbook aims to provide comprehensive, state-of-the-art information about the various uro-oncologic cancers in a simplified manner so that it can be easily understood and followed by its readership ranging from residents, fellows, urologists, and medical fraternity. I would like to congratulate the editors Singh, Nayak, and Panaiyadiyan who are well-established physicians in the field of uro-oncology and to all the individual contributors for their insightful contributions toward this book. Knowing editors personally, especially Dr. Singh and Dr. Nayak, who are senior professors at All India Institute of Medical Sciences, New Delhi, India, which I always consider as a Temple of education, as I have had an opportunity to learn and work there. By editing this book, they have done their duty not only as surgeon-scientists but also as educators disseminating knowledge. Of course, for the editors, this has been a huge work but for sure it has been a labor of love, although laborious. This book is a tremendous compendium in the field of uro-oncology, and I look forward to using it in my practice while taking care of patients and in educational opportunities with all of you.

Ashok K. Hemalas, MD, MCh, MAMS, FAMS, FACS, FRCS (Glas)
Professor, Department of Urology
Wake Forest School of Medicine

Chief of Uro-oncology, Comprehensive Cancer Center of Atrium
Health Wake Forest Baptist

Professor, Wake Forest Institute for Regenerative Medicine

Chair, Robotics Committee, Wake Forest Baptist Medical Center

Fellowship Director, Advance Robotics and Minimally
Invasive Surgery, Fellowship Co-Director, Endourology,
Wake Forest Baptist Medical Center &
Wake Forest School of Medicine
Winston-Salem, NC, USA

Ex-Professor of Urology,
All India Institute of Medical Sciences
New Delhi, India

Padma Shri and Dr. B. C. Roy National Awardee
by Honorable President of India

Foreword

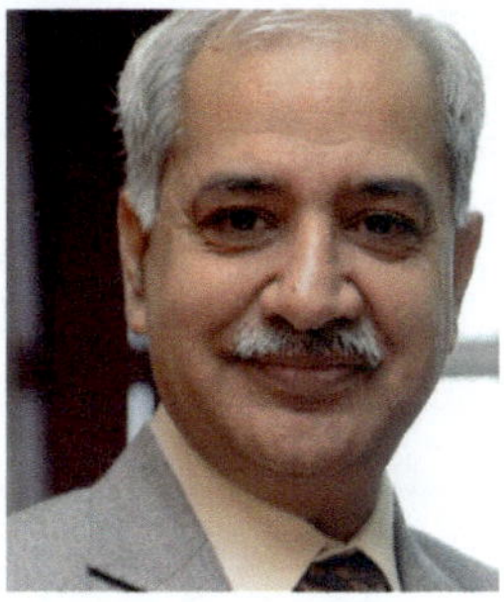

It gives me a great pleasure writing this foreword for this book *A Guide to Management of Urological Cancers*. The field of uro-oncology has been growing very rapidly over the last few decades. It is expected to continue to grow at a similar or even more rapid pace. A new book every few years is required. At the present time, this book will singularly provide a reference resource for the management of all the common urological cancers. Rather than being a guide, the book is a comprehensive and contemporary textbook on urological cancers. All the authors are from major academic centers from across the globe, providing a balanced perspective regarding management of these cancers from different countries. Each chapter is multi-authored. This provides an opportunity for elimination of an individual bias. Experience wise, each author is a consultant with at least a few years of experience in clinical practice as well as teaching and research in the field of uro-oncology. I wish a great success to this book, the success that it deserves. I wish and hope that further editions of this book are brought out every few years.

Amlesh Seth
Professor and Head
Department of Urology
All India Institute of Medical Sciences
New Delhi, India

Member, Governing Council, World Uro-Oncology Federation

Member, Executive Committee, Urological Society of India

Preface

It is an absolute pleasure as editors of this book A Guide to Management of Urological Cancers to write the preface. The inaugural edition of this book encompasses contributions from eminent uro-oncologists, medical oncologists, and radiation oncologists across the globe who share their expertise in managing urological cancers discussing the diagnosis, management, and recent updates in the treatment guidelines. Contribution of such eminent leaders of these fields is essential to our readers.

This edition of the book is a comprehensive review on evaluation and management of all urological cancers. Experts in the field have reviewed the current state of the knowledge on etiology, diagnosis, staging, treatment options, and follow-up strategies of all urological cancers. We have tried to maintain a uniform pattern in creating the chapters on each cancer which will help the readers in better understanding and maintaining the flow while studying.

We hope the contents of this book will immensely help the readers and health care providers for managing urological cancer patients. We have learned a lot while editing the book and hope the same for our readers.

We would like to take this opportunity to thank all our authors for their hard work and contribution for this book and hope this inaugural edition will serve as a reference for urologists to evaluate, treat, and follow urological cancer patients. We would like to thank Springer Nature for their constant support and understanding about this academic endeavor.

New Delhi, India

Prabhjot Singh
Brusabhanu Nayak
Sridhar Panaiyadiyan

Contents

Part I Renal Cell Carcinoma

1 **Diagnosis and Clinical Staging** 3
Aditya Prakash Sharma, Murali Krishna, and Sudheer Kumar Devana

2 **Pathology and Staging** 17
Meenakshi Rao and Balamurugan Thirunavukkarasu

3 **Management of Localized and Locally Advanced RCC** 27
Ravimohan Suryanarayan Mavuduru

4 **Management of Metastatic Renal Cell Carcinoma** 41
Rohit K. Jain, Humaira Sarfraz, Muhammad Z. Farooq, and Guru Sonpavde

5 **Adjuvant Treatment and Follow-Up of Clinically Localized Renal Cell Carcinoma** 53
Jan K. Rudzinski, Benjamin B. Beech, Betty Wang, Guru Sonpavde, and Logan W. Zemp

Part II Upper Tract Urothelial Carcinoma

6 **Diagnosis and Clinical Staging** 73
Utsav Shailesh Shah, Sanjoy Kumar Sureka, and Uday Pratap Singh

7 **Pathology and Staging** 79
Seema Kaushal and Shivangi Dagar

8 **Management** 89
Rahul Jena and Gautam Ram Choudhary

Part III Carcinoma Urinary Bladder

9 **Diagnosis and Clinical Staging** 113
Sammy Gharbieh, Kawa Omar, Ramesh Thurairajah, Muhammed S. Khan, and Rajesh Nair

10 **Pathology and Staging** 125
Gauri Deshpande, Santosh Menon, and Sangeeta Desai

11 **Management of Non-Muscle Invasive Bladder Cancer** 141
Subodh K. Regmi

12 **Management of MIBC** 153
John Hayes, Saachi Chhaya, Harry Manning, Kenrick Ng, Anand Sharma, and Nikhil Vasdev

13 **Metastatic Carcinoma Urinary Bladder, Adjuvant Treatment and Follow-Up** 169
Shuvadeep Ganguly, Sindhu Chitikela, and Atul Batra

Part IV Prostate Cancer

14 **Diagnosis and Clinical Staging** 187
Harshit Garg, Dharam Kaushik, and Michael A. Liss

15 **Pathology and Staging** 209
Moushumi Suryavanshi and Garima Durga

16 **Management of Localized and Locally Advanced Prostate Cancer** 229
Siddharth Yadav and Anup Kumar

17 **Metastatic Prostate Cancer** 241
Sindhu Chitikela, Shuvadeep Ganguly, and Atul Batra

18 **Adjuvant Treatment and Follow Up after Radical Prostatectomy in Prostate Cancer** 257
K. P. Haresh and V. R. Anjali

Part V Penile Cancer

19 **Diagnosis and Clinical Staging** 269
Jyoti Mohan Tosh, Vikas Kumar Panwar, and Ankur Mittal

20 **Pathology and Staging** 279
Subhash Yadav, Santosh Menon, and Sangeeta Desai

21 **Management** 291
Kevin Arulraj, Brusabhanu Nayak, Prabhjot Singh, and Sridhar Panaiyadiyan

22 **Adjuvant Treatment and Follow Up** 303
Kevin Arulraj, Sridhar Panaiyadiyan, Prashant Gupta, Prabhjot Singh, and Brusabhanu Nayak

Part VI Testicular Cancer

23 **Diagnosis and Clinical Staging** 315
Ravi Teja Sepuri and Gagan Prakash

24 Pathology and Staging 325
Pavithra Ayyanar and Suvendu Purkait

25 Management 341
Praful Pandey and Ranjit Kumar Sahoo

26 Retroperitoneal Lymph Node Dissection 359
Ajit Gujela and Gagan Prakash

About the Editors

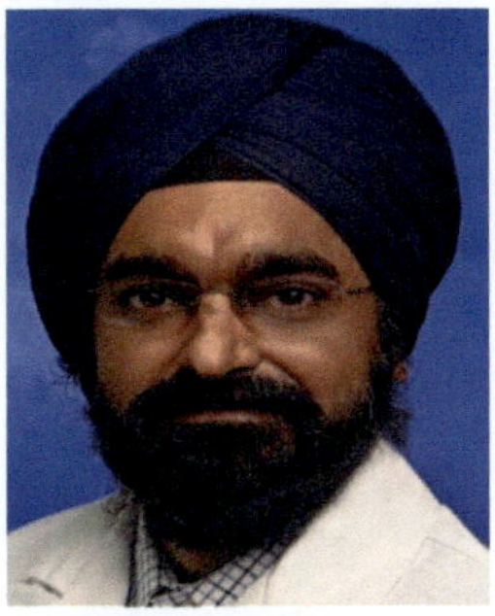

Prabhjot Singh is currently working as a Professor in the department of Urology at All India Institute of Medical Sciences (AIIMS), New Delhi, India. He has completed his surgical residency in Postgraduate Institute of Medical Education and Research, Chandigarh, and received his Urology training at AIIMS, New Delhi. He has a teaching experience of more than 13 years and trained residents in general Urology including Uro-oncology subspecialty. He has published more than 120 researches in various peer-reviewed national and international journals. He also has 15 chapters in edited books to his credit. His core interests include Uro-oncology and Reconstructive Urology subspecialties and has completed many projects related to urological malignancies under Institute intramural and Indian Council of Medical Research grants. He has received many academic awards and fellowships including Best Research award (AIIMS, New Delhi), AUA/IAUA Chakraborty fellowship, IACA travel fellowship, Hargovind Memorial Travel Fellowship, etc. He is an active reviewer and member of Editorial Board for various reputed national and international journals. He has presented research papers, chaired academic sessions, and delivered lectures in various national conferences. He is a member of many urological societies.

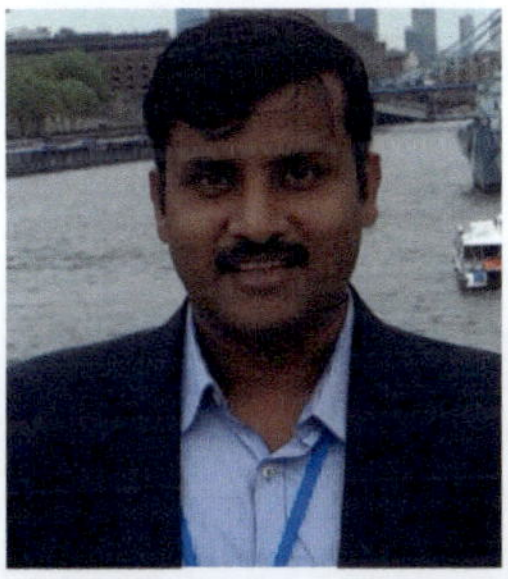

Brusabhanu Nayak is currently working as Additional Professor (Uro-oncology) in the department of Urology at AIIMS, New Delhi, India. He has completed his surgical residency and urological training at AIIMS, New Delhi. He has done his clinical fellowship on Advanced Robotics and Laparoscopy from Clinic St Augustine, Bordeaux, France. He has teaching experience of more than 12 years and has guided many urology trainees in their thesis. He has more than 100 published papers in many national and international journals of repute. He has also authored five chapters in edited books to his credit. He has received many academic awards and fellowships including DUSCON Gold medal for best basic research, Best oncology research award (AIIMS, New Delhi), European Urology Scholarship, JUA fellowship, MIUC International and National Fellowship, AIIMS International Fellowship, Hargovind Memorial Travel Fellowship, etc. Uro-oncology has been his core area of interest and he has completed many intramural and extramural (ICMR)-funded projects in the same. He has contributed many researches focusing on various prognostic and predictive biomarkers applied in the subspecialty of Uro-oncology. He has chaired academic sessions, presented papers, and delivered lectures in various national and international conferences. He is a reviewer of many reputed journals besides being an active member of many urological societies.

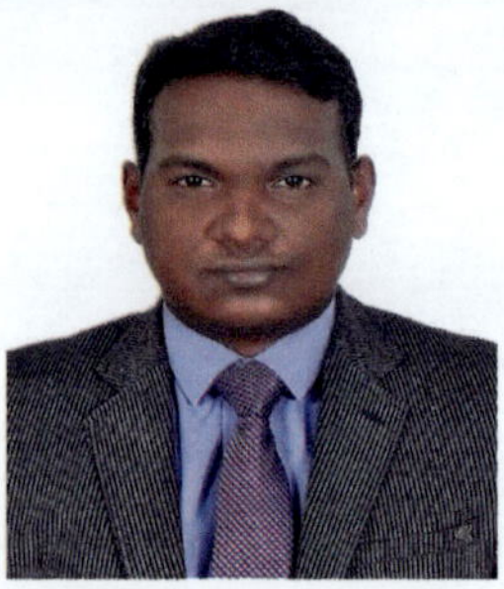

Sridhar Panaiyadiyan is currently working as an Assistant Professor in the department of Uro-oncology at the National Cancer Institute (NCI), Jhajjar campus under AIIMS, New Delhi, India. He has completed his general surgery and urological training at AIIMS, New Delhi. He has completed a fellowship in Minimal Invasive Urology at the same institute. He has 6 years of teaching experience and has published more than 30 research papers in various national and international journals to his credit. This includes many researches in Uro-oncology subspecialty. He has received many academic awards including Marudhara Jodhpur best paper, USI Best paper award, etc. He has also contributed to three chapters in edited books. He has presented many research papers in national conferences and has won many awards for his clinical research. He is an active member of many urological societies.

Part I

Renal Cell Carcinoma

Diagnosis and Clinical Staging

1

Aditya Prakash Sharma, Murali Krishna, and Sudheer Kumar Devana

1.1 Introduction

Renal cell carcinoma (RCC) is the eighth most common cancer worldwide. It continues to be predominantly a surgical disease where radical nephrectomy or nephron-sparing surgery being the most frequently performed procedure worldwide. Even in advanced stages of renal cancer, surgery in the form of cytoreductive nephrectomy is performed to decrease the tumor burden. Diagnosis based on symptomatology and imaging helps to stage the disease preoperatively. Staging helps to decide the best surgical option and also predicts the surgical outcome. It also helps to predict the final oncological outcome.

1.2 Diagnosis of Renal Cancer

1.2.1 Clinical Diagnosis of Renal Cancer

RCC was earlier described by the characteristic clinical triad of lump abdomen, flank pain, and hematuria. Currently, patients are often detected incidentally (up to 50%) to have renal mass on imaging done for evaluation of other pathology or during routine medical checkup. In the other half of patients, hematuria and flank pain continue to be the predominant presenting symptoms. The presence of palpable mass occurs in less than 10% patients of RCC. Other symptoms like lower limb edema, ascites due to venacaval obstruction, generalized weakness, loss of weight, and appetite are seen in patients with advanced metastatic RCC.

Physical examination is essentially normal in most cases. Clinical findings may include a palpable lump in the flank or varicocele. A nonreducible varicocele is a surrogate marker for RCC, which usually happens in case of a large renal mass causing obstruction of the gonadal vein.

Urine analysis may be helpful in detecting microscopic hematuria in patients of renal mass.

1.2.2 Paraneoplastic Syndromes

Totally, 10–40% patients of RCC may develop paraneoplastic syndromes [1]. It may also be a presenting symptom in some patients of RCC. The syndromes may be classified as endocrine and nonendocrine (Table 1.1). The most common para-neoplastic syndrome associated with RCC is hypercalcemia [2]. Most patients with hypercalcemia have advanced-stage malignancy. The pathophysiology behind hypercalce-

A. P. Sharma (✉) · M. Krishna · S. K. Devana
Department of Urology, Postgraduate Institute of Medical Education and Research, Chandigarh, India

P. Singh et al. (eds.), *A Guide to Management of Urological Cancers*,
https://doi.org/10.1007/978-981-99-2341-0_1

Table 1.1 Paraneoplastic syndromes

Endocrine	Nonendocrine
Hypercalcemia	Amyloidosis
Hypertension	Anemia
Polycythaemia	Neuromyopathies
Nonmetastatic hepatic dysfunction	Vasculopathy
Galactorrhea	Nephropathy
Cushing's syndrome	Coagulopathy
Alterations in glucose metabolism	Prostaglandin elevation

mia has been suggested to be the secretion of *parathormone-related peptide* (PTHrP). PTHrP acts on PTH receptors and leads to increased bone resorption and decreased renal calcium clearance [3]. Hypercalcemia can also be a result of extensive bone metastasis; however, this does not qualify as a paraneoplastic syndrome.

Another common paraneoplastic syndrome is hypertension [4]. Potential mechanism involves secretion of renin, parenchymal compression, presence of arterio-venous fistula, and polycythaemia [5]. Polycythaemia is also noted in 1–8% of patients with RCC. This commonly occurs secondary to the secretion of erythropoietin (EPO). Stauffer's syndrome characterized by hepatic dysfunction is another peculiar paraneoplastic syndrome associated with RCC [5]. Various nonmetastatic hypotheses for hepatic dysfunction include secretion of hepatotoxins by tumor and aberrant production of IL-6 leading to liver injury.

1.3 Imaging Diagnosis

Various imaging techniques are available to better characterize the renal masses whether benign or malignant, presence of necrosis, number of renal vessels, extent of tumor thrombus in renal vein and IVC, local invasion to surrounding structures, associated lymphadenopathy, and metastasis.

1.4 Ultrasound

In most cases of renal mass, ultrasound is often the first modality of investigation a patient has undergone. At times, the patient undergoes ultrasound abdomen for some other complaints and is incidentally detected to have a renal mass. RCC may appear hyper-echoic, iso-echoic, or hypo-echoic in comparison to the surrounding renal parenchyma. Tumor pseudo-capsule may be visualized as hypoechoic halo. Ultrasound helps in differentiating between a solid or cystic renal mass. Detection of renal vein thrombus or inferior vena caval thrombus is another area where USG with color doppler is particularly helpful. The advantages of easy availability and noninvasiveness are, however, offset by nonreproducibility and poor sensitivity.

1.4.1 Contrast-Enhanced Ultrasound

Contrast-enhanced ultrasound (CEUS) is a newer modality utilizing contrast-containing micro-bubbles injected before ultrasound to visualize blood perfusion in real time. RCC in particular has neo-angiogenesis with new capillary formation. CEUS features of renal cancer include quick take-up of contrast agent during cortical phase with enhancement more or equal to renal parenchyma. In late medulla or delayed phase, there is quick drainage of contrast agent from the lesion. As per literature, the sensitivity and specificity of CEUS in diagnosing renal cancer are 97% and 86%, respectively [6]. Other advantages of CEUS over conventional USG are the display rate of pseudo-capsule and detection of hemorrhagic or necrotic foci are higher. Advantages over CT scan are lack of radiation exposure, real-time imaging, and better appreciation of smaller blood vessels. Disadvantages of CEUS include inability to detect distant metastasis and inter-observer variability.

A particularly important application of CEUS is in further characterization of cystic renal masses. Traditionally, contrast-enhanced CT scan has been used for diagnosis and risk stratification of these masses. Bosniak classification discussed later gives an idea regarding the malignant potential of cystic renal masses. Bosniak grades IIF and III, however, need further characterization as the risk of malignancy in this group ranges from 5 to 60%. The higher spatial and temporal resolution allows better detection of contrast enhancement of thin cyst walls and septa thus allowing for better characterization [7]. Use of CEUS for follow-up on Bosniak IIF lesions is also described. On follow-up CEUS, 7.1% of Bosniak IIF lesions showed upstaging [8]. The rate of malignancy in CEUS-characterized Bosniak III cyst was 66%, which was relatively high as compared to other imaging modalities [9].

1.5 Contrast-Enhanced Computerized Tomography (CECT)

Multiphasic CECT is the investigation of choice for the evaluation of renal masses. The stages of a renal-specific CT include unenhanced phase, corticomedullary phase (25–70 s), nephrographic phase (80–180 s), and excretory phase (>180 s) [10]. Majority of RCCs present as a solid mass on imaging with attenuation values of ≥20 HU on unenhanced CT (Fig. 1.1). Small tumors may have a homogeneous appearance, while larger tumors appear heterogeneous due to hemorrhage or necrosis. During the cortico-medullary phase, renal cortex enhances more due to contrast in cortical capillaries and peritubular spaces. Opacification of renal vasculature also occurs in this phase. This is important in understanding the arterial anatomy in cases planned for nephron-sparing surgery and to rule out the presence of tumor thrombus in the renal vein [11]. During the nephrographic phase, the renal parenchyma enhances homogeneously and helps in easy differentiation between tumor and normal tissue. The different CT characteristics of various renal masses are given in Table 1.2.

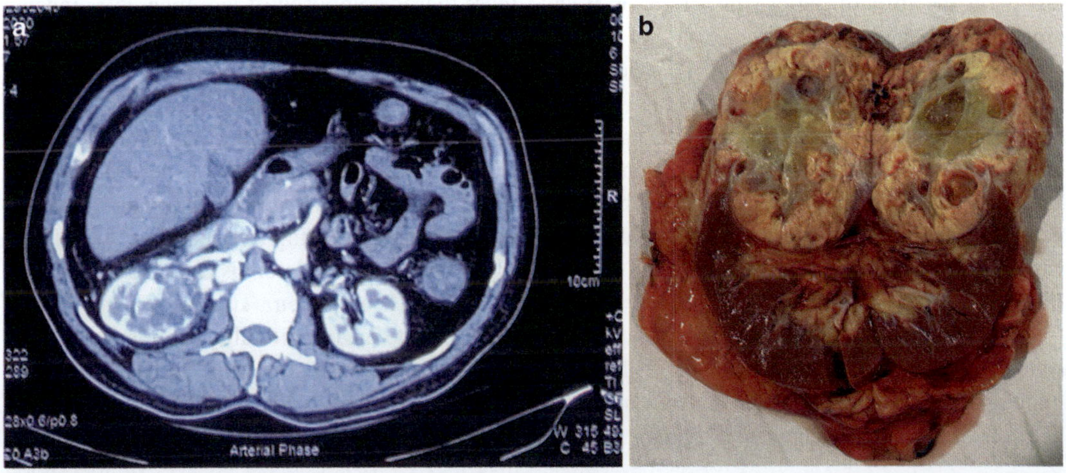

Fig. 1.1 (**a**) Contrast-enhanced computerized tomogram showing enhancing mass lesion suggestive of renal cell carcinoma. (**b**) Cross-section examination of radical nephrectomy specimen showing RCC

Table 1.2 CT characteristics of renal space occupying lesions

Renal pathology	CT characteristics
Angiomyolipoma	−10 HU or less on unenhanced CT (Fig. 1.2)
Cysts	Homogenous lesion with smooth wall
	Attenuation between −10 HU and +20 HU
	Attenuation >70 HU suggestive of hemorrhagic cyst
Clear cell RCC	Strong enhancement in cortico-medullary phase (114 ± 44 HU) and washout effect during nephrographic phase (66 ± 24 HU)
Papillary RCC	Contrast enhancement up to 20 HU in cortico-medullary phase compared to unenhanced phase

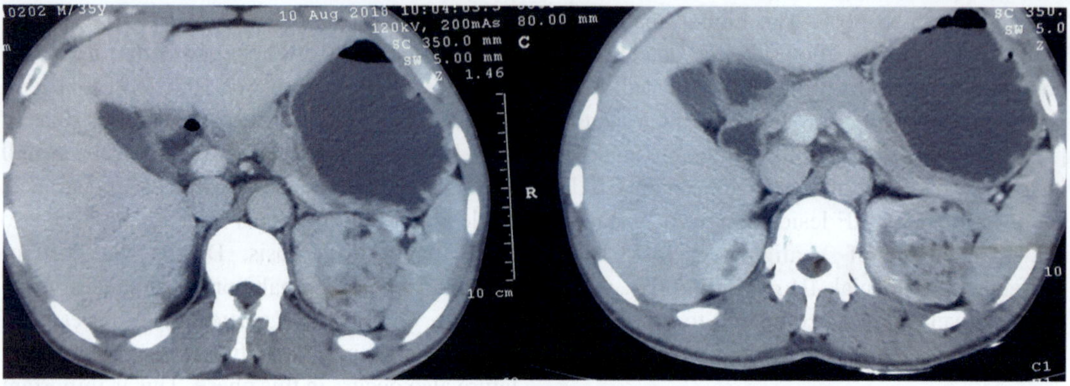

Fig. 1.2 CECT showing mass lesion with fatty attenuation suggestive of angiomyolipoma

The sensitivity and specificity of CT scan in prediction of RCC range from 60–79% to 44–100%, respectively [12]. The size of the tumor is another major predicting factor with 1 cm increase in tumor size leading to 16% increase in risk of malignancy [13].

A useful strategy is to categorize renal masses based on the growth pattern into Ball or Bean type (Figs. 1.3 and 1.4). Ball type of renal mass is commonly encountered on CECT, where the mass while growing compresses the surrounding structures like the calyceal system with a pseudocapsule formation and deformation of renal contour. Hence, these masses can be seen both on unenhanced and contrast-enhanced images. This is classically seen in RCC or other benign masses (Fig. 1.3). Bean types of renal masses are infiltrative in nature without any definitive pseudocapsule, and the reniform shape of kidney is maintained. Bean type of renal masses may not be seen clearly on unenhanced CT images. This is classically seen in urothelial carcinoma of pelvis or calyces (Fig. 1.4).

Cystic renal masses are commonly encountered during imaging. To better stratify the risk of malignancy in cystic tumor, Bosniak classification w s introduced which has been recently updated in 2019. A cystic renal mass is defined as mass that is composed of less than 25% enhancing component. Renal abscess may at times mimic complex a renal cysts (Fig. 1.5).The updated Bosniak classification is given in Table 1.3. In addition to detection of renal masses, CT scan is also able to assess the loco-regional status of the disease. Information such as presence of enlarged lymph nodes, liver metastasis, renal vein, or IVC thrombus can also be obtained from CECT abdomen. The advantages of CT scan include easy availability, easy reproducibility, ability to reformat images, and a quick acquisition time. The disadvantages are radiation exposure and use of iodinated contrast.

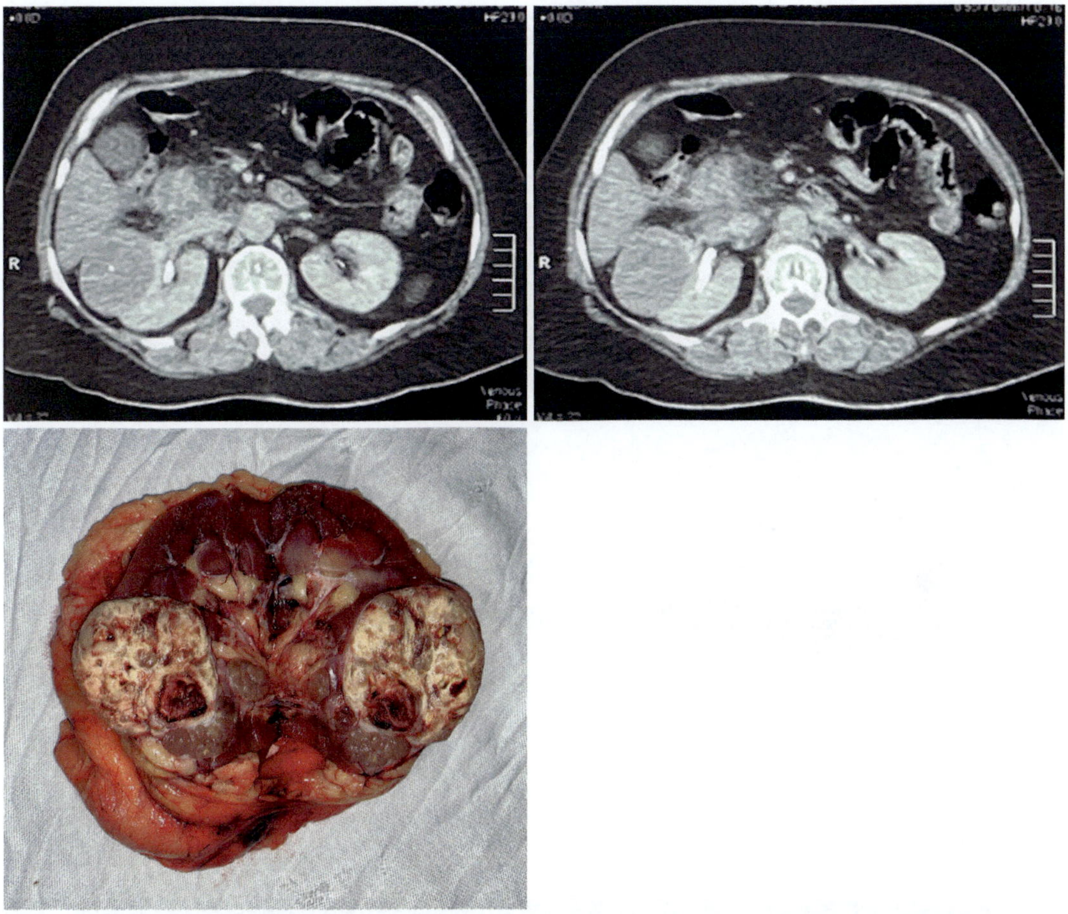

Fig. 1.3 Classical ball-shaped pattern of renal mass. The patient underwent nephrectomy, and the pathology was clear cell carcinoma

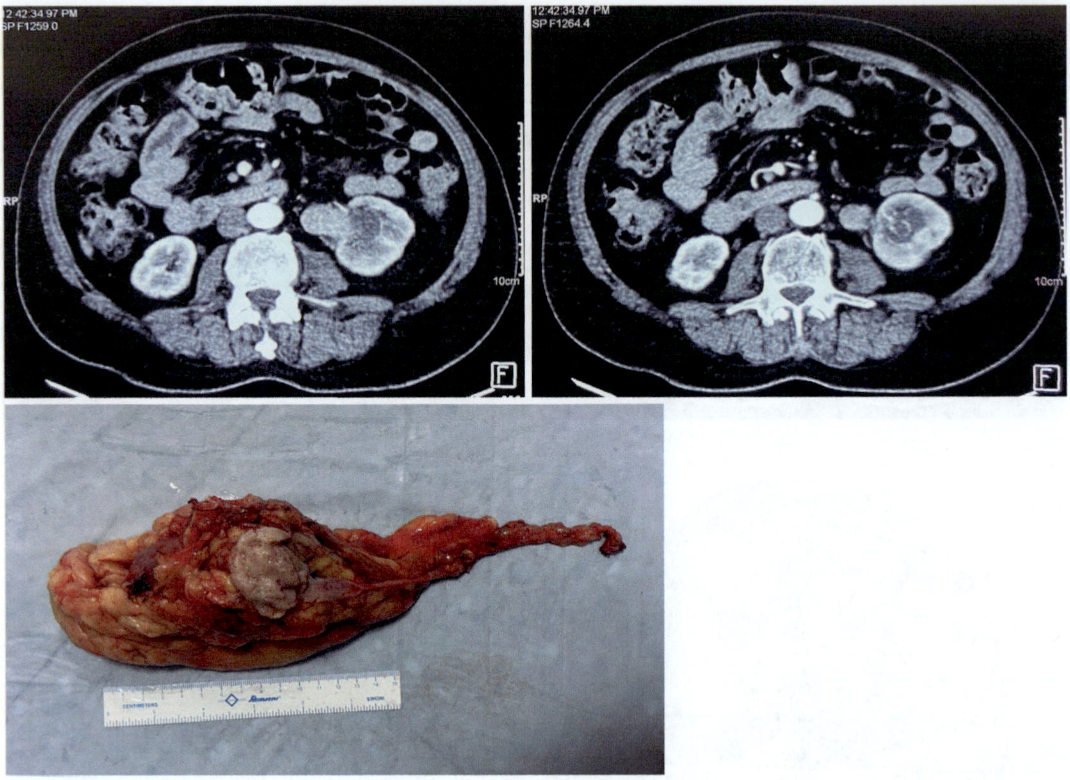

Fig. 1.4 Classical bean-shaped pattern of renal mass. The patient underwent radical nephrouretrectomy, and pathology was urothelial carcinoma

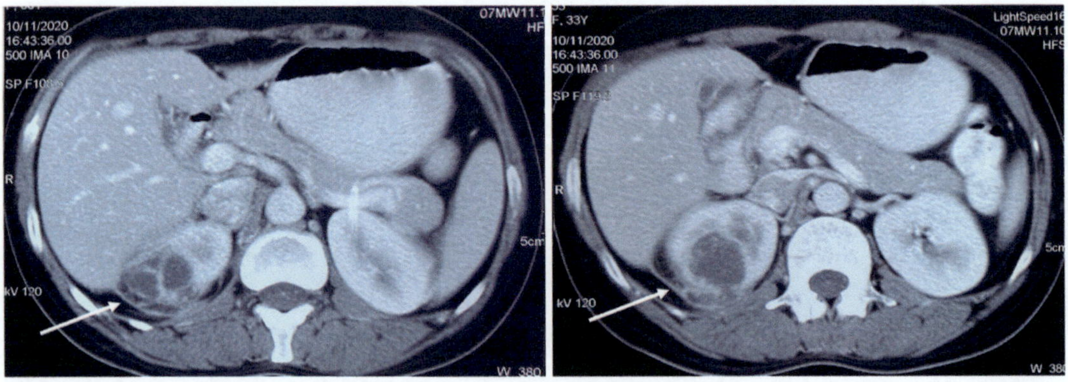

Fig. 1.5 Renal abscess may mimic complex renal cysts at times. History and examination findings help in clinching the diagnosis in such cases

Table 1.3 Bosniak classification of renal cysts on CT scan

Class	Bosniak classification 2019
I	Well-defined, thin (≤2 mm) smooth wall; homogeneous simple fluid (−9 to 20 HU); no septa or calcifications; the wall may enhance
II	Six types, all well defined with thin (≤2 mm) smooth walls:
	1. Cystic masses with thin (≤2 mm) and few (one to three) septa; septa and wall may enhance; may have calcification of any type
	2. Homogenous hyperattenuating (≥70 HU) cystic masses at noncontrast CT
	3. Homogeneous nonenhancing cystic masses >20 HU at renal mass protocol CT, may have calcification of any type
	4. Homogeneous cystic masses −9 to 20 HU at noncontrast CT
	5. Homogeneous cystic masses 21 to 30 HU at portal venous phase CT
	6. Homogeneous low attenuation cystic masses that are too small to characterize
IIF	Cystic masses with a smooth minimally thickened (3 mm) enhancing wall or smooth minimal thickening (3 mm) of one or more enhancing septa, or many (≥4) smooth thin (≤2 mm) enhancing septa
III	One or more enhancing thick (≥4 mm width) or enhancing irregular (displaying ≤3 mm obtusely margined convex protrusions) walls or septa
IV	One or more enhancing nodules (≥4 mm convex protrusion with obtuse margins, or a convex protrusion of any size that has acute margins)

1.6 Magnetic Resonance Imaging

Though CT scan is the imaging modality of choice for characterization of renal masses, the requirement of use of iodinated contrast makes it not suitable for patients with compromised renal function. In such cases, magnetic resonance imaging (MRI) with gadolinium contrast is a safer alternative. Caution should be exercised in patients with GFR <30 mL/min/1.73 m^2 as use of gadolinium contrast risks the occurrence of nephrogenic systemic fibrosis [14]. MRI can also be used as an add-on investigation in tumors that appear indeterminate on USG or CT. The recommended sequences in a renal protocol MRI are T2W single-shot fast spin, T1W gradient echo in/out, T1W SPGR with fat saturation precontrast, and T1WSPGR with fat saturation post contrast. Delayed post-contrast sequence and diffusion-weighted imaging sequences are optional [15]. MRI is also useful in situations where there is any doubt in invasion of inferior venacava by the tumor thrombus in locally advanced RCC.

The various MRI characteristics of renal lesions are described in Table 1.4 [16].

Table 1.4 MRI characteristics of renal lesions

Renal pathology	MRI characteristics
Clear cell RCC	T1W: Isointense to surrounding parenchyma
	T2W: Hyperintense/heterogenous signal
	Heterogeneous enhancement post contrast
Papillary RCC	Well circumscribed and homogeneous
	T2W: Low signal intensity
	Less avidity and slower enhancement post contrast
Chromophobe RCC	Well circumscribed and homogeneous
	T2W: Intermediate to low signal intensity
	Enhancement pattern less avid than ccRCC but more avid than pRCC
Angiomyolipoma	T1W: High signal intensity
	Fat suppressed sequence: Low signal intensity
	T2W: Signal intensity as per fat content
Oncocytoma	T1W: Low signal intensity
	T2W: High and heterogeneous signal intensity

ccRCC clear cell renal cell carcinoma, *pRCC* papillary renal cell carcinoma

Table 1.5 Bosniak classification for renal cysts on MRI

Class	Bosniak classification 2019
I	Well-defined, thin (≤2 mm) smooth wall; homogeneous simple fluid (signal intensity similar to CSF); no septa or calcifications; the wall may enhance
II	Three types, all well-defined with thin (≤2 mm) smooth walls:
	1. Cystic masses with thin (≤2 mm) and few (one to three) enhancing septa; any nonenhancing septa; may have calcification of any type
	2. Homogenous masses markedly hyperintense at T2-weighted imaging (similar to CSF) at noncontrast MRI
	3. Homogeneous masses markedly hyperintense on T1-weighted imaging (approximately × 2.5 normal parenchymal signal intensity) at noncontrast MRI
IIF	Two types:
	1. Cystic masses with a smooth minimally thickened (3 mm) enhancing wall or smooth minimal thickening (3 mm) of one or more enhancing septa, or many (≥4) smooth thin (≤2 mm) enhancing septa
	2. Cystic masses that are heterogeneously hyperintense at noncontrast fat saturated T1-weighted imaging
III	One or more enhancing thick (≥4 mm width) or enhancing irregular (displaying ≤3 mm obtusely margined convex protrusions) walls or septa
IV	One or more enhancing nodules (≥4 mm convex protrusion with obtuse margins, or a convex protrusion of any size that has acute margins)

Similar to CT scan, cystic lesions on MRI are also classified according to Bosniak classification which has been modified for MRI. The advantages of MRI are absence of ionizing radiation and use of safer contrast in the form of gadolinium. The disadvantages are longer acquisition time and risk of nephrogenic systemic fibrosis in patients of CKD Table 1.5.

1.7 FDG PET/CT

FDG PET/CT has a limited role in management of RCC. Physiological excretion of FDG in urine limits visualization of renal masses. Though several protocols such as forced diuresis with hydration to increase clearance of FDG from kidney have been tried, and the pooled sensitivity remains at 50–60%. Studies have shown that quantification of SUVmax may play a role in predicting the biological behavior of the renal lesion. Higher SUVmax is associated with poorer prognosis and increased risk of metastasis. Another important role of FDG PET is in the detection of metastasis during the follow-up period. Around 30% patients develop metastasis after undergoing nephrectomy for localized disease. PET CT was able to diagnose local recurrence and metastatic disease with a sensitivity of 90% and specificity of 91%. FDG PET is also useful in differentiating tumor thrombus versus bland thrombus in inferior vena cava (IVC).

With the advent of tyrosine kinase inhibitors and immune check point inhibitors, management of metastatic RCC has undergone tremendous changes. Tumor response evaluation following these therapies has been done conventionally using CT scan and following the RECIST criteria. Using PET scan change in SUVmax value of metastatic lesions following systemic therapy is used as a marker of future oncological outcome. A recent study showed that reduction in SUVmax posttreatment was associated with increased overall survival and progression-free survival.

1.8 Renal Mass Biopsy

The role of renal mass biopsy (RMB) for diagnosing renal cancer is controversial. In the era of radical nephrectomy and partial nephrectomy, presurgery biopsy did not impact the final surgical procedure. Added concerns regarding the safety in terms of tumor seeding or implantation and diagnostic accuracy of RMB led to this procedure being used less often in clinical practice.

In the current era, most renal masses are detected incidentally on imaging. With the advances in imaging technology, renal malignancy can be diagnosed with high sensitivity and specificity in almost all cases. However, some cases may still pose a clinical dilemma. Differentiation between RCC and benign tumors such as fat poor AML or oncocytoma is still not possible with sufficient accuracy.

RMB can affect treatment decisions especially if active surveillance is being considered for a suspected benign renal mass. The median diagnostic yield for malignancy on RMB was 92% in a systematic review. Also in small renal masses, the sensitivity and specificity were 99.7% and 98.2%, respectively [17]. Concordance between tumor grade and renal biopsy ranges between 62.5% and 87%. Nondiagnostic biopsy can also occur and is most commonly due to inaccurate targeting of the lesion. Use of core biopsy needle and imaging-guided biopsy can help in decreasing the rate of nondiagnostic biopsy. Serious complications after renal mass biopsy are a rare occurrence. The most common complication is minor bleeding. Tumor tract seeding is extremely rare.

The indications for renal mass biopsy are as follows [18] in a patient with a known extrarenal malignancy, caused by an inflammatory process such as infection, findings suggestive of unresectable cancer, severe medical comorbidities considered for surgery, considered for percutaneous ablation or stereotactic radiotherapy, multiple or bilateral masses, masses in a solitary kidney or transplant kidney, and clinical T1a (≤4 cm) RCC.

1.9 Staging of Renal Cell Cancer

Robson provided the first ever staging for renal masses in 1963 [19, 20]. The four stages were divided as follows: Stage 1: Tumor within capsule. Stage 2: Tumor invasion of perinephric fat, confined to the gerota fascia. Stage 3: Tumor involvement of regional lymph nodes, renal vein, or vena cava. Stage 4: Adjacent organ involvement or distant metastases [19, 20]. This staging had lot of drawbacks such as it combined the poor prognostic lymph node involvement with a potentially curable renal vein involvement. The tumor size was not accounted for, and the extent of the venous thrombus was not mentioned [20]. The TNM system proposed by AJCC/UICC was adopted and brought succinct anatomic delineation of the disease and reflected the tumor biology and prognosis more accurately [21]. In the case of bilateral renal masses, both masses are staged separately (Fig. 1.6).

The TNM staging of renal cell cancer is used for all histopathological variants of RCC as given in AJCC/UICC [21]. The T stage is shown in Fig. 1.7. For nodal staging, N0 denotes: no regional lymph node metastasis and N1 denotes metastasis in regional lymph node(s). In M

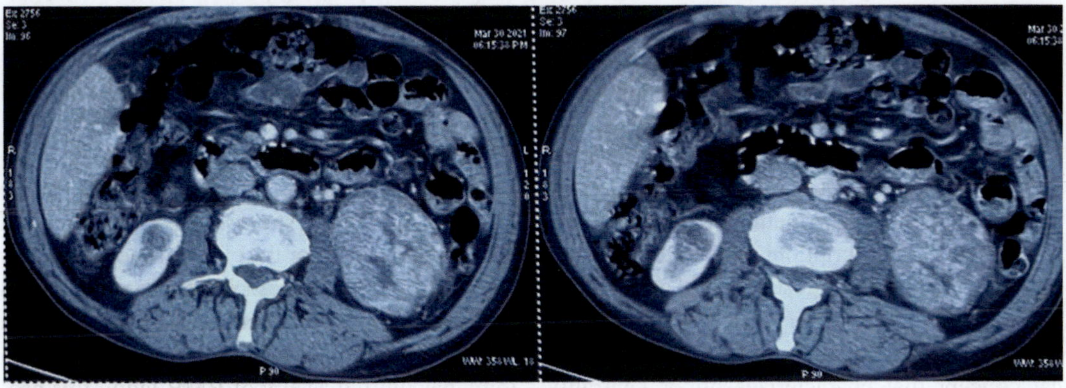

Fig. 1.6 CECT showing bilateral renal masses which may pose a challenge while staging

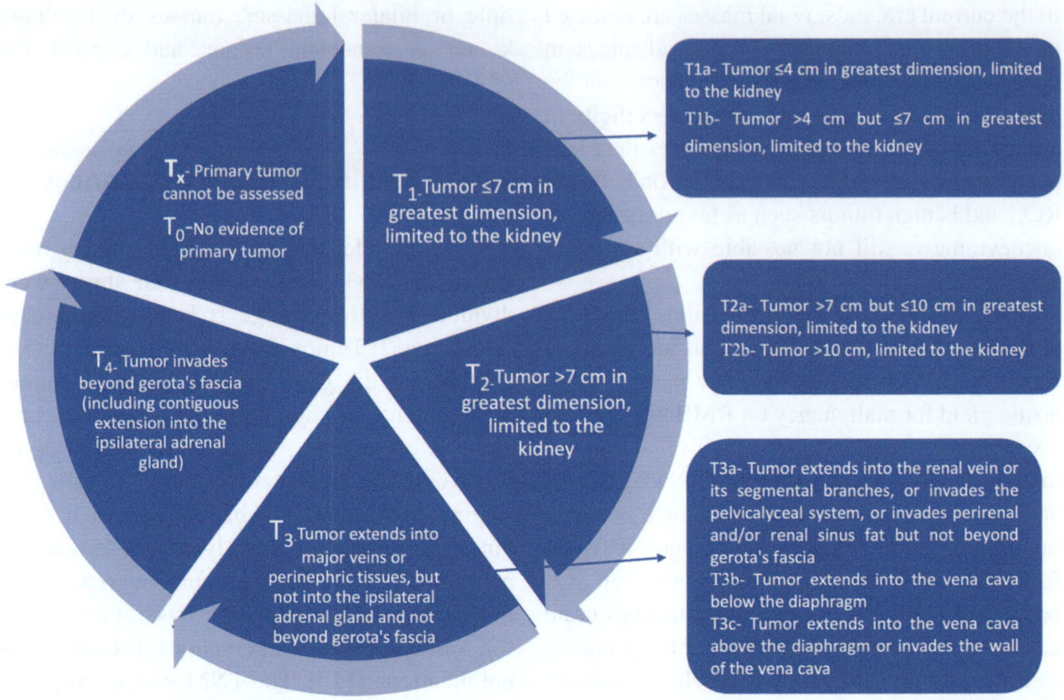

Fig. 1.7 AJCC T staging of renal cancer

staging, M0 denotes No distant metastasis, whereas M1 denotes presence of distant metastasis.

1.10 Nephrometry Scores

Although not a part of staging process, the tumor complexity is one of the prime factors deciding the management strategy for RCC [22, 23]. There are several scoring systems available for determining the tumor complexity and thereby guiding the surgeon regarding decision making whether a partial nephrectomy would be feasible and in deciding the approach to the surgery [23–27]. Two most commonly used scoring systems are RENAL and PADUA scores, which involve similar components and methodology, enabling a comprehensive description of the tumor size, polarity, location, and closeness to the collecting system [23, 24]. Other index such as the C-INDEX score involves a complex mathematical concept that characterizes tumor centrality based on the ratio of the distance between the tumor and kidney center and tumor radius [24]. Other nephrometry scores that have been used are arterial-based complexity [28]. This score was based on whether the tumor is involving the cortex or medulla or reaching upto the sinus fat or to the collecting system and the branches of the arterial tree involved. The Mayo Adhesive Probability score was developed to predict whether the sticky perinephric fat is going to cause difficulty during partial nephrectomy [29].

The scoring systems have also been used to predict the perioperative outcomes especially the combined outcomes such as Trifecta and Pentafecta outcomes after partial nephrectomy [30]. However, none of the scores have been found to be superior to the other [24]. The prime utility of scoring systems is now to provide a standard language for the clinicians to communicate about the tumor complexity. Even the initial premise that low-complexity tumors need partial and high-complexity tumor need radical nephrectomy has blurred as even higher complex tumors

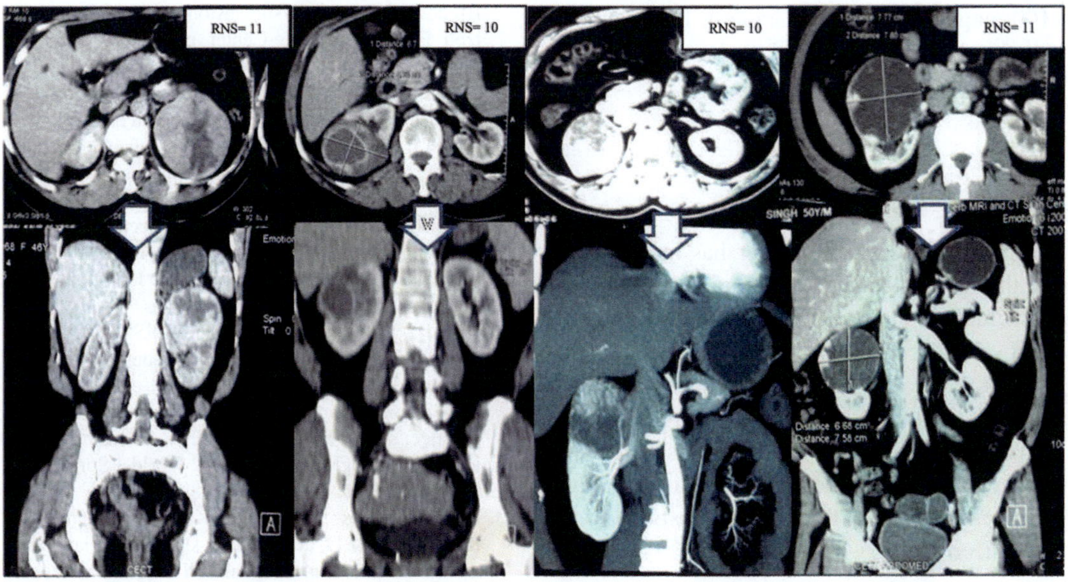

Fig. 1.8 RENAL nephrometry scoring system for scoring tumor complexity. CT images of highly complex renal masses. RNS, RENAL nephrometry score

Table 1.6 Nephrometry scoring

RENAL	1 point	2 points	3 points
R (radius, maximal diameter) (cm)	≤4	>4 but <7	≥7
E (exophytic/endophytic)	≥50% exophytic	<50% exophytic	Completely endophytic
N (nearness to collecting system/renal sinus) (mm)	≥7	>4 but <7	≤4
A (anterior/posterior locator)	No points given. Descriptor of "a," "p," or "x" assigned to describe mass location		
L (location relative to polar lines)	Entirely below lower polar or above upper polar line	Mass crosses polar line	50% of mass is across polar line or mass is entirely between polar lines or mass crosses axial midline

are being managed with partial nephrectomy (Fig. 1.8). The details of these scoring systems are discussed later in Table 1.6.

1.11 Grading of Renal Cell Carcinoma

The International Society of Uropathology Pathology (ISUP) grading is used to grade the histopathology of tumor. The new system replaces the older system of Fuhrman grading for clear cell carcinoma [31]. The ISUP proposed this novel grading system based on the evaluation of the nucleoli. These grading systems also bear the prognostic significance on outcomes of RCC especially recurrence-free survival and overall survival.

Grade 1: inconspicuous nucleoli and basophilic at ×400 magnification. Grade 2: nucleoli that are clearly visible at ×400 magnification and eosinophilic; Grade 3: clearly visible nucleoli at

×100 magnification; and Grade 4: have extreme pleomorphism or rhabdoid and/or sarcomatoid morphology.

1.12 Conclusions

Diagnosis of renal cell cancer has moved from one that at as advanced symptoms to that being an incidental diagnosis. Imaging modality has improved over the years, and a categorical diagnosis of RCC can be made preoperatively and need for tissue diagnosis before surgery is seldom needed. TNM staging of RCC as per AJCC/UICC entails both clinical and pathological stage, and it remains one of the best prognostic tools for this cancer.

References

1. Palapattu GS, Kristo B, Rajfer J. Paraneoplastic syndromes in urologic malignancy: the many faces of renal cell carcinoma. Rev Urol. 2002;4(4):163–70.
2. Chasan SA, Pothel LR, Huben RP. Management and prognostic significance of hypercalcemia in renal cell carcinoma. Urology. 1989;33(3):167–70.
3. Goldberg MF, Tashjian AH Jr, Order SE, Dammin GJ. Renal adenocarcinoma containing a parathyroid hormone-like substance and associated with marked hypercalcemia. Am J Med. 1964;36:805–14.
4. Kirchner FK Jr, Braren V, Smith C, Wilson JP, Foster JH, Hollifield JW, et al. Renal carcinoma discovered incidentally by arteriography during evaluation for hypertension. J Urol. 1976;115(6):643–5.
5. Dahl T, Eide I, Fryjordet A. Hypernephroma and hypertension. Two case reports. Acta Med Scand. 1981;209(1-2):121–4.
6. Pan KH, Jian L, Chen WJ, Nikzad AA, Kong FQ, Bin X, et al. Diagnostic performance of contrast-enhanced ultrasound in renal cancer: a meta-analysis. Front Oncol. 2020;10:586949.
7. Quaia E, Bertolotto M, Cioffi V, Rossi A, Baratella E, Pizzolato R, et al. Comparison of contrast-enhanced sonography with unenhanced sonography and contrast-enhanced CT in the diagnosis of malignancy in complex cystic renal masses. AJR Am J Roentgenol. 2008;191(4):1239–49.
8. Defortescu G, Cornu JN, Bejar S, Giwerc A, Gobet F, Werquin C, et al. Diagnostic performance of contrast-enhanced ultrasonography and magnetic resonance imaging for the assessment of complex renal cysts: a prospective study. Int J Urol. 2017;24(3):184–9.
9. Schwarze V, Rubenthaler J, Cecatka S, Marschner C, Froelich MF, Sabel BO, et al. Contrast-enhanced ultrasound (CEUS) for the evaluation of Bosniak III complex renal cystic lesions-a 10-year specialized European Single-Center experience with histopathological validation. Medicina (Kaunas). 2020;56(12):692.
10. Birnbaum BA, Jacobs JE, Ramchandani P. Multiphasic renal CT: comparison of renal mass enhancement during the corticomedullary and nephrographic phases. Radiology. 1996;200(3):753–8.
11. Welch TJ, LeRoy AJ. Helical and electron beam CT scanning in the evaluation of renal vein involvement in patients with renal cell carcinoma. J Comput Assist Tomogr. 1997;21(3):467–71.
12. Kim JH, Sun HY, Hwang J, Hong SS, Cho YJ, Doo SW, et al. Diagnostic accuracy of contrast-enhanced computed tomography and contrast-enhanced magnetic resonance imaging of small renal masses in real practice: sensitivity and specificity according to subjective radiologic interpretation. World J Surg Oncol. 2016;14(1):260.
13. Thompson RH, Kurta JM, Kaag M, Tickoo SK, Kundu S, Katz D, et al. Tumor size is associated with malignant potential in renal cell carcinoma cases. J Urol. 2009;181(5):2033–6.
14. Bauerle T, Saake M, Uder M. Gadolinium-based contrast agents: what we learned from acute adverse events, nephrogenic systemic fibrosis and brain retention. Rofo. 2021;193(9):1010–8.
15. Rouviere O, Cornelis F, Brunelle S, Roy C, Andre M, Bellin MF, et al. Imaging protocols for renal multiparametric MRI and MR urography: results of a consensus conference from the French Society of Genitourinary Imaging. Eur Radiol. 2020;30(4):2103–14.
16. Lopes Vendrami C, Parada Villavicencio C, DeJulio TJ, Chatterjee A, Casalino DD, Horowitz JM, et al. Differentiation of solid renal tumors with multiparametric MR imaging. Radiographics. 2017;37(7):2026–42.
17. Marconi L, Dabestani S, Lam TB, Hofmann F, Stewart F, Norrie J, et al. Systematic review and meta-analysis of diagnostic accuracy of percutaneous renal tumour biopsy. Eur Urol. 2016;69(4):660–73.
18. Lim CS, Schieda N, Silverman SG. Update on indications for percutaneous renal mass biopsy in the era of advanced CT and MRI. AJR Am J Roentgenol. 2019;212(6):1187–96.
19. Robson CJ. Radical nephrectomy for renal cell carcinoma. J Urol. 1963;89:37–42. https://doi.org/10.1016/s0022-5347(17)64494-x.
20. Guinan P, Saffrin R, Stuhldreher D, Frank W, Rubenstein M. Renal cell carcinoma: comparison of the TNM and Robson stage groupings. J Surg Oncol. 1995;59(3):186–9. https://doi.org/10.1002/jso.2930590310.
21. Amin MB, Edge SB, Greene FL, et al. AJCC cancer staging manual. 8th ed. New York: Springer; 2017.
22. Kutikov A, Uzzo RG. The R.E.N.A.L. nephrometry score: a comprehensive standardized system for quantitating renal tumor size, location and depth. J Urol. 2009;182:844–53.
23. Bora GS, Mavuduru RS, Sharma AP, Devana SK, Kakkar N, Lal A, Singh SK, Mandal AK. Initial

experience of robotic nephron sparing surgery in cases of high renal nephrometry scores. Indian J Urol. 2017;33(3):230–5. https://doi.org/10.4103/iju.IJU_331_16.
24. Sharma AP, Mavuduru RS, Bora GS, Devana SK, Palani K, Lal A, Kakkar N, Singh SK, Mandal AK. Comparison of RENAL, PADUA, and C-index scoring systems in predicting perioperative outcomes after nephron sparing surgery. Indian J Urol. 2018;34(1):51–5. https://doi.org/10.4103/iju.IJU_247_17.
25. Ficarra V, Novara G, Secco S, et al. Preoperative aspects and dimensions used for an anatomical (PADUA) classification of renal tumours in patients who are candidates for nephron-sparing surgery. Eur Secur. 2009;56:786–93.
26. Okhunov Z, Rais-Bahrami S, George AK, Waingankar N, Duty B, Montag S, Rosen L, Sunday S, Vira MA, Kavoussi LR. The comparison of three renal tumor scoring systems: C-index, P.A.D.U.A., and R.E.N.A.L. nephrometry scores. J Endourol. 2011;25(12):1921–4.
27. Sharma G, Tyagi S, Mavuduru R, Bora GS, Sharma AP, Devana SK, Gorsi U, Kakkar N, Singh SK. External validation of SPARE nephrometery score in predicting overall complications, trifecta and pentafecta outcomes following robot-assisted partial nephrectomy. Minerva Urol Nephrol. 2022;74(1):63–71. https://doi.org/10.23736/S0393-2249.20.03972-7.
28. Spaliviero M, Poon BY, Karlo CA, Guglielmetti GB, Di Paolo PL, Beluco Corradi R, Martin-Malburet AG, Campos-Juanatey F, Escudero-Fontano E, Sjoberg DD, Russo P, Coleman JA, Akin O, Touijer KA. An arterial based complexity (ABC) scoring system to assess the morbidity profile of partial nephrectomy. Eur Urol. 2016;69(1):72–9. https://doi.org/10.1016/j.eururo.2015.08.008.
29. Franquet Q, Matillon X, Terrier N, Rambeaud JJ, Crouzet S, Long JA, Fassi-Fehri H, Codas-Duarte R, Poncet D, Jouve T, Noble J, Malvezzi P, Rostaing L, Descotes JL, Badet L, Fiard G. The Mayo adhesive probability score can help predict intra- and postoperative complications in patients undergoing laparoscopic donor nephrectomy. World J Urol. 2021;39(7):2775–81. https://doi.org/10.1007/s00345-020-03513-4.
30. Tyagi S, Sharma G, Bora GS, Mavuduru RS, Sharma AP, Devana SK, Gorsi U, Kakkar N, Singh SK. Trifecta and pentafecta outcomes following robot-assisted partial nephrectomy for hilar versus nonhilar tumors: a propensity-matched analysis. Indian J Urol. 2021;37(4):318–24. https://doi.org/10.4103/iju.iju_136_21.
31. Moch H. WHO-ISUP-Graduierungssystem für Nierenkarzinome [The WHO/ISUP grading system for renal carcinoma]. Pathologe. 2016;37(4):355–60. https://doi.org/10.1007/s00292-016-0171-y.

Pathology and Staging

2

Meenakshi Rao and
Balamurugan Thirunavukkarasu

2.1 Introduction

Renal cell carcinoma (RCC) ranks as the seventh most common cancer in men and tenth most common cancer in women. It amounts for 2% of global cancers and 2% of deaths related to cancer. It is primarily a disease of the elderly usually presenting at sixth and seventh decades. The incidence is higher in males than in females, high-income countries, and African Americans. One study on Indian population showed one-third of renal tumors presenting less than 50 years of age [1, 2]. The *risk factors* include obesity, smoking, hypertension, occupational exposure (exposure to trichloroethylene, a chemical additive, and solvent used in metal degreasing), and acquired cystic disease [3, 4].

2.1.1 Genetic Susceptibility

Renal carcinomas may be sporadic (no associated genetic predisposition) or genetic (familial/hereditary). The tumor syndromes associated with RCC are Von Hippel-Lindau syndrome, Birt–Hogg–Dube syndrome, hereditary leiomyomatosis and RCC syndrome, succinate-dehydrogenase-deficient tumor syndromes, hereditary papillary RCC (familial papillary RCC syndrome), and BAP1 tumor predisposition syndrome [5–14].

2.2 Classification of Renal Carcinomas

The traditional classification is based on dominant architectural and cytological features (clear cell and papillary renal cell carcinoma), location of the tumors (medullary and collecting duct carcinoma), background renal diseases (acquired cystic disease), and molecularly defined entities. The recent 5th edition of WHO classification of renal tumors, 2022 [15] emphasizess on molecularly defined entities such as *TFE3*, *TFEB* rearranged RCC, succinate dehydrogenase-deficient RCC, fumarate hydratase-deficient RCC, *ALK*-rearranged RCC, SMARCB-1-deficient renal cell carcinoma, etc.

A brief overview of the WHO classification of renal cell carcinomas (RCCs) is mentioned in Table 2.1:

In addition, mixed epithelial and stromal renal tumors, renal mesenchymal tumors, neuroendocrine tumors, and hematolymphoid tumors are also included in the classification. Since they comprise a minority of renal tumors, this chapter focuses on renal carcinomas.

M. Rao (✉)
Department of Pathology & Lab Medicine, AIIMS, Jodhpur, India
e-mail: raom@aiimsjodhpur.edu.in

B. Thirunavukkarasu
Department of Pathology, AIIMS, Delhi, India

P. Singh et al. (eds.), *A Guide to Management of Urological Cancers*,
https://doi.org/10.1007/978-981-99-2341-0_2

Table 2.1 Brief overview of the WHO classification of renal cell carcinomas

1. Clear cell renal tumors
Clear cell RCC
Multilocular cystic renal neoplasm of low malignant potential
2. Papillary renal tumors
Papillary adenoma
Papillary RCC
3. Oncocytic and chromophobe renal tumors
Oncocytoma
Chromophobe RCC
Other tumors—hybrid oncocytic tumors, low-grade oncocytic tumors
4. Collecting duct carcinoma
5. Other renal tumors
Eosinophilic solid and cystic renal cell carcinoma
Clear cell papillary renal cell tumor
Mucinous tubular and spindle cell carcinoma
Tubulocystic renal cell carcinoma
Acquired cystic disease-associated renal cell carcinoma
6. Molecularly defined renal carcinoma
TFE3-rearranged RCC
TFEB-rearranged RCC
Succinate dehydrogenase-deficient RCC
Fumarate hydratase-deficient RCC
ALK-rearranged RCC
SMARCB-1-deficient medullary-like/ undifferentiated/dedifferentiated RCC
ELOC-mutated RCC

The pertinent morphologic features of the commoner and newer RCCs are discussed below:

2.2.1 Clear Cell RCC

Clear cell carcinoma is a heterogeneous malignant tumor comprising of clear cells and occasional eosinophilic cytoplasm. It is the commonest sporadic RCC amounting to 60–75% of all RCC. The cell of origin is renal tubular epithelial cell. The underlying molecular event is loss of chromosome 3p and inactivation of *VHL* gene by methylation or mutation. It leads to increase in hyphypoxia-inducible factor alpha and expression of target genes [16].

Grossly, the tumor cut surface is golden yellow to brown with hemorrhage and necrosis, which imparts a variegated appearance (Fig. 2.1).

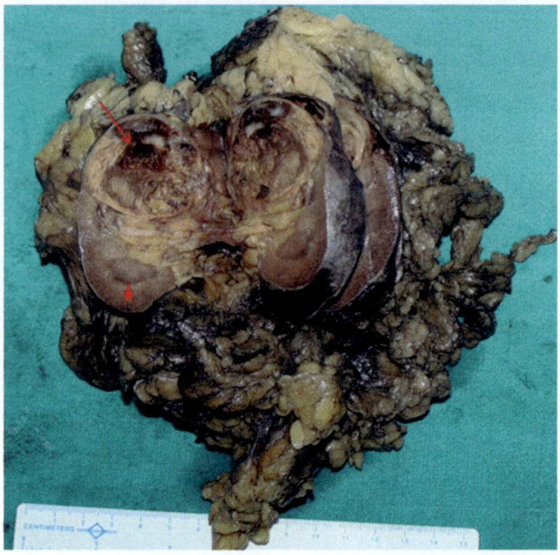

Fig. 2.1 A radical nephrectomy specimen showing a tumor in the upper pole with the classical gross appearance of renal cell carcinoma, depicting a variegated cut surface with areas of hemorrhage and necrosis (tumor indicated with red arrow). Normal renal parenchyma is identified in the lower pole (red asterisk). The renal capsule and the perinephric fat have a black appearance since the specimen has been inked prior to cut opening for staging purpose

Microscopy comprises of clear cells in nests and an alveolar pattern with a rich capillary network surrounding each nest. It may have eosinophilic cytoplasm and papillary areas. Higher grades can show nucleolar prominence and rhabdoid and/or sarcomatoid areas (Fig. 2.2). Clear cell carcinoma, eosinophilic variant may have diagnostic conundrum with other oncocytic renal tumors, due to the abundant eosinophilic cytoplasm.

2.2.2 Papillary RCC

It is the second most common RCC, amounting to 13–20% of the RCCs. It is characterized by trisomy and tetrasomy of chromosomes 7 and 17 and loss of the Y chromosome. Low-grade papillary RCC carries *MET* germline mutation. Cut surface of the tumor is variable, with yellow, red-brown color depending on the microscopic components. Microscopy shows papillary structures lined by cuboidal to columnar cells with scant basophilic cytoplasm. Foamy histiocytes and psammoma bodies can be seen in these tumors.

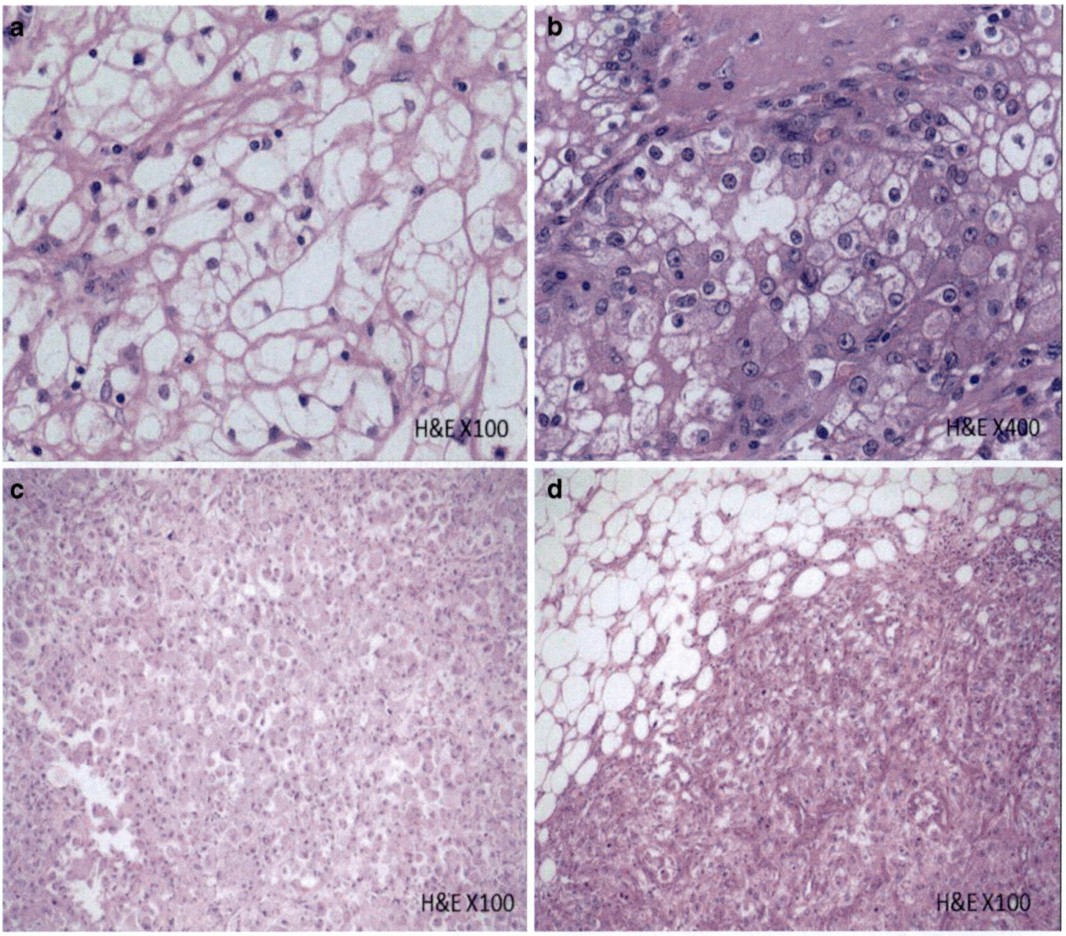

Fig. 2.2 Image depicting the WHO/ISUP histologic grading in renal cell carcinomas. Panel (**a**) shows a grade 1 tumor with small nuclei and inconspicuous nucleoli at high-power view (400× magnification). Panel (**b**) shows a grade 2 tumor with mild enlarged nucleus with conspicuous nucleoli at high-power view (400× magnifications). In grade 3 tumors, the nucleoli are conspicuous at low-power view (100× magnification). Panel (**c**) shows rhabdoid features in form of cells having abundant eosinophilic cytoplasm, eccentric nuclei, and prominent nucleoli. Panel (**d**) shows sarcomatoid features in form of spindling of the pleomorphic tumor cells. The tumor has invaded the perirenal fat, as indicated by the surrounding adipose tissue. Presence of sarcomatoid or rhabdoid features in a renal cell carcinoma signifies a grade 4 tumor

High-grade tumors have a variety of differentials, including fumarate hydratase-deficient RCC. It generally has a better prognosis than clear cell RCC [17].

2.2.3 Chromophobe RCC

Chromophobe RCC accounts for 5–7% of all RCCs. It shows multiple chromosomal losses of chromosome 1, 2, 6, 10, 13, or Y chromosome. Some cases are associated with Birt–Hogg–Dube syndrome, harboring Folliculin gene mutation. Cut surface of the tumor is tan, brown color, or classic mahogany color (Fig. 2.3). Microscopy is characterized by sheets, nests separated by hyalinized septa composed of pale large cells with prominent cell membrane imparting a plant cell-like appearance. There is perinuclear halo with hyperchromatic rasinoid nuclei (Fig. 2.4). The close differential diagnoses include succinate dehydrogenase-deficient-RCC and oncocytic tumors. It has a favorable prognosis compared to clear cell RCC and papillary RCC [18].

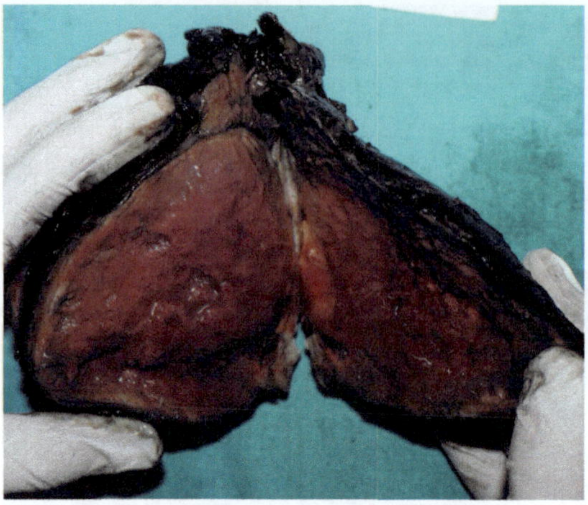

Fig. 2.3 Gross appearance of chromophobe renal cell carcinoma in a partial nephrectomy specimen. These tumors have a homogeneous brown cut surface. Compare with conventional clear cell carcinoma in Fig. 2.1, which has a variegated appearance

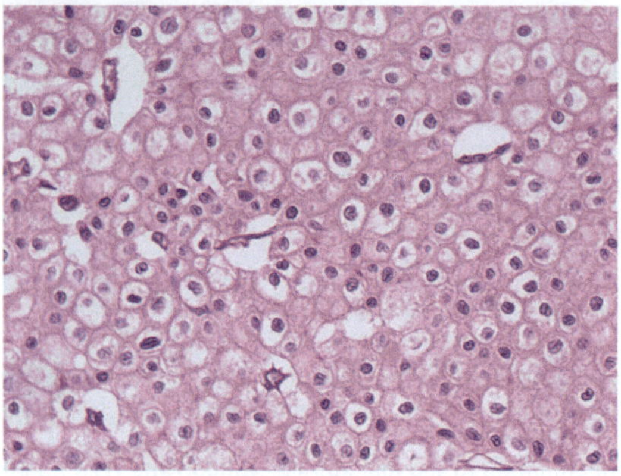

Fig. 2.4 Microscopic appearance of chromophobe renal cell carcinoma. The tumor cells have abundant granular eosinophilic cytoplasm with pleomorphic wrinkled nuclei and perinuclear halo. (H&E, 400×) Currently chromophobe renal cell carcinomas are not graded

2.2.4 Clear Cell Papillary Renal Cell Tumor

Previously called clear cell papillary renal cell carcinoma, these tumors have been renamed clear cell papillary renal cell tumor because of their indolent nature. The tumors are mostly detected incidentally. Unlike clear cell RCC, these tumors are positive for cytokeratin (CK) 7, alpha-methylacyl-CoA racemase (AMACR) and show a unique "cup-like" positivity for CAIX, while they are negative for CD10 [19].

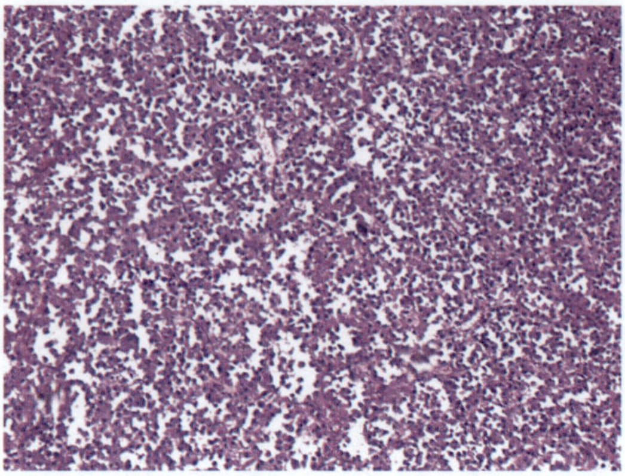

Fig. 2.5 Low power microscopic appearance of the recently included morphological type of renal cell carcinoma, eosinophilic solid and cystic renal cell carcinoma. Note the hobnailing of the tumor cells. (H&E, 100×)

2.2.5 Eosinophilic Solid and Cystic RCC

A newly included morphological entity in the classification, this tumor is composed of cystic and solid areas with voluminous eosinophilic cytoplasm, basophilic stippling (Leishmania body-like), and variable CK20 positivity. They are characterized by biallelic mutation of *TSC1* or *TSC2* genes [20, 21]. Cystic areas frequently show hob nailing (Fig. 2.5).

2.2.6 Mucinous Tubular and Spindle Cell Renal Cell Carcinoma

Mucinous tubular and spindle cell carcinoma (quite a mouthful!) is composed of anastomotic tubules with low-grade cuboidal cells and bland spindle cells in a myxoid stroma. There can be morphological variation among the different components. The histology and immunohistochemical profile overlaps with papillary RCC [22].

2.2.7 Collecting Duct Carcinoma

These are rare tumors located in the medullary region, with infiltrating glandular morphology, high-grade cytology, and desmoplastic stromal response. It is a diagnosis of exclusion after considering urothelial carcinoma, SDH-deficient RCC, and metastasis [23].

2.2.8 Molecularly Defined Renal Cell Carcinomas

Fumarate hydratase (FH) deficient RCCs are morphologically heterogeneous but have characteristic eosinophilic macronucleoli. These tumors show FH loss and/or with 2-succinocysteine (SC) expression. Previously, these tumors were classified as hereditary leiomyomatosis and RCC-associated renal cell carcinoma. However, since not all cases are syndromic, and a few sporadic cases are also seen, these tumors are now called as FH-deficient RCCs. These are aggressive tumors and are important to recognize for genetic counselling [24].

***TFE3*-rearranged RCC** are characterized by TFE3 gene fusion with one or many gene partners like *ASPL*, *PRCC*, and *NONO*. Nearly one-third of them occur in the pediatric population. They have papillary architecture with voluminous clear cytoplasm and numerous psammoma bodies. Strong TFE3 nuclear positivity can help with diagnosis. Fluorescent in situ hybridization (FISH) and RNA sequencing may be needed for definite diagnosis. *TFEB*-rearranged RCCs have a biphasic morphology comprising of large epithelioid cells and small cells around basement membrane-like material [25].

Succinate dehydrogenase (SDH)-deficient RCCs have bland cells with pale, eosinophilic flocculent material and loss of SDHB on immunohistochemistry. Germ line testing and long-term surveillance testing for other SDH-deficient neoplasms are required [26].

***ALK*-rearranged RCC** has polygonal cells with eosinophilic, vacuolated cytoplasm and are often associated with Sickle cell trait.

SMARCB1-deficient medullary carcinoma *(previously called renal medullary carcinoma)* is a high-grade carcinoma with Integrase Interactor 1 (INI-1) deficiency on immunohistochemistry, medullary location, and sickle cell trait. These tumors are associated with very poor prognosis [27].

2.2.9 Proposed Entities in the New WHO Classification of Renal Carcinomas

A few emerging entities have been mentioned in the WHO classification of urinary and male genital tumors, 5th edition, 2022 [28]. However, due to lack of sufficient evidence, these have not yet been incorporated as specific tumor types:

1. Thyroid-like follicular carcinoma (currently not classified in the WHO classification)
2. Eosinophilic vacuolated tumor (currently classified as other oncocytic tumors in the WHO classification)
3. Papillary neoplasm with reverse polarity (currently classified as a subtype of papillary RCC)
4. Biphasic hyalinizing psammomatous RCC (currently not classified in the WHO classification)
5. Low-grade oncocytic tumor (currently classified as other oncocytic tumors in the WHO classification)

2.3 Immunohistochemistry

Although many of the RCCs can be diagnosed on morphology, immunohistochemistry (IHC) is essential for diagnosis of RCCs, especially in ambiguous morphology. Majority of RCC can be diagnosed with a limited immunohistochemical panel [29, 30] as depicted in Table 2.2.

Table 2.2 Immunohistochemical panel for diagnosis of RCCs

	CD10	CK7	CD117	Vimentin	AMACR	CAIX	Other
Clear cell RCC	++	–	–	++	+	++	
Papillary RCC	+	++	–	++	++	–	
Chromophobe RCC	+/–	++	++	–	+/–	–	
Translocation- associated RCC	+	–	–	–	++	–	TFE3, TFEB, Melan A
SMARCB1- deficient medullary carcinoma							INI 1 loss on IHC
FH-deficient RCC	–	–	–	–	–	–	Negative FH, aberrant staining for 2-SC
SDH-deficient RCC	–	–	–	–	–	–	SDHB loss

CD cluster of differentiation, *AMACR* α-methylacyl-coenzyme A racemase, *CAIX* carbonic anhydrase IX

2.4 Pathologic Prognostic Factors

Apart from the stage of the tumor (discussed in the following section), the following factors are also essential to assess the prognosis.

1. **Grade of RCCs**

   Grading is validated for clear cell RCC and papillary RCC. Grading is not applicable in chromophobe RCC, and TFE3-rearranged RCC is not useful in inherently aggressive tumors (like collecting duct carcinoma and SMARCB-1-deficient renal medullary carcinoma) and can be misleading in certain tumors due to high nuclear grade despite indolent tumor behavior (tubulocystic carcinoma, eosinophilic solid and cystic RCC, acquired cystic disease-associated RCC). Low WHO/ISUP grade is necessary for accurate classification (like clear cell papillary renal cell tumor) [31].

   The World Health Organisation/International Society of Urological Pathology (WHO/ISUP) grading is given in Table 2.3 and shown in Fig. 2.2:
2. **Histological subtype**

   Type 1 papillary RCC (previous classification, now papillary RCC) has better prognosis. Collecting duct carcinoma and medullary carcinoma have inherent poor prognosis.
3. **Sarcomatoid/rhabdoid areas:** It is essential to mention the percentage of Grade 4 component, as >50% carry worse prognosis compared to <10% [32].
4. **Lympho-vascular invasion:** Presence of microscopic lympho-vascular invasion is a poor prognostic factor.
5. **Coagulative tumor necrosis:** Granular necrosis lacking nuclear features, characterized by sheets of dead cells is an independent poor prognostic factor [33].

Table 2.3 WHO/ISUP grading of renal carcinomas

Grade	Description
1	Tumor nucleoli absent or inconspicuous and basophilic at 400× magnification
2	Nucleoli conspicuous and eosinophilic at 400× and visible but not prominent at 100×
3	Nucleoli conspicuous and eosinophilic at 100×
4	Extreme nuclear pleomorphism, multinucleate giant cells, and/or rhabdoid/sarcomatoid differentiation

2.5 Pathologic Staging of Renal Carcinomas

Staging of renal carcinomas is performed as per the latest (8th edition) Union for International Cancer Control (UICC) Tumour, Node, Metastasis (TNM) Classification of Malignant Tumours [34]. Involvement of perirenal fat and renal sinus is depicted in Figs. 2.6 and 2.7, respectively, and involvement of the adrenal gland is depicted in Figs. 2.8 and 2.9 and Table 2.4.

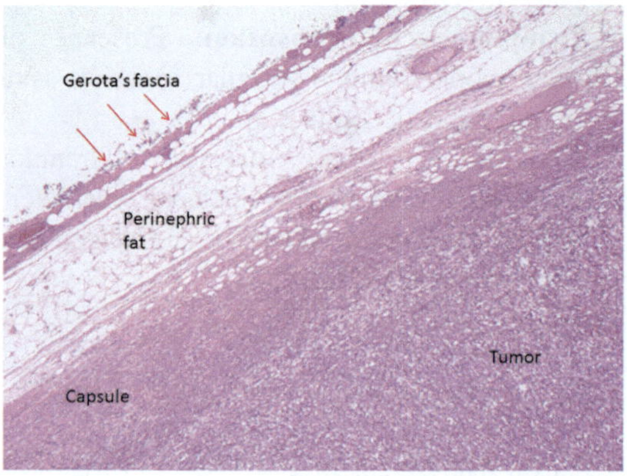

Fig. 2.6 Scanner view showing renal tumor with tumor capsule, perirenal fat, and Gerota's fascia (marked with arrows). The tumor has invaded the capsule and is involving the perinephric fat; however, the Gerota's fascia is not involved by the tumor. This indicates a pathologic stage pT3a tumor. The gerota's fascia is marked with red arrows and black ink can also be appreciated at the fascia. (H&E, 40×)

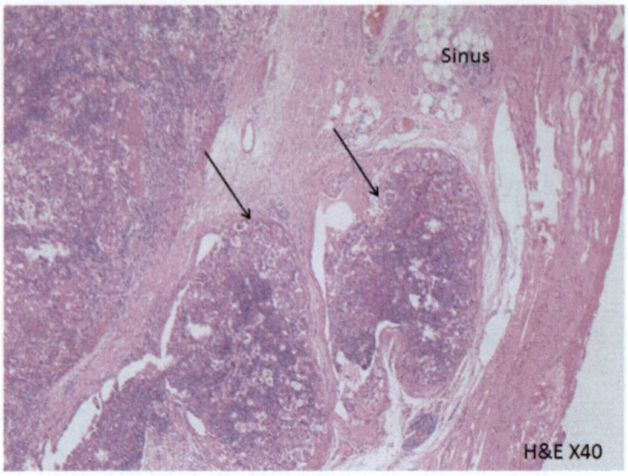

Fig. 2.7 Scanner power view showing sinus vessel involvement by the renal carcinoma (marked with arrows). Adjacent main tumor and perinephric fat can also be identified. Invasion of renal sinus fat or vessels indicates a pathologic stage pT3a tumor. (H&E, 40×)

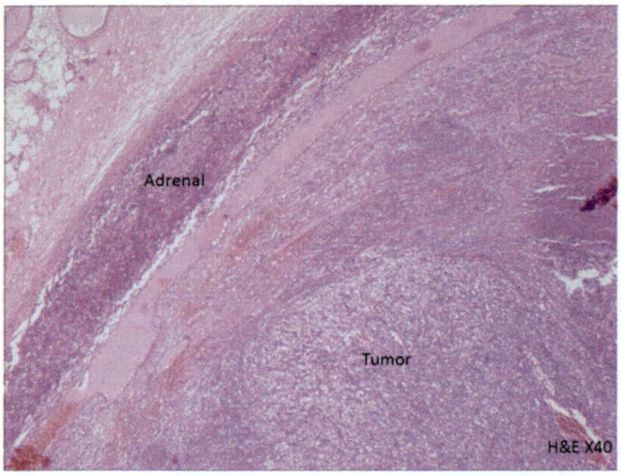

Fig. 2.8 Scanner view of the adrenal gland showing involvement by tumor. Ipsilateral, contiguous involvement of the adrenal gland signifies pathologic stage pT4 and noncontiguous (discontinuous) tumor deposit in the adrenal gland signifies pathologic stage pM1 (metastatic)

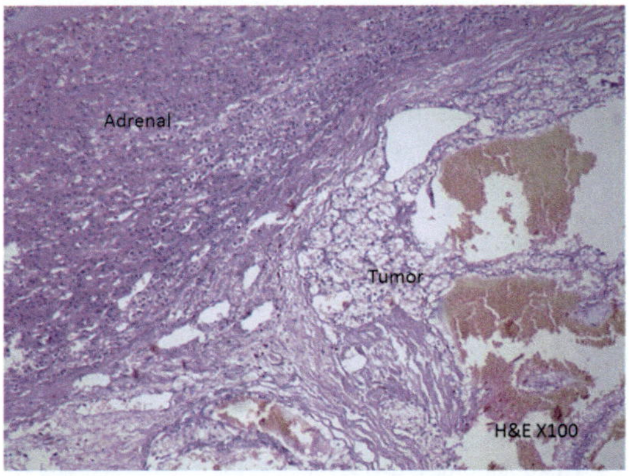

Fig. 2.9 Low-power view of the adrenal gland showing involvement by tumor. Ipsilateral, contiguous involvement of the adrenal gland signifies pathologic stage pT4 and noncontiguous (discontinuous) tumor deposit in the adrenal gland signifies pathologic stage pM1 (metastatic)

Table 2.4 Pathological staging of RCCs [34]

T category	Criteria
T1 (limited to kidney)	T1a—tumor size <4 cm
	T1b—tumor size 4–7 cm
T2 (limited to kidney)	T2a—tumor size 7–10 cm
	T2b—tumor size >10 cm
T3	T3a—extends to renal vein, segmental branches or pelvicalyceal system or perirenal and/or renal sinus fat not beyond Gerota's fascia (Figs. 2.6 and 2.7)
	T3b—IVC invasion below the diaphragm
	T3c—IVC invasion above the diaphragm or invades the wall of vena cava
T4	Invasion beyond Gerota's fascia (including extension into ipsilateral adrenal gland)[a] (Fig. 2.8)
N category	N0—no regional nodes
	N1—metastasis in regional nodes
M category	M0—no distal metastasis
	M1—Distant metastasis (Fig. 2.9)

[a]Ipsilateral, contiguous involvement of the adrenal gland signifies pathologic stage pT4 and noncontiguous (discontinuous) tumor deposit in the adrenal gland signifies pathologic stage pM1 (metastatic)

References

1. Moch H, et al. The 2022 World Health Organization classification of tumours of the urinary system and male genital organs—part A: renal, penile, and testicular tumours. Eur Urol. 2022;82(5):458–68.
2. Agnihotri S, et al. Renal cell carcinoma in India demonstrates early age of onset & a late stage of presentation. Indian J Med Res. 2014;140(5):624–9.
3. Kabaria R, et al. Renal cell carcinoma: links and risks. Int J Nephrol Renovasc Dis. 2016;9:45–52.
4. Chow WH, et al. Epidemiology and risk factors for kidney cancer. Nat Rev Urol. 2010;7(5):245–57.
5. Neumann HP, et al. Prevalence, morphology and biology of renal cell carcinoma in von Hippel-Lindau disease compared to sporadic renal cell carcinoma. J Urol. 1998;160:1248–54.
6. Przybycin CG, et al. Hereditary syndromes with associated renal neoplasia: a practical guide to histologic recognition in renal tumor resection specimen. Adv Anat Pathol. 2013;20(4):245–63.
7. Farley MN, et al. A novel Germline mutation in BAP-1 predisposes to familial clear-cell renal cell carcinoma. Mol Cancer Res. 2013;11(9):1061–71.
8. Glasker S, et al. Von Hippel-Lindau disease: current challenges and future prospects. Onco Targets Ther. 2020;13:5669–90.
9. Kennedy JM, et al. Clinical and morphologic review of 60 hereditary renal tumors from 30 hereditary renal cell carcinoma syndrome patients: lessons from a comtemporary single institution series. Med Oncol. 2019;36(9):74. https://doi.org/10.1007/s12032-019-1297-6.
10. Toro JR, et al. Birt-Hogg-Dube syndrome: a novel marker of kidney neoplasia. Arch Dermatol. 1999;135(10):1195–202.
11. Schmidt L, et al. Molecular genetics and clinical features of Birt-Hogg-Dube syndrome. Nat Genet. 1997;16(1):68–73.
12. Menko FH, et al. Hereditary leiomyomatosis and renal cell cancer (HLRCC): renal cancer risk, surveillance and treatment. Familial Cancer. 2014;13(4):637–44.
13. Abdel-Rahman MH, et al. Germline BAP1 mutation predisposes to uveal melanoma, lung adenocarcinoma, meningioma and other cancers. J Med Genet. 2011;48(12):856–9.
14. Yang Y, et al. Characterization of genetically defined sporadic and hereditary type 1papillary renal cell carcinoma cell lines. Genes Chromosomes Cancer. 2021;60(6):434–46.
15. WHO Classification of Tumours Editorial Board. Urinary and male genital tumours, vol. 8. 5th ed. Lyon: International Agency for Research on Cancer; 2022.
16. Mitchell TJ, et al. Timing the landmark events in the evolution of clear cell renal cell cancer: TRACERx renal. Cell. 2018;173(3):611–623.e17.
17. Pitra T, et al. Chromosomal numerical aberration pattern in papillary renal cell carcinoma: review article. Ann Diagn Pathol. 2019;40:189–99.
18. Garje R, et al. Comprehensive review of chromophobe renal cell carcinoma. Crit Rev Oncol Hematol. 2021;160:103287.
19. Williamson SR. Clear cell papillary renal cell carcinoma: an update after 15 years. Pathology. 2021;53(1):109–19.

20. Trpkov K, et al. Eosinophilic, solid, and cystic renal cell carcinoma. Am J Surg Pathol. 2016;40(1):60–71.
21. Sharma R, et al. Eosinophilic solid and cystic renal cell carcinoma: from unclassified to classified, a case report. Turk Patoloji Derg. 2022;38(1):60–5.
22. Nathany S, Monappa V. Mucinous tubular and spindle cell carcinoma: a review of histopathology and clinical and prognostic implications. Arch Pathol Lab Med. 2020;144(1):115–8.
23. Seo AN, et al. Clinicopathologic and molecular pathology of collecting duct carcinoma and related renal cell carcinomas. Adv Anat Pathol. 2017;24(2):65–77.
24. Muller M, et al. Pattern multiplicity and fumarate hydratase (FH)/S-(2-succino)-cysteine (2SC) staining but not eosinophilic nucleoli with perinucleolar halos differentiate hereditary leiomyomatosis and renal cell carcinoma-associated renal cell carcinomas from kidney tum. Mod Pathol. 2018;31(6):974–83.
25. Argani P. Translocation carcinomas of the kidney. Genes Chromosom Cancer. 2022;61(5):219–27.
26. Kuroda N, et al. Review of succinate dehydrogenase-deficient renal cell carcinoma with focus on clinical and pathobiological aspects. Pol J Pathol. 2016;1:3–7.
27. Cheng JX, et al. Renal medullar carcinoma:rhabdoid features and the absence of INI1 expression as markers of aggressive behaviour. Mod Pathol. 2008;21(6):647–52.
28. Trpkov K, et al. New developments in existing WHO entities and evolving molecular concepts: the genitourinary pathology society (GUPS) update on renal neoplasia. Mod Pathol. 2021;34(7):1392–424.
29. Truong LD, Shen SS. Immunohistochemical diagnosis of renal neoplasms. Arch Pathol Lab Med. 2011;135(1):92–109.
30. Akgul M, Williamson SR. Immunohistochemistry for the diagnosis of renal epithelial neoplasms. Semin Diagn Pathol. 2022;39(1):1–16.
31. Delahunt B, et al. Grading of renal cell carcinoma. Histopathology. 2019;74(1):4–17.
32. Dagher J, et al. Percentage grade 4 tumor predicts outcome for clear cell renal cell carcinoma. Pathology. 2019;51(4):349–52.
33. Samaratunga H, et al. Granular necrosis: a distinctive form of cell death in malignant tumors. Pathology. 2020;52(5):507–14.
34. Amin MB, et al. The eighth edition AJCC cancer staging manual: continuing to build a bridge from a population-based to a more "personalized" approach to cancer staging. CA Cancer J Clin. 2017;67(2):93–9.

Management of Localized and Locally Advanced RCC

3

Ravimohan Suryanarayan Mavuduru

3.1 Introduction

Renal cell carcinoma (RCC) management is one of the most evolving domains in urooncology care. The tumour is typically labelled as internist tumour and most often they are detected incidentally on a routine screening. RCCs typically arise from the proximal tubular epithelium of the nephron and hence mostly are cortical in location. RCCs grow slowly and can present as localized or locally advanced or even metastatic stage. RCCs located within the covering layer of kidney, i.e., renal capsule are localized RCC. Locally advanced RCCs are the ones having any of the following characteristics: extending into major veins, invading the adrenal gland, extending into the peri-renal or peri-pelvic fat, or invading beyond the Gerota fascia. To understand this, let us first briefly revise the anatomical coverings of kidneys (Fig. 3.1). The fat pad outside the Gerota fascia is known as pararenal fat. The fat pad between the Gerotafascia and renal capsule is known as perirenal fat. The fat pad in the renal hilum and the sinus spaces is known as peripelvic or sinus fat pad. Invasion by a renal mass of anyone of these spaces and/or contiguous involvement of an adrenal gland qualifies as a locally advanced tumour.

R. S. Mavuduru (✉)
Department of Urology, PGIMER, Chandigarh, India

P. Singh et al. (eds.), *A Guide to Management of Urological Cancers*,
https://doi.org/10.1007/978-981-99-2341-0_3

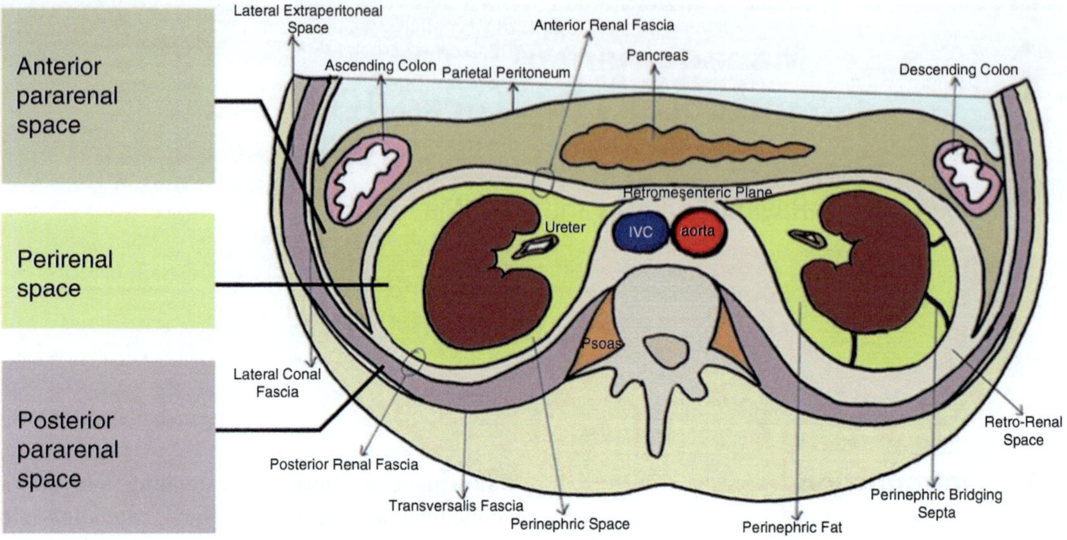

Fig. 3.1 Diagrammatic cross-sectional representation of the fascial coverings of kidneys

3.2 Why Is It Essential to Differentiate Localized and Locally Advanced RCC?

Because prognostically they are different. In a study, it was shown that the 5-year survival rate of localized RCC was 92% versus 68% for locally advanced and 12% for metastatic stage [1]. Moreover, the preferred treatment approach varies which will be discussed in the subsequent sections of the chapter. Let us first revise the TNM staging of RCC.

3.3 TNM Staging of RCCs

Traditionally, RCCs were staged using Robson staging [2], which had a lot of shortcomings. Currently, TNM staging is used to stage renal masses (Table 3.1). TNM original version in 2002 was modified in 2009, 2012 and 2017. These modifications included subcategorizing T2 tumours, inclusion of renal sinus fat and perirenal fat, distinguishing between contiguous and non-contiguous involvement of adrenal gland and any nodal involvement.

Table 3.1 TNM staging

T—Primary tumour	
TX	Primary tumour cannot be assessed
T0	No evidence of primary tumour
T1	Tumour <7 cm or less in greatest dimension, limited to the kidney
T1a	Tumour <4 cm or less
T1b	Tumour >4 cm but <7 cm
T2	Tumour >7 cm in greatest dimension, limited to the kidney
T2a	Tumour >7 cm but <10 cm
T2b	Tumours >10 cm, limited to the kidney
T3	Tumour extends into major veins or perinephric tissues but not into the ipsilateral adrenal gland and not beyond Gerota fascia
T3a	Tumour extends into the renal vein or its segmental branches, or invades the pelvicalyceal system or invades perirenal and/or renal sinus fat, but not beyond Gerota fascia[a]
T3b	Tumour grossly extends into the vena cava below diaphragm
T3c	Tumour grossly extends into vena cava above the diaphragm or invades the wall of the vena cava
T4	Tumour invades beyond Gerotafascia (including contiguous extension into the ipsilateral adrenal gland)
N—regional lymph nodes	
NX	Regional lymph nodes cannot be assessed

Table 3.1 (continued)

T—Primary tumour			
TX	Primary tumour cannot be assessed		
N0	No regional lymph node metastasis		
N1	Metastasis in regional lymph node(s)		
M—Distant metastasis			
M0	No distant metastasis		
M1	Distant metastasis		
pTNM stage grouping			
Stage I	T1	N0	M0
Stage II	T2	N0	M0
Stage III	T3	N0	M0
	T1, T2, T3	N1	M0
Stage IV	T4	Any N	M0
	Any T	Any N	M1

[a]Adapted based on the American Joint Committee on Cancer (AJCC), 8th edn. 2017 [3]

3.4 Evaluation of Renal Mass

80–90% of the renal masses are incidentally detected. In symptomatic patient's abdominal lump, hematuria, flank pain is the most usual presenting symptoms. The classic triad of pain hematuria and lump is seen in only about 6–10% of patients [4, 5]. Occasionally (approx. 30%), they may present with one of the paraneoplastic syndromes such as anemia and hypercalcemia [6]. Constitutional symptoms at presentation are rare. Syndromic association is seen in 5–8% and can rarely be the presenting symptoms (Fig. 3.2) [7]. About 15% localized RCC are symptomatic as against 60% of locally advanced RCCs. Thus, if a patient of RCC presents with symptoms, then they are more likely to be locally advanced.

Ultrasound forms the basis of initial suspicion. Typically, ultrasound description of an RCC is solid cystic hypoechoic lesion arising from the kidney. Contrast-enhanced CT (CECT) is the most common investigation performed for staging and surgical planning. The specific protocol for CT evaluation of a renal mass involves an unenhanced phase, an early arterial phase and a parenchymal phase with contrast typically known as triphasic CT. An enhancement of more than 15 Hounsfeild units in a solid renal mass is considered significant. Sometimes there might be a cystic renal mass, and it becomes difficult to differentiate benign versus malignant masses. Bosniak classification was developed essentially to characterize the cystic renal masses [8]. This system classifies renal cysts into five categories (Table 3.2), based on CT imaging appearance, to predict malignancy risk [9].

Renal masses with Bosniak type 4 definitely merit treatment like any malignant lesion. The most difficult to differentiate are the BII and BIII lesions (Fig. 3.3) [9]. The accuracy of CT in such lesions low with a reported sensitivity of 36% and specificity of 76% [10]. An advancement in the ultrasound, namely contrast-enhanced ultrasound (CEUS) improves the diagnostic accuracy in such indeterminate lesions. In the same study, CEUS showed high sensitivity (100%) and specificity (97%), with a negative predictive value of 100% (κ = 0.95) [10]. MRI is also a preferred modality in the evaluation of indeterminate renal masses, especially the cystic renal masses. Patients with contrast allergy, renal dysfunction and pregnancy are other preferred indications of MRI. Even in young patients who are worried about the radiation exposure of frequent CT scans, MRI is a preferred alternative. One clear area where MRI is preferred over CT is MR venography for renal masses with inferior vena cava thrombus (IVCT) both to determine the extent and the caval wall invasion (Fig. 3.4) [11]. Diffusion-weighted (DWI) and perfusion-weighted imaging are being explored for renal mass assessment [12]. Multiparametric MRI (mpMRI) based scoring has been developed and validated in clear cell RCC patients and has been shown to be accurate [13] This score is known as clear cell likelihood score (ccLS) and was developed for evaluation of small renal masses. The ccLS is a 5-tier classification that denotes the likelihood of a mass representing ccRCC, ranging from 'very unlikely' to 'very likely'. However, this scoring needs further validation.

FDG-PET has a limited role in evaluation of renal masses [14]. 3D printing is another emerging modality in management of renal mass especially the complex RCC planned for nephron-sparing surgery (NSS) [15].

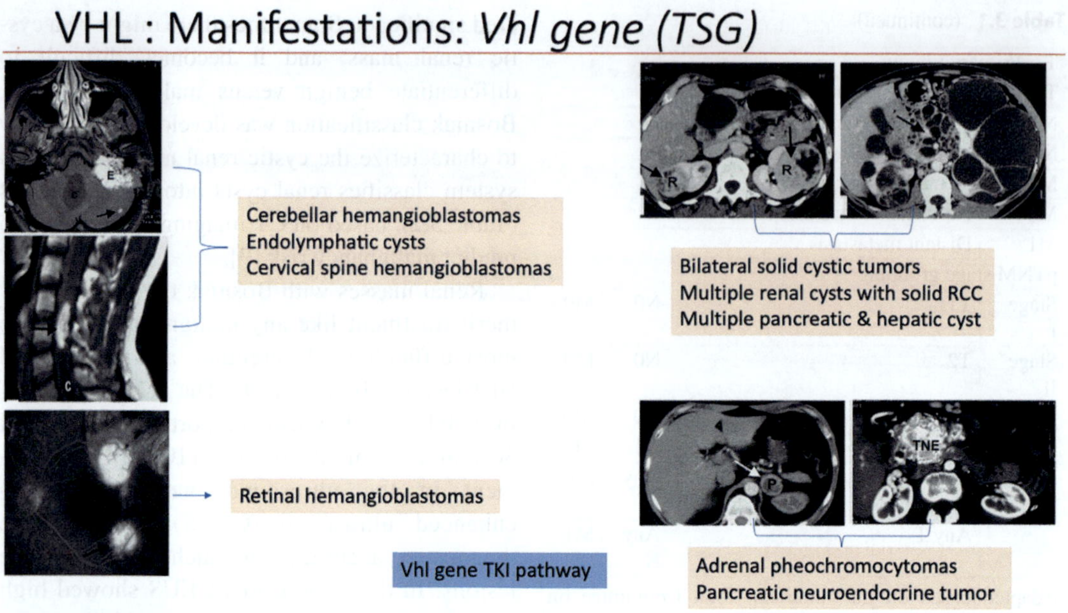

Fig. 3.2 Von Hippel Lindau disease manifestation

Table 3.2 Bosniak classification

Bosniak category	Features	Work-up
I	Simple benign cyst with a hairline-thin wall without septa, calcification, or solid components. Same density as water and does not enhance with contrast medium	Benign
II	Benign cyst that may contain a few hairline-thin septa. Fine calcification may be present in the wall or septa. Uniformly high-attenuation lesions <3 cm in size, with sharp margins without enhancement	Benign
IIF	These may contain more hairline-thin septa. Minimal enhancement of a hairline-thin septum or wall. Minimal thickening of the septa or wall. The cyst may contain calcification, which may be nodular and thick, with no contrast enhancement. No enhancing soft-tissue elements. This category also includes totally intra-renal, nonenhancing, high attenuation renal lesions >3 cm. Generally well-marginated	Follow-up, up to 5 years. Some are malignant.
III	These are indeterminate cystic masses with thickened irregular walls or septa with enhancement	Surgery or active surveillance. Over 50% are malignant
IV	Clearly containing soft tissue-enhancing components	surgery. Most are malignant

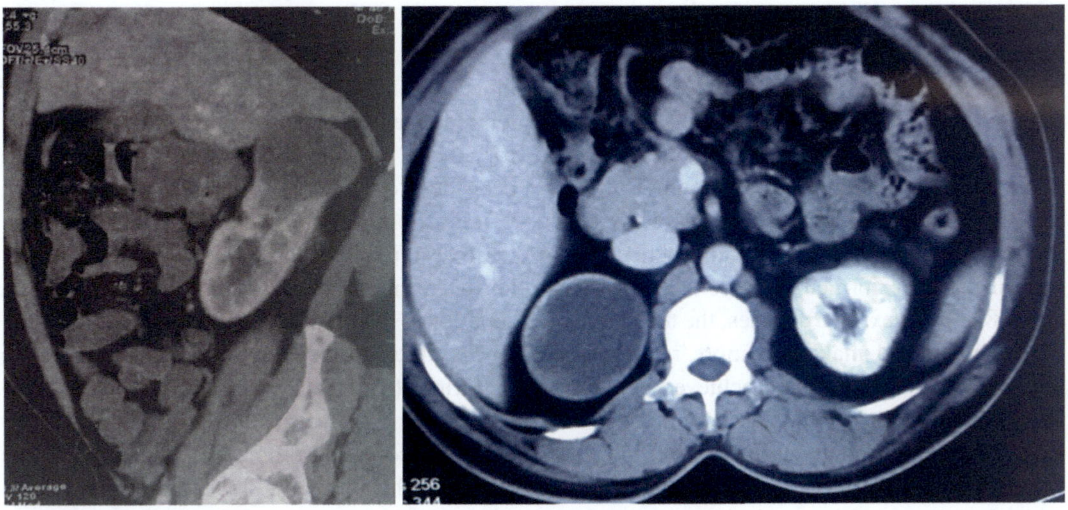

Fig. 3.3 : CECT axial and sagittal cuts showing Type 3 Bosniak cyst. Histopathology of partial nephrectomy was cystic renal cell cancer

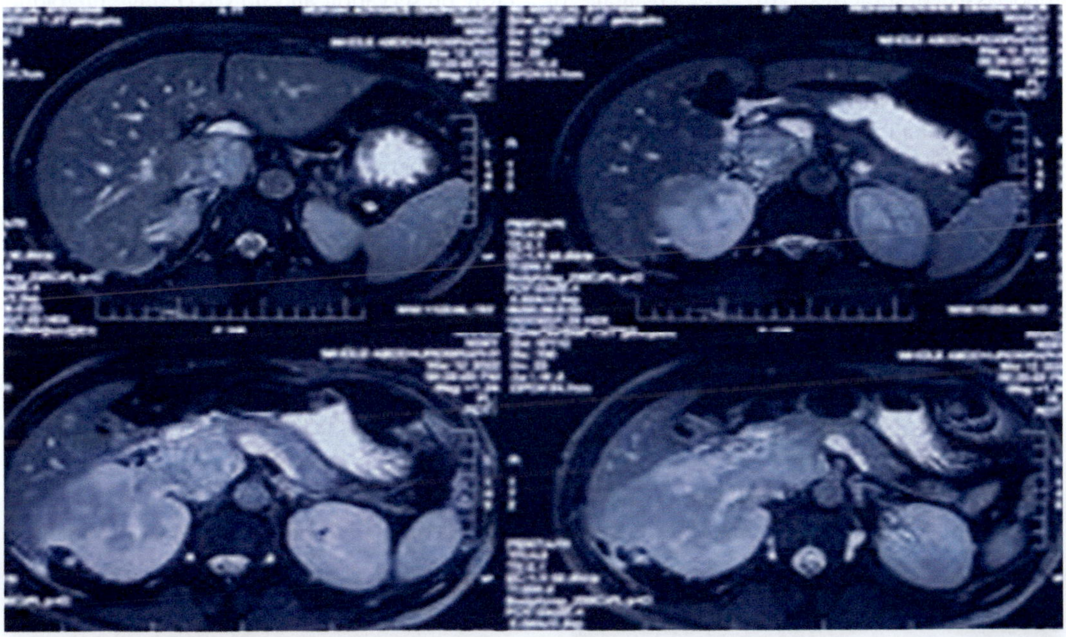

Fig. 3.4 MRI T1W with contrast showing right renal mass and IVC thrombus. There is suspicious wall invasion at the level of renal hilum based on the neovascularity and lack of delineation of IVC wall

3.5 Management

RCCs are unique in that they are relatively radio-resistant and chemo-resistant [16]. Also the pattern of spread for the classic RCCs, i.e., clear cell type is different, in that they tend to have hematogenous spread, while the lymphatic spread is usually associated with metastatic disease [17]. The management philosophy in localized RCC and locally advanced RCC are quite different. While in localized RCC, the aim of treatment is to maximize the renal function preservation, in locally advanced RCCs, it is to prevent the risk of local recurrence and progression by removing the entire tumour along with adjacent organs if required.

For maximal preservation of functional renal parenchyma maintaining the oncological outcomes partial nephrectomy (PN) or NSS techniques have been developed and practiced. The first NSS was performed by more than 100 years ago [18]. Over next two decades, the technique of NSS has evolved making it more reproducible and less complicated. This is achieved by clamping the renal hilum, dissecting the tumour with a rim of normal parenchyma and renorraphy. All this must be accomplished in 25–30 min times, which is the proposed warm ischaemia time [19]. NSS can be performed by open or minimal invasive (MIS) methods such as laparoscopic or robot-assisted surgeries [20]. The advantage of open technique is that one can do cooling of the kidney using ice slush, which allows for more surgical resection time. Traditionally, using an ice slush around the mobilized kidneys immediately after clamping the renal vessels for 10 min ensures a core temperature of the kidney to about 15–20 C, allowing a resection time of up to 3 h, without compromising the renal functional outcomes [21]. The advantage of minimally invasive surgery such as laparoscopy is smaller incision and thus an earlier convalescence with equivalent oncological outcomes [22]. However, achieving all the steps of partial nephrectomy remains a challenge during laparoscopic procedure. Robot-assisted partial nephrectomy (RAPN) overcomes this challenge due to better hand dexterity with 7° of freedom and motion scaling. RAPN has shown to have shorter warm ischaemia times and lesser blood loss than laparoscopic NSS [23]. In order to predefine the feasibility of partial nephrectomy for a renal mass, various scoring systems have been developed such as RENAL, PADUA and C-index [24]. It is beyond the scope of this chapter to describe the details of each scoring system; however, no scoring system has been shown superior to the other [25, 26]. With robotic assistance, more and more complex NSSs were being performed [27]. It is imperative to standardize the outcomes of NSS especially in the high nephrometry scores. The outcome comparisons are usually done using the Trifecta and Pentafecta outcomes. Negative surgical margin, no postoperative complications and WIT of <25 min are defined as trifecta. Additionally, >90% estimated GFR preservation and no CKD stage upgrading at 1 year constitute the Pentafecta outcomes [28]. The scoring systems as a guide for the level of difficulty and the trifecta and pentafecta parameters for outcome measures are being used to compare in between the studies across the globe. Even in patients with high nephrometry scores, the trifecta and pentafecta parameters are well maintained [29]. Further advancements such as use of intraoperative ultrasound, use of indigocyanine green dye (ICG) and image overlay technologies have improved the outcomes during minimal invasive treatments. So the question arises should NSS be performed in all patients? NSS should be performed in imperative indications such as a solitary functioning kidney (Fig. 3.5). There is no benefit of performing NSS

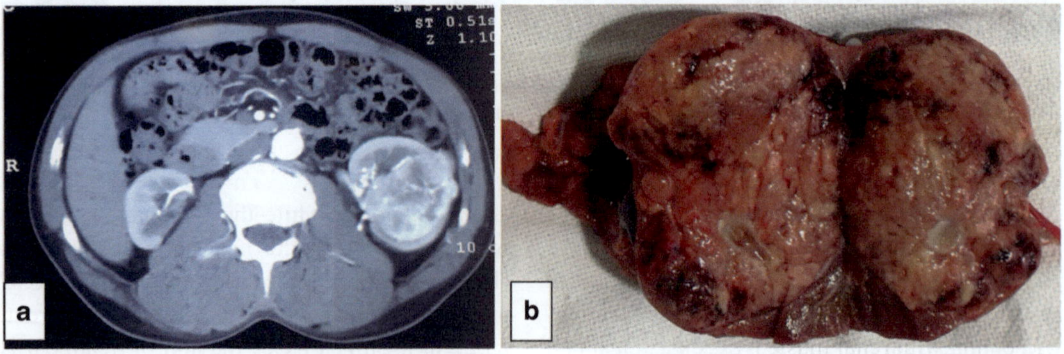

Fig. 3.5 (**a**) CECT showing a locally advanced RCC. Patient underwent partial nephrectomy since the other kidney was small with compromised renal function. (**b**) Cut section of the specimen

for patients >75 years of age where it has been shown to have no OS benefit [30]. PN is associated with better quality of life and better preservation of renal function especially in patients with CKD. However, when the GFR is <15 mL/min, then NSS can be avoided.

Radical nephrectomy (RN) in localized RCC is considered for T1b, T2, T3 and T4 tumours where NSS is likely to result in less amount of functional parenchyma or there may be compromise in oncological outcomes. However, contemporary series have shown equivalent benefit of PN with respect to overall survival and cancer-specific survival as compared to RN [31, 32]. RN can be performed by open or minimal invasive (MIS) methods such as laparoscopic or robot-assisted surgeries. Open RN can be performed by flank incision, anterior subcostal incision and long midline incision. For large upper polar tumour extending high up, thoracoabdominal approach is more suitable particularly for left-sided large upper polar tumour.

3.6 Role of Renal Biopsy

Weather localized or locally advanced, indeterminate renal masses should be dealt with core biopsies. It is typically done under ultrasound guidance and rarely under CT guidance [33]. Although theoretical risk of tumour seeding is present, but it has been largely overcome by using coaxial technique of biopsy. In a series, it was found that the fine-needle biopsies are associated with a specificity and sensitivity of 99.1% and 99.7%, respectively [34].

3.7 Role of Genetic Testing in RCC

Although hereditary tumours account for 5–8% of RCCs, but genetic abnormalities are found to be present in about 38% of patients of metastatic RCC [35]. Hence, it is imperative to offer genetic testing in younger patients (<45 years of age) presenting with renal masses, patients with bilateral cysts or multiple renal masses, first- or second-degree relatives of patients of RCCs or even a close relative with a known pathological variant. Some of the histological variants are associated with hereditary syndromes such as papillary RCC (hereditary papillary RCC), multiple chromophobe RCCs, oncocytomas and angiomyolipomas. More importantly, their management should involve a multidisciplinary team with proper work-up and guidance for the patients and their family members [7].

Locally advanced RCC (LA-RCC) is typically dealt with radical nephrectomy. This can be performed by open or laparoscopic/robot-assisted techniques. Some issues pertaining to LA-RCC need to be understood. These are the role of lymphadenectomy and its template, role of multi-organ resections, role of neoadjuvant and adjuvant therapies to downsize the lesions and tumour extension into the inferior vena (IVC).

3.8 Role of Lymphadenectomy

The role of lymph node dissection (LND) in RCC is controversial. Some retrospective studies have shown some benefit in overall survival (OS), while others failed to show any OS benefit [36, 37]. A single RCT on this subject also failed to show any OS benefit of LND; however, it was underpowered since majority of the patients were having small tumours [38]. All these studies are fraught with heterogeneity [39]. Moreover, morbidity of LND ranges between 17 and 35% [40]. Hence, routine LND is not performed except in clinically palpable/intraoperatively visible nodes. Presence of necrosis >50% in the tumour on imaging or the size of tumour >10 cm on imaging is also considered as additional parameters where LND can be considered [41]. The exact template for LND is another unresolved area [42]. Typically for right-sided tumour, the paracaval and the inter-aorto-caval nodes and for left-sided tumours the pre and paraaortic nodes are harvested. It has been seen that nonclear cell variants of RCC (nc-RCC) especially the papillary RCCs have higher chance of lymph-node metastasis than clear cell histology, hence performing LND in those suspected to have nc-RCC based on imaging or proven on core biopsy may be beneficial [40]. Adjacent organs involved by the renal masses must be excised whenever feasible [43].

3.9 Renal Mass with Inferior Vena Caval Thrombus (IVCT)

This entity needs special description. The oncological outcomes of surgery in a non-metastatic setting are good when complete resection with thrombectomy is performed [44, 45]. But presence of thrombus adds to the surgical risk. Due to obstruction to the venous outflow, there are various collaterals, which open up and carry risk of torrential bleed during surgery. Apart from this, there is a potential risk of thromboembolism. Left-sided renal masses with IVCT carry added risk of renal functional deterioration due to venous outflow obstruction of the functional right kidney. IVCT has been divided into various levels based on extent of thrombus (Fig. 3.6). Higher the level of thrombus higher is the recurrence rate and poorer 5-year survival [45, 46]. Also the surgical difficulty increases with the increase in the level of thrombus.

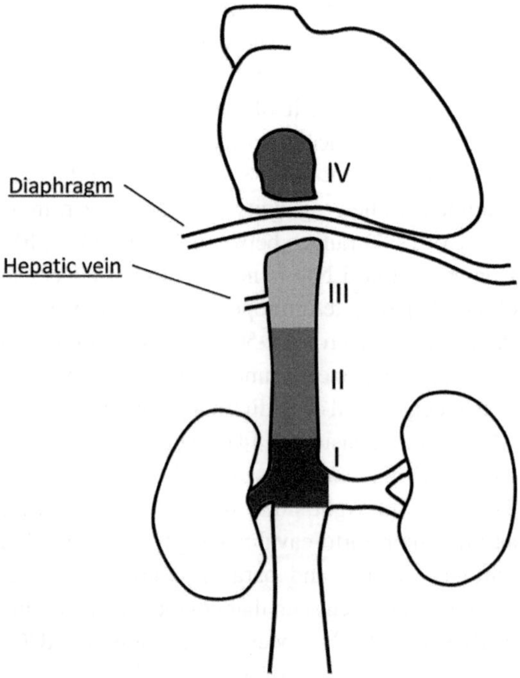

Fig. 3.6 Diagrammatic representation of classification of IVC thrombus

Level 1 and 2 thrombus can be managed in a urological suite. Level 3 and 4 thrombus typically requires surgical team with multiple specialties such as gastrosurgeon for liver mobilization, and a cardiothoracic surgeon for cardiac bypass. The preoperative workup for a level 4 thrombus must include a 2D-ECHO and coronary artery evaluation. If coronaries show significant block, then IVC thrombectomy and coronary artery bypass surgeries should be combined. Typical steps in managing IVCT are preoperative angiembolization of the kidney especially there are large nodes sitting in the hilum or big collaterals (Fig. 3.7). Angioembolization would minimize the venous blood pressure in the collaterals thus decreasing the blood loss and also allows the surgeon to directly reach the IVC. Alternatively the renal artery can be ligated intraoperatively as a first step by going into the inter-aorto-caval groove for right renal artery and paraaortic space for left renal artery. Inferior mesenteric vein serves as a good landmark to reach directly onto the aorta. The second step is isolation of the infrahilar cava, the opposite renal vein and the cava above the thrombus. Care should be taken to identify and ligate the lumbar veins, which may cause torrential bleed when the cava is opened. For left-sided tumours, both the renal artery and vein are isolated and clamped. In level 3 IVCT, the caval control can be achieved by mobilizing the liver; the piggy-bag technique.

If a suprahepatic control is taken for level 3 thrombus, Pringle's maneuverer is performed in order to control the portal vein and hepatic arteries for preventing hepatic congestion while on clamp.

For level 4 thrombus, typically the patient had to be taken on a cardiopulmonary bypass and the thrombus is continuously monitored intraoperatively using a transoesophageal ECHO cardiography (Fig. 3.8). The order of clamping the cava is first the infrahilar then the opposite renal vein and then the supra thrombal cava. While declamping reverse order if followed, the thrombus is delivered intact. Any wall of IVC with infiltration should be excised. Once on clamp, the IVC is

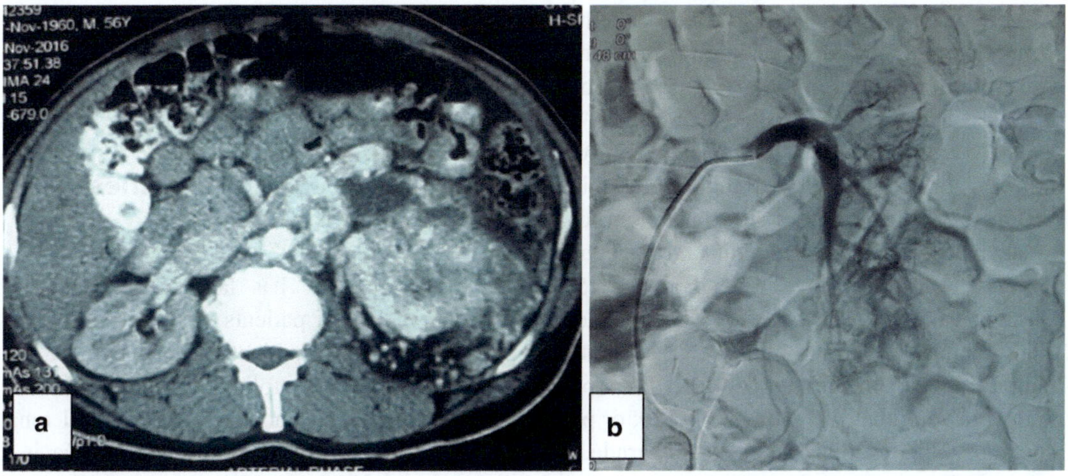

Fig. 3.7 (**a**) Contrast-enhanced CT showing a locally advanced RCC with level 1 IVC thrombus multiple venous collaterals and multiple enlarged lymphnodes encasing the renal artery; (**b**) main left renal artery embolization through transfemoral route using gelfoam and coils

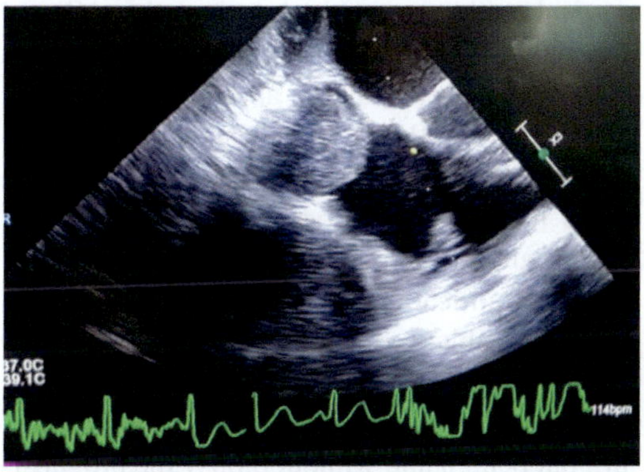

Fig. 3.8 Intraoperative trans-esophageal echo showing the tumour thrombus inside the atrium

opened at the junction of renal vein and IVC. Care should be taken to deliver the thrombus intact to prevent tumour thromboembolism. Once the thrombus is delivered out, then a vascular side clamp is applied on the IVC for repair using 5-0-6-0 proline sutures. This would limit the IVC clamp time and the antecedent hemodynamic instabilities. In general, care should be taken to prevent IVC luminal narrowing upto 50%. If the IVC lumen is severely compromised, then a patch graft can be used to repair IVC. Material for patch reconstruction includes bovine and autologous pericardium, Dacron, PTFE and autologous saphenous vein. There are small series where IVCT has been managed by laparoscopic or robot-assisted minimally invasive surgical options [47, 48]. OS in patients of IVCT is comparable to any LA-RCC [46].

3.10 Role of Neoadjuvant/ Adjuvant Therapy LA-RCC

RCCs especially those with clear cell histology are immune-responsive. With better understanding of the molecular pathways especially the vascular–endothelial growth factor (VEGF) inhibitors, myriad of agents such as sunitinib, pazopanib, sorafenib, cabozantinib and bevacizumab have been studied and approved for use in the past. Further with the advent of checkpoint inhibitors (CPIs), various studies have shown benefit of these agents such as Ipilumumab, Nevolumab, Pembrolizumab and Atezolizumab in management of clear cell RCCs. However, these agents were used and approved in metastatic settings only with or without cytoreductive nephrectomy (CTN) [49, 50]. It is beyond the scope of this chapter to cover all the trials of various drugs and their approvals. Based on beneficial survival outcomes in metastatic settings, these agents were explored for its beneficial effects in locally advanced RCCs. S-TRAC trial showed a disease-free survival (DFS) benefit of 12 months for sunitinib when administered in an adjuvant setting for high-risk (pT3, pT4 or node-positive), localized clear cell RCC but no OS benefit [51, 52]. A similar study on adjuvant sunitinib and sorafenib compared to placebo in high-risk clear cell RCC did not show any significant 5-year DFS [53]. Similarly, adjuvant pazopanib has also not shown any DFS advantage [54]. Thus, TKI failed to show any significant benefit. What about CPIs? In a study evaluating Pembrolizumab in intermediate-high risk (pT2, grade 4 or sarcomatoid features, N0 M0; or pT3, any grade, N0 M0), high risk (pT4, any grade, N0 M0; or pT any state, any grade, node-positive M0) or M1 clear cell RCC found that with 24 months of follow-up, adjuvant pembrolizumab led to a statistically significant and clinically meaningful disease-free survival benefit versus placebo in the intent-to-treat population ($p = 0.001$) [55]. Various ongoing trials exploring the role of CPI alone or in combinations with another CPI or TKI are underway in the adjuvant settings and have the potential to become the new standard of care. CPIs are also being studied in the neoadjuvant setting of LA-RCC. The future landscape in this area is exciting and rapidly evolving.

3.11 Is There a Role of Downsizing the Tumour Before Surgery with These Agents?

Neoadjuvant therapy generally 2 cycles of sunitinib have shown to result in 25–30% of unresectable tumours becoming resectable with equal proportion of patients experiencing cancer progression on therapy [56]. More than 2 cycles of sunitinib have shown to be associated with an undesirable increase in operative adhesions. Also there is no data currently available suggesting that neoadjuvant therapy and completion of nephrectomy have an impact, either positive or negative, on cancer-specific outcomes [57]. Hence, the use of neoadjuvant therapies to downsize tumour may be reserved for patients with large tumour with solitary kidney who otherwise would have required RN. Lack of sufficient evidence in this regard makes this approach experimental.

3.12 Therapeutic Approaches Other Than Surgery

Treatment of RCC has largely been surgical extirpation. But in patients not desirous of surgery or an old frail patients not suitable for surgery or recurrence following PN alternative options need to be understood. For small renal masses <4 cm (SRM), active surveillance is a viable concept especially for older individuals [58]. The average rate of growth of a renal mass has shown to be 0.09 cm/year [59]. There are other competing causes of mortality in older individuals than SRM. The OS and cancer-specific survival are comparable between the AS and intervention with an acceptable quality of life, hence AS is considered appropriate in older patients with SRM [60]. Clear cell RCCs are known to be growing rapidly than papillary RCC, hence it may be imperative to perform biopsy before putting the patients on AS for better follow-up stratification [61]. Apart from AS, there are various ablative techniques available for managing SRMs. A renal biopsy is mandatory before any tumour ablation. One 30% of the SRMs may turn out benign and without biopsy the prognosis and survival outcome comparisons can never be made [62]. The ablative techniques which are well studied are the cryoablation and radiofrequency ablation [63]. These ablative techniques can be performed through percutaneous or laparoscopic approaches. The most preferred technique is the percutaneous approach using ultrasound guidance. Tumours located close to the renal sinus, renal vasculature, pelvicalyceal system or large renal masses are relative contraindications for these ablative techniques. In such situations, there is a risk of leaving behind the margin of the tumour in order to prevent inadvertent injury to vital structures within the kidney [64]. The short-term outcomes are comparable with PN, but long-term outcomes are debatable and favor PN with respect to risk of recurrence and disease progression [65]. Hence, these ablative techniques are reserved for frail patient who are unfit for surgery or an extremely select group of patients available expertise [66]. Other ablative techniques are stereotactic ablative radiotherapy, microwave ablation, high-intensity focussed ultrasound ablation or irreversible electroporation. These techniques are not well studied yet and largely experimental [67].

References

1. Vergho DC, Loeser A, Kocot A, et al. Tumor thrombus of inferior vena cava in patients with renal cell carcinoma—clinical and oncological outcome of 50 patients after surgery. BMC Res Notes. 2012;5:5.
2. Gaillard F. Robson staging system of renal cell carcinoma. https://radiopaedia.org/articles/robson-staging-system-of-renal-cell-carcinoma.
3. Rosiello G, Larcher A, Fallara G, Giancristofaro C, Martini A, Re C, Cei F, Musso G, Tian Z, Karakiewicz PI, Mottrie A. Head-to-head comparison of all the prognostic models recommended by the European Association of Urology guidelines to predict oncologic outcomes in patients with renal cell carcinoma. Urol Oncol. 2022;40(6):271.e19.
4. Vasudev NS, Wilson M, Stewart GD, Adeyoju A, Cartledge J, Ķimuli M, Datta S, Hanbury D, Hrouda D, Oades G, Patel P. Challenges of early renal cancer detection: symptom patterns and incidental diagnosis rate in a multicentre prospective UK cohort of patients presenting with suspected renal cancer. BMJ Open. 2020;10(5):e035938.
5. Lee CT, Katz J, Fearn PA, Russo P. Mode of presentation of renal cell carcinoma provides prognostic information. Urol Oncol. 2002;7(4):135–40.
6. Kim HL, Belldegrun AS, Freitas DG, Bui MH, Han KR, Dorey FJ, Figlin RA. Paraneoplastic signs and symptoms of renal cell carcinoma: implications for prognosis. J Urol. 2003;170(5):1742–6.
7. Mucci LA, Hjelmborg JB, Harris JR, Czene K, Havelick DJ, Scheike T, Graff RE, Holst K, Möller S, Unger RH, McIntosh C. Familial risk and heritability of cancer among twins in Nordic countries. JAMA. 2016;315(1):68–76.
8. Warren KS, McFarlane J. The Bosniak classification of renal cystic masses. BJU Int. 2005;95(7):939–42.
9. Schoots IG, Zaccai K, Hunink MG, Verhagen PC. Bosniak classification for complex renal cysts reevaluated: a systematic review. J Urol. 2017;198(1):12–21.
10. Defortescu G, Cornu JN, Béjar S, Giwerc A, Gobet F, Werquin C, Pfister C, Nouhaud FX. Diagnostic performance of contrast-enhanced ultrasonography and magnetic resonance imaging for the assessment of complex renal cysts: a prospective study. Int J Urol. 2017;24(3):184–9.
11. Mueller-Lisse UG, Mueller-Lisse UL. Imaging of advanced renal cell carcinoma. World J Urol. 2010;28(3):253–61.
12. Giannarini G, Petralia G, Thoeny HC. Potential and limitations of diffusion-weighted magnetic resonance imaging in kidney, prostate, and bladder cancer including pelvic lymph node staging: a critical analysis of the literature. Eur Urol. 2012;61(2):326–40.
13. Steinberg RL, Rasmussen RG, Johnson BA, Ghandour R, De Leon AD, Xi Y, Yokoo T, Kim S, Kapur P, Cadeddu JA, Pedrosa I. Prospective performance of clear cell likelihood scores (ccLS) in renal masses evaluated with multiparametric magnetic resonance imaging. Eur Radiol. 2021;31(1):314–24.
14. Liu Y. The place of FDG PET/CT in renal cell carcinoma: value and limitations. Front Oncol. 2016;6:201.
15. Gyftopoulos K, Zagkou S. Personalized 3D model printing and better surgical and oncological outcomes: the kidney tumor paradigm. Clin Oncol. 2021;6:1881.
16. Porter JR. The role of lymphadenectomy for renal cell carcinoma: are we any closer to an answer? Eur Urol. 2017;71(4):568–9.
17. Johnsen JA, Hellsten S. Lymphatogenous spread of renal cell carcinoma: an autopsy study. J Urol. 1997;157(2):450–3.
18. Herr HW. A history of partial nephrectomy for renal tumors. J Urol. 2005;173(3):705–8.
19. Thompson RH, Lane BR, Lohse CM, Leibovich BC, Fergany A, Frank I, Gill IS, Blute ML, Campbell SC. Renal function after partial nephrectomy: effect of warm ischemia relative to quantity and quality of preserved kidney. Urology. 2012;79(2):356–60.
20. Soisrithong C, Sirisreetreerux P, Sangkum P, Kijvikai K, Viseshsindh W, Kongchareonsombat W, Leenanupunth C, Kochakarn W, Jenjitranant P. Comparative outcomes and predictive assessment of trifecta in open, laparoscopic, and robotic-assisted partial nephrectomy cases with renal cell carcinoma: a 10-year experience at Ramathibodi hospital. Res Rep Urol. 2021;13:425.
21. Uzzo RG, Novick AC. Nephron sparing surgery for renal tumors: indications, techniques and outcomes. J Urol. 2001;166(1):6–18.
22. Porpiglia F, Volpe A, Billia M, Scarpa RM. Laparoscopic versus open partial nephrectomy: analysis of the current literature. Eur Urol. 2008;53(4):732–43.
23. Benway BM, Bhayani SB, Rogers CG, Dulabon LM, Patel MN, Lipkin M, Wang AJ, Stifelman MD. Robot assisted partial nephrectomy versus laparoscopic partial nephrectomy for renal tumors: a multi-institutional analysis of perioperative outcomes. J Urol. 2009;182(3):866–73.
24. Ellison JS, Montgomery JS, Hafez KS, Miller DC, He C, Wolf JS Jr, Weizer AZ. Association of RENAL nephrometry score with outcomes of

minimally invasive partial nephrectomy. Int J Urol. 2013;20(6):564–70.
25. Wang YD, Huang CP, Chang CH, Wu HC, Yang CR, Wang YP, Hsieh PF. The role of RENAL, PADUA, C-index, CSA nephrometry systems in predicting ipsilateral renal function after partial nephrectomy. BMC Urol. 2019;19(1):1–7.
26. Sharma AP, Mavuduru RS, Bora GS, Devana SK, Palani K, Lal A, Kakkar N, Singh SK, Mandal AK. Comparison of RENAL, PADUA, and C-index scoring systems in predicting perioperative outcomes after nephron sparing surgery. Indian J Urol. 2018;34(1):51.
27. Bora GS, Mavuduru RS, Sharma AP, Devana SK, Kakkar N, Lal A, Singh SK, Mandal AK. Initial experience of robotic nephron sparing surgery in cases of high renal nephrometry scores. Indian J Urol. 2017;33(3):230.
28. Sri D, Thakkar R, Patel HR, Lazarus J, Berger F, McArthur R, Lavigueur-Blouin H, Afshar M, Fraser-Taylor C, Le Roux P, Liban J. Robotic-assisted partial nephrectomy (RAPN) and standardization of outcome reporting: a prospective, observational study on reaching the "trifecta and Pentafecta". J Robot Surg. 2021;15(4):571–7.
29. Sharma G, Sharma AP, Tyagi S, Bora GS, Mavuduru RS, Devana SK, Singh SK. Robot-assisted partial nephrectomy for moderate to highly complex renal masses. A systematic review and meta-analysis. Indian J Urol. 2022;38(3):174.
30. Sun M, Bianchi M, Trinh QD, Hansen J, Abdollah F, Hanna N, Tian Z, Shariat SF, Montorsi F, Perrotte P, Karakiewicz PI. Comparison of partial vs. radical nephrectomy with regard to other-cause mortality in T1 renal cell carcinoma among patients aged $\geq$ 75 years with multiple comorbidities. BJU Int. 2013;111(1):67–73.
31. Shah PH, Moreira DM, Patel VR, Gaunay G, George AK, Alom M, Kozel Z, Yaskiv O, Hall SJ, Schwartz MJ, Vira MA. Partial nephrectomy is associated with higher risk of relapse compared with radical nephrectomy for clinical stage T1 renal cell carcinoma pathologically up staged to T3a. J Urol. 2017;198(2):289–96.
32. Liu H, Kong QF, Li J, Wu YQ, Pan KH, Xu B, Wang YL, Chen M. A meta-analysis for comparison of partial nephrectomy vs. radical nephrectomy in patients with pT3a renal cell carcinoma. Transl Androl Urol. 2021;10(3):1170.
33. Schmidbauer J, Remzi M, Memarsadeghi M, Haitel A, Klingler HC, Katzenbeisser D, Wiener H, Marberger M. Diagnostic accuracy of computed tomography-guided percutaneous biopsy of renal masses. Eur Urol. 2008;53(5):1003–12.
34. Marconi L, Dabestani S, Lam TB, Hofmann F, Stewart F, Norrie J, Bex A, Bensalah K, Canfield SE, Hora M, Kuczyk MA. Systematic review and meta-analysis of diagnostic accuracy of percutaneous renal tumour biopsy. Eur Urol. 2016;69(4):660–73.
35. Bratslavsky G, Mendhiratta N, Daneshvar M, Brugarolas J, Ball MW, Metwalli A, Nathanson KL, Pierorazio PM, Boris RS, Singer EA, Carlo MI. Genetic risk assessment for hereditary renal cell carcinoma: clinical consensus statement. Cancer. 2021;127(21):3957–66.
36. Sullivan LD, Westmore DD, McLoughlin MG. Surgical management of renal cell carcinoma at the Vancouver general hospital: 20-year review. Can J Surg. 1979;22(5):427–31.
37. Ristau BT, Manola J, Haas NB, Heng DY, Messing EM, Wood CG, Kane CJ, DiPaola RS, Uzzo RG. Retroperitoneal lymphadenectomy for high risk, nonmetastatic renal cell carcinoma: an analysis of the ASSURE (ECOG-ACRIN 2805) adjuvant trial. J Urol. 2018;199(1):53–9.
38. Blom JH, van Poppel H, Maréchal JM, Jacqmin D, Schröder FH, de Prijck L, Sylvester R. Radical nephrectomy with and without lymph-node dissection: final results of European Organization for Research and Treatment of cancer (EORTC) randomized phase 3 trial 30881. Eur Urol. 2009;55(1):28–34.
39. Bekema HJ, MacLennan S, Imamura M, Lam TB, Stewart F, Scott N, MacLennan G, McClinton S, Griffiths TL, Skolarikos A, MacLennan SJ. Systematic review of adrenalectomy and lymph node dissection in locally advanced renal cell carcinoma. Eur Urol. 2013;64(5):799–810.
40. Kroeger N, Pantuck AJ, Wells JC, et al. Characterizing the impact of lymph node metastases on the survival outcome for metastatic renal cell carcinoma patients treated with targeted therapies. Eur Urol. 2015;68:506–15.
41. Crispen PL, Breau RH, Allmer C, Lohse CM, Cheville JC, Leibovich BC, Blute ML. Lymph node dissection at the time of radical nephrectomy for high-risk clear cell renal cell carcinoma: indications and recommendations for surgical templates. Eur Urol. 2011;59(1):18–23.
42. Campi R, Sessa F, Di Maida F, et al. Templates of lymph node dissection for renal cell carcinoma: a systematic review of the literature. Front Surg. 2018;5:76.
43. Castellanos-Hernández H, Solares-Sánchez ME, Sánchez-Turati JG, et al. Multiple organ resection in renal cancer. Rev Mex Urol. 2012;72(3):131–5.
44. Blute ML, Leibovich BC, Lohse CM, Cheville JC, Zincke H. The Mayo Clinic experience with surgical management, complications and outcome for patients with renal cell carcinoma and venous tumour thrombus. BJU Int. 2004;94(1):33–41.
45. Martínez-Salamanca JI, Huang WC, Millán I, Bertini R, Bianco FJ, Carballido JA, Ciancio G, Hernández C, Herranz F, Haferkamp A, Hohenfellner M. Prognostic impact of the 2009 UICC/AJCC TNM staging system for renal cell carcinoma with venous extension. Eur Urol. 2011;59(1):120–7.
46. Abel EJ, Masterson TA, Karam JA, et al. Predictive Nomogram for recurrence following surgery for nonmetastatic renal cell cancer with tumor thrombus. J Urol. 2017;198:810–6.

47. Chopra S, Simone G, Metcalfe C, et al. Robot-assisted level II–III inferior vena cava tumor thrombectomy: step-by-step technique and 1-year outcomes. Eur Urol. 2017;72:267–74.
48. Wang B, Huang Q, Liu K, et al. Robot-assisted level III-IV inferior vena cava thrombectomy: initial series with step-by-step procedures and 1-yr outcomes. Eur Urol. 2020;78:77–86.
49. Choueiri TK, Motzer RJ. Systemic therapy for metastatic renal-cell carcinoma. N Engl J Med. 2017;376:354–66.
50. Lara PN Jr, Evans CP. Cytoreductive nephrectomy in metastatic renal cell cancer: not all that it's cut out to be. JAMA Oncol. 2019;5:171–2.
51. Ravaud A, Motzer RJ, Pandha HS, George DJ, Pantuck AJ, Patel A, Chang YH, Escudier B, Donskov F, Magheli A, Carteni G. Adjuvant sunitinib in high-risk renal-cell carcinoma after nephrectomy. N Engl J Med. 2016;375(23):2246–54.
52. Staehler M, Motzer RJ, George DJ, Pandha HS, Donskov F, Escudier B, Pantuck AJ, Patel A, DeAnnuntis L, Bhattacharyya H, Ramaswamy K. Adjuvant sunitinib in patients with high-risk renal cell carcinoma: safety, therapy management, and patient-reported outcomes in the S-TRAC trial. Ann Oncol. 2018;29(10):2098–104.
53. Haas NB, Manola J, Uzzo RG, Flaherty KT, Wood CG, Kane C, Jewett M, Dutcher JP, Atkins MB, Pins M, Wilding G. Adjuvant sunitinib or sorafenib for high-risk, non-metastatic renal-cell carcinoma (ECOG-ACRIN E2805): a double-blind, placebo-controlled, randomised, phase 3 trial. Lancet. 2016;387(10032):2008–16.
54. Motzer RJ, Haas NB, Donskov F, Gross-Goupil M, Varlamov S, Kopyltsov E, Lee JL, Melichar B, Rini BI, Choueiri TK, Zemanova M. Randomized phase III trial of adjuvant pazopanib versus placebo after nephrectomy in patients with localized or locally advanced renal cell carcinoma. J Clin Oncol. 2017;35(35):3916.
55. Choueiri TK, Tomczak P, Park SH, Venugopal B, Ferguson T, Chang YH, Hajek J, Symeonides SN, Lee JL, Sarwar N, Thiery-Vuillemin A. Adjuvant pembrolizumab after nephrectomy in renal-cell carcinoma. N Engl J Med. 2021;385(8):683–94.
56. Amin C, Wallen E, Pruthi RS, et al. Preoperative tyrosine kinase inhibition as an adjunct to debulking nephrectomy. Urology. 2008;72:864–8.
57. Tomita Y. Treatment strategies for advanced renal cell carcinoma: a new paradigm for surgical treatment. Int J Urol. 2016;23:13–21.
58. Pierorazio PM, Johnson MH, Ball MW, Gorin MA, Trock BJ, Chang P, Wagner AA, McKiernan JM, Allaf ME. Five-year analysis of a multi-institutional prospective clinical trial of delayed intervention and surveillance for small renal masses: the DISSRM registry. Eur Urol. 2015;68(3):408–15.
59. Uzosike AC, Patel HD, Alam R, Schwen ZR, Gupta M, Gorin MA, Johnson MH, Gausepohl H, Riffon MF, Trock BJ, Chang P. Growth kinetics of small renal masses on active surveillance: variability and results from the DISSRM registry. J Urol. 2018;199(3):641–8.
60. Vartolomei L, Cotruş A, Stanciu C, Delcea C, Tozzi M, Lievore E, Crocetto F, Del Giudice F, Lucarelli G, Muto M, Ferro M. Quality of life and psychological distress among patients with small renal masses. J Clin Med. 2022;11(14):3944.
61. Finelli A, Cheung DC, Al-Matar A, Evans AJ, Morash CG, Pautler SE, Siemens DR, Tanguay S, Rendon RA, Gleave ME, Drachenberg DE. Small renal mass surveillance: histology-specific growth rates in a biopsy-characterized cohort. Eur Urol. 2020;78(3):460–7.
62. Widdershoven CV, Aarts BM, Zondervan PJ, Henderickx MM, Klompenhouwer EG, van Delden OM, Prevoo W, Montauban van Swijndregt AD, van Moorselaar RJ, Bex A, Lagerveld BW. Renal biopsies performed before versus during ablation of T1 renal tumors: implications for prevention of overtreatment and follow-up. Abdom Radiol. 2021;46(1):373–9.
63. Atwell TD, Schmit GD, Boorjian SA, Mandrekar J, Kurup AN, Weisbrod AJ, Chow GK, Leibovich BC, Callstrom MR, Patterson DE, Lohse CM. Percutaneous ablation of renal masses measuring 3.0 cm and smaller: comparative local control and complications after radiofrequency ablation and cryoablation. Am J Roentgenol. 2013;200(2):461–6.
64. Zargar H, Atwell TD, Cadeddu JA, Jean J, Janetschek G, Kaouk JH, Matin SF, Polascik TJ, Zargar-Shoshtari K, Thompson RH. Cryoablation for small renal masses: selection criteria, complications, and functional and oncologic results. Eur Urol. 2016;69(1):116–28.
65. Andrews JR, Atwell T, Schmit G, Lohse CM, Kurup AN, Weisbrod A, Callstrom MR, Cheville JC, Boorjian SA, Leibovich BC, Thompson RH. Oncologic outcomes following partial nephrectomy and percutaneous ablation for cT1 renal masses. Eur Urol. 2019;76(2):244–51.
66. Ljungberg B, Albiges L, Bensalah K, Bex A, Giles RH, Hora M, Kuczyk MA, Lam T, Marconi L, Merseburger AS, Powles T, et al. EAU guidelines on renal cell carcinoma. Arnhem: EAU Central Office; 2019.
67. Zhou W, Herwald SE, McCarthy C, Uppot RN, Arellano RS. Radiofrequency ablation, cryoablation, and microwave ablation for T1a renal cell carcinoma: a comparative evaluation of therapeutic and renal function outcomes. J Vasc Interv Radiol. 2019;30(7):1035–42.

Management of Metastatic Renal Cell Carcinoma

4

Rohit K. Jain, Humaira Sarfraz, Muhammad Z. Farooq, and Guru Sonpavde

4.1 Introduction

Kidney cancer is the 14th most common cancer worldwide. It is the ninth most common cancer in men and the 14th most common cancer in women [1]. It is estimated that there will be 79,000 new cases of kidney cancer and an estimated 13,920 people will die of this disease in 2022 in the United States [2]. Approximately 90% of kidney tumors are renal-cell carcinoma (RCC), 80% of which is composed of clear-cell histology (ccRCC). Other less common cell types include papillary, chromophobe, and collecting duct tumors. Approximately, 16% patients are diagnosed with de-novo metastatic disease (mRCC) with most common sites being lung, bone, liver, and brain [3].

The treatment landscape of mRCC has significantly changed improving the overall prognosis of this disease. High-dose interleukin-2 yielded durable survival in a small subset of metastatic ccRCC, while interferon alpha prolonged median survival modestly. However, the median survival remained ~1 year [4]. Subsequently, first-line vascular endothelial growth factor (VEGF)-targeted tyrosine kinase inhibitor (TKI) monotherapy employing sunitinib or pazopanib led to doubling of survival to ~2 years [5, 6]. While everolimus, an mTOR inhibitor had demonstrated improved progression-free survival (PFS) compared to placebo post-VEGF inhibitor, cabozantinib improved overall survival (OS) versus everolimus in the same setting [7]. Following the emergence of immune checkpoint inhibitors, nivolumab, a programmed cell death protein (PD)-1 inhibitor, extended OS when compared with everolimus in the post-VEGF inhibitor setting, which was characterized by highly durable responses [8]. Thereafter, the development of combination T-cell immune checkpoint inhibitors (ICIs) with PD-1 and cytotoxic T-lymphocyte-associated antigen 4 (CTLA-4) antibodies (Abs) has shown acceptable safety, extended OS, and exhibited durable antitumor activity compared to first-line sunitinib in poor- and intermediate-risk metastatic ccRCC. Multiple phase III randomized clinical trials have compared PD-1 inhibitors combined with a VEGF inhibitor and demonstrated improved OS against sunitinib, which has resulted in a major shift in front-line treatment strategies [9]. VEGF inhibitors and ICIs have also provided more modest improved outcomes in nonclear cell (ncc)-RCC. The emerging class of hypoxia-inducible factor (HIF) inhibitors promises to provide another increment in outcomes. In this chapter, we summarize these developments and the evolution of systemic therapy for metastatic RCC.

R. K. Jain · H. Sarfraz · M. Z. Farooq
H. Lee Moffitt Cancer Center, Tampa, FL, USA

G. Sonpavde (✉)
Dana Farber Cancer Institute, Boston, MA, USA

Advent Health Cancer Institute, Orlando, FL, USA
e-mail: gurup_sonpavde@dfci.harvard.edu

P. Singh et al. (eds.), *A Guide to Management of Urological Cancers*,
https://doi.org/10.1007/978-981-99-2341-0_4

4.2 Prognostic Models for Metastatic Disease

Prognostic scoring systems have been developed to define risk groups for patients with mRCC [10, 11]. The first prognostic factor model to be widely applied was from the Memorial Sloan Kettering Cancer Center (MSKCC) [10]. This model was derived from patients treated with interferon and included five prognostic factors for multivariable analysis: interval from diagnosis to treatment of less than 1 year; Karnofsky Performance Status (KPS) less than 80%; serum LDH greater than 1.5 times the upper limit of normal (ULN); corrected serum calcium greater than the ULN; and serum hemoglobin less than the lower limit of normal (LLN). Patients with none of these factors are considered low risk or with good prognosis, those with one or two factors present are considered intermediate risk, and patients with three or more of the factors are considered poor risk.

International metastatic RCC Database Consortium (IMDC) was derived from a population of patients with mRCC treated with VEGF-targeted therapy [11]. Six clinical parameters were included in this model; hemoglobin less than the LLN, serum-corrected calcium greater than the ULN, KPS less than 80%, and time from initial diagnosis to initiation of therapy of less than 1 year, absolute neutrophil count (ANC) greater than ULN and platelets greater than ULN. Patients with no adverse factors were in the favorable-risk category in which an mOS was not reached and a 2-year OS was 75% (95% CI, 65–82%). Patients with 1–2 adverse factors were in the intermediate-risk category in which an mOS was 27 months and a 2-year OS was 53% (95% CI, 46–59%). Finally, those patients with 3–6 adverse factors were in the poor-risk category in which an mOS was 8.8 months and a 2-year OS was 7% (95% CI, 2–16%).

4.3 Cytoreductive Nephrectomy

Cytoreductive nephrectomy (CN) is removal of primary tumor in metastatic setting. CN before systemic therapy is recommended in select patients with a potentially surgically resectable primary tumor mass. Initial data was from clinical trials in which CN + interferon was compared to interferon alone. Although addition of CN did show improve OS and time to disease progression, however, the yield maybe lower as these trials were conducted prior to development of IMDC risk criteria's [12, 13].

With newer VEGF-directed therapies, retrospective data did suggest that CN is clinically significant in mRCC patients that are being treated with these agents [14, 15]. Based on these findings prospective trials were conducted including noninferiority CARMENA trial [16]. This trial had 450 participants who were intermediate or poor risk and assigned to either CN + sunitinib arm or sunitinib alone arm. The mOS was 18.4 months in the sunitinib monotherapy arm that was noninferior to the mOS of 13.9 months for patients who had CN prior to sunitinib therapy (HR: 0.89; 95% CI 0.71–1.10). However, many of the patients in this trial had poor-risk features, underscoring the importance of patient selection to obtain the greatest benefit from nephrectomy or targeted therapy. A post hoc analysis of the CARMENA trial reported that for patients with only one IMDC risk factor, OS was longer following nephrectomy (31.4 vs. 25.2 months) [17]. Another trial named SURTIME was conducted in which patients either had CN followed by sunitinib or a deferred approach where they received 3 cycles of sunitinib followed by CN [18]. Patients who had deferred CN did not have improved 28 week PFS which was the primary end point (43% vs. 42%, $p = 0.61$). The intention to treat OS hazard ratio of deferred versus immediate CN was 0.57 (95% CI 0.34–0.95; $p = 0.03$) with a median OS of 32.4 months (95% CI, 14.5–65.3 months) in the deferred CN arm and 15 months (95% CI, 9.3–29.5 months) in the immediate CN arm. In the deferred CN arm, 98% patients got sunitinib compared to 80% in the immediate arm. Systemic progression before planned CN in the deferred approach resulted in recommendation of not undergoing nephrectomy in 29% patients.

Thus, CARMENA and SURTIME trials did inform that the subset of patients can be treated with upfront CN, however, is not SOC for all patients. However, patient selection is critical, and upfront CN is only reserved in patients with favorable procedures such as minimal extra-renal disease and favorable risk patients, while deferred approach maybe more suitable for patients that had excellent response to systemic therapy. At this point in time, there are ongoing prospective clinical trials such as PROBE trial (NCT04510597) and NORDIC-SUN trial (NCT03977571) defining the role of cytoreductive nephrectomy in patients who subsequently receive checkpoint antibody therapy. Further study will better define the role of cytoreductive nephrectomy in the rapidly evolving treatment landscape for RCC [19].

4.4 First-Line Treatment for Metastatic ccRCC

4.4.1 Combination of VEGF-TKI Plus ICI

4.4.1.1 Axitinib + Pembrolizumab

In a phase III randomized trial KEYNOTE-426, the doublet of axitinib (VEGF-TKI) 5 mg twice daily orally plus pembrolizumab (PD-1) monoclonal antibody 200 mg IV every 3 weeks was compared to sunitinib 50 mg orally, 4 weeks on and 2 weeks off in 861 patients with metastatic ccRCC in the first-line setting [20]. In the updated analyses at a median follow-up of 42.8 months, the mOS was 45.7 months (95% CI, 43.6–not reached) with pembrolizumab plus axitinib compared with 40.1 months (95% CI, 34.3–44.2) with sunitinib (HR 0.73; 95% CI 0.60–0.88; $p < 0.001$). The mPFS was 15.7 months (95% CI, 13.6–20.2) versus 11.1 months (95% CI, 8.9–12.5), respectively (HR 0.68; 95% CI, 0.58–0.80; $p < 0.0001$) [20, 21]. Of 432 patients who received pembrolizumab + axitinib, 103 (23.8%) completed 2 years of therapy without progression [21]. The treatment efficacy was consistent across the International Metastatic Renal Cell Carcinoma Database Consortium (IMDC) risk groups (favorable, intermediate, and poor risk) and irrespective of tumor PD-L1 protein expression. In terms of treatment-related adverse events (TRAE), 75.8% patients receiving pembrolizumab plus axitinib developed grade 3 or higher TRAEs in contrast to 70.6% patients in the sunitinib group. In both groups, the most frequently observed adverse effects were diarrhea and hypertension. However, diarrhea and transaminase elevation were more notable in the pembrolizumab plus axitinib group, while palmar plantar erythrodysesthesia syndrome was more pronounced in the sunitinib group [20].

4.4.1.2 Cabozantinib + Nivolumab

The CheckMate 9ER studied the combination of cabozantinib 40 mg once a day plus nivolumab 240 mg every 2 weeks versus sunitinib 50 mg orally, 4 weeks on and 2 weeks off in 651 patients with mRCC in the first-line setting. Thus, this trial employed a dose of cabozantinib that was lower than the monotherapy dose of 60 mg once daily that was previously approved in the first-line and post-VEGF inhibitor settings [22]. Per the last updated analyses at median follow-up of 32.9 months, the combination showed improved mPFS of 16.6 (95% CI, 12.8–19.8) with nivolumab plus cabozantinib and 8.3 months (95% CI, 7.0–9.7) with sunitinib (HR 0.56; 95% CI, 0.46–0.68). The mOS was also prolonged with cabozantinib plus nivolumab versus sunitinib 37.7 versus 34.3 months (HR 0.70, 95% CI, 0.55–0.90) [23]. RR was high in combination at 55.7% versus 27.1% with sunitinib. Totally, 75% patients on the combination arm developed grade 3 or higher TRAE. The most common toxicities noted with cabozantinib and nivolumab were diarrhea, palmar–palmar erythrodysesthesia, and hypertension, seen in 63.8%, 40.0%, and 34.7% of patients [22].

4.4.1.3 Lenvatinib + Pembrolizumab

The CLEAR trial was a Phase III, multicomparison, randomized study which explored efficacy and safety of lenvatinib 20 mg/pembrolizumab 200 mg versus lenvatinib 18 mg/everolimus 5 mg versus sunitinib monotherapy 50 mg orally, 4 weeks on and 2 weeks off for 1069 patients with treatment-naïve mRCC [22]. Notably, the starting dose of lenvatinib was relatively high in the lenvatinib-pembrolizumab group, which may have contributed to the greater ORR, PFS as well as toxicities with this particular combination when comparing with other similar combinations across trials. Relative to sunitinib, higher mPFS was seen with the combination of lenvatinib/pembrolizumab treatment arms (22.1 vs. 11.1 months; HR 0.38; 95% CI, 0.23–0.62). The ORR for lenvatinib/pembrolizumab, lenvatinib/everolimus, and sunitinib was reported as 71.0%, 55.3%, and 36.1%, respectively. In both arms, median OS was not reached (HR for OS 0.71, 95% CI, 0.30–1.71). However, ORR was significantly improved in combination group versus monotherapy with sunitinib (65.3% vs. 49.2%; odds ratio 2.14, 95% CI, 1.07–4.28). Grade 3 or higher TRAE was seen in 88.0% in lenvatinib/pembrolizumab and 79.7% on sunitinib. The most common toxicities noted among patients in the lenvatinib/pembrolizumab treatment arm were diarrhea, hypertension, hypothyroidism, and decreased appetite [22, 24].

4.4.1.4 Axitinib + Avelumab

The JAVELIN Renal 101 trial evaluated first-line treatment combination of axitinib 5 mg BID plus avelumab 10 mg/kg every 2 weeks versus sunitinib in mRCC. One of the co-primary endpoints, PFS among PD-L1-positive patients was improved by the combination at 13.8 versus 8.4 months with sunitinib (HR 0.61, 95% CI, 0.47–0.79, $p < 0.001$). PFS also improved in the overall intention to treat group. The ORR in PD-L1-positive patients was 55.2% with avelumab plus axitinib and 25.5% with sunitinib. The other co-primary endpoint, OS in the overall group was not attained with axitinib plus avelumab (42.2 months—not estimable) as compared to the sunitinib group (37.8 months; 31.4 months—not estimable). Although this regimen has received FDA approval, because of a lack of a defined OS advantage, it does not currently represent a preferred front-line treatment option. Grade 3 or higher TRAE were seen in 71.2% in the axitinib plus avelumab arm with diarrhea, hypertension, and fatigue being the most common [25].

4.4.2 Dual Checkpoint Inhibitors

4.4.2.1 Ipilimumab + Nivolumab

A multicenter Phase III trial CheckMate 214 trial investigated combination of ipilimumab 1 mg/kg nivolumab 3 mg/kg versus sunitinib 50 mg orally, 4 weeks on and 2 weeks off in 1096 patients. The trial primarily targeted patients with previously untreated IMDC intermediate-risk or poor-risk patients (although good risk patients were also recruited to evaluate as secondary endpoints) and demonstrated that the nivolumab and ipilimumab doublet was superior to sunitinib [26]. At a median follow-up of 67.7 months, the study has continued to show the survival benefit of ipilimumab/nivolumab combination compared to sunitinib, demonstrating an mOS of 47.0 versus 26.6 months for the intermediate/poor-risk population (HR 0.68; 95% CI, 0.58–0.81; $p < 0.0001$). The mPFS was also noted to be superior in the intermediate/poor-risk population (11.6 vs. 8.3 months; HR 0.73; 95% CI, 0.61–0.87; $p = 0.0004$) as was response rate (42.0% vs. 27.0%). Notably, prolonged treatment-free intervals were possible while maintaining a response, which is anticipated to confer benefits to quality of life [27]. However, in the favorable-risk group, the PFS probabilities appeared to favor sunitinib (median 12.4 vs. 28.9 months; HR 1.60; 95% CI, 1.13–2.26; $p = 0.0073$) [28]. These data have been used to support VEGF inhibitor monotherapy as first-line therapy for good-risk patients. Commonly observed grade 3–4 adverse events noted in the ipilimumab and nivolumab included elevated lipase (10%), amylase (6%), and high alanine aminotransferase (5%). 29% patients required corticosteroids for immune-mediated toxicities. An ongoing randomized phase III trial COSMIC-313 is evaluating the combination of cabozantinib with ipilimumab + nivolumab versus the combination of nivolumab and ipilimumab in patients with previously untreated advanced intermediate- or poor-risk mRCC. COSMIC-313 met its primary endpoint, demonstrating significant improvement in PFS at the primary analysis. At a prespecified interim analysis for the secondary endpoint of OS, the combination of cabozantinib, nivolumab, and ipilimumab versus the combination of nivolumab and ipilimumab did not demonstrate a significant benefit awaiting next analysis of OS [29].

4.4.3 VEGF-TKI Monotherapy

4.4.3.1 Cabozantinib

Cabozantinib, a vascular endothelial growth factor 2, MET and AXL inhibitor, was initially approved for standard second-line therapy for mRCC where improved OS was demonstrated versus everolimus (HR 0.66, $p = 0.00026$) [7]. Subsequently, the use of this agent was approved in the first-line setting following a randomized phase II multicenter study CABOSUN. In this trial, patients with IMDC intermediate- or poor-risk categories were randomly assigned cabozantinib 60 mg once daily or sunitinib 50 mg daily orally, 4 weeks on, and 2 weeks off. Treatment with cabozantinib significantly improved overall response rate to 33% (95% CI, 23–44) versus 12% (95% CI, 5.4–21) with Sunitinib. Also, median progression-free survival (PFS), the primary endpoint, was noted to be longer at 8.2 months in cabozantinib versus 5.6 months in suntinib group (HR 0.48, 95% CI, 0.31–0.74, $p = 0.0008$). With a median follow-up of 34.5 months, the secondary endpoint, OS was not statistically better with an mPFS of 26.6 months (95% CI, 14.6–not estimable) with cabozantinib and 21.2 months (95% CI, 16.3–27.4) with sunitinib (HR 0.80, 95% CI, 0.53–1.21). Grade 3 or higher TRAE was noted in 68% for cabozantinib and 65% for sunitinib. These included fatigue (6% vs. 15%), diarrhea (10% vs. 11%), hypertension (28% vs. 22%), palmar-plantar erythrodysesthesia (8% vs. 4%), and hematological adverse events (3% vs. 22%) [30, 31].

4.4.3.2 Sunitinib

Sunitinib was the first tyrosine kinase inhibitor approved by FDA for mRCC as upfront therapy after a trial comparing it with the standard of care at that time, interferon alpha. As monotherapy, taken as 50 mg orally once daily for 4 weeks on and 2 weeks off, the median PFS was significantly prolonged in the Sunitinib arm (11 months) versus the interferon arm (5 months). Also, objective response rate was higher with Sunitinib 31% versus 6% with interferon alpha. Among the grade 3 or 4 treatment-related adverse events, fatigue was more frequent in the interferon group, while diarrhea was more common in the sunitinib group [32].

4.4.3.3 Pazopanib

In COMPARZ trial, pazopanib 800 mg daily oral dose was found to be noninferior to sunitinib 50 mg orally once daily for 4 weeks on 2 weeks off with regard to PFS and OS. Patients receiving sunitinib had higher incidence of fatigue (63% vs. 55%), palmar-plantar erythrodysesthesia (50% vs. 29%), and thrombocytopenia (78% vs. 41%) compared to pazopanib. On the contrary, patients treated with pazopanib had a greater incidence of increased liver enzymes (60% vs. 43%) with sunitinib. The trial showed that while both the drugs have comparable efficacy; the safety and quality of life metrics suggest Pazopanib is better tolerated than Sunitinib [6]. The PISCES study was a randomized cross over study involving 169 patients with mRCC received pazopanib 800 mg daily for 10 weeks, a 2-week washout and then sunitinib 50 mg daily (4 weeks on, 2 weeks off, and 4 weeks on) for 10 weeks versus the opposite sequence. The study showed that 70% patients preferred pazopanib over 22% patients favoring sunitinib due to less fatigue, better overall quality of life, hand/foot, or moth/throat soreness with pazopanib, while less diarrhea was reported as the most common reason favoring sunitinib [33].

4.4.3.4 Cytokine Therapy

High-dose interleukin-2 was historically employed in well-selected fit patients mostly predicated on durable complete responses in ~10% of patients. An analysis of 255 patients in seven phase II trials showed a 14% response rate, with 5% complete responses, with a major subset of these responses being extremely durable. However, this therapy is generally administered in an inpatient intensive care unit setting and can be associated with significant acute toxicities notably the capillary leak syndrome and cardiovascular events [34]. While the role of high-dose IL-2 has significantly receded, the agent should continue to figure in shared decision-making with selected patients and has the benefit of a very brief duration of therapy, which may be associated with durable responses and cures.

4.4.3.5 Surveillance

mRCC is known to be a disease with extreme heterogeneity of course of disease. Hence, active surveillance has been pursued. In a prospective trial, 48 asymptomatic patients included in analysis with mRCC underwent surveillance imaging until initiation of systemic therapy for a median follow-up 38.1 months. The median time until start of systemic therapy was 14.9 months (95% CI, 10.6–25.0). Decreased surveillance period was noted in patients with increased metastatic sites ($p = 0.0414$) and higher IMDC adverse risk factors ($p = 0.0403$) [35].

4.5 Second and Subsequent Lines of Therapy for Metastatic ccRCC

Optimal frontline treatment option in mRCC is very important in the management as they have the greatest potential to achieve complete remission. Once disease progresses after first-line regimen, management options in the refractory setting are limited with suboptimal outcomes. Patients that progress after first-line ipilimumab + nivolumab or VEGF inhibitor + PD-1/L1 inhibitor therapy are usually managed with VEGF-targeted monotherapies that patients have not been exposed to, e.g., cabozantinib or axitinib. Also, there is an option to use a combination regimen with lenvatinib and everolimus in those not exposed to prior lenvatinib or nivolumab monotherapy in those with progression following prior VEGF inhibitor monotherapy.

4.5.1 Axitinib

Axitinib is used in the second-line setting as it showed improved PFS in the Axis trial comparing the safety and efficacy of axitinib 5 mg BID versus sorafenib 400 mg BID following prior cytokine or VEGF inhibitor therapy. Although the OS did not differ between the two groups, the mPFS was longer for axitinib (HR 0.656, 95% CI, 0.552–0.779). In a subgroup analysis, patients with either prior cytokine or VEGF inhibitor treatment were observed to have longer mPFS with axitinib. Common grade 3–4 adverse events seen in this trial were hypertension (17%), diarrhea (11%), and fatigue (10%) in axitinib-treated patients and hand-foot syndrome (17%), hypertension (12%), and diarrhea (8%) in sorafenib-treated patients [36].

4.5.2 Cabozantinib

The Meteor trial compared cabozantinib 60 mg once daily and everolimus 10 mg once daily following progression on prior VEGF inhibitor. Cabozantinib improved PFS (HR 0.51, 95% CI, 0.41–0.62) and ORR (17% vs. 3%). Most importantly, the OS was prolonged with a mOS of 21.4 months for cabozantinib versus 16.5 months for everolimus (HR 0.66; 95% CI, 0.53–0.83). Grade 3–4 adverse events occurred in 39% of the cabozantinib group and 40% of patients treated with everolimus. Most common grade 3–4 events in the cabozantinib group were hypertension 15%, diarrhea 13%, fatigue 11%, hand-foot syndrome 8%, anemia 6%, and hypomagnesemia 5%. The dose reduction was effective in managing toxicities in this trial and required in 60% of the affected cohort in the Meteor trial [7].

4.5.3 Lenvatinib + Everolimus

A randomized phase 2 trial was conducted to include patients with ccRCC that had progressed after first-line VEGF inhibitor therapy in the metastatic setting [37]. Patients in this trial were randomized to combination of Lenvatinib 18 mg + everolimus 5 mg versus single-agent lenvatinib 24 mg versus everolimus 10 mg daily monotherapy. Trial concluded that a combination regimen of lenvatinib + everolimus significantly prolonged the PFS compared with single agent everolimus (HR 0.40, 95% CI, 0.24–0.68; $p = 0.0005$). The mPFS was 14.6 months (95% CI, 5.9–20.1) for lenvatinib + everolimus and 5.5 months (95% CI, 3.5–7.1) for everolimus. Patient treated with single-agent lenvatinib had a PFS of 7.4 months (95% CI, 5.6–10.2), which was also longer as compared to everolimus (HR 0.61, 95% CI, 0.38–0.98; $p = 0.048$). The PFS did not differ for patients allocated lenavatinib plus everolimus compared to monotherapy with lenvatinib (HR 0.66, 0.39–1.10; $p = 0.12$). The ORR was seen in 43% in combination regimen of lenvatinib + everolimus compared to single-agent everolimus (6%) (RR 7.2, 95% CI, 2.3–22.5; $p < 0.0001$) and 27% in single-agent lenvatinib group (RR 1.6, 95% CI, 0.9–2.8; $p = 0.10$). The mOS was 18.5 months for combination lenvatinib + everolimus versus 17.8 months for single-agent lenvatinib versus 16.5 months for single-agent everolimus. Grade 3–4 adverse events were fewer in single-agent everolimus 50%, compared to 79% in lenvatinib monotherapy and 71% in lenvatinib + everolimus combination arm. Most common grade 3–4 events that were seen are diarrhea, fatigue, and hypertension. Thus, combination of lenvatinib + everolimus was included in the management of relapsed/refractory metastatic ccRCC.

4.5.4 Nivolumab

Nivolumab 3 mg/kg IV every 2 weeks prolonged OS compared to everolimus 10 mg orally daily for metastatic ccRCC following progression on a VEGF inhibitor in a pivotal phase III trial CheckMate 025 that led to its approval. The median OS was 25 months with nivolumab compared with 19.6 months with everolimus. The hazard ratio for death with nivolumab versus everolimus was 0.73 (98.5% CI, 0.57–0.93; $p = 0.002$). The ORR was greater with nivolumab than with everolimus 25% versus 5%. Grade 3–4 adverse events occurred in 19% of the patients in the nivolumab arm compared to 37% in the everolimus arm. Thus, nivolumab is a valid option in those progressing after first-line VEGF inhibitor monotherapy [8].

4.5.5 Tivozanib

Tivozanib is a newer potent and relatively selective VEGFR-inhibiting agent that has been recently approved by FDA on March 10, 2021. This approval was based on TIVO-3 trial [38], a randomized phase III study in which tivozanib was compared to sorafenib for patients with relapsed/refractory RCC following at least 2 lines of prior therapy with one prior agent including a VEGF inhibitor. In this study, patients were randomized to get either tivozanib 1.34 mg orally once daily for 21/28-day cycle compared to sorafenib 400 mg twice daily. Tivozanib was superior to sorafenib with improvement of PFS (HR 0.73; 95% CI 0.56–0.95; $p = 0.016$) with notably, benefit also seen in those who were also exposed to prior ICI. The estimated median PFS was 5.6 months in the tivozanib arm compared to 3.9 months in the sorafenib arm. No OS benefit was achieved (HR 0.97; 95% CI, 0.75–1.24). Most common grade 3–4 adverse events seen with tivozanib were hypertension (24%). Compared to sorafenib, tivozanib had lower incidence of grade 3–4 rash, diarrhea, and palmar-plantar erythrodysesthesia. Thus, tivozanib is another viable and tolerable option as salvage therapy of mRCC.

4.5.6 Belzutifan

Based on the nearly ubiquitous presence of somatic VHL-inactivating mutations, which leads to upregulation of HIF, a major transcription factor involved in promoting the genesis of ccRCC, rational agents have been pursued to target HIF-2α. One such agent, belzutifan was shown to be safe and active (ORR 25%) as late-line salvage therapy of mRCC [39]. The major toxicity was anemia. A nonrandomized expansion cohort evaluating belzutifan in patents with germline VHL mutations (VHL disease) and a VHL-associated malignancy (RCC, central nervous system hemangioblastoma, pancreatic neuroendocrine tumor) showed activity for this agent with ORR 49% and highly durable responses [40]. Belzutifan was approved in this setting or VHL disease and these associated malignancies. Phase III trials are evaluating belzutifan for conventional ccRCC as late salvage therapy (vs. everolimus) and as a component of first-line therapy (with lenvatinib-pembrolizumab).

4.6 Therapy for Metastatic Nonclear Cell RCC (nccRCC)

Therapy for nccRCC has not been evaluated in phase III trials. Upto 20% of patients with RCC are subtypes of nonclear cell RCC. Various subtypes of nccRCC include papillary, chromophobe, unclassified, and others.

For metastatic papillary RCC, the PAPMET trial demonstrated that cabozantinib is the preferred TKI likely because of its MET-inhibitory properties. In this trial, patients were randomized into four groups: sunitinib 50 mg, cabozantinib 60 mg, crizotinib 250 mg BID, or savolitinib 600 mg orally daily. PFS was seen to be longer in the cabozantinib group (median 9 months) versus sunitinib (5.6 months). Response rate for cabozantinib was 23% versus 4% for sunitinib. Savolitinib and crizotinib did not improve PFS compared to sunitinib. Grade 3–4 adverse events were seen in 69% of patients receiving sunitinib versus 74% of patients receiving cabozantinib. Thus, cabozantinib is the preferred agent for use in papillary RCC [41].

A phase 2 KEYNOTE 427 study by McDermott et al. used pembrolizumab 200 mg IV every 3 weeks for <2 years in advanced nccRCC. In this study, 71.5% had confirmed papillary, 12.7% had chromophobe, and 15.8% with unclassified RCC histology. In all patients, ORR was 26.7%. The median duration of response was 29 months. ORR according to subtype was 28.8% for papillary versus 9.5% for chromophobe and 30.8% for unclassified. The median OS was 28.9 months. Treatment-related adverse events were seen in 69.7% of patients with the most common adverse event being pruritis (20%) and hypothyroidism (14.5%) [42].

Nivolumab has also been used in nccRCC, and data was presented by Albiges et al. Nivolumab was given 240 mg IV every 2 weeks. The 12-week ORR was 6%, and stable disease was seen in 49% of patients. Median PFS was 3.9 months. Thus, single-agent nivolumab demonstrated limited activity in nccRCC patients [25]. Combination of ipilimumab and nivolumab in nccRCC was reported by Gupta et al. and showed median PFS of 7.1 months. Sixty-one percent patients had TRAE with colitis (22%) and hepatotoxicity (16%) being the most common [43].

Cosmic-021 study enrolled 30 patients with nccRCC with 15 having papillary and 7 with chromophobe subtype. Patients were given a combination of cabozantinib and atezolizumab. ORR was noted in 33% of patients. PR was seen in six patients with papillary subtype and one with chromophobe subtype. In total, 30% of patients had grade 3–4 treatment related events with hypophosphatemia (13%) being most common [44].

4.7 Conclusion

The approval of a doublet ICI combination and multiple VEGF-TKI plus ICI combinations for previously untreated mRCC patients has brought a major shift in the front-line setting which was previously dominated by VEGF-TKI monotherapy. All the VEGF-TKI plus ICI combinations have shown high ORR, PFS, and OS benefit against sunitinib except avelumab and axitinib which has only extended PFS. However, none of them are compared against each other, and there is no biomarker to help us in choosing the appropriate regimen. As per NCCN guidelines for favorable-risk patients, any of the three approved VEGF-TKI plus ICI combination (pembrolizumab/axitinib, nivolumab/cabozantinib, lenvatinib/pembrolizumab) can be used, although VEGF TKI monotherapy is also reasonable in select patients. Moreover, active surveillance and high-dose IL-2 are reasonable in selected patients after informed and shared decision making. In intermediate- and poor-risk patients along with

Table 4.1 Sequence of preferred treatment options for metastatic clear cell renal cell carcinoma patients

Treatment	First line	Second line	Third line
Good risk	• Axitinib + Pembrolizumab	• Cabozanitnib	• Tivozanib
	• Cabozantinib + Nivolumab	• Axitinib	• Other agents if not used previously.
	• Lenvatinib + Pembrolizumab	• Lenvatinib/ everolimus	
	• Cabozantinib	• Nivolumab	
	• Pazopanib		
	• Sunitinib		
	• Active surveillance		
	• High-dose IL-2		
Intermediate/poor risk	• Nivolumab + Ipilimumab		
	• Axitinib + pembrolizumab		
	• Cabozantinib + Nivolumab		
	• Lenvatinib + Pembrolizumab		
	• Cabozantinib		
Adjuvant	• Pembrolizumab		
	• Sunitinib		

these three regimens, ipilimumab/nivolumab and cabozantinib are also appropriate options (Table 4.1) [45].

Quhal et al. in their systematic metanalysis suggested that VEGF-TKI plus ICI has higher likelihood of conferring superior PFS and OS as compared to doublet ICI, and thus recommended the use of VEGF-TKI plus ICI combinations regardless of IMDC risk group and PD-L1 expression status [46]. However, it must be noted that retrospective analyses of some of the aforementioned trials have demonstrated that benefit with VEGF plus ICI combinations appears more robust in the intermediate and poor risk groups as opposed to the good risk group [21, 23]. Aeppli et al. reported that among cancer experts, IMDC risk stratification and ICI contraindication were most important in decision making and most of the cancer experts use pembrolizumab/axitinib for favorable-risk and ipilimumab/nivolumab for intermediate- or poor-risk patients [21, 23, 42].

Once the patient progresses on doublet ICI combination or VEGF-TKI plus ICI combination, then VEGF-TKI monotherapy or lenvatinib/everolimus may be considered. In those progressing on VEGF-TKI first-line monotherapy, nivolumab may be considered as conventional second-line therapy. McKay et al. in OMNIVORE trial showed that initial nivolumab monotherapy followed by two doses of ipilimumab in those with suboptimal response to nivolumab resulted in no CRs and a low PR/CR conversion [47]. Conversely, Gul et al. studied the role of salvage ipilimumab/nivolumab after prior ICI exposure and reported ORR of 20% [48]. Tivozanib is the only agent specifically approved for third or later-line therapy. The emerging role of belzutifan should be noted. Overall, the most important thing to consider in making treatment decision is to consider the side-effect profile of these combinations and tailoring according to individual patient comorbidities and physician expertise. The role of metastatectomy is still important in select patients with oligometastatic disease and long time from prior disease. The role of delayed cytoreductive nephrectomy is undergoing evaluation in the setting of first-line ICI-based therapy. As effective agents are discovered for metastatic disease, they will then be evaluated in the adjuvant and perioperative settings. Indeed, adjuvant pembrolizumab and sunitinib are approved in the USA based on improved disease-free survival, and other ongoing trials may radically alter the adjuvant landscape [49, 50]. Other important factors contributing to decision making will include comorbidities, performance status, treatment cost, biomarker selections, and patient preference. Finally, all patients should be offered clinical trials investigating new agents since the vast majority of patients are still incurable.

References

1. World Cancer Research Fund International. Kidney cancer statistics. https://www.wcrf.org/cancer-trends/kidney-cancer-statistics/
2. Siegel RL, Miller KD, Fuchs HE, Jemal A. Cancer statistics, 2022. CA Cancer J Clin. 2022;72(1):7–33.
3. Kane CJ, Mallin K, Ritchey J, Cooperberg MR, Carroll PR. Renal cell cancer stage migration: analysis of the National Cancer Data Base. Cancer. 2008;113(1):78–83.
4. Negrier S, Escudier B, Lasset C, Douillard JY, Savary J, Chevreau C, et al. Recombinant human interleukin-2, recombinant human interferon alfa-2a, or both in metastatic renal-cell carcinoma. Groupe Francais d'Immunotherapie. N Engl J Med. 1998;338(18):1272–8.
5. Escudier B, Eisen T, Stadler WM, Szczylik C, Oudard S, Siebels M, et al. Sorafenib in advanced clear-cell renal-cell carcinoma. N Engl J Med. 2007;356(2):125–34.
6. Motzer RJ, Hutson TE, Cella D, Reeves J, Hawkins R, Guo J, et al. Pazopanib versus sunitinib in metastatic renal-cell carcinoma. N Engl J Med. 2013;369(8):722–31.
7. Choueiri TK, Escudier B, Powles T, Mainwaring PN, Rini BI, Donskov F, et al. Cabozantinib versus Everolimus in advanced renal-cell carcinoma. N Engl J Med. 2015;373(19):1814–23.
8. Motzer RJ, Escudier B, McDermott DF, George S, Hammers HJ, Srinivas S, et al. Nivolumab versus Everolimus in advanced renal-cell carcinoma. N Engl J Med. 2015;373(19):1803–13.
9. Jain RK, Lara P. Evolving frontline treatment landscape for advanced or metastatic renal cell carcinoma. Kidney Cancer. 2020;4(2):71–9.
10. Motzer RJ, Mazumdar M, Bacik J, Berg W, Amsterdam A, Ferrara J. Survival and prognostic stratification of 670 patients with advanced renal cell carcinoma. J Clin Oncol. 1999;17(8):2530.
11. Heng DYC, Xie W, Regan MM, Warren MA, Golshayan AR, Sahi C, et al. Prognostic factors for overall survival in patients with metastatic renal cell carcinoma treated with vascular endothelial growth factor–targeted agents: results from a large, multicenter study. J Clin Oncol. 2009;27(34):5794–9.
12. Flanigan RC, Salmon SE, Blumenstein BA, Bearman SI, Roy V, McGrath PC, et al. Nephrectomy followed by interferon alfa-2b compared with interferon alfa-2b alone for metastatic renal-cell cancer. N Engl J Med. 2001;345(23):1655–9.
13. Mickisch GH, Garin A, van Poppel H, de Prijck L, Sylvester R. Radical nephrectomy plus interferon-alfa-based immunotherapy compared with interferon alfa alone in metastatic renal-cell carcinoma: a randomised trial. Lancet. 2001;358(9286):966–70.
14. Heng DY, Wells JC, Rini BI, Beuselinck B, Lee JL, Knox JJ, et al. Cytoreductive nephrectomy in patients with synchronous metastases from renal cell carcinoma: results from the international metastatic renal cell carcinoma database consortium. Eur Urol. 2014;66(4):704–10.
15. Poprach A, Holanek M, Chloupkova R, Lakomy R, Stanik M, Fiala O, et al. Cytoreductive nephrectomy and overall survival of patients with metastatic renal cell carcinoma treated with targeted therapy—data from the National Renis Registry. Cancers (Basel). 2020;12(10):2911.
16. Méjean A, Ravaud A, Thezenas S, Colas S, Beauval JB, Bensalah K, et al. Sunitinib alone or after nephrectomy in metastatic renal-cell carcinoma. N Engl J Med. 2018;379(5):417–27.
17. Mejean A, Ravaud A, Thezenas S, Chevreau C, Bensalah K, Geoffrois L, et al. Sunitinib alone or after nephrectomy for patients with metastatic renal cell carcinoma: is there still a role for cytoreductive nephrectomy? Eur Urol. 2021;80(4):417–24.
18. Bex A, Mulders P, Jewett M, Wagstaff J, van Thienen JV, Blank CU, et al. Comparison of immediate vs. deferred cytoreductive nephrectomy in patients with synchronous metastatic renal cell carcinoma receiving sunitinib: the SURTIME randomized clinical trial. JAMA Oncol. 2019;5(2):164–70.
19. Deferred cytoreductive nephrectomy in synchronous metastatic renal cell carcinoma: the NORDIC-SUN-trial. https://classic.clinicaltrials.gov/ct2/show/NCT03977571
20. Rini BI, Plimack ER, Stus V, Gafanov R, Hawkins R, Nosov D, et al. Pembrolizumab plus Axitinib versus Sunitinib for advanced renal-cell carcinoma. N Engl J Med. 2019;380(12):1116–27.
21. Rini BI, Plimack ER, Stus V, Waddell T, Gafanov R, Pouliot F, et al. Pembrolizumab (pembro) plus axitinib (axi) versus sunitinib as first-line therapy for advanced clear cell renal cell carcinoma (CcRCC): results from 42-month follow-up of KEYNOTE-426. J Clin Oncol. 2021;39:4500.
22. Choueiri TK, Powles T, Burotto M, Escudier B, Bourlon MT, Zurawski B, et al. Nivolumab plus cabozantinib versus sunitinib for advanced renal-cell carcinoma. N Engl J Med. 2021;384(9):829–41.
23. Powles TCT, Burotto M, Escudier M, et al. Final overall survival analysis and organ-specific target lesion

assessments with two-year follow up in CheckMate 9ER: nivolumab plus cabozantinib versus sunitinib for patients with advanced renal cell carcinoma. J Clin Oncol. 2022;40(6_Suppl):350.
24. Rha SYCT, Matveev VB, et al. Efficacy and safety of lenvatinib (LEN) plus pembrolizumab (PEMBRO) versus sunitinib (SUN) in the East Asian subset of patients with advanced renal cell carcinoma (aRCC) from the phase 3 CLEAR trial. J Clin Oncol. 2022;40(6_Suppl):338.
25. Motzer RJ, Penkov K, Haanen J, Rini B, Albiges L, Campbell MT, et al. Avelumab plus axitinib versus sunitinib for advanced renal-cell carcinoma. N Engl J Med. 2019;380(12):1103–15.
26. Motzer RJ, Tannir NM, McDermott DF, Aren Frontera O, Melichar B, Choueiri TK, et al. Nivolumab plus ipilimumab versus sunitinib in advanced renal-cell carcinoma. N Engl J Med. 2018;378(14):1277–90.
27. Motzer RJCT, McDermott DF, et al. Biomarker analysis from CheckMate 214: nivolumab plus ipilimumab versus sunitinib in renal cell carcinoma. J Immunother Cancer. 2022;10:e004316.
28. Motzer RJ, McDermott DF, Escudier B, Burotto M, Choueiri TK, Hammers HJ, et al. Conditional survival and long-term efficacy with nivolumab plus ipilimumab versus sunitinib in patients with advanced renal cell carcinoma. Cancer. 2022;128(11):2085–97.
29. Exelixis announces cabozantinib in combination with nivolumab and ipilimumab significantly improved progression-free survival in phase 3 COSMIC-313 pivotal trial in patients with previously untreated advanced Kidney Cancer [press release]. 2022. https://ir.exelixis.com/news-releases/news-release-details/exelixis-announces-cabozantinib-combination-nivolumab-and
30. Choueiri TK, Hessel C, Halabi S, Sanford B, Michaelson MD, Hahn O, et al. Cabozantinib versus sunitinib as initial therapy for metastatic renal cell carcinoma of intermediate or poor risk (Alliance A031203 CABOSUN randomised trial): progression-free survival by independent review and overall survival update. Eur J Cancer. 2018;94:115–25.
31. Choueiri TK, Halabi S, Sanford BL, Hahn O, Michaelson MD, Walsh MK, et al. Cabozantinib versus Sunitinib as initial targeted therapy for patients with metastatic renal cell carcinoma of poor or intermediate risk: the Alliance A031203 CABOSUN trial. J Clin Oncol. 2017;35(6):591–7.
32. Motzer RJ, Hutson TE, Tomczak P, Michaelson MD, Bukowski RM, Rixe O, et al. Sunitinib versus interferon alfa in metastatic renal-cell carcinoma. N Engl J Med. 2007;356(2):115–24.
33. Escudier B, Porta C, Powles T, et al. Randomized, controlled, double-blind, cross-over trial assessing treatment preference for pazopanib versus sunitinib in patients with metastatic renal cell carcinoma: PISCES study. J Clin Oncol. 2014;32(14):1412–8.
34. Fyfe G, Fisher RI, Rosenberg SA, Sznol M, Parkinson DR, Louie AC. Results of treatment of 255 patients with metastatic renal cell carcinoma who received high-dose recombinant interleukin-2 therapy. J Clin Oncol. 1995;13(3):688–96.
35. Rini BI, Dorff TB, Elson P, et al. Active surveillance in metastatic renal-cell carcinoma: a prospective, phase 2 trial. Lancet Oncol. 2016;17(9):1317–24.
36. Escudier B, Michaelson MD, Motzer RJ, Hutson TE, Clark JI, Lim HY, et al. Axitinib versus sorafenib in advanced renal cell carcinoma: subanalyses by prior therapy from a randomised phase III trial. Br J Cancer. 2014;110(12):2821–8.
37. Motzer RJ, Hutson TE, Glen H, Michaelson MD, Molina A, Eisen T, et al. Lenvatinib, everolimus, and the combination in patients with metastatic renal cell carcinoma: a randomised, phase 2, open-label, multicentre trial. Lancet Oncol. 2015;16(15):1473–82.
38. Rini BI, Pal SK, Escudier BJ, Atkins MB, Hutson TE, Porta C, et al. Tivozanib versus sorafenib in patients with advanced renal cell carcinoma (TIVO-3): a phase 3, multicentre, randomised, controlled, open-label study. Lancet Oncol. 2020;21(1):95–104.
39. Choueiri TK, Bauer TM, Papadopoulos KP, Plimack ER, Merchan JR, McDermott DF, et al. Inhibition of hypoxia-inducible factor-2alpha in renal cell carcinoma with belzutifan: a phase 1 trial and biomarker analysis. Nat Med. 2021;27(5):802–5.
40. Jonasch E, Donskov F, Iliopoulos O, Rathmell WK, Narayan VK, Maughan BL, et al. Belzutifan for renal cell carcinoma in von Hippel-Lindau disease. N Engl J Med. 2021;385(22):2036–46.
41. Pal SK, Tangen C, Thompson IM Jr, Balzer-Haas N, George DJ, Heng DYC, et al. A comparison of sunitinib with cabozantinib, crizotinib, and savolitinib for treatment of advanced papillary renal cell carcinoma: a randomised, open-label, phase 2 trial. Lancet. 2021;397(10275):695–703.
42. Aeppli S, Schmaus M, Eisen T, Escudier B, Grunwald V, Larkin J, et al. First-line treatment of metastatic clear cell renal cell carcinoma: a decision-making analysis among experts. ESMO Open. 2021;6(1):100030.
43. Gupta R, Ornstein MC, Li H, Allman KD, Wood LS, Gilligan T, et al. Clinical activity of Ipilimumab plus Nivolumab in patients with metastatic non-clear cell renal cell carcinoma. Clin Genitourin Cancer. 2020;18(6):429–35.
44. McGregor BA, Agarwal N, Suarez C, Tsao CK, Kelly W, Pagliaro L, et al. 709P Cabozantinib (C) in combination with atezolizumab (a) in non-clear cell renal cell carcinoma (nccRCC): results from cohort 10 of the COSMIC-021 study. Ann Oncol. 2020;31:S558.
45. NCCN. NCCN guidelines version 4. 2022 Kidney Cancer. 2022. https://www.nccn.org/guidelines/category_1
46. Quhal F, Mori K, Bruchbacher A, Resch I, Mostafaei H, Pradere B, et al. First-line immunotherapy-based combinations for metastatic renal cell carcinoma: a systematic review and network meta-analysis. Eur Urol Oncol. 2021;4(5):755–65.

47. McKay RR, McGregor BA, Xie W, Braun DA, Wei X, Kyriakopoulos CE, et al. Optimized management of nivolumab and ipilimumab in advanced renal cell carcinoma: a response-based phase II study (OMNIVORE). J Clin Oncol. 2020;38(36):4240–8.
48. Gul A, Stewart TF, Mantia CM, Shah NJ, Gatof ES, Long Y, et al. Salvage ipilimumab and nivolumab in patients with metastatic renal cell carcinoma after prior immune checkpoint inhibitors. J Clin Oncol. 2020;38(27):3088–94.
49. Choueiri TK, Tomczak P, Park SH, Venugopal B, Ferguson T, Chang YH, et al. Adjuvant pembrolizumab after nephrectomy in renal-cell carcinoma. N Engl J Med. 2021;385(8):683–94.
50. Ravaud A, Motzer RJ, Pandha HS, George DJ, Pantuck AJ, Patel A, et al. Adjuvant sunitinib in high-risk renal-cell carcinoma after nephrectomy. N Engl J Med. 2016;375(23):2246–54.

5 Adjuvant Treatment and Follow-Up of Clinically Localized Renal Cell Carcinoma

Jan K. Rudzinski, Benjamin B. Beech, Betty Wang, Guru Sonpavde, and Logan W. Zemp

Abbreviations

AE	Adverse events
ccRCC	Clear cell renal cell carcinoma
CSS	Cancer-specific survival
DFS	Disease-free survival
ECOG	Eastern Cooperative Oncology Group
HR	High risk
ICI	Immune checkpoint inhibitor(s)
IR	Intermediate risk
ITT	Intention to treat
LR	Low risk
MAMs	Multiarm multistage
MSK	Memorial Sloan Kettering
OS	Overall survival
PDGF	Platelet-derived growth factor
RCC	Renal cell carcinoma
SSIGN	The stage, size, grade, and necrosis
TCGA	The cancer genome atlas
TKI	Tyrosine kinase inhibitor(s)
UISS	University of California Los Angeles Integrated Staging System
VEGF	Vascular endothelial growth factor
VHL	Von Hippel-Lindau

5.1 Introduction

Renal cell carcinoma (RCC) is a highly vascularized malignancy, comprising approximately 4% of all newly diagnosed cancers, and commonly occurring in the seventh and eighth decade of life [1, 2]. Clear cell RCC (ccRCC) is the most common subtype, accounting for 75% of malignant renal tumors and 90% of metastatic RCC [2–4]. Significant prognostic factors for RCC include tumor stage and grade, as well as the presence of nodal or distant metastases at initial presentation [5–7]. RCC has the propensity to metastasize to

Jan K. Rudzinski and Benjamin B. Beech contributed equally with all other contributors.

J. K. Rudzinski
The University of Texas MD Anderson Cancer Center, Houston, TX, USA

B. B. Beech
Memorial Sloan Kettering Cancer Center, New York, NY, USA

B. Wang
Faculty of Medicine and Dentistry, Division of Urology, University of Alberta, Edmonton, AB, Canada

G. Sonpavde
Dana-Farber Cancer Institute, Genitourinary Cancer Section, Boston, MA, USA

L. W. Zemp (✉)
Department of Genitourinary Oncology, Moffit Cancer Center, Tampa, FL, USA
e-mail: Logan.Zemp@moffitt.org

P. Singh et al. (eds.), *A Guide to Management of Urological Cancers*, https://doi.org/10.1007/978-981-99-2341-0_5

locoregional lymph nodes or distant sites such as the adrenal gland, lung, liver, bone, as well as the brain [8]. Once metastatic, few patients have durable response to systemic therapies, and the therapeutic paradigm is centered around controlling the disease burden to prolong overall survival (OS).

The 5-year survival for localized RCC ranges from 88.4–92.6% for early and 7.3–11.7% for stage 3 and 4 disease [2, 9]. The estimated 5-year relapse rate for patients with advanced disease is approximately 40% with a median time to relapse of 18 months from time of surgery [10, 11]. There is currently limited high-level evidence to support the routine use of adjuvant therapy despite the high risk of recurrence [2]. Therefore, adjuvant therapy remains an unmet need for those with advanced disease and significant risk of recurrence.

Ideally, adjuvant therapy can be used to select high-risk patients, in order to reduce disease recurrence and prolong survival, with an acceptable toxicity profile. This chapter provides an overview of the existing literature for adjuvant therapies in RCC, ongoing clinical trials, and future directions in this disease space.

5.2 Postoperative Predictive Models for Clinically Localized RCC

To predict postoperative outcomes for patients with localized RCC, several prognostic risk classifications and nomograms have been published, as summarized in Table 5.1. In general, nomograms compute predictive probability for individual patients based on prespecified variables,

Table 5.1 Summary of clinical predictive models for clinically localized renal cell carcinoma

Study	Year of publication	Number of patients included	Components	Oncologic outcomes
Nomograms				
Sorbellini et al. [12]	2005	701	2002 TNM pathologic stage	5-year RFS
			Tumor size	
			Necrosis	
			Furham grade	
			Vascular invasion	
			Clinical presentation	
Karakiewicz et al. [13]	2017	2500	2002 TNM stage	1, 2, 5, and 10-year CSS
			Histologic subtype	
			Tumor size	
			Furham grade	
			Symptom classification	
Risk classifications				
Frank et al. [14]	2002	1801	1997 TNM stage	1, 3, 5, 7, and 10-year CSS
			Tumor size	
			Necrosis	
			Furham grade	
Leibovich et al. [15]	2003	1671	2002 TNM stage	1, 3, 5, 7, 10-year MFS
			Tumor size	
			Necrosis	
			Furham grade	
Patard et al. [16]	2004	4000	1997 TNM stage	1–5-year DFS and OS
			Furham grade	
			Vascular invasion	
			ECOG PS	

whereas risk stratification models group patients with similar characteristics into distinct clusters to help predict outcomes. Accurate clinical predictive models could aid in adjuvant therapy trial design, postoperative counseling, and risk-adapted surveillance strategies [17]. However, further prospective validation is required to incorporate these into routine clinical practice.

The Memorial Sloan Kettering (MSK) postoperative nomogram published by Sorbellini et al. incorporates tumor size, pathologic stage, Fuhrman grade, presence of necrosis, vascular invasion, and clinical presentation (incidental vs. local or systemic symptoms) to predict 5-year freedom from recurrence following radical surgery in patients with ccRCC. This nomogram was derived from clinicopathological data of 701 patients through Cox proportional hazards regression at a single center and was externally validated [12]. More recently, the Karakiewicz nomogram was derived from variables such as the 2002 TNM stage, tumor size, Fuhrman grade, histologic subtype, age, as well as symptom classification. This series included approximately 2500 patients with an external validation cohort to help predict 1-, 2-, 5-, and 10-year cancer specific survival (CSS) for patients who underwent radical nephrectomy for clinically localized RCC of all stages [13]. For both predictive models, the sum of points achieved for each predictor is used to compute a total score and determine the probability of either remaining recurrence free or CSS.

Patard et al. published The University of California Los Angeles Integrated Staging System (UISS), which is based on collaborative effort from eight international academic centers incorporating over 4000 patients [16]. This classification system is based on 1997 TNM staging, Fuhrman grade, and Eastern Cooperative Oncology Group performance status (ECOG) which then stratifies patients into low (LR), intermediate (IR), and high-risk (HR) cohorts to estimate postoperative 1–5-year OS. The estimated 5-year survival rates were 92% for LR, 67% for IR, and 44% for HR. The high-risk population for recurrence includes those with T3 N0 or Nx, Fuhrman grade ≥ 2, ECOG ≥ 1, and T4 and/or N+, for whom the risk of recurrence at 5 years was demonstrated to be as high as 60% within 10 months postoperatively [16]. The Stage, Size, Grade, and Necrosis (SSIGN) score proposed by Frank et al. was derived from 1801 patients who underwent radical nephrectomy for clinically localized ccRCC [14]. This algorithm incorporates the 1997 TNM classification, tumor size (≤ or ≥10 cm), nuclear grade, as well as presence or absence of tumor necrosis to predict CSS. In this classification, each of the individual categories is assigned a specific score, and the sum of these points is used to predict estimated CSS based on Kaplan–Meier estimates. Subsequently, the Leibovich score was designed to predict disease-free survival (DFS) and progression to metastasis after surgery and stratifies patients into three risk groups (LR, IR, HR) based on tumor stage, regional lymph node status, nuclear grade, and the presence or absence of necrosis [15]. This risk-classification system was based on data from 1671 patients who underwent unilateral nephrectomy for clinically localized ccRCC. The mean estimated time to disease progression for the LR group who developed metastatic disease was 7.4 years, 4 years for IR, and 1.7 years for HR disease.

Overall, in a comparative analysis by Tan et al., the Karakiewicz nomogram demonstrated superior accuracy for predicting survival compared to the MSK and Leibovich models [17].

5.2.1 Integration of Genomic Signatures into Risk-Predictive Models

One of the most common genetic alterations associated with ccRCC development is the loss of short arm of chromosome 3 [18]. More specifically, gene alterations in VHL, PBRM-1, SETD2, BAP-1, and MTOR have also been strongly implicated in pathogenesis of ccRCC [19, 20]. With further advances in understanding the biology of the disease, integration of genomic signatures into the risk stratification algorithms has been proposed as summarized in Table 5.2. However, due to their relative novelty, along with lack of prospective validation, these nomograms have not yet been widely adopted.

Table 5.2 Summary of genomic signatures incorporated into risk-predictive models

Author (nomogram name)	Year of publication	Number of patients with localized ccRCC	Genomic analysis	Oncologic outcomes	Genes of interest	Nomogram integration
Rinni et al. [21] (16 gene assay)	2015	942	RNA expression profile of 732 genes from FFPE samples	Time to recurrence	**Vascular**	Leibovich
					APOLD1	
					EDNRB	
					NOS3	
					PPAP2B	
					Immune	
					CEACAM1	
					CX3CL1	
					CCL5	
					Inflammation	
					IL-6	
					Cell growth	
					EIF4EBP1	
					TUBB2A	
					LMNB1	
Brooks et al. [22] (ClearCode34)	2012	72	RNA expression profile of 34 genes from FFPE[a] samples	Risk of recurrence, DSM, OS	**ccA (high-risk)**	Leibovich
					MAPT, STK32B, FZD1, RGS5, GIPC2, PDGFD, EPAS1, MAOB, CDH5, TCEA3, LEPROTL1, BNIP3L, EHBP1, VCAM1, PHYH, PRKAA2, SLC4A4, ESD, TLR3, NRP1, C11orf1, ST13, ARNT, C13orf1	
					ccB (low-risk)	
					SERPINA3, SLC4A3, MOXD1, KCNN4, ROR2, FLJ23867, FOXM1, UNG2, GALNT10, GALNT4	
Morgan et al. [23] (CCP)	2018	565[b]	RNA expression profile of 31 genes from FFPE[a] samples	DSM	*FOXM1, CDC20, CDKN3, CDC2, KIF11, KIAA0101, NUSAP1, CENPF, ASPM, BUB1B, RRM2, DLGAP5, BIRC5, KIF20A, PLK1, TOP2A, TK1, PBK, ASF1B, C18orf24, RAD54L, PTTG1, CDCA3, MCM10, PRC1, DTL, CEP55, RAD51, CENPM, CDCA8, ORC6L*	Karakiewicz

[a]FFPE denotes formalin fixed, paraffin embedded
[b]Morgan 2018 study included patients with clear cell, papillary, and chromophobe RCC

Rini et al. investigated the integration of 16-gene expression signature (11 cancer-related and five reference genes) representing vascular, immune response, inflammation, cell cycle, and cell growth, into the recurrence score following nephrectomy for localized RCC [21]. This was derived from a retrospective cohort of 942 patients from Cleveland Clinic with stage I–III ccRCC through real-time polymerase chain reaction (PCR) analysis. Overall, this recurrence score was associated with risk of tumor recurrence following stratification by stage and adjustment for tumor size, nuclear grade, and the Leibovich score to provide accurate and individualized risk assessment. In a subsequent validation study with a cohort of patients from adjuvant sunitinib (S-TRAC) trial, higher recurrence score was associated with worse recurrence-free survival (RFS), DFS, and CSS in both sunitinib and placebo groups [24].

The ClearCode34 proposed by Brooks et al. utilized 72 samples of localized RCC to develop a 34-gene expression panel to stratify patients into high-risk (ccA) and low-risk (ccB) cohorts [22]. The predictive accuracy of the ClearCode34 was tested using a set of 380 patients with non-metastatic ccRCC from The Cancer Genome Atlas (TCGA) and formalin-fixed institutional samples. Contrary to the author's hypothesis, ccB subtype demonstrated higher risk of tumor recurrence and an increased risk of death from RCC compared to ccA tumors [22].

Morgan et al. developed an RNA-based cell cycle progression (CCP) score derived from 565 patient samples and 31 cell cycle genes to determine if a multigene proliferation signature could help predict long-term oncologic outcomes for patients with localized RCC post radical nephrectomy [23]. The CCP score was shown to be an independent predictor of long-term recurrence and disease-specific mortality after adjusting for clinical variables. With further validation, the CCP score could allow for accurate individualized risk stratification to guide clinical decisions.

5.3 Risk-Adapted Follow-Up After Treatment of Clinically Localized RCC

Following surgical treatment of clinically localized RCC, there is no unified consensus on the optimal follow-up strategy. Postoperative monitoring is critical for early identification of cancer recurrence, renal impairment, and cardiovascular events. Current clinical practice guidelines recommend risk-stratified and individualized approach to postoperative follow-up as summarized in Table 5.3 [27]. In a recent study by Powles et al., the authors demonstrated survival benefit for patients who were followed within a structured surveillance protocol in comparison to those who were not [28].

The European Association Urology RCC Guidelines Panel recommends postoperative risk stratification based on the 2003 Leibovich model for ccRCC and the UISS for non-ccRCC [25]. Given the poor sensitivity of chest radiography and ultrasound for the detection of small metastatic deposits, the EAU recommends CT imaging of the chest and abdomen as their preferred imaging modality. Possible discontinuation of oncologic imaging, with the discussion centered on patient age, comorbidities, and life expectancy, can be considered for low-risk patients >3 years and intermediate-risk patients >5 years of follow-up [25].

The American Urological Association (AUA) recently published an updated guideline for localized RCC, which encourages individualized follow-up based on the risk of disease recurrence and possible sequelae from treatment [26]. Their proposed follow-up schedule presents four different risk levels: LR, IR, HR, and very high risk (VHR) based on primary disease T and N stage, Fuhrman grade, surgical margin status, and variant tumor pathology. In addition to interval imaging, the AUA recommends periodic laboratory testing including serum creatinine, eGFR, and urinalysis for all patients, as well as complete blood count, lactate dehydrogenase, liver function tests, alkaline phosphatase, and calcium level, to be obtained if advanced disease is suspected. Abdominal imaging is preferred with MRI or CT and contrast-enhancement; however, US can be used in addition to cross-sectional imaging for the LR/IR patient. Similarly, CT is the preferred chest imaging modality; however, CXR may be used for the LR/IR risk group. In select cases, targeted imaging can be considered as clinically indicated (i.e., bone scan, CT head/spine). After 5 years of risk-stratified follow-up, clinicians may re-evaluate the need for further

Table 5.3 Summary of risk-adapted follow-up after treatment of clinically localized RCC

Guideline	Year of publication (updated results)	Risk stratification	Risk definition	Follow-up protocl
European Association of Urology (eau) [25]	2022	High	ccRCC: Leibovicg≥6	CT at 3, 6, 12, and 18 months, 2 and 3 years, every 1 year until year 5 years, then CT once every 2 years
			Non-ccRCC: pT2–4, or any pT any grade with N1	
		Intermediate	ccRCC Leibovich: Leibovich 3–5	CT at 6 and 12 months, 2 and 3 years, then every 1 year, after 5 years, CT once every 2 years
			Non-ccRCC: pT1b, grade 3–4	
		Low	ccRCC: Leibovich 0–2	CT at 6 and 18 months, 3 years, then CT once every 2 years
			Non-ccRCC: pT1Nx-0, grade 1–2	
American association of urology (AUA)[a] [26]	2021	Very high	pT4 or pN1 or sarcomatoid/rhabdoid differentiation, or macroscopic PSM	3, 6, 9, 12, 18, 24, 30, 36, 48, 60, 72–84, and 96–120 months
		High	pT3 any grade	6, 12, 18, 24, 30, 36, 48, 60, 72–84, and 96–120 months
		Intermediate	pT1 and grade 3/4, or pT2 any grade	6, 12, 24, 36, 48, 60, 72–84, and 96–120 months
		Low	pT1 and grade 1/2	12, 24, 48, 60, 72–84, and 96–120 months
National Comprehensive Cancer Network (NCCN) [2]	2022	Stage IV	T4, any N, M0	H & P every 6–16 weeks
				CT/MRI every 6–16 weeks
		Stage III	T1–2, N1, M0 or T3, NX, N0–1, M0	Same as stage II
		Stage II	T2, N0, M0	H & P every 3–6 months for 3 years, then annually up to 5 years.
				Comprehensive metabolic panel every 3–6 months for 3 years, then annually up to 5 years
				CT/MRI within 3–6 months of surgery, then every 3–6 months for at least 3 years annually up to 5 years
				Baseline CT chest within 3–6 months, then every 3–6 months for at least 3 years, then annually up to 5 years
		Stage I	T1, N0, M0	H & P annually
				Laboratory tests annually
				CT/MRI or US within 3–12 months of surgery, then annually for 3 years or longer
				CXR or CT chest annually for 5 years

[a]AUA recommends history &and physical exam (H & P), laboratory testing, and abdominal and chest CT at each follow-up internal—informed and shared decision-making guide surveillance beyond 60 months

imaging and its modality-based disease and patient characteristics, using a shared decision-making model.

The NCCN guidelines for kidney cancer follow-up are similar to the AUA guidelines. Follow-up of patients beyond 5 years after nephrectomy should be at the discretion of the physician and patient, acknowledging that a subset of patients may recur after 5 years from surgery [2].

5.3.1 Implications for Clinical Practice

- The standard-of-care treatment for patients with clinically localized RCC is partial or radical nephrectomy, however, up to 40% are at risk of recurrence.
- Clinical practice guidelines such as the EAU, AUA, and NCCN advocate for structured postoperative follow-up for early detection of cancer recurrence, renal impairment, and cardiovascular events.
- To accurately predict postoperative outcomes, several risk predictive models have been established.
- Among the existing models, the Karakiewicz nomogram and the Leibovich score may become increasingly utilized in adjuvant RCC clinical trials.
- With accumulating knowledge on RCC biology, integration of genomic signatures has been suggested to improve the accuracy of predictive algorithms.
- Further prospective validation is required to incorporate these risk predictive models into routine clinical practice.

5.4 Angiogenesis Pathway Inhibitors

Von Hippel-Lindau (VHL) tumor suppressor gene alterations play a pivotal role in the development of ccRCC [18]. It is estimated that in >50% of patients with sporadic ccRCCs, there is an abnormality in VHL gene resulting in overexpression of VEGF receptors [29]. In an effort to target this pathway, small molecules TKIs were developed to inhibit the activation of the VEGF and platelet-derived growth factor (PDGF) receptors on the surface of endothelial cells [30]. These agents were initially trialed in the metastatic setting where they showed significant activity. Given this, they were also explored in the adjuvant setting with the goal of improving DFS and OS as summarized in Table 5.4 [31, 32, 36, 37].

The ASSURE trial was a double-blind, placebo-controlled randomized clinical trial which enrolled 1943 patients with completely resected, pT1b or greater, high-grade (G3–4), N0–N1, nonmetastatic (M0) RCC confirmed on central pathologic review. Eligible participants were randomized (1:1:1) to receive 54 weeks of sunitinib 50 mg daily on 6-week therapeutic cycles (4 weeks on treatment with a 2 weeks break), sorafenib 400 mg twice daily continuously, or placebo for 1 year [38]. High discontinuation rate due to TKI-associated adverse events (AE) was noted among patients randomized to sunitinib (44%) and sorafenib (45%) compared to placebo (11%). To account for this, the study was amended to decrease the starting doses of sunitinib to 37.5 mg daily (4 weeks on therapy and 2 weeks off) and sorafenib to 400 mg once daily with gradual dose titration. Further dose reduction of sunitinitb to 25 mg daily and sorafenib 400 mg daily every other week were also permitted. The most frequently reported grade 3–4 AEs within the TKI cohort were hypertension (17% sunitinib, 16% sorafenib), hand-foot syndrome (15% sunitinib, 33% sorafenib), rash (2% sunitinib, 15% sorafenib, and fatigue (18% sunitinib patients, 7% sorafenib patients). The primary outcome for this trial was DFS, and there was no significant difference between treatment groups (median DFS 5.8 years, 6.1 years, 6.6 years for sunitinib, sorafenib, and placebo, respectively). In an updated analysis published in 2018, the reported 5-year DFS rates were 47.7%, 49.9%, and 50.0%, respectively for sunitinib, sorafenib, and placebo, with 5-year OS of 75.2%, 80.2%, and 76.5% (HR 1.06; 97.5% CI: 0.78–1.45; p = 0.66, sunitinib vs. placebo; and HR 0.80; 97.5% CI: 0.58–1.11; p = 0.12 for sorafenib

Table 5.4 Summary of adjuvant tyrosine kinase inhibitortrials (2016–2021)

Study	Year of publication (updated results)	Number of patients included	Oncologic eligibility	Treatment	Control	Oncologic outcomes	Adverse events
S-TRAC [31]	2016 (**2018**)	615	T3/4, N0/Nx, or Tany with local nodal involvement	Sunitinib	Placebo	Improvement in DFS on central radiological review, no improvement in OS	Grade ≥ 3 in63.4%
ASSURE [32]	2016 (**2017**)	1943	≥pT1b, nonmetastatic RCC	Sunitinib or sorafenib	Placebo	No improvement in DFS or OS	Grade ≥ 3 in >55% in both sunitinib and sorafenib groups
PROTECT [33]	2017 (**2021**)	1538	pT2G3–4 N0, pT3-T4G_{any}N0 or $pT_{any}G_{any}$N1,clearcell or predominant clearcell RCC	Pazopanib 800 mg or Pazopanib 600 mg	Placebo	Improved DFS in ITT pazopanib 800 mg, no improvement in DFS ITT pazopanib 600 mg. No improvement in OS	Grade ≥ 3 in 60%
ATLAS [34]	2018	724	>pT2 and/or N+, any Fuhrman grade/ECOG, predominant clearcell nonmetastatic RCC	Axitinib	Placebo	No improvement in DFS or OS (trial stopped for futility at preplanned interim analysis and OSdata not mature at interim analysis)	Grade ≥ 3 in 61%
SORCE [35]	2020	1656	Clear-cell or nonclear cell RCC at intermediate or high risk or relapse, as per Leibovich risk model	Sorafenib 1 year or Sorafenib 3 year	Placebo	No improvement in DFS or OS	Grade ≥ 3 in 58.6% for sorafenib 1 year, 63.9% for sorafenib 3 years

Patients included in the above trials had completely resected primary tumors vs. placebo) [33]. The ASSURE investigators concluded that adjuvant TKI therapy did not improve survival and that substantial discontinuation rates occurred due to excessive toxicity despite dose reductions.

The S-TRAC trial was an international double-blind, phase 3 randomized clinical trial which enrolled 615 patients with loco-regional, high risk, nonmetastatic ccRCC to sunitinib 50 mg daily or placebo on a 6 weeks cycle (4 weeks on therapy and 2 weeks off) for 1 year or until disease recurrence [39]. The trial permitted for dose reduction to sunitinib 37.5 mg daily on the same 6-weeks cycle. The primary endpoint was DFS using central radiological review, while secondary endpoints included investigator assessed DFS, OS, and toxicity profile. The median durations of DFS were 6.8 years (95% CI: 5.8—not reached) in the sunitinib group and 5.6 years (95% CI: 3.8–6.6) in the placebo group (HR 0.76; 95% CI: 0.59–0.98; $p = 0.03$). However, the difference in DFS was not confirmed on investigator radiological review (HR 0.81; 95% CI: 0.64–1.02; $p = 0.08$). The overall survival data was not mature at the time of initial publication, and an updated analysis failed to show a significant difference (HR 0.92; 95% CI: 0.66–1.28; $p = 0.6$) [34]. Safety profile analysis demonstrated that grade 3 and 4 AEs occurred more frequently in the sunitinib group (Gr 3: 48.4% vs. 15.4%; Gr 4: 12.1% vs. 3.6%). Dose interruptions and discontinuations were also more common in the sunitinib group. Given the improvement in DFS, the US Food and Drug Administration approved sunitinib as adjuvant treatment for high-risk ccRCC in 2017 which also led to its adoption into the National Comprehensive Cancer Network Guidelines [2, 35].

The PROTECT trial randomized 1538 patients with nonmetastatic (M0) pT2G3–4N0, pT3–4G_{any}N0, or p$T_{any}G_{any}$N1 ccRCC patients, post radical nephrectomy, to pazopanib or placebo in a 1:1 fashion for 1 year. Four hundred and three patients received the planned pazopanib starting dose of 800 mg daily with subsequent dose reduction to 600 mg daily due to toxicity [40]. The primary endpoint was DFS in an intention to treat (ITT) analysis within the cohort receiving the reduced dose, while DFS in an ITT analysis of the full cohort (full and reduced dose) was a secondary endpoint. In the reduced dose cohort, DFS was not significantly different compared to placebo (HR 0.86; 95% CI: 0.70–1.06; $p = 0.16$). However, patients treated with 800 mg of pazopanib did have improved DFS on ITT analysis (HR 0.69; 95% CI: 0.51–0.94; $p = 0.02$), which contributed to improved DFS on ITT analysis of the entire cohort (HR 0.80; 95% CI: 0.68–0.95; $p = 0.01$). Furthermore, a recently updated analysis failed to demonstrate an OS benefit for pazopanib compared to placebo (HR 1.0, 95% CI: 0.80–1.26; $p > 0.9$) [41]. Within the cohort treated with pazopanib, only 49% patients completed 12 months of treatment compared to 72–75% in the placebo safety groups. Dose reductions were experienced in the 51% of patients in the 600 mg group and 66% in the 800 mg group. The most common reason for discontinuations was hepatotoxicity with elevations in alanine aminotransferase (16% in the 600 mg group and 18% in the 800 mg group).

The ATLAS trial randomized 724 patients who had undergone radical nephrectomy with ≥pT2 and/or N+, G_{any}, ccRCC, and an ECOG performance status of 0 or 1 to either axitinib 5 mg twice daily or placebo for 1–3 years [42]. The primary endpoint was DFS per an independent review committee (IRC) in the ITT population. A prespecified efficacy analysis was also conducted in the highest-risk subpopulation (pT3, G 3–4 or pT4, and/or N+, T_{any}, G_{any}). At a preplanned interim analysis by IRC, the trial was terminated early due to lack of difference in DFS between the two groups (HR 0.87; 95% CI: 0.66–1.15; $p = 0.3$). However, within the highest-risk cohort, risk reduction of DFS events was identified in patients receiving axitinib compared to placebo on investigator analysis (HR 0.64; 95% CI: 0.47–0.88; $p = 0.005$) but not on IRC analysis (HR 0.74; 95% CI: 0.53–1.03; $p = 0.07$). Patients treated with axitinib reported higher rates of treatment-related AEs compared to those in placebo arm (91% vs. 56%), as well as higher grade 3–4 AEs (49% vs. 12%). The most reported AEs were hypertension (40%), diarrhea (47%), dysphonia (42%), and hand-foot syndrome (32%). Furthermore, the number of patients experiencing dose reductions, interruptions, and permanent discontinuations was significantly higher in those who received axitinib.

Lastly, the SORCE trial was an international, double-blind, three-arm randomized clinical trial involving 1711 participants randomized (2:3:3) to receive 1 year of sorafenib followed by 2 years of placebo, 3 years of sorafenib, or 3-years of placebo [43]. Eligible participants had completely resected M0 RCC with an intermediate (score 3–5) or high (score 6–11) relapse risk according to the Leibovich model [15]. Due to high discontinuation rates, the initial starting dose of 400 mg twice daily was reduced to 400 mg daily. Dose escalation was permitted to 400 mg twice daily at the discretion of the physician. The primary endpoint was DFS, with secondary endpoints of OS. The median DFS was not reached for 3 years of sorafenib or for placebo (HR 1.01; 95% CI: 0.83–1.23; $p = 0.95$). Similar to other trials, grade ≥ 3 AEs were reported (58.6–63.9%) among patients randomized to sorafenib compared to placebo (29.2%).

A recent systematic review and meta-analysis published in 2021 provide an update on the use of adjuvant TKI therapy for localized and locally advanced RCC [44]. In total, five trials (S-TRAC, ASSURE, PROTECT, ATLAS, and SORCE) were included in the meta-analysis comprising of 6521 patients. Pooled data for all-risk populations demonstrated a significantly longer DFS associated with TKI therapy compared to placebo, with a HR of 0.88 (95% CI: 0.81–0.96, $p = 0.004$). When subgroup analyses were performed for patients with higher and lower risk of tumor recurrence, TKI therapy was not associated with a longer DFS compared to placebo in either group, the pooled DFS HR was 0.98 (95% CI: 0.82–1.18, $p = 0.9$) and 0.91 (95% CI: 0.82–1.02, $p = 0.1$), respectively. Despite promising results for DFS, adjuvant TKI was not associated with an improvement in OS when compared to placebo, with a pooled HR of 0.93 (95% CI: 0.83–1.04, $p = 0.2$). Furthermore, TKI therapy was associated with significantly higher rates of all grade and high-grade treatment-related AE compared to placebo (OR 5.20, 95% CI: 4.10–6.59) and (OR 3.85, 95% CI: 1.22–12.17), respectively.

5.5 Immunotherapy

5.5.1 Interleukin and Interferon

Immunotherapy has long been used in the treatment of advanced RCC. Some of the earliest effective treatments for metastatic RCC were interferon-α and interleukin-2 (IL-2). Interferon-α has a response rate in the range of 10–15%, but durable complete response is rare [45, 46]. IL-2 has a slightly improved response rate of 15–20%, but importantly up to 10% of patients experience a complete response which was typically durable over long-term follow-up [47, 48]. However, this came at the cost of significant toxicity, including the risk of vascular leak syndrome, which could be life threatening. Given this level of severe toxicity and the relatively small proportion of patients who will benefit, IL-2 was largely displaced as novel-targeted therapies were developed for the treatment of metastatic RCC.

Given its activity in the metastatic setting, immunotherapy was also explored in the adjuvant space as summarized in Table 5.5. Messing et al. reported a randomized trial of 283 patients with pT3/4a and/or node-positive RCC who were randomized post nephrectomy to either observation or interferon-α. They did not identify any significant improvement in RFS or OS in the active treatment arm and noted that over 11% of patients in the interferon group experienced severe (grade 4) toxicities [49]. Clark et al. reported a trial of 69 patients who had locally advanced (pT3b-T4 or pN+) or metastatic RCC, which was fully resected with no evidence of residual disease. Patients were randomized to 1 course of high-dose IL-2 or observation. Given the toxicities of high dose IL-2, a small randomized trial was designed and powered to demonstrate a large improvement in 2-year disease-free survival (DFS) from 40% for the observation group to 70% for the treatment group. The trial was closed early for futility-based on prespeci-

Table 5.5 Summary of historical trials of adjuvant interferon-α and interleukin-2 (2003–2014)

Authors	Year of publication	Number of patients included	Oncologic eligibility	Treatment	Control	Oncologic outcomes	Adverse events
Messing et al. [45]	2003	283	pT3/4a or pN+	Interferon-α	Observation	No improvement in RFS or OS	Grade 4 in 11.4%
Clark et al. [46]	2003	69	pT3b-T4 or pN+ or M1 (resected)	High dose IL-2	Observation	No improvement in RFS or OS	Grade ≥ 3 in 88%
Atzpodien et al. [47]	2005	203	pT3b-T4 or pN+, or M1 (resected)	SC interferon-α + SC IL-2 + IV 5FU[a]	Observation	No improvement in RFS or OS	Not reported
Passalacqua et al. [48]	2014	303	pT2-T3b or pN0–3	SC Interferonα+ SC IL-2	Observation	No improvement in RFS or OS	Grade ≥ 3 in >9%
Aitchison et al. [49]	2014	305	pT3b-T4 or pN+ or PSM[b]	SC interferon-α + SC IL-2 + IV 5FU	Observation	No improvement in RFS or OS	Grade ≥ 3 in 41%

[a]5-FU denotes 5-fluorouracil
[b]PSM denotes positive surgical margin

fied interim analysis, and no difference in RFS or OS was noted between arms. Further, 88% of patients treated with IL-2 experienced grade 3 or 4 toxicity, most commonly hypotension [50]. A German cooperative group trial enrolled 203 patients with high-risk RCC post nephrectomy (pT3b-4 or pN+ or resected solitary metastasis) and randomized them to observation or combination treatment with subcutaneous IL-2, subcutaneous interferon-α, and IV 5-fluorouracil (5FU). They found no difference in RFS and that OS was actually worse in the treatment arm [51]. The Italian Oncology Group for Clinical Research performed a trial of 303 patients with fully resected RCC, stage pT2-3b pN0–3M0 who were randomized to observation or a combination of low-dose subcutaneous IL-2 and interferon-α. They also identified no improvement in RFS or OS in the treatment arm [52]. Lastly, Aitchison et al. enrolled 305 patients with fully resected RCC who had stage pT3b-4 or pN+ or positive surgical margins and no metastases. They were randomized to observation or treatment with combined subcutaneous IL-2, subcutaneous interferon-α, and IV 5FU. No significant difference in RFS or OS was detected between the arms, and importantly 35% of patients did not complete treatment due to toxicity [53]. In sum, across several trials of interferon-α and IL-2 in the adjuvant setting, including different routes of administration, different doses, and as monotherapy or in combination, no improvement in RFS or OS has been demonstrated, and high-grade toxicities leading to treatment discontinuation were common.

5.6 Immune Checkpoint Inhibitors

The development of immune checkpoint inhibitors (ICIs) was a revolution in the treatment of metastatic RCC. These agents target immune cell signaling to stimulate an enhanced immune response toward malignant cells. The most common agents include antibodies against cytotoxic T-lymphocyte-associated antigen 4 (CTLA-4) and programmed cell death protein 1/programmed cell death protein ligand 1 (PD-1/PDL-1). The initial approved ICIs for metastatic RCC were the combination of ipilimumab and nivolumab, targeting CTLA-4, and PD-1, respectively [54]. Since then, several further combinations have been approved for use in the metastatic setting, including some pairing ICIs with TKIs such as axitinib, lenvatinib, and cabozantinib [55–57]. All have shown improved survival as compared to sunitinib alone and as such now make up the standard of care first-line treatment options for metastatic clear cell RCC [58]. Given the efficacy of these immune checkpoint inhibitors in the metastatic setting, there was interest in moving them earlier in the disease paradigm and into the adjuvant setting. Thus far, a single positive trial has been reported, with further trials underway.

The Keynote-564 trial was a double-blind, phase 3 trial which compared pembrolizumab monotherapy to placebo for patients with ccRCC at high risk of recurrence after nephrectomy with or without metastasectomy [59]. Patients were considered high risk if they met any of the following criteria: pathologic tumor stage 2 with nuclear grade 4 or sarcomatoid differentiation; or pathologic tumor stage 3 or higher; or regional lymph-node metastasis; or stage M1 with no evidence of disease postoperatively. Eligible participants were those with negative surgical margins and no prior exposure to systemic therapy for RCC. Randomization was 1:1 to pembrolizumab or placebo and was stratified by metastatic status. Pembrolizumab was administered at a dose of 200 mg IV every 3 weeks for a maximum of 17 cycles (approximately 1 year). The primary outcome was DFS, which was defined as the time from randomization to the first documented local or distant recurrence or death. Secondary endpoints included OS, safety, andpatient-reportedd outcomes.

A total of 994 patients were randomized to receive either adjuvant pembrolizumab (n = 496) or placebo (n = 498). At the time of prespecified interim analysis, the median time from randomization was 24 months. Pembrolizumab was associated with significantly longer DFS compared to placebo (DFS at 24 months, 77.3% vs.

68.1%; HR for recurrence or death, 0.68; 95% CI: 0.53–0.87; $p = 0.002$), which appeared more robust following an updated analysis after longer follow-up of 30 months (HR for DFS 0.63, 95% CI 0.50–0.80; $p < 0.0001$) [60]. The benefit was consistent across subgroups regardless of risk groups and PD-L1 expression and appeared particularly robust in the small subgroup of M1 NED (HR 0.28, 95% CI 0.12–0.66). The estimated DFS rate at 24 months was 78.3% with pembrolizumab versus 67.3% with placebo. The OS analysis was not mature but was trending in favor of pembrolizumab (HR 0.52, 95% CI 0.31–0.86; $p = 0.0048$), and the p-value did not cross the statistical hypothesis testing boundary. Grade 3 or higher AE related to treatment occurred in 18.6% of the patients who received pembrolizumab and in 1.2% of those who received placebo. Thus, no prohibitive and excessive toxicities were observed, and there were no deaths related to pembrolizumab therapy. Based on this trial, adjuvant pembrolizumab has been added to the NCCN guidelines for patients with high-risk clear cell RCC.

Despite this, there has been some controversy over establishing pembrolizumab as a standard of care for all comers with high-risk RCC. Concerns have been raised over the high cost of therapy, and the significant rate of AE, which can be irreversible, as well as severe and life threatening in some cases [61]. Additionally, there have been calls for improved risk stratification to better identify those who will benefit most from this therapy. Finally, given the lack of OS benefit at this point (pending longer follow-up), it may be challenging to justify the routine use of ICI in the adjuvant setting at this time [62].

5.7 Ongoing Trials and Future Directions

Currently, there are three active trials examining the role of ICIs in the adjuvant setting for RCC. The IMmotion010 trial is no longer recruiting but has yet to be reported. This is a phase III RCT of atezolizumab versus placebo for patients with resected RCC at high risk for recurrence and with a clear cell or sarcomatoid component [63]. Patients will receive 1200 mg of atezolizumab IV every 3 weeks for 16 cycles (approximately 1 year). The primary outcome is DFS, while secondary outcomes include OS and AE profile. The study design largely mirrors that of Keynote-564.

Additionally, there are three further trials that are currently recruiting as summarized in Table 5.6. The CheckMate 914 trial is a phase 3 trial of adjuvant nivolumab alone, or in combination with ipilimumab for patients with RCC and predominantly clear cell histology [64]. This trial will enroll patients with high-grade pT2a, any grade pT2b-4, or N1 disease. Eligible participants will be randomized to nivolumab and ipilimumab, versus nivolumab and placebo, versus placebo alone. The primary outcome is DFS, with secondary outcomes OS and AE. This will be the first trial of combination ICIs in the adjuvant setting, which is the standard in the first-line metastatic setting. The PROSPER RCC trial (NCT03055013) is evaluating a different innovative strategy of priming the immune system prior to nephrectomy with one dose of neoadjuvant nivolumab 480 mg followed by nine doses of adjuvant nivolumab 480 mg every 4 weeks in patients with high-risk RCC compared to surgery alone.

The RAMPART trial has been designed by the Medical Research Council in the UK and uses a multiarm multistage design (MAMS), which allows the addition of new treatment arms over time, as well as the ability to update the control arm should the standard of care change over time [65]. Currently, the control arm, Arm A is observation alone (no placebo), while Arm B is monotherapy with the PDL-1 inhibitor durvalumab, and Arm C is durvalumab in combination with the CTLA-4 inhibitor tremelimumab. The population will include patients with resected RCC (both clear cell and nonclear cell subtypes), no macroscopic residual disease, and intermediate to high risk of recurrence based on the Leibovitch score (scores 3–11 will be accrued). The primary endpoints are DFS and OS, while secondary endpoints include safety and quality of life. Biospecimens will also be collected for translational research. This trial is unique both for the

Table 5.6 Summary of RCC adjuvant therapy trials currently recruiting (per clinicaltrials.gov)

Name (trial identifier)	Location	Phase	Oncologic eligibility	Treatment
IMmotion010: A study of Atezolizumab as adjuvant therapy in participants with renal cell carcinoma (RCC) at high risk of developing metastasis following Nephrectomy (NCT03024996) [57]	186 international sites	III	– Histologically confirmed RCC with either clear cell or sarcomatoid component at high risk of recurrence (T2 grade 4, T3a grade 3–4, T3b/c any grade. T4 any grade or TxN+ any grade)	Atezolizumab vs. Placebo
			– Complete resection (no evidence of residual disease& tumor specimen evaluable for PD-L1	
			– Absence of metastasis with ECOG-PS ≤ 1	
RAMPART: Renal adjuvant MultiPle arm randomised Trial (NCT03288532) [59]	35 sites across the United Kingdom	III	– Histologically proven RCC (excluding oncocytoma, collecting duct, and medullary)	Durvalumab vs. Durvalumab + Tremelimumab vs. Active monitoring
			– Completely resected (no evidence of disease on postoperative imaging)	
			– Microscopically positive surgical margins on radical nephrectomy acceptable, if no macroscopic disease on postoperative imaging	
			– Leibovitch score 3–11	
Checkmate 914: A study comparing Nivolumab, Nivolumab in combination with Ipilimumab and placebo in participants with localized kidney cancer who underwent surgery to remove part of a kidney (NCT03138512) [58]	228 international sites	III	– RCC with predominantly clear cell histology (sarcomatoid included)	Nivolumab + Ipilimumab vs. Nivolumab + placebo vs. Placebo
			– complete resection with negative surgical margins	
			– no evidence of macroscopic disease on postoperative imaging	
			– TNM staging meeting one of the following:	
			– pT2a, G3/4, N0 M0	
			– pT2b, G any, N0 M0	
			– pT3, G any, N0 M0	
			– pT4, G any, N0 M0	
			– pT any, G any, N1 M0	

MAMS design as well as the use of Leibovitch score to risk stratify patients which other trials have not done in this space.

To improve adjuvant trial design with a precision medicine approach, several studies are underway focused on developing novel blood and urine-based DNA biomarkers to detect minimal residual disease (MRD) and better risk stratify patients and identify those best suited for adjuvant therapy. However, compared to other urologic malignancies, one of the main challenges with ccRCC is its propensity to shed very small amounts of circulating free DNA (cfDNA) [66] [67, 68]. To circumvent this problem, cell-free methylated DNA immunoprecipitation and high-throughput sequencing (cfMeDIP-seq) is an emerging technique, which could help identify high-risk genomic signatures with superior sensitivity, lower DNA requirement, lower cost, and with an ability to enrich for cancer-specific DNA signatures [66]. Going forward, clinical trials may integrate this methodology into their design to better select which patients may benefit most from adjuvant therapy. Ultimately, the combination of markers of MRD and predictive biomarkers for benefit will enable precision medicine in the adjuvant setting.

Looking to the future, novel immune therapies beyond ICI are also being investigated, including T-cell agonists, tumor vaccines, T-regulatory antagonists, and adoptive cell therapy [69]. Despite continued advances in novel therapies, appropriate patient selection with the help of accurate predictive biomarkers and models will be of paramount importance [70]. Furthermore, accumulating knowledge on molecular subtypes of RCC with next-generation sequencing could pave the wave for the establishment of genomic signatures to help guide therapy selection.

Acknowledgments None.

Disclosures Rudzinski JK[1], Beech BB[2], Wang B[3], and Zemp LW[5] have no conflicts or disclosures. Sonpavde GP[4] has following conflicts & disclosures in the past 36 months:

1. *Advisory Board:* BMS, Genentech, EMD Serono, Merck, Sanofi, Seattle Genetics/Astellas, Astrazeneca, Exelixis, Janssen, Bicycle Therapeutics, Pfizer, Gilead, Scholar Rock, G1 Therapeutics, Eli Lilly/Loxo Oncology, Infinity Pharmaceuticals
2. *Research Support:* Sanofi, Astrazeneca, Gilead, QED, Lucence, Predicine, BMS, EMD Serono
3. *Steering committee of studies*: BMS, Bavarian Nordic, Seattle Genetics, QED, G1 Therapeutics (all unpaid), and Astrazeneca, EMD Serono, Debiopharm (paid)
4. *Data safety monitoring committee*: Mereo
5. *Employment:* Spouse employed by Myriad
6. *Travel costs*: BMS, Astrazeneca.
7. *Writing/Editor fees*: Uptodate, Editor of Elsevier Practice Update Bladder Cancer Center of Excellence.
8. *Speaking fees*: Physicians Education Resource (PER), Onclive, Research to Practice, Medscape, Cancer Network, Masters Lecture Series (MLS).

Conflicts of Interest None of the authors have any relevant disclosures, and none of the authors have any financial or nonfinancial interests that may be relevant to the submitted work.

Funding None.

References

1. Siegel RL, Miller KD, Fuchs HE, Jemal A. Cancer statistics, 2021. CA Cancer J Clin. 2021;71(1):7–33.
2. Motzer RJ, Jonasch E, Agarwal N, Alva A, Baine M, Beckermann K, et al. Kidney cancer, version 3.2022, NCCN clinical practice guidelines in oncology. J Natl Compr Cancer Netw. 2022;20(1):71–90.
3. Lipworth L, Morgans AK, Edwards TL, Barocas DA, Chang SS, Herrell SD, et al. Renal cell cancer histological subtype distribution differs by race and sex. BJU Int. 2016;117(2):260–5.
4. Leibovich BC, Lohse CM, Crispen PL, Boorjian SA, Thompson RH, Blute ML, et al. Histological subtype is an independent predictor of outcome for patients with renal cell carcinoma. J Urol. 2010;183(4):1309–15.

5. Dall'Oglio MF, Ribeiro-Filho LA, Antunes AA, Crippa A, Nesrallah L, Goncalves PD, et al. Microvascular tumor invasion, tumor size and Fuhrman grade: a pathological triad for prognostic evaluation of renal cell carcinoma. J Urol. 2007;178(2):425–8; discussion 8.
6. Lam JS, Shvarts O, Said JW, Pantuck AJ, Seligson DB, Aldridge ME, et al. Clinicopathologic and molecular correlations of necrosis in the primary tumor of patients with renal cell carcinoma. Cancer. 2005;103(12):2517–25.
7. Sengupta S, Lohse CM, Leibovich BC, Frank I, Thompson RH, Webster WS, et al. Histologic coagulative tumor necrosis as a prognostic indicator of renal cell carcinoma aggressiveness. Cancer. 2005;104(3):511–20.
8. Bianchi M, Sun M, Jeldres C, Shariat SF, Trinh QD, Briganti A, et al. Distribution of metastatic sites in renal cell carcinoma: a population-based analysis. Ann Oncol. 2012;23(4):973–80.
9. Leibovich BC, Lohse CM, Cheville JC, Zaid HB, Boorjian SA, Frank I, et al. Predicting oncologic outcomes in renal cell carcinoma after surgery. Eur Urol. 2018;73(5):772–80.
10. Janzen NK, Kim HL, Figlin RA, Belldegrun AS. Surveillance after radical or partial nephrectomy for localized renal cell carcinoma and management of recurrent disease. Urol Clin North Am. 2003;30(4):843–52.
11. Janowitz T, Welsh SJ, Zaki K, Mulders P, Eisen T. Adjuvant therapy in renal cell carcinoma-past, present, and future. Semin Oncol. 2013;40(4):482–91.
12. Sorbellini M, Kattan MW, Snyder ME, Reuter V, Motzer R, Goetzl M, et al. A postoperative prognostic nomogram predicting recurrence for patients with conventional clear cell renal cell carcinoma. J Urol. 2005;173(1):48–51.
13. Karakiewicz PI, Briganti A, Chun FK, Trinh QD, Perrotte P, Ficarra V, et al. Multi-institutional validation of a new renal cancer-specific survival nomogram. J Clin Oncol. 2007;25(11):1316–22.
14. Frank I, Blute ML, Cheville JC, Lohse CM, Weaver AL, Zincke H. An outcome prediction model for patients with clear cell renal cell carcinoma treated with radical nephrectomy based on tumor stage, size, grade and necrosis: the SSIGN score. J Urol. 2002;168(6):2395–400.
15. Leibovich BC, Blute ML, Cheville JC, Lohse CM, Frank I, Kwon ED, et al. Prediction of progression after radical nephrectomy for patients with clear cell renal cell carcinoma: a stratification tool for prospective clinical trials. Cancer. 2003;97(7):1663–71.
16. Patard JJ, Kim HL, Lam JS, Dorey FJ, Pantuck AJ, Zisman A, et al. Use of the University of California los Angeles integrated staging system to predict survival in renal cell carcinoma: an international multicenter study. J Clin Oncol. 2004;22(16):3316–22.
17. Tan MH, Li HH, Choong CV, Chia KS, Toh CK, Tang T, et al. The Karakiewicz nomogram is the most useful clinical predictor for survival outcomes in patients with localized renal cell carcinoma. Cancer. 2011;117(23):5314–24.
18. Nabi S, Kessler ER, Bernard B, Flaig TW, Lam ET. Renal cell carcinoma: a review of biology and pathophysiology. F1000Res. 2018;7:307.
19. Hsieh JJ, Purdue MP, Signoretti S, Swanton C, Albiges L, Schmidinger M, et al. Renal cell carcinoma. Nat Rev Dis Primers. 2017;3:17009.
20. Beroukhim R, Brunet JP, Di Napoli A, Mertz KD, Seeley A, Pires MM, et al. Patterns of gene expression and copy-number alterations in von-hippel Lindau disease-associated and sporadic clear cell carcinoma of the kidney. Cancer Res. 2009;69(11):4674–81.
21. Rini B, Goddard A, Knezevic D, Maddala T, Zhou M, Aydin H, et al. A 16-gene assay to predict recurrence after surgery in localised renal cell carcinoma: development and validation studies. Lancet Oncol. 2015;16(6):676–85.
22. Brooks SA, Brannon AR, Parker JS, Fisher JC, Sen O, Kattan MW, et al. ClearCode34: a prognostic risk predictor for localized clear cell renal cell carcinoma. Eur Urol. 2014;66(1):77–84.
23. Morgan TM, Mehra R, Tiemeny P, Wolf JS, Wu S, Sangale Z, et al. A multigene signature based on cell cycle proliferation improves prediction of mortality within 5 years of radical nephrectomy for renal cell carcinoma. Eur Urol. 2018;73(5):763–9.
24. Rini BI, Escudier B, Martini JF, Magheli A, Svedman C, Lopatin M, et al. Validation of the 16-gene recurrence score in patients with locoregional, high-risk renal cell carcinoma from a phase III trial of adjuvant sunitinib. Clin Cancer Res. 2018;24(18):4407–15.
25. Ljungberg B, Albiges L, Abu-Ghanem Y, Bedke J, Capitanio U, Dabestani S, et al. European Association of Urology Guidelines on renal cell carcinoma: the 2022 update. Eur Urol. 2022;82(4):399–410.
26. Campbell SC, Clark PE, Chang SS, Karam JA, Souter L, Uzzo RG. Renal mass and localized renal cancer: evaluation, management, and follow-up: AUA guideline: part I. J Urol. 2021;206(2):199–208.
27. Capitanio U, Larcher A, Cianflone F, Trevisani F, Nini A, Mottrie A, et al. Hypertension and cardiovascular morbidity following surgery for kidney cancer. Eur Urol Oncol. 2020;3(2):209–15.
28. Powles T, Albiges L, Staehler M, Bensalah K, Dabestani S, Giles RH, et al. Updated European Association of Urology guidelines: recommendations for the treatment of first-line metastatic clear cell renal cancer. Eur Urol. 2018;73(3):311–5.
29. Kaelin WG Jr. The von Hippel-Lindau tumor suppressor gene and kidney cancer. Clin Cancer Res. 2004;10(18 Pt 2):6290S–5S.
30. Rini BI, Campbell SC, Escudier B. Renal cell carcinoma. Lancet. 2009;373(9669):1119–32.
31. Motzer RJ, Hutson TE, Tomczak P, Michaelson MD, Bukowski RM, Oudard S, et al. Overall survival and updated results for sunitinib compared with interferon alfa in patients with metastatic renal cell carcinoma. J Clin Oncol. 2009;27(22):3584–90.

32. Escudier B, Eisen T, Stadler WM, Szczylik C, Oudard S, Siebels M, et al. Sorafenib in advanced clear-cell renal-cell carcinoma. N Engl J Med. 2007;356(2):125–34.
33. Haas NB, Manola J, Dutcher JP, Flaherty KT, Uzzo RG, Atkins MB, et al. Adjuvant treatment for high-risk clear cell renal cancer: updated results of a high-risk subset of the ASSURE randomized trial. JAMA Oncol. 2017;3(9):1249–52.
34. Motzer RJ, Ravaud A, Patard JJ, Pandha HS, George DJ, Patel A, et al. Adjuvant sunitinib for high-risk renal cell carcinoma after nephrectomy: subgroup analyses and updated overall survival results. Eur Urol. 2018;73(1):62–8.
35. George DJ, Martini JF, Staehler M, Motzer RJ, Magheli A, Donskov F, et al. Phase III trial of adjuvant sunitinib in patients with high-risk renal cell carcinoma: exploratory pharmacogenomic analysis. Clin Cancer Res. 2019;25(4):1165–73.
36. Greef B, Eisen T. Medical treatment of renal cancer: new horizons. Br J Cancer. 2016;115(5):505–16.
37. Rini BI, Escudier B, Tomczak P, Kaprin A, Szczylik C, Hutson TE, et al. Comparative effectiveness of axitinib versus sorafenib in advanced renal cell carcinoma (AXIS): a randomised phase 3 trial. Lancet. 2011;378(9807):1931–9.
38. Haas NB, Manola J, Uzzo RG, Flaherty KT, Wood CG, Kane C, et al. Adjuvant sunitinib or sorafenib for high-risk, non-metastatic renal-cell carcinoma (ECOG-ACRIN E2805): a double-blind, placebo-controlled, randomised, phase 3 trial. Lancet. 2016;387(10032):2008–16.
39. Ravaud A, Motzer RJ, Pandha HS, George DJ, Pantuck AJ, Patel A, et al. Adjuvant sunitinib in high-risk renal-cell carcinoma after nephrectomy. N Engl J Med. 2016;375(23):2246–54.
40. Motzer RJ, Haas NB, Donskov F, Gross-Goupil M, Varlamov S, Kopyltsov E, et al. Randomized phase III trial of adjuvant pazopanib versus placebo after nephrectomy in patients with localized or locally advanced renal cell carcinoma. J Clin Oncol. 2017;35(35):3916–23.
41. Motzer RJ, Russo P, Haas N, Doehn C, Donskov F, Gross-Goupil M, et al. Adjuvant pazopanib versus placebo after nephrectomy in patients with localized or locally advanced renal cell carcinoma: final overall survival analysis of the phase 3 PROTECT trial. Eur Urol. 2021;79(3):334–8.
42. Gross-Goupil M, Kwon TG, Eto M, Ye D, Miyake H, Seo SI, et al. Axitinib versus placebo as an adjuvant treatment of renal cell carcinoma: results from the phase III, randomized ATLAS trial. Ann Oncol. 2018;29(12):2371–8.
43. Eisen T, Frangou E, Oza B, Ritchie AWS, Smith B, Kaplan R, et al. Adjuvant sorafenib for renal cell carcinoma at intermediate or high risk of relapse: results from the SORCE randomized phase III intergroup trial. J Clin Oncol. 2020;38(34):4064–75.
44. Laukhtina E, Quhal F, Mori K, Motlagh RS, Pradere B, Schuettfort VM, et al. Adjuvant therapy with tyrosine kinase inhibitors for localized and locally advanced renal cell carcinoma: an updated systematic review and meta-analysis. Urol Oncol. 2021;39(11):764–73.
45. deKernion J, Sarna G, Figlin R, Lindner A, Smith R. The treatment of renal cell carcinoma with human leukocyte alpha-interferon. J Urol. 1983;130(6):1063–6.
46. Minasian L, Motzer R, Gluck L, Mazumdar M, Vlamis V, Krown S. Interferon alfa-2a in advanced renal cell carcinoma: treatment results and survival in 159 patients with long-term follow-up. J Clin Oncol. 1993;11(7):1368–75.
47. Dutcher J, Atkins M, Fisher R, Weiss G, Margolin K, Aronson F, et al. Interleukin-2-based therapy for metastatic renal cell cancer: the Cytokine Working Group experience, 1989–1997. Cancer J Sci Am. 1997;3(Suppl 1):S73–8.
48. Fisher R, Rosenberg S, Fyfe G. Long-term survival update for high-dose recombinant interleukin-2 in patients with renal cell carcinoma. Cancer J Sci Am. 2000;6(Suppl 1):S55–7.
49. Messing E, Manola J, Wilding G, Propert K, Fleischmann J, Crawford E, et al. Phase III study of interferon alfa-NL as adjuvant treatment for resectable renal cell carcinoma: an eastern cooperative oncology group/intergroup trial. J Clin Oncol. 2003;21(7):1214–22.
50. Clark J, Atkins M, Urba W, Creech S, Figlin R, Dutcher J, et al. Adjuvant high-dose bolus interleukin-2 for patients with high-risk renal cell carcinoma: a cytokine working group randomized trial. J Clin Oncol. 2003;21(16):3133–40.
51. Atzpodien J, Schmitt E, Gertenbach U, Fornara P, Heynemann H, Maskow A, et al. Adjuvant treatment with interleukin-2- and interferon-alpha2a-based chemoimmunotherapy in renal cell carcinoma post tumour nephrectomy: results of a prospectively randomised trial of the German cooperative renal carcinoma Chemoimmunotherapy group (DGCIN). Br J Cancer. 2005;92(5):843–6.
52. Passalacqua R, Caminiti C, Buti S, Porta C, Camisa R, Braglia L, et al. Adjuvant low-dose interleukin-2 (IL-2) plus interferon-α (IFN-α) in operable renal cell carcinoma (RCC): a phase III, randomized, multicentre trial of the Italian Oncology Group for Clinical Research (GOIRC). J Immunother. 2014;37(9):440–7.
53. Aitchison M, Bray C, Van Poppel H, Sylvester R, Graham J, Innes C, et al. Adjuvant 5-flurouracil, alpha-interferon and interleukin-2 versus observation in patients at high risk of recurrence after nephrectomy for renal cell carcinoma: results of a phase III randomised European Organisation for Research and Treatment of Cancer (Genito-Urinary Cancers Group)/National Cancer Research Institute trial. Eur J Cancer. 2014;50(1):70–7.
54. Motzer R, Tannir N, McDermott D, Arén Frontera O, Melichar B, Choueiri T, et al. Nivolumab plus ipilimumab versus sunitinib in advanced renal-cell carcinoma. N Engl J Med. 2018;378(14):1277–90.

55. Rini B, Plimack E, Stus V, Gafanov R, Hawkins R, Nosov D, et al. Pembrolizumab plus axitinib versus sunitinib for advanced renal-cell carcinoma. N Engl J Med. 2019;380(12):1116–27.
56. Choueiri T, Powles T, Burotto M, Escudier B, Bourlon M, Zurawski B, et al. Nivolumab plus cabozantinib versus sunitinib for advanced renal-cell carcinoma. N Engl J Med. 2021;384(9):829–41.
57. Motzer R, Choueiri TK. Lenvatinib plus pembrolizumab for renal cell carcinoma. Reply. N Engl J Med. 2021;385(3):287.
58. Tran J, Ornstein M. Clinical review on the management of metastatic renal cell carcinoma. JCO Oncol Pract. 2022;18(3):187–96.
59. Choueiri T, Tomczak P, Park S, Venugopal B, Ferguson T, Chang Y, et al. Adjuvant pembrolizumab after nephrectomy in renal-cell carcinoma. N Engl J Med. 2021;385(8):683–94.
60. Choueiri TK, Tomczak P, Park SH, Venugopal B, Ferguson T, Symeonides SN, et al. Pembrolizumab as post nephrectomy adjuvant therapy for patients with renal cell carcinoma: Results from 30-month follow-up of KEYNOTE-564. J Clin Oncol. 2022;40(6_Suppl):290.
61. Bleyer A. Adjuvant pembrolizumab after nephrectomy in renal-cell carcinoma. N Engl J Med. 2021;385(20):1919–20.
62. Magee D, Kutikov A. Re: adjuvant pembrolizumab after nephrectomy in renal-cell carcinoma. Eur Urol. 2022;81(3):317–8.
63. Uzzo R, Bex A, Rini B, Albiges L, Suarez C, Donaldson F, et al. A phase III study of atezolizumab (atezo) vs. placebo as adjuvant therapy in renal cell carcinoma (RCC) patients (pts) at high risk of recurrence following resection (IMmotion010). J Clin Oncol. 2017;35(15_Suppl):TPS4598.
64. Bex A, Russo P, Tomita Y, Grünwald V, Ramirez L, McHenry B, et al. A phase III, randomized, placebo-controlled trial of nivolumab or nivolumab plus ipilimumab in patients with localized renal cell carcinoma at high-risk of relapse after radical or partial nephrectomy (CheckMate 914). J Clin Oncol. 2020;38(15_Suppl):TPS5099.
65. Oza B, Frangou E, Smith B, Bryant H, Kaplan R, Choodari-Oskooei B, et al. RAMPART: a phase III multi-arm multi-stage trial of adjuvant checkpoint inhibitors in patients with resected primary renal cell carcinoma (RCC) at high or intermediate risk of relapse. Contemp Clin Trials. 2021 Sep;108:106482.
66. Nuzzo PV, Berchuck JE, Korthauer K, Spisak S, Nassar AH, Alaiwi SA, et al. Detection of renal cell carcinoma using plasma and urine cell-free DNA methylomes. Nat Med. 2020;26(7):1041–3.
67. Zill OA, Banks KC, Fairclough SR, Mortimer SA, Vowles JV, Mokhtari R, et al. The landscape of actionable genomic alterations in cell-free circulating tumor DNA from 21,807 advanced cancer patients. Clin Cancer Res. 2018;24(15):3528–38.
68. Pal SK, Sonpavde G, Agarwal N, Vogelzang NJ, Srinivas S, Haas NB, et al. Evolution of circulating tumor DNA profile from first-line to subsequent therapy in metastatic renal cell carcinoma. Eur Urol. 2017;72(4):557–64.
69. Carlo MI, Voss MH, Motzer RJ. Checkpoint inhibitors and other novel immunotherapies for advanced renal cell carcinoma. Nat Rev Urol. 2016;13(7):420–31.
70. Barata PC, Rini BI. Treatment of renal cell carcinoma: current status and future directions. CA Cancer J Clin. 2017;67(6):507–24.

Part II

Upper Tract Urothelial Carcinoma

Diagnosis and Clinical Staging

6

Utsav Shailesh Shah, Sanjoy Kumar Sureka, and Uday Pratap Singh

6.1 Introduction

Five to ten percent of urothelial carcinomas originate in the upper tract, in contrast to bladder urothelial carcinomas which account for more than 90% of the cases [1]. The diagnosis of upper tract TCC is based on multiple factors which shall be discussed in this chapter. Urine cytology and imaging play a dominant role in diagnosis. Staging is routinely based on tumor, nodes, and metastasis (TNM) classification [2].

6.2 Diagnosis

6.2.1 Symptoms

The diagnosis of upper tract TCC is made generally in patients undergoing workup for hematuria. Macroscopic or microscopic hematuria is the commonest symptom seen in 70–80% of cases with upper tract TCC [3]. About 20–30% patients have pain in the flank region as a result of clot or tumor tissue resulting in obstruction. The incidence of flank pain as a result of malignant obstruction or clot is much more prevalent in upper tract TCC than bladder TCC [4]. Upper tract TCC is also present with abdominal mass, weight loss, anorexia and bone pain.

6.2.2 Urine Cytology

Urinary tract cytology plays a pivotal role in diagnosis and decision-making in case of a suspected upper tract TCC. The overall sensitivity of urine cytology for upper tract TCC is 55–92% [5]. As compared to bladder tumors, this sensitivity of cytology is less [6]. Studies have shown that the performance of urine cytology in upper tract is better when done for high-grade tumors. The European Association of Urology (EAU) guidelines recommend urinary cytology as a part of the standard diagnostic workup (grade A recommendation). If a high-grade tumor is found in cytology, the European Association of Urology (EAU) guidelines recommends doing a radical nephroureterectomy (grade B recommendation) [7]. Routinely, the Paris system for urinary cytology reporting is used.

Other options apart from voided urine cytology are barbotages or washings of the upper tract, which can be obtained using a ureteral catheter while performing a cystoscopy of these patients. Obtaining a specimen from the renal cavities and ureteral lumina is preferred before doing retrograde pyelography (RGP) as the contrast used during RGP can result in distortion of cytological

U. S. Shah · S. K. Sureka · U. P. Singh (✉)
Department of Urology and Renal Transplantation, Sanjay Gandhi Postgraduate Institute of Medical Sciences, Lucknow, India

P. Singh et al. (eds.), *A Guide to Management of Urological Cancers*,
https://doi.org/10.1007/978-981-99-2341-0_6

specimens [8]. Urothelial tissue fragments can be seen in barbotage specimens, which are indicative of exfoliated normal urothelium and/or neoplastic fragments [9].

6.2.3 Imaging

Computed tomography urography (CTU) is the preferred modality for diagnosing upper tract TCCs owing to their high accuracy and is often considered to be the 'Gold standard' imaging study for these tumors. In patients with renal insufficiency, an MR Urogram can be obtained. CTU is more sensitive and specific for the diagnosis and staging of UTUC as compared to MR urography [10]. Gadolinium-based contrast agents for MRU should be restricted in patients with <30 mL/min creatinine clearance.

In CTU, a three-phase image acquisition is obtained, which includes an unenhanced phase, a corticomedullary phase, and an excretory phase for a suspected upper tract TCC following injection of an intravenous contrast agent [11]. Findings that are suggestive of upper tract TCC include filling defects (Fig. 6.1), which are radiolucent, obstruction (Fig. 6.2), improper visualization of the pelvicalyceal system, or incomplete filling of a part of the ureter. The average Hounsfield unit (HU) density of transitional cell carcinomas ranges from 10 to 70 HU [12].

In upper tract TCC, distal ureter is the most common site of involvement in the ureter, accounting for 73% of all lesions, followed by 24% in the mid ureter and 3% in the proximal ureter. Bilateral ureteral involvement is seen in 2–5% of patients with upper tract TCCs [13].

CT of the thorax, abdomen, and pelvis are generally obtained concomitantly to rule out lung and abdominal spread. It is mandatory to rule out metastases before embarking upon treatment with a curative intent. The role of ^{18}F-Fluorodeoxglucose positron emission tomography/computed tomography(FDG-PET/CT) in

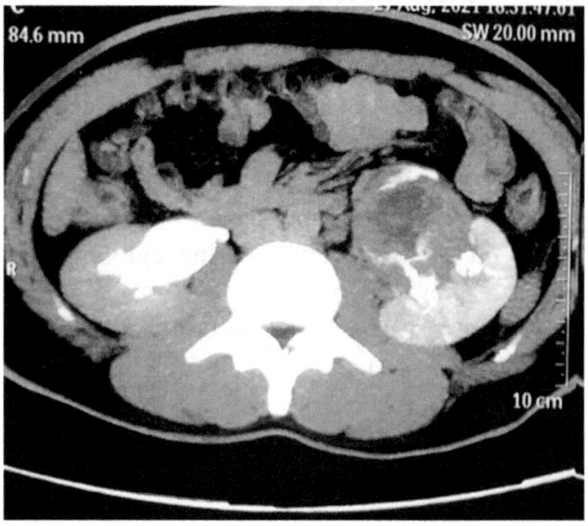

Fig. 6.1 Axial section of CT urogram shows a large left renal pelvic tumor as filling defects

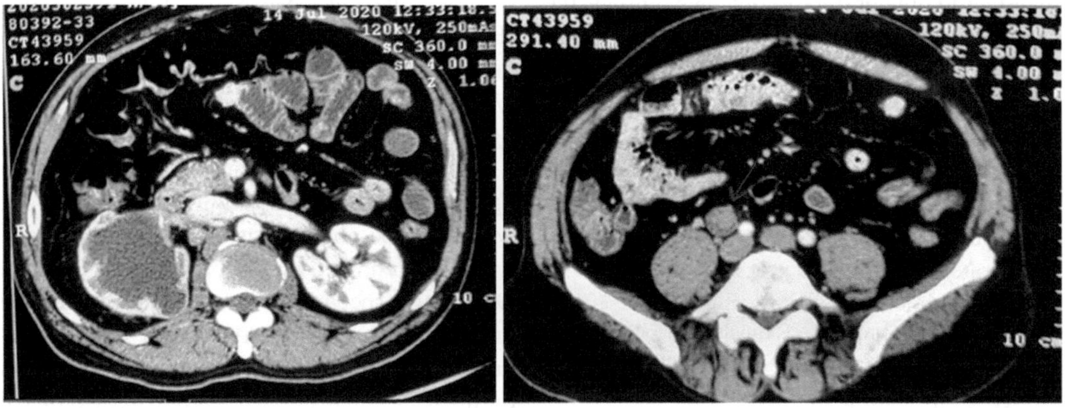

Fig. 6.2 Axial section of CT urogram shows marked right hydroureteronephrosis with distended ureter upto mid-ureteric level and hyperdense content within it (Red Arrow)

bladder cancer is currently in the scenario when CT is contraindicated. The deterrent to widespread adoption of ^{18}F-FDG PET/CT as an imaging modality in upper tract TCC is due to the lack of prospective studies with high level of evidence regarding the same [14].

6.2.4 Cystoscopy

Cystoscopy is mandatory in patients with upper tract TCC's to rule out concomitant bladder lesions [15]. It is generally performed under anaesthesia when a definitive procedure for the upper tract TCC is planned.

6.2.5 Endoscopy of the Upper Tract

Endoscopic assessment of the upper tract can be done either using a retrograde or an antegrade approach.

6.2.5.1 Ureterorenoscopy

Epithelial flat lesions of the upper tract without mass effect or urothelial thickening are generally not visible on imaging [16]. Guidelines have recommended using diagnostic ureteroscopy (URS) and biopsy if imaging and cytology are insufficient for the diagnosis and/or risk stratification of the tumor.

URS can be done using a semi-rigid or preferably a flexible ureteroscope to visualize the ureter and pelvicalyceal system in patients with upper tract lesions. The appearance, number, size, and other features of the tumor can be determined by doing a ureteroscopy. Also, tumor biopsies can be obtained during URS. Tumor grading in diagnostic URS biopsy is accurate; however, as the amount of tissue obtained is limited, stage assessment is often inaccurate [17]. This is because mostly, URS biopsy specimens do not include deep layers of ureter or renal pelvis. Thus, a more definitive and accurate prediction of tumor stage as well as risk stratification requires a combination of urine cytology, cross-sectional imaging, visual inspection of tumor, and tumor grade [18]. Such stratification helps in decision making with regard to management (radical nephroureterectomy vs. kidney sparing approach) of upper tract TCC [17].

Narrow band imaging, photodynamic diagnosis and IMAGE 1S™ (Karl Storz, Germany) are in experimental phase for use in upper tract TCC. Using optical coherence tomography and confocal laser endomicroscopy, there have been attempts to evaluate tumor grade and stage in vivo and from preliminary results it appears to be a promising technique [19].

In conclusion, URS can be readily used when there is a diagnostic uncertainty, in patients with a solitary renal unit or when a renal-sparing treatment is being considered.

6.2.5.2 Antegrade Endoscopic Evaluation

Over the years, percutaneous antegrade access has been abandoned as a result of the development of flexible ureterorenoscopes. However, in select cases where retrograde access is not easy, an antegrade approach for evaluation of the upper tract might be required. Antegrade nephroscopy, URS, urography, biopsy, and even tumor resection can be done using this approach. Low-risk tumors inaccessible or difficult to manage with flexible URS can be treated using this technique [16]. But the risk of implantation of tumor cells in the retroperitoneum should be kept in mind by the operating surgeon [20].

6.3 Clinical Staging of Upper Tract TCC

6.3.1 TNM (Tumor, Nodes, Metastasis) Classification of Upper Tract TCC

The TNM classification for upper tract TCC has undergone various changes over the years. Currently, the 2017 TNM classification is used for staging upper tract TCC (Table 6.1). The regional lymph nodes for pelvic and upper ureteral tumors are the hilar and retroperitoneal lymph nodes. For lesions of the mid and lower

Table 6.1 TNM classification for upper tract TCC [2]

T—primary tumor	
TX	Primary tumor cannot be assessed
T0	No evidence of primary tumor
Ta	Noninvasive papillary carcinoma
Tis	Carcinoma in situ
T1	Tumor invades subepithelial connective tissue
T2	Tumor invades muscularis
T3	– renal pelvis: Tumor invades beyond muscularis into peripelvic fat or renal parenchyma
	– ureter: Tumor invades beyond muscularis into periureteric fat
T4	Tumor invades adjacent organs or through the kidney into perinephric fat
N—Regional lymph nodes	
NX	Regional lymph nodes cannot be assessed
N0	No regional lymph node metastasis
N1	Metastasis in a single lymph node 2 cm or less in the greatest dimension
N2	Metastasis in a single lymph node more than 2 cm, or multiple lymph nodes
M—Distant metastasis	
M0	No distant metastasis
M1	Distant metastasis

TNM tumor, node, metastasis (classification)

ureter, pelvic lymph nodes are the regional lymph nodes. Laterality does not affect node classification.

6.3.2 American Joint Committee on Cancer (AJCC) Staging of Upper Tract TCC

The AJCC 8th edition staging system can be used to stage these tumors [21].

6.3.3 Tumor Grading

In 1973, the World Health Organization (WHO) classification for tumor grading of upper tract TCC was defined. For decades, the same classification was used wherein the tumors were graded from Grade 1 (G1) to Grade 3 (G3) [16]. In recent years, the 2004/2016 WHO classification was described. The 2004/2016 WHO classification distinguishes between noninvasive tumors: papillary urothelial neoplasia of low malignant potential and low- and high-grade carcinomas based on histologic characteristics (low grade vs. high grade) [16].

6.3.4 Genomic Characterization of Upper Tract TCC

Recent attempts have aimed at characterization of genomic landscape of upper tract TCC. In patients suffering from upper tract TCC, mutations have been identified in FGFR3, KMT2D, PIK3CA, and TP53. Further studies are needed to validate these findings [22].

References

1. Siegel R, Miller K, Jemal A. Cancer statistics, 2017. CA Cancer J Clin. 2017;67(1):7–30.
2. Brierley JD, Gospodarowicz MK, Wittekind C. TNM classification of malignant tumours. 8th ed. Hoboken, NJ: Wiley-Blackwell; 2017.
3. Inman B, Tran V, Fradet Y, Lacombe L. Carcinoma of the upper urinary tract. Cancer. 2009;115(13):2853–62.
4. Cowan N. CT urography for hematuria. Nat Rev Urol. 2012;9(4):218–26.
5. Potretzke A, Knight B, Vetter J, Anderson B, Hardi A, Bhayani S, et al. Diagnostic utility of selective upper tract urinary cytology: a systematic review and meta-analysis of the literature. Urology. 2016;96:35–43.
6. Messer J, Shariat S, Brien J, Herman M, Ng C, Scherr D, et al. Urinary cytology has a poor performance for predicting invasive or high-grade upper-tract urothelial carcinoma. BJU Int. 2011;108(5):701–5.
7. Zhang M, VandenBussche C, Hang J, Miki Y, McIntire P, Peyton S, et al. A review of urinary cytology in the setting of upper tract urothelial carcinoma. J Am Soc Cytopathol. 2021;10(1):29–35.
8. Messer J, Terrell J, Herman M, Ng C, Scherr D, Scoll B, et al. Multi-institutional validation of the ability of preoperative hydronephrosis to predict advanced pathologic tumor stage in upper-tract urothelial carcinoma. Urol Oncol. 2013;31(6):904–8.
9. Zhang M, Zhou A, Rosenthal D, VandenBussche C. Urinary tract washing specimens containing atypical urothelial tissue fragments are significantly associated with urothelial neoplasia. Diagn Cytopathol. 2017;45(9):795–9.
10. Razavi SA, et al. Comparative effectiveness of imaging modalities for the diagnosis of upper and lower urinary tract malignancy: a critically appraised topic. Acad Radiol. 2012;19:1134.

11. Jinzaki M, Matsumoto K, Kikuchi E, Sato K, Horiguchi Y, Nishiwaki Y, et al. Comparison of CT urography and excretory urography in the detection and localization of Urothelial carcinoma of the upper urinary tract. Am J Roentgenol. 2011;196(5):1102–9.
12. Lantz EJ, Hattery RR. Diagnostic imaging of urothelial cancer. Urol Clin North Am. 1984;11(4):567–83.
13. Melamed MR, Reuter VE. Pathology and staging of urothelial tumors of the kidney and ureter. Urol Clin N Am. 1993;29:333–47.
14. Girard A, Vila Reyes H, Shaish H, Grellier J, Dercle L, Salaün P, et al. The role of 18F-FDG PET/CT in guiding precision medicine for invasive bladder carcinoma. Front Oncol. 2020;10:565086.
15. Soria F, et al. Epidemiology, diagnosis, preoperative evaluation and prognostic assessment of upper-tract urothelial carcinoma (UTUC). World J Urol. 2017;35:379.
16. Rouprêt M, Babjuk M, Compérat E, Zigeuner R, Sylvester R, Burger M, et al. European Association of Urology guidelines on upper urinary tract Urothelial carcinoma: 2017 update. Eur Urol. 2018;73(1):111–22.
17. Ishikawa S, et al. Impact of diagnostic ureteroscopy on intravesical recurrence and survival in patients with urothelial carcinoma of the upper urinary tract. J Urol. 2010;184:883.
18. Clements T, Messer JC, Terrell JD, et al. High-grade ureteroscopic biopsy is associated with advanced pathology of upper-tract urothelial carcinoma tumors at definitive surgical resection. J Endourol. 2012;26(4):398–402.
19. Breda A, et al. Correlation between confocal laser Endomicroscopy (Cellvizio((R))) and histological grading of upper tract Urothelial carcinoma: a step forward for a better selection of patients suitable for conservative management. Eur Urol Focus. 2018;4:954.
20. Huang A, Low RK. deVere white R. nephrostomy tract tumor seeding following percutaneous manipulation of a ureteral carcinoma. J Urol. 1995;153(3 Pt 2):1041–2.
21. Amin MB, Edge SB, Greene FL, et al., editors. AJCC cancer staging manual. 8th ed. NewYork: Springer; 2017.
22. Moss TJ, et al. Comprehensive genomic characterization of upper tract urothelial carcinoma. Eur Urol. 2017;72:641.

Pathology and Staging

7

Seema Kaushal and Shivangi Dagar

7.1 Introduction

Urothelial carcinoma is the most common cancer of the urothelial tract. Upper urinary tract comprises of the renal pelvis and ureter. Upper tract urothelial carcinomas (UTUC) are uncommon and constitute only 5–10% of urothelial carcinoma [1].

7.2 Epidemiology

An estimated annual incidence of UTUC in Western countries is almost two cases per 100,000 population, while there is paucity of data for Indian population. UTUC is three times more common in men [2]. UTUC in renal pelvis is twice as common as ureteral tumors. Concurrent bladder cancer may be present in 17% of cases [3]. Recurrence is more common in bladder occurring in 22–47% of UTUC patients [4], compared with only 2–6% in the contralateral upper tract [5]. UTUC is an aggressive malignancy, and about two-thirds of cases are invasive at diagnosis. 3–5% of patients are known to develop a metachronous UTUC after having undergone radical cystectomy for muscle-invasive bladder cancer. Familial or hereditary UTUCs are linked to hereditary nonpolyposis colorectal carcinoma (HNPCC) [6]. The Amsterdam criteria are a set of diagnostic criteria used to help identify families that are likely to have Lynch syndrome [7].

7.3 Etiology

Various risk factors have been implicated as causal agents of UTUC, the main ones being tobacco smoking, aristolochic acid, and occupational exposure to carcinogenic aromatic amines including benzidine and b-naphthalene. Specific risk factors include Chinese herb nephropathy and Balkan endemic nephropathy [8]. There can be interindividual susceptibility variations depending on genetic polymorphism and the hosts' ability to counteract the carcinogenic stimuli.

7.4 Macroscopy

Macroscopically, the tumor can be located in renal pelvis or ureter or both. Most of these tumors are papillary. They may be polypoidal, nodular, or even ulcerated. They may invade into renal parenchyma and resemble a primary renal neoplasm.

S. Kaushal (✉) · S. Dagar
Department of Pathology, All India Institute of Medical Sciences, New Delhi, India

P. Singh et al. (eds.), *A Guide to Management of Urological Cancers*,
https://doi.org/10.1007/978-981-99-2341-0_7

7.5 Histopathology

Histologically, epithelial tumors of upper urinary tract resemble bladder urothelial neoplasms and the entire gamut of morphological spectra of bladder tumors can be encountered. Renal pelvis urothelial tumors may occur as papillary [i.e., papillary urothelial neoplasm of low malignant potential, low-grade papillary carcinoma, or high-grade papillary carcinoma], urothelial carcinoma in situ, and invasive urothelial carcinoma (Fig. 7.1).

UTUCs with pure nonurothelial histology are very rare; however, divergent differentiation

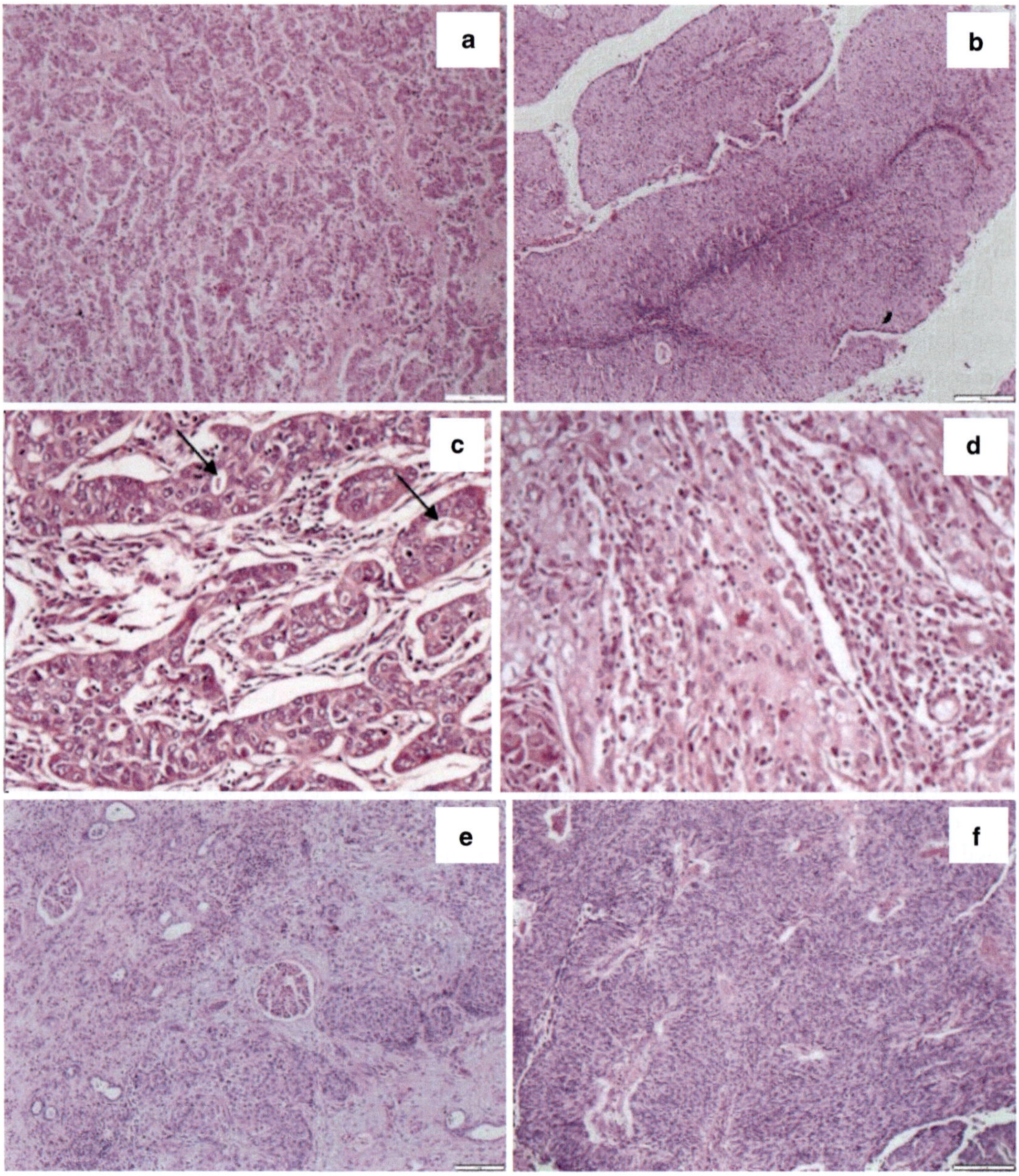

Fig. 7.1 High-grade urothelial carcinoma (**a–e**), conventional histology (**a**), papillary architecture (**b**), glandular differentiation (**c**), squamous differentiation (**d**), infiltrating into renal pelvis (**e**), low-grade urothelial carcinoma (**f**)

[glandular and squamous], unusual morphology (nested, plasmacytoid, microcystic, micropapillary, and clear cell), and poorly differentiated carcinoma (lymphoepithelial like, sarcomatoid, and giant cell) have been reported [9–13].

Any other tumor that can develop in the bladder has been reported in the upper tract, with similar histopathological features.

7.6 Cytology of UTUCs

Diagnostic workup for UTUCs includes cytologic examination of voided urine (VU) or washings (barbotages) obtained from the upper urinary tract. Owing to their higher sensitivity, instrumented and/or selective upper tract specimens (i.e., catheterized, washings/barbotages, and brushings) are superior to VU for the detection of UTUC. A bilateral upper tract cytology is likely to be useful to exclude high-grade urothelial carcinoma (HGUC) of upper tract for patients with serially indeterminate VU specimens and negative cystoscopic findings [14].

The diagnostic criteria defined by The Paris System of Reporting Urinary cytology have been recommended for similar use in both upper and lower urinary tract cytology specimens irrespective of the collection method [15, 16]. One exception is the number of cells required to diagnose high grade urothelial carcinoma (HGUC), which is ≥10 cells meeting the cytomorphological criteria for HGUC in upper tract, while it is ≥5 cells for lower tract.

Presently, the diagnostic utility of cytological examination for upper urinary tract is limited, and the value of performing cell blocks on upper urinary tract specimens is not well defined and requires further investigation.

7.7 Molecular Landscape of UTUCs

7.7.1 Mutational Profile of UTUCs

Our understanding of the distinct molecular alterations present in UTUC and bladder cancer has been broadened and transformed with the advent of next-generation sequencing (NGS) technologies, thus opening new horizons for application of precision oncology to match the therapies to the molecular alterations present in a given tumor to improve clinical outcomes. Testing for the presence of these molecular drivers acts as an adjunct to the classical approach of deciding on cancer treatment based solely on clinicopathological and histological aspects [17].

The current practice of stratifying UTUCs into low and high risk incorporates only the clinical and pathological factors. These clinicopathological factors comprise uni−/multifocal disease, tumor size, low/high-grade cytology or biopsy, and the presence of hydronephrosis or variant histology [18].

However, with the advent of newer molecular techniques in the past few decades, more emphasis is being given to characterize molecular alterations specific to UTUC, which can aid in therapeutically significant stratification of patients so as to provide targeted therapy and aid in clinical decision making.

Recent genomic and gene expression studies have enhanced our understanding of the UTUC biology. UTUC displays different molecular and genetic features as compared to bladder cancer despite their histological similarities [19–21]. TCGA has classified bladder UC into five molecular subtypes: luminal-papillary, luminal-infiltrated, luminal, basal/squamous, and neuronal [22, 23]. However, UTUC was not included in this analysis. In the past few years, several studies have focused on the molecular characterization of UTUC using next-generation sequencing [19, 20, 24–27]. The most frequently mutated genes reported are FGFR3 (40–80%), KMT2D (35–56%), KMT2A (32–47%), and TP53 (18–26%) [19, 20, 24, 28]. Other common mutations involving oncogenes or tumor suppressor genes, such as HRAS, NRAS, KRAS, ARID1A, PIK3CA, and CDKN2A have also been described.

Alteration of TP53/MDM2 has been associated with more aggressive disease and worse outcomes, whereas FGFR3 alterations are linked to a better prognosis [20, 29].

7.7.2 Genetic Predisposition to UTUC

UTUC can occur in the setting of Lynch syndrome due to germline mutations in the DNA mismatch repair (MMR) genes MLH1, MSH2, MSH6, or PMS2 [30–32]. It is particularly associated with MSH2 mutations. An inherited mutation or a sporadic event causes loss of function of MMR system, resulting in microsatellite instability (MSI). The frequency of MSI has been reported to be between 3.9% and 20% in UTUC as compared to <1% in bladder cancer [33, 34].

High MSI is correlated with a better prognosis, particularly in younger patients with non-metastatic disease [35]. Furthermore, high MSI is associated with a higher tumor mutational burden (TMB) and correlated to a higher response rate with immune checkpoint (ICI) treatment [36].

7.7.3 Molecular Subtyping of UTUCs

Due to its rarity, the attempt to subtype UTUC has taken a backseat in comparison to the more prevalent bladder cancer. Until recently, there was very little information available on whether UTUC recapitulates the same molecular subtypes as bladder cancer.

Various studies attempting molecular subtyping of UTUC have almost unanimously concluded luminal-like subtype to be the most common among UTUCs and they are T cell depleted as compared to bladder cancers. Table 7.1 summarizes the recent studies aiming to develop a system for molecular subtyping of UTUC.

A recent study identified two epigenetic subtypes of UTUC based on methylation profiling, namely EpiC-low and EpiC-high. EpiC-low is hypomethylated, immune depleted, and enriched for FGFR3 mutations, the latter are hypermethylated, immune infiltrated, and associated with SWI/SNF genes somatic mutations (Fig. 7.4) [38].

Our knowledge of the molecular pathogenesis of UTUC still remains limited despite several genomic studies of UTUC having been published. More recently, Fujii et al. conducted a comprehensive molecular study of UTUC patients by sequencing of urine sediment-derived DNA and reported five molecular subtypes, namely hypermutated, TP53/MDM2, RAS, FGFR3, and triple negative that correlate with clinicopathological features. Most of the tumors were luminal like, concurring with the findings of previous studies [37].

This promising attempt may pave way to defining clinicopathologically significant molecular subtypes of UTUC as it helps in correlating the DNA-based molecular subtypes with specific clinical outcomes and provides a high-quality resource for future investigation. Each of the sub-

Table 7.1 Summary of recent studies exploring the molecular subtypes of UTUC

Author	Year	Results
Fuiji et al. [37]	2021	Classified UTUC into five subgroups according to alteration status of TP53, MDM2, RAS, and FGFR3 and the presence/absence of hypermutation
		71.5% were luminal-like tumors (Fig. 7.2)
Su et al. [38]	2021	Two epigenetic UTUC subtypes identified based on methylation profiling, namely EpiC-low and EpiC-high (Fig. 7.3)
Robinson et al. [19]	2019	62.5% UTUC are luminal-papillary; majority of others also express luminal profile
Moss et al. [28]	2017	Clustered UTUCs into four molecular subgroups, correlating with clinical and pathological features (Fig. 7.4)
Sanford et al. [39]	2015	UTUCs express genes consistent with luminal subtype

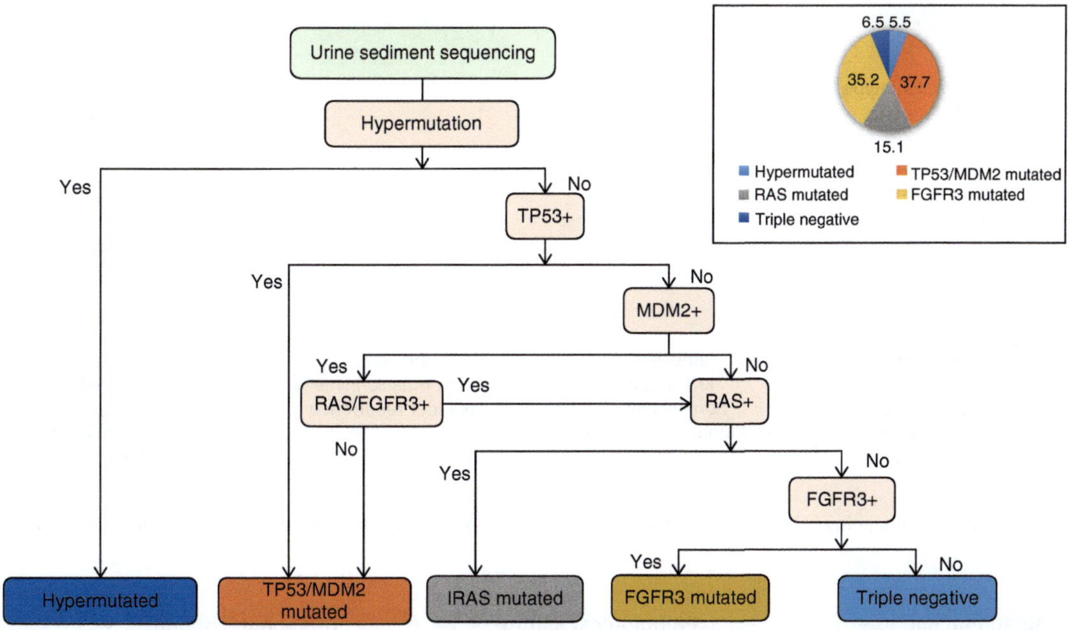

Fig. 7.2 Flow chart showing classification of UTUC into five subgroups according to alteration status of *TP53*, *MDM2*, *RAS*, and *FGFR3* and also to the presence/absence of hypermutation. Adapted from Yoichi Fujii et al. [37]

Fig. 7.3 Proposal of molecular subtypes classification of upper tract urothelial carcinomas. Adapted from Su et al. [38]

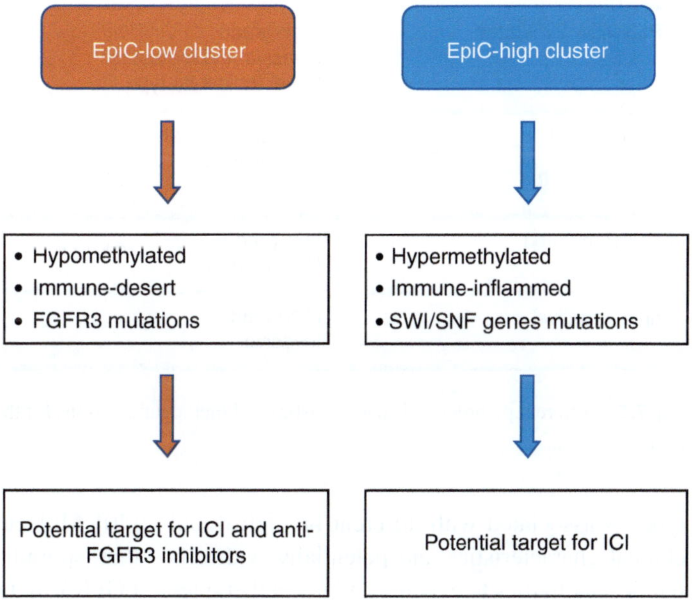

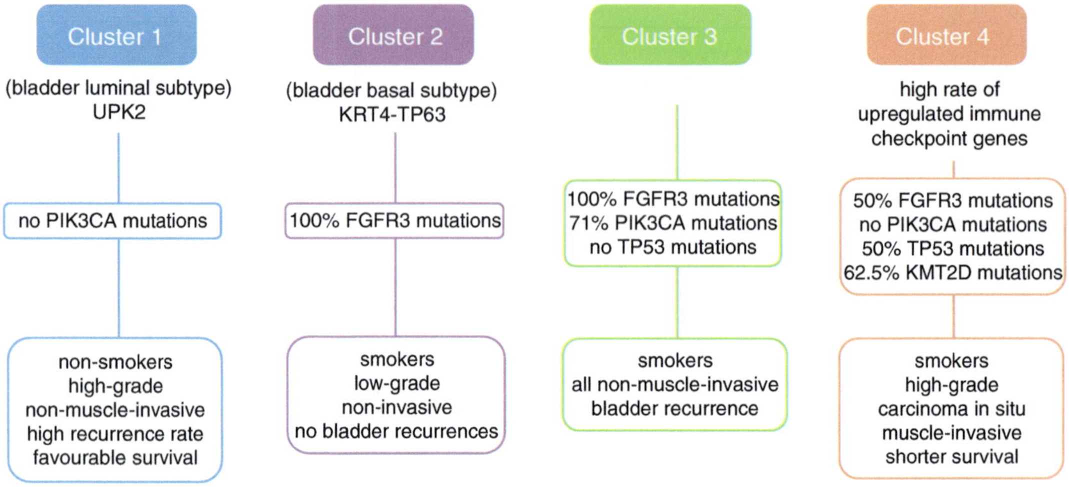

Fig. 7.4 RNA sequencing UTUC molecular subtypes and their correlation with clinical variables. Adapted from Moss et al. [28]

Mutational subtype	Pathological feature	Therapeutic option
Hypermutated	Non-invasive Lynch syndrome	FGFR inhibitors Chemotherapy? Immunotherapy?
TP53/MDM2 mutated	High grade Invasive and metastatic Basal molecular type	Chemotherapy or Immunotherapy
RAS mutated	Exclusively renal pelvis Non-invasive	?
FGFR3 mutated	Low grade Non-invasive	FGFR inhibitors
Triple negative	High grade Invasive	Chemotherapy or Immunotherapy

Fig. 7.5 Different pathological characteristics and therapeutic options for the molecular subtypes defined by Fuiji et al. [37]

types is associated with different biological and clinical characteristics and potentially with different sensitivities to existing and novel therapies as indicated (Figs. 7.2 and 7.5) [37].

7.7.4 Immune Microenvironment of UTUCs

The immune milieu of tumors plays an important role in determining host's antitumoral response [40]. Molecular profiling studies have established that sporadic UTUC displays a high rate of FGFR3 mutations [19, 20, 24, 28]. Also, it has been shown that upper tract tumors with FGFR3 alterations express lower CD8 T-cell gene signatures [19, 41]. Sporadic UTUC with FGFR3 mutations might be considered immune cold tumors, while UTUC developing in a Lynch syndrome setting because of an MMR loss of function could be considered immune hot tumors [42].

Correlations have been observed between PD-L1 positivity on tumoral cells and outcomes in UTUC patients, although PD-L1 expression rate varies between 20 and 25% depending on the cutoff used [43, 44]. PD-L1 can serve as a useful prognostic tool to help select appropriate adjuvant treatment.

7.8 Staging and Grading

TNM staging differs for upper and lower urinary tract urothelial carcinoma. Tables 7.2, 7.3, and 7.4 summarize the definitions of TNM staging for urothelial carcinoma of renal pelvis and ureter as defined by AJCC (American Joint Committee on Cancer), 8th edition.

In urothelial carcinoma, muscularis propria invasion carries particular clinical significance. Urothelial tumors of upper tract are graded same as the urothelial tumors of bladder using the same WHO/ISUP (World Health Organisation/ International Society of Urologic pathologists) system into low grade and high grade [45, 46]. Modern therapy for UTUC encompasses a multimodal approach with surgical, chemotherapeutic, and radiotherapeutic modalities. Treatment options depend on the risk stratification of the patients. Immune checkpoint inhibitors represent a novel-targeted therapeutic option.

Table 7.2 Definition of primary tumor (T)

T category	T criteria
TX	Primary tumor cannot be assessed
T0	No evidence of primary tumor
Ta	Papillary noninvasive carcinoma
Tis	Carcinoma in situ
T1	Tumor invades subepithelial connective tissue
T2	Tumor invades the muscularis
T3	For renal pelvis only: Tumor invades beyond muscularis into peripelvic fat or into the renal parenchyma
	For ureter only: Tumor invades beyond muscularis into periureteric fat
T4	Tumor invades adjacent organs, or through the kidney into the perinephric fat

Table 7.3 Definition of regional lymph nodes (N)

N category	N criteria
NX	Regional lymph nodes cannot be assessed
N0	No regional lymph node metastasis
N1	Metastasis ≤2 cm in greatest dimension, in a single lymph node
N2	Metastasis >2 cm, in a single lymph node; or multiple lymph nodes

Table 7.4 Definition of distant metastasis (M)

M category	M criteria
M0	No distant metastasis
M1	Distant metastasis

7.9 Summary

UTUC represents a rare entity whose clinical and molecular landscape has not fully been explored till date and much of the clinical decision making has been based on data extrapolated from the relatively much common bladder cancer. There has been a growing body of evidence suggesting significant differences between the two, thus necessitating the further characterization of UTUC to optimize precision oncology-based treatment and improve clinical outcomes in patients.

References

1. Siegel RL, et al. Cancer statistics, 2019. CA Cancer J Clin. 2019;69:7.
2. Shariat SF, et al. Gender differences in radical nephroureterectomy for upper tract urothelial carcinoma. World J Urol. 2011;29:481.
3. Cosentino M, et al. Upper urinary tract urothelial cell carcinoma: location as a predictive factor for concomitant bladder carcinoma. World J Urol. 2013;31:141.
4. Xylinas E, et al. Prediction of intravesical recurrence after radical nephroureterectomy: development of a clinical decision-making tool. Eur Urol. 2014;65:650.
5. Li WM, et al. Oncologic outcomes following three different approaches to the distal ureter and bladder cuff in nephroureterectomy for primary upper urinary tract urothelial carcinoma. Eur Urol. 2010;57:963.
6. Roupret M, Yates DR, Comperat E, Cussenot O. Upper urinary tract urothelial cell carcinomas and other urological malignancies involved in the heredi-

tary nonpolyposis colorectal cancer (lynch syndrome) tumor spectrum. Eur Urol. 2008;54:1226–36.
7. Umar A, Boland CR, Terdiman JP, et al. Revised Bethesda guidelines for hereditary nonpolyposis colorectal cancer (Lynch syndrome) and microsatellite instability. J Natl Cancer Inst. 2004;96:261–8.
8. Visser O, Adolfsson J, Rossi S, Verne J, Gatta G, Maffezzini M, Franks KN, RARECARE Working Group. Incidence and survival of rare urogenital cancers in Europe. Eur J Cancer. 2012;48(4):456–64.
9. Gupta R, Paner GP, Amin MB. Neoplasms of the upper urinary tract: a review with focus on urothelial carcinoma of the pelvicalyceal system and aspects related to its diagnosis and reporting. Adv Anat Pathol. 2008;15:127–39.
10. Holmang S, Johansson SL. Urothelial carcinoma of the upper urinary tract: comparison between the WHO/ISUP 1998 consensus classification and WHO 1999 classification system. Urology. 2005;66:274–8.
11. Olgac S, Mazumdar M, Dalbagni G, Reuter VE. Urothelial carcinoma of the renal pelvis: a clinicopathologic sludy of 130 cases. Am J Surg Pathol. 2004;28:1545–52.
12. Perez-Montiel D, Wakely PE, Hes O, Michal M, Suster S. High-grade urothelial carcinoma of the renal pelvis: clinicopathologic study of 108 cases with emphasis on unusual morphologic variants. Mod Pathol. 2006;1(9):494–503.
13. Rink M, Robinson BD, Green DA, Cha EK, Hansen J, et al. Impact of histological variants on clinical outcomes of patients with upper urinary tract urothelial carcinoma. J Urol. 2012;188:393–404.
14. Zhang ML, VandenBussche CJ, Hang J-F, Miki Y, McIntire PJ, Peyton S, Vohra P. A review of urinary cytology in the setting of upper tract urothelial carcinoma. J Am Soc Cytopathol. 2021;10(1):29–35. https://doi.org/10.1016/j.jasc.2020.06.011.
15. VandenBussche CJ, Allison DB, Gupta M, Ali SZ, Rosenthal DL. A 20-year and 46,000-specimen journey to Paris reveals the influence of reporting systems and passive peer feedback on pathologist practice patterns. Cancer Cytopathol. 2018;126:381e389.
16. Cowan ML, VandenBussche CJ. The Paris system for reporting urinary cytology: early review of the literature reveals successes and rare shortcomings. J Am Soc Cytopathol. 2018;7:185e194.
17. Sailer V, Eng KW, Zhang T, et al. Integrative molecular analysis of patients with advanced and metastatic cancer. JCO Precis Oncol. 2019;3:PO.19.00047.
18. Rouprêt M, Babjuk M, Compérat E, et al. European Association of Urology guidelines on upper urinary tract urothelial carcinoma: 2017 update. Eur Urol. 2018;73:111–22.
19. Robinson BD, Vlachostergios P, Bhinder B, Liu W, Li K, Moss TJ, Bareja R, Park K, Tavassoli P, Cyrta J, et al. Upper tract urothelial carcinoma has a luminal-papillary T-cell depleted contexture and activated FGFR3 signaling. Nat Commun. 2019;10:1–11.
20. Audenet F, Isharwal S, Cha EK, Donoghue MTA, Drill EN, Ostrovnaya I, Pietzak EJ, Sfakianos JP, Bagrodia A, Murugan P, et al. Clonal relatedness and mutational differences between upper tract and bladder urothelial carcinoma. Clin Cancer Res. 2018;25:967–76.
21. Atlas NCG. The cancer genome atlas research network comprehensive molecular characterization of urothelial bladder carcinoma. Nature. 2014;507:315–22.
22. Robertson AG, Kim J, Al-Ahmadie H, Bellmunt J, Guo G, Cherniack AD, Hinoue T, Laird PW, Hoadley K, Akbani R, et al. Comprehensive molecular characterization of muscle-invasive bladder cancer. Cell. 2017;171:540–556.e25.
23. Kamoun A, de Reyniès A, Allory Y, Sjödahl G, Robertson AG, Seiler R, Hoadley KA, Groeneveld CS, Al-Ahmadie H, Choi W, et al. A consensus molecular classification of muscle-invasive bladder cancer. Eur Urol. 2019;77:420–33.
24. Sfakianos JP, Cha EK, Iyer G, Scott SN, Zabor EC, Shah R, Ren Q, Bagrodia A, Kim PH, Hakimi AA, et al. Genomic characterization of upper tract urothelial carcinoma. Eur Urol. 2015;68:970–7.
25. Hassler MR, Bray F, Catto JW, Grollman AP, Hartmann A, Margulis V, Matin SF, Roupret M, Sfakianos JP, Shariat SF, et al. Molecular characterization of upper tract urothelial carcinoma in the era of next-generation sequencing: a systematic review of the current literature. Eur Urol. 2020;78:209–20.
26. Hoang ML, Chen C-H, Sidorenko VS, He J, Dickman KG, Yun BH, Moriya M, Niknafs N, Douville C, Karchin R, et al. Mutational signature of aristolochic acid exposure as revealed by whole-exome sequencing. Sci Transl Med. 2013;5:197ra102.
27. Castells X, Karanović S, Ardin M, Tomić K, Xylinas E, Durand G, Villar S, Forey N, Le Calvez-Kelm F, Voegele C, et al. Low-coverage exome sequencing screen in formalin-fixed paraffin-embedded tumors reveals evidence of exposure to carcinogenic aristolochic acid. Cancer Epidemiol Biomark Prev. 2015;24:1873–81.
28. Moss TJ, Qi Y, Xi L, Peng B, Kim T-B, Ezzedine NE, Mosqueda ME, Guo CC, Czerniak BA, Ittmann M, et al. Comprehensive genomic characterization of upper tract urothelial carcinoma. Eur Urol. 2017;72:641–9.
29. Bagrodia A, Audenet F, Pietzak EJ, Kim K, Murray KS, Cha EK, Sfakianos JP, Iyer G, Singla N, Arcila M, et al. Genomic profile of urothelial carcinoma of the upper tract from ureteroscopic biopsy: feasibility and validation using matched radical nephroureterectomy specimens. Eur Urol Focus. 2019;5(3):365–8.
30. Engel C, Loeffler M, Steinke V, Rahner N, Holinski-Feder E, Dietmaier W, Schackert HK, Goergens H, Doeberitz MVK, Goecke TO, et al. Risks of less common cancers in proven mutation carriers with lynch syndrome. J Clin Oncol. 2012;30:4409–15.
31. Van Der Post RS, Kiemeney L, Ligtenberg MJL, Witjes JA, De Kaa CAH-V, Bodmer D, Schaap L, Kets CM, Van Krieken JHJM, Hoogerbrugge N. Risk of urothelial bladder cancer in Lynch syndrome is increased, in particular among MSH2 mutation carriers. J Med Genet. 2010;47:464–70.

32. Watson P, Vasen H, Mecklin J-P, Bernstein I, Aarnio M, Järvinen HJ, Myrhøj T, Sunde L, Wijnen JT, Lynch HT. The risk of extra-colonic, extra-endometrial cancer in the lynch syndrome. Int J Cancer. 2008;123:444–9.
33. Rao A, McGrath JE, Xiu J, de Souza AL, Gulati S, Abuali I, Sagaram S, Nabhan C, Korn WM, Ryan CJ, et al. Characterization of microsatellite instability (dMMR/MSI-H) and mutational landscape in a large contemporary cohort of upper tract urothelial cancer (UTUC) patients. J Clin Oncol. 2021;39:465.
34. Bonneville R, Krook MA, Kautto E, Miya J, Wing MR, Chen H-Z, Reeser JW, Yu L, Roychowdhury S. Landscape of microsatellite instability across 39 cancer types. JCO Precis Oncol. 2017;1:1–15.
35. Rouprêt M, Fromont G, Azzouzi A-R, Catto JW, Vallancien G, Hamdy FC, Cussenot O. Microsatellite instability as predictor of survival in patients with invasive upper urinary tract transitional cell carcinoma. Urology. 2005;65:1233–7.
36. Luchini C, Bibeau F, Ligtenberg M, Singh N, Nottegar A, Bosse T, Miller R, Riaz N, Douillard J-Y, Andre F, et al. ESMO recommendations on microsatellite instability testing for immunotherapy in cancer, and its relationship with PD-1/PD-L1 expression and tumour mutational burden: a systematic review-based approach. Ann Oncol. 2019;30:1232–43.
37. Fujii Y, Sato Y, Suzuki H, Kakiuchi N, Yoshizato T, Lenis AT, Maekawa S, Yokoyama A, Takeuchi Y, Inoue Y, Ochi Y. Molecular classification and diagnostics of upper urinary tract urothelial carcinoma. Cancer Cell. 2021;39(6):793–809.
38. Su X, Lu X, Bazai SK, Compérat E, Mouawad R, Yao H, Rouprêt M, Spano J-P, Khayat D, Davidson I, et al. Comprehensive integrative profiling of upper tract urothelial carcinomas. Genome Biol. 2021;22:1–25.
39. Sanford T, Porten S, Meng MV. Molecular analysis of upper tract and bladder urothelial carcinoma: results from a microarray comparison. PLoS One. 2015;10:e0137141.
40. Wellenstein MD, De Visser KE. Cancer-cell-intrinsic mechanisms shaping the tumor immune landscape. Immunity. 2018;48:399–416.
41. Wang L, Gong Y, Saci A, Szabo PM, Martini A, Necchi A, Siefker-Radtke A, Pal S, Plimack ER, Sfakianos JP, et al. Fibroblast growth factor receptor 3 alterations and response to PD-1/PD-L1 blockade in patients with metastatic urothelial cancer. Eur Urol. 2019;76:599–603.
42. Donahue TF, Bagrodia A, Audenet F, Donoghue MT, Cha EK, Sfakianos JP, Sperling D, Al-Ahmadie H, Clendenning M, Rosty C, et al. Genomic characterization of upper-tract urothelial carcinoma in patients with lynch syndrome. JCO Precis Oncol. 2018;2018:1–13.
43. Chen C-H, Tsai M-Y, Chiang P-C, Sung M-T, Luo H-L, Suen J-L, Tsai E-M, Chiang P-H. Prognostic value of PD-L1 combined positive score in patients with upper tract urothelial carcinoma. Cancer Immunol Immunother. 2021;70:1–10.
44. Lu Y, Kang J, Luo Z, Song Y, Tian J, Li Z, Wang X, Liu L, Yang Y, Liu X. The prevalence and prognostic role of PD-L1 in upper tract urothelial carcinoma patients underwent radical nephroureterectomy: a systematic review and meta-analysis. Front Oncol. 2020;10:1400.
45. Epstein JI, Amin MB, Reuter VR, Mostofi FK, Bladder Consensus Conference Committee. The World Health Organization/International Society of Urological Pathology consensus classification of urothelial (transitional cell) neoplasms of the urinary bladder. Am J Surg Pathol. 1998;22:1435–48.
46. Genega EM, Kapali M, Torres-Quinones M, Huang WC, Knauss JS, Wang LP, et al. Impact of the 1998 World Health Organization/International Society of Urological Pathology classification system for urothelial neoplasms of the kidney. Mod Pathol. 2005;18:11–8.

8 Management

Rahul Jena and Gautam Ram Choudhary

8.1 Introduction

The entire urinary tract, including the proximal urethra, the bladder, the ureters and the pelvicalyceal system (PCS), is lined by transitional cell epithelium also called the urothelium. Urothelial carcinomas are the most common malignant neoplasms arising from this epithelium and urothelial cancers of the bladder are the tenth most common form of cancer in the world and the sixth most common cancer in developed countries [1, 2]. However, upper tract urothelial carcinomas (UTUC), i.e., tumours involving the ureters and the PCS of the kidneys are relatively rare, although their detection rates are increasing with a better understanding of the follow-up of bladder cancer and also increased survival [3]. In the following sections, we will give an overview of the epidemiology, risk factors, histopathology, diagnosis and staging of UTUCs. This shall be followed by contemporary evidence-based recommendations on the management of UTUCs, including neoadjuvant or adjuvant therapies, surgical treatment and follow-up. We will also attempt to provide a brief summary of the recent advances in targeted therapy for UTUCs.

R. Jena · G. R. Choudhary (✉)
Department of Urology, All India Institute of Medical Sciences, Jodhpur, Rajasthan, India
e-mail: jenar@aiimsjodhpur.edu.in; choudharygr@aiimsjodhpur.edu.in

8.2 Epidemiology

Upper tract urothelial carcinomas comprise 5–10% of all urothelial carcinomas [1]. They are more common in men between the ages of 70 and 90 years with the highest geographical concentration observed in the northern European region of Balkan [4]. African Americans develop UTUCs twice more often than Caucasians. Up to 5% of UTUCs can have bilateral renal involvement and tumours involving the PCS are twice as common as ureteral tumours, with 10–20% of the cases having multifocal tumours [5]. Concurrent carcinoma in situ (CIS) is present in 11–36% of cases and concurrent bladder cancer in 17% [5, 6]. Prior history of bladder cancer varies with race, being 41% in American men and 4% in Asian Chinese men [7]. Reports of metachronous UTUC after treatment for bladder cancer vary from 7.5 to 25% for non-muscle invasive bladder cancer patients undergoing BCG therapy and 3–5% in patients who have undergone radical cystectomy for muscle invasive disease [8–10]. After treatment of ipsilateral UTUC, recurrences involve the bladder occurs in 22–47% of the cases and the contralateral upper tract in 2–4% of the cases [11, 12]. Most of these upper tract recurrence involve the PCS. Up to 60% of UTUCs are invasive at diagnosis and 7% metastatic at presentation [13].

P. Singh et al. (eds.), *A Guide to Management of Urological Cancers*,
https://doi.org/10.1007/978-981-99-2341-0_8

8.3 Risk Factors

- ***Genetic factors:*** The familial form of UTUC (10–20% of the cases) is linked to hereditary nonpolyposis colorectal carcinoma (HNPCC) also called Lynch syndrome [14]. Patients with this condition have mutations in the DNA mismatch repair genes MLH1, MSH2, MSH6 and PMS2 and have a higher likelihood of developing colonic, ovarian, sebaceous, gastric, pancreatic, uterine and UTUCs. Patients with UTUC and HNPCC are generally younger than 60 years and have a greater female preponderance than sporadic tumours. The Amsterdam criteria should be used to identify patients with Lynch syndrome [15]. The European association of Urology guidelines recommend that any person aged less than 65 years with UTUC should be probed about personal history of any other HNPCC spectrum cancer or presence of first-degree relative with HNPCC-related cancer at less than 50 years of age or any two first-degree relatives with history of HNPCC-related cancer at any age [16]. If any of the above factors is present, then the individual should undergo genetic testing for the above-mentioned mutations along with evaluation and follow-up for other HNPCC-related cancers and familial genetic counselling.
- ***Tobacco use:*** Cigarette smoking is the single most important modifiable risk factor for UTUC. Routine tobacco use increases the relative risk of UTUC from 2.5 to 7 [17, 18]. This risk also depends on the number of cigarettes consumed daily. Genetic polymorphisms in the enzymes that neutralize the aromatic amines present in cigarette smoke reflect the susceptibility to carcinogenesis. Smoking cessation leads to a decrease in the relative risk with a risk reduction of 60–70% at 10 years. Interestingly, the ureter is at greater risk of carcinogenesis compared to the PCS in this subpopulation [19].
- ***Aristocholic acid nephropathy:*** Aristocholic acid is found in the plants *Aristolochia fangchi* and *Aristolochia clematitis*, which grow as weed in the wheat fields of the Balkan countries and possibly contaminate the food source [20]. Exposure to this compound leads to development of Balkan endemic nephropathy (BEN). The characteristic of this nephropathy is proximal tubular dysfunction with a dense glomerular fibrosis [21]. Metabolites of aristocholic acid cause mutations in the TP53 gene. The UTUCs that develop in this form of nephropathy has an incidence almost 50–100 times more compared to the rest of the world and has a strong predisposition for early age at diagnosis, higher stage at presentation, presence of bilateral disease and lack of gender predominance. A similar geographic clustering of such UTUCs is seen in Taiwan where there is a high incidence of traditional herbal medicine containing aristocholic acid [22].
- ***Occupational factors:*** Workers with exposure to aromatic amines in dye, petroleum, textiles, rubber, plastics and chemical industries have a higher relative risk of developing UTUC [23].
- ***Analgesic abuse:*** Patients with pelvic and ureteral tumours have been reported to have a history of analgesic abuse in 22% and 11% of the cases, respectively [23].
- ***Arsenic:*** Arsenic has been postulated to be a risk factor for UTUC in Taiwan due to contamination of drinking water, but a definite association has not been proven [24].
- ***Miscellaneous factors:*** The use of coffee, tea and yerba mate has been postulated to lead to an increased incidence of UTUC. Chronic irritation with stones has also been found to be associated with development of UTUC.

8.4 Pathology

The ureter and the renal pelvis are derived from the mesoderm in contrast to the bladder, which is endodermal in origin. However, the urothelium lining these structures is the same as the one lining the bladder. An important thing to note here is the fact that the ureter and the renal pelvis have a relatively thinner muscle layer beneath the otherwise abundant urothelium compared to the bladder. Theoretically, this can lead to faster spread of any malignant process outside the organ. The benign lesions of the upper tract include von Brunn's nests, papillomas and inverted papillomas. The malignant potential of these lesions is truly unknown and some series have demonstrated that upto 18% go on to develop metachronous UTUCs [25]. Therefore, surveillance for at least 2 years after diagnosis is recommended [26]. A gradual progression from dysplasia to hyperplasia to CIS is observed in a large number of cases of UTUC, and the presence of CIS and urothelial dysplasia should be viewed as markers of worse prognosis [27].

Urothelial carcinomas comprise more than 90% of upper tract urothelial tumours. These lesions could be flat, papillary or sessile and may be unifocal or multifocal. The propensity of muscle invasion is higher in the upper ureter and renal pelvic compared to the lower ureter and often there is significant associated CIS. Up to 25% of all UTUCs show variant histological differentiation in the form of squamous cell, micropapillary, glandular, sarcomatoid, neuroendocrine and lymphoepithelioid morphology [28]. While these variant histologies are usually thought to be associated with aggressive disease, it is the micropapillary variant, which is associated with advanced stage at presentation in most cases and inferior cancer specific and progression-free survival [29].

Non urothelial malignant tumours of the upper tract are usually very rare and comprise mainly of pure squamous cell carcinoma and adenocarcinoma of the renal pelvis [30]. These tumours are usually at an advanced stage at presentation and are associated with dismal outcomes.

8.5 Diagnosis

8.5.1 Clinical Features

Gross or microscopic hematuria is the most common symptom of UTUC, occurring in 56–98% of cases [31, 32]. Flank pain is the next most common symptom seen in 20–30% of patients. Flank pain may be dull aching and gradual in onset when associated with obstructed system and hydronephrosis. Acute pain of the flank is usually associated with clot colic and maybe present in 10–40% of the cases [33]. Approximately 10% of the patients may have a flank lump palpable [33]. About 15% of the patients are asymptomatic at presentation and are incidentally diagnosed on radiology. Anorexia, weight loss and bone pains are usually associated with advanced disease and should prompt an evaluation for metastatic disease. There are reports of patients presenting with renoalimentary fistula also [34]. UTUC is a rare finding at autopsy.

8.5.2 Radiological Imaging

Contrast-enhanced computed tomography (CECT) with CT urography (CTU) is the cross-sectional imaging of choice for evaluation of UTUC with a sensitivity and specificity of 92% and 95%, respectively [35, 36]. Multiplanar acquisitions and 3D reconstruction of thin slices make it easy to delineate even small filling defects inside the ureter. Flat lesions are relatively more difficult to pick up on CECT. The typical appearance of an UTUC may range from a large locally advanced mass in the kidney (Fig. 8.1a), a hydronephrotic and obstructed kidney showing enhancing solid masses inside the PCS (Fig. 8.1b) to small polypoidal lesions inside the PCS and ureter, which may appear as filling defects on urography sequences (Fig. 8.1c). Differential diagnosis of filling defects includes blood clot, stones, overlying bowel gas, external compression, sloughed papilla and fungus ball. Urothelial cancers have an average density of 46 Hounsfield units (HU) and range between 10 and 70 HU. The average density of a radiolucent uric acid stone is 100 HU with a range of 80 to 250 HU. Measurements of the HUs in a CT could be useful in differentiating two common causes of radiolucent filling defects on excretory or retrograde urography. UTUC has also been reported to mimic xanthogranulomatous pyelonephritis on CECT [37]. Magnetic res-

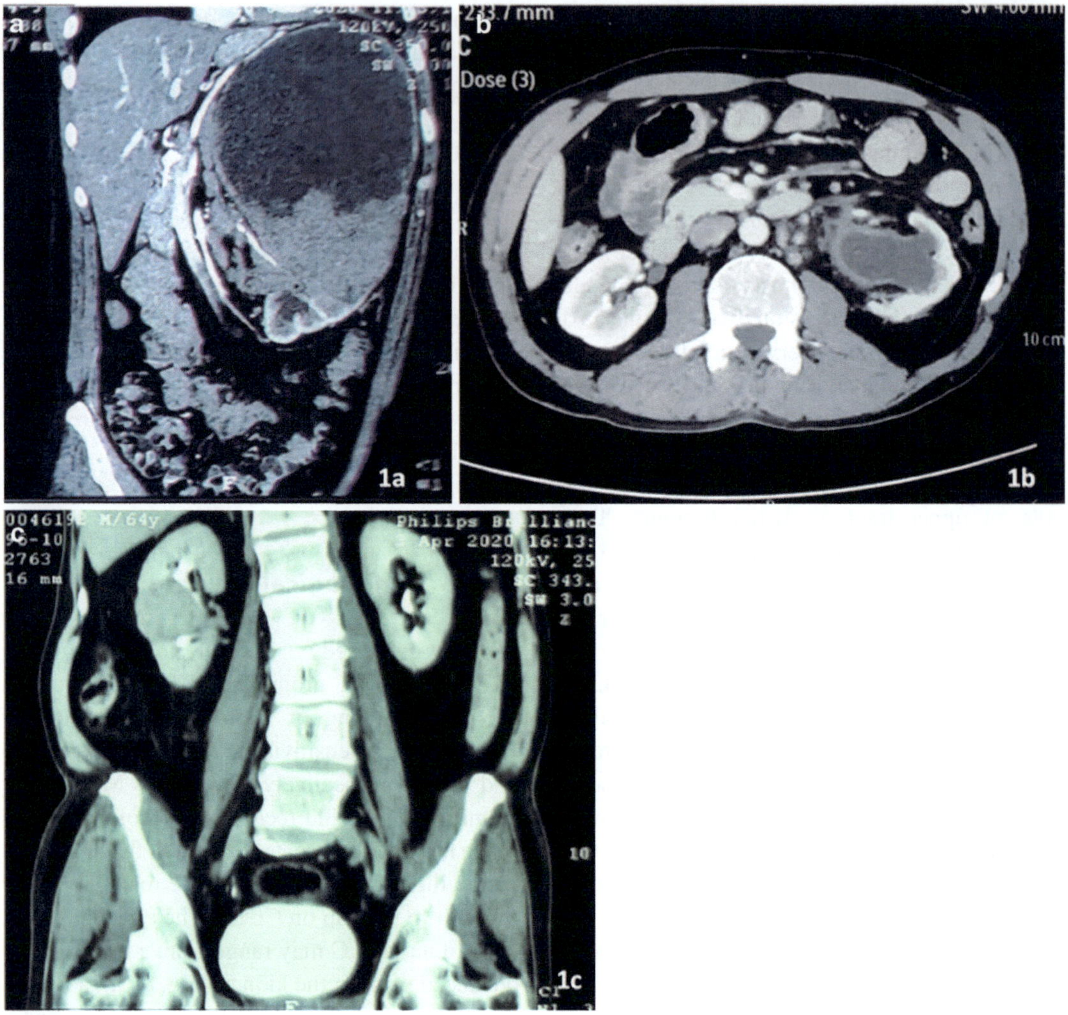

Fig. 8.1 (**a**) Large locally advanced TCC of the left kidney. Patient did not have any hematuria and presented only with complaints of lethargy and weight loss. (**b**) Hydronephrotic obstructed kidney showing thickening of the renal pelvis on the left side. Patient was a smoker and had presented with history of gross total painless hematuria of 1 month duration. (**c**) Poorly enhancing midpolar mass presenting as a filling defect and causing splaying of the calyces on urography phase of the right kidney. Patient had presented with gross total painless hematuria of 15 days duration

onance (MR) urography is indicated in patients to whom the radiation or iodinated contrast media are contraindicated and cannot undergo CT urography [38]. Cross sectional either by CT or MR has the added advantage of evaluating the contralateral kidney and also the whole abdomen for evidence of metastatic disease. Both the EAU and the NCCN guidelines also recommend chest imaging by either chest X-ray or CT scan in select patients [16, 39].

8.5.3 Cytological Evaluation

Abnormal cytology in the absence of bladder findings may point towards high-grade UTUC. The sensitivity of voided urine sample in detecting UTUC remains low, in fact lower than the sensitivity for bladder tumours [40]. Hence, it is recommended that cytology be done of the ureteral washings obtained via ureteric catheter or during diagnostic ureterorenoscopy [41]. The sensitivity of fluorescence in situ hybridisation (FISH) for molecular abnormalities characteristic of UTUCs is approximately 50% and therefore its use in clinical practice remains unproven [42, 43].

8.5.4 Endoscopic Evaluation of the Bladder and Upper Tracts

Urethrocystoscopy is a mandatory part of evaluation of UTUC to tule out concomitant bladder cancer. Flexible ureterorenoscopy (URS) can be used to visualise the ureter and the pelvicalyceal system and can reliably detect the presence, size and appearance of the tumour. Tumour grade can also be reliably detected in combination with ureteroscopic biopsies [44]. Under grading may occur and thus intensive follow-up is necessary if kidney-sparing treatment is chosen [45]. In addition, ureteroscopy also helps in sampling of ureteral urine and in brush biopsies. Flexible ureteroscopy in combination with techniques like narrow band imaging, confocal laser endomicroscopy (Cellvizio) and optical coherence tomography have shown promising results in the detection of flat epithelial lesions also [46–49]. A combination of ureteroscopic biopsy, cross-sectional imaging findings like hydronephrosis and findings of urine cytology help in the decision-making process of whether to do a radical surgery or go for kidney-sparing surgery [50, 51]. Whether diagnostic URS increases the chances of intravesical recurrence after radical nephroureterectomy is still controversial, and the EAU guidelines and the NCCN guidelines recommend that diagnostic URS and biopsy be done whenever imaging and cytology findings are not sufficient for the diagnosis and/or risk stratification and staging of the tumour [16, 39].

8.6 Staging, Prognosis and Risk Stratification

UTUC is classified the same way as bladder cancer. The 2004/2016 WHO classification divides non-invasive carcinomas into papillary urothelial neoplasms of low malignant potential and high- and low-grade papillary urothelial carcinomas in addition to CIS and invasive carcinomas [52, 53]. The TNM classification system is the most commonly used to stage UTUC (Table 8.1) [54]. The regional lymph nodes (LNs) for pelvic and upper ureteral tumours are the hilar and retroperitoneal LNs and pelvic LNs for mid and distal ureteral tumours. The laterality of the LNs does not affect N classification. Almost 70% of the ureteral tumours are in the distal ureter, 25% in the mid ureter and 5% in the upper ureter [55]. Synchronous or metachronous bilateral disease has an incidence of 1.6–6.0% of the cases [56]. Patients with ureteral or multifocal tumours have a worse prognosis than renal pelvic tumours [57, 58]. Upper tract recurrence after bladder cancer has an incidence of 2–6% [59]. The estimated risk of recurrence in the bladder after treatment of UTUC varies from 15 to 75% within 5 years [56]. There are several theories for this including downstream seeding, longer exposure time to carcinogens in the bladder and greater number of urothelial cells in the bladder that are subject to

Table 8.1 TNM classification of upper tract urothelial carcinoma

T—Primary tumour	
Tx	Primary tumour cannot be assessed
T0	No evidence of primary tumour
Ta	Non-invasive papillary carcinoma
Tis	Carcinoma in situ
T1	Tumour invades subepithelial connective tissue
T2	Tumour invades muscularis
T3	(Renal pelvis) tumour invades beyond muscularis into peripelvic fat or renal parenchyma
	(Ureter) tumour invades beyond muscularis propria into periureteric fat
T4	Tumour invades adjacent organs or through kidney into perinephric fat
N—Regional lymph nodes	
Nx	Regional lymph nodes cannot be assessed
N0	No regional lymph node metastasis
N1	Metastasis in a single lymph node 2 cm in diameter or less in the greatest dimension
N2	Metastasis in a single lymph node more than 2 cm or multiple lymph nodes
M—Distant metastasis	
M0	No distant metastasis
M1	Distant metastasis.

random carcinogenic events. The most widely accepted theory is the downstream seeding, which is further supported by the fact that the bladder tumour recurrences after UTUC are monoclonal and occur at the site of previous bladder trauma due to ureterectomy. Predictors of bladder recurrence include patient-specific factors: male gender, previous bladder cancer, smoking and preoperative chronic kidney disease; tumour-specific factors: positive preoperative urinary cytology, ureteral location, multifocality, invasive pT stage and necrosis; treatment-specific factors: laparoscopic approach, extravesical bladder cuff removal and positive surgical margins [60, 61].The presence of CIS increases the incidence of multifocality and panurothelial disease. UTUCs have significant metastatic potential. Non-organ confined disease is the most significant predictor followed by vascular and lymphatic invasion [13]. In addition to the distant spread, UTUC also demonstrates epithelial spread, probably as a result of the "field change" effect of the urothelium and leads to the development of pan urothelial disease [62].

The prognostic factors for UTUC can be patient-related factors and tumour-related factors. Patient-related factors include

8.6.1 Age and Gender

An older age is an independent risk factor for decreased cancer-specific survival [63]. However, age is not a contraindication to treatment [64]. Gender has no effect on prognosis [63].

8.6.2 Race

African Americans have worse prognosis compared to other population groups.

8.6.3 Tobacco Use

Tobacco use is an independent predictor of poor prognosis. It increases the risk of recurrence, mortality and also recurrence within the bladder after treatment [17, 18].

8.6.4 Surgical Delay

A delay of greater than 12 weeks since diagnosis confers a worse prognosis [65].

8.6.5 Other Factors

A higher American Society of Anaesthesiologists score, poor performance status, higher BMI, high neutrophil–lymphocyte ratio, low albumin, higher fibrinogen levels, elevated liver enzymes, altered renal function and higher C-reactive protein levels before treatment confer a worse prognosis [16].

Tumour-related factors that confer a worse prognosis included higher stage, higher grade, presence of carcinoma is in situ, distal ureteric tumours, lymph node involvement and extranodal extension, presence of lymphovascular invasion, extensive tumour necrosis, positive surgical margins and presence of variant histology (Table 8.2) [63]. Based on the above factors, the European Association of Urology (EAU) guidelines have divided UTUC into high-risk or low-risk tumours (Table 8.3) [16]. A low-risk UTUC must have all of the following features: unifocal disease, tumour size less than

Table 8.2 Prognostic factors for UTUC

Pre-operative factors	Post-operative factors
• Multifocality	• Stage
• Grade (biopsy, cytology)	• Grade
• Advanced age	• Carcinoma in situ
• Tobacco consumption	• Distal ureter management
• ECOG PS 1	• Lymphovascular invasion
• ASA score	• Lymph node involvement
• Systemic symptoms	• Tumour architecture
• Hydronephrosis	• Positive surgical margins
• Delay in surgery >3 months	• Variant histology
• Tumour location	
• BMI > 30	
• Neutrophil to lymphocyte ratio	

Table 8.3 Risk stratification of non-metastatic UTUC

Low risk (all factors need to be present)	High risk (any one of the factors to be present)
• Unifocal disease	• Multifocal disease
• Tumour size <2 cm	• Tumour size >2 cm
• Negative for high-grade cytology	• High-grade cytology
• Low-grade URS biopsy	• High-grade URS biopsy
• No invasive aspect on CT	• Local invasion on CT scan
	• Hydronephrosis
	• Previous radical cystectomy for high grade cancer
	• Variant histology

2 cm, low-grade cytology, low-grade URS biopsy and non-invasive features on CT urography. However, to be classified a high-risk UTUC, the tumour needs to have only one of the following features: presence of hydronephrosis, size greater than 2 cm, high-grade cytology, high-grade URS biopsy, history of previous radical cystectomy, presence of multifocal disease or variant histology.

8.7 Management of Localised UTUC: Kidney-Sparing Surgery

Historically, the gold standard treatment for UTUC has been radical nephroureterectomy (RNU) with bladder cuff excision with regional lymph node dissection. The risk stratification system proposed by EAU guidelines helps to choose patients suitable for kidney-sparing surgery. For patients with low-risk UTUC, this significantly reduces the morbidity associated with radical surgery while providing similar oncological outcomes and survival as RNU [66]. Kidney-sparing surgery may be considered in certain high-risk patients also after weighing the risks of cancer control with risks of renal deterioration, especially in patients with solitary kidneys, bilateral tumours, severe renal insufficiency and those who are poor surgical candidates. Kidney-sparing surgery can be broadly divided into endoscopic management and open/minimally invasive techniques.

8.7.1 Endourological Techniques

The basic steps involve access to the tumour by ureteroscopy and/or pyeloscopy. Now access can be obtained by either retrograde route or antegrade route. Small diameter rigid and flexible ureteroscopes have made location and size of the tumour less of an issue. But broadly speaking, for low-volume ureteral and sometimes renal tumours, a retrograde ureteroscopy is preferred and for larger tumours of the kidney or upper ureter or difficult locations like in the lower calyx, an antegrade percutaneous access if preferred. In patients with previous urinary diversions also, antegrade approach is preferred. A combined antegrade and retrograde approach may be considered in select patients. Similar to endoscopic management of bladder tumours, the goal is to resect the urothelial tumour completely and obtain adequate tissue for histopathological examination of grade and stage. Staged resection may be tried for certain cases of high-volume disease when there are doubts that the tumour may be high grade or that the patient may ultimately require a RNU. In such cases, the goal is only to obtain biopsies.

8.7.1.1 Ureteroscopy

This avoids the need for a percutaneous puncture of the kidney thus maintaining a closed channel and preventing potential exposure of non-urothelial surfaces by malignant cells. The disadvantage is that smaller instruments limit the field of vision and often limit the ability to completely ablate a tumour or obtain tissue for grading and accurate staging. Access to the lower and middle ureter may be readily obtained using rigid ureteroscopes, while upper ureteric and pyelocaliceal masses necessitate the use of a flexible ureteroscope (Fig. 8.2). Usually, modern ureteroscopes do not require pre-procedural ureteric dilatation for adequate access. The use of a

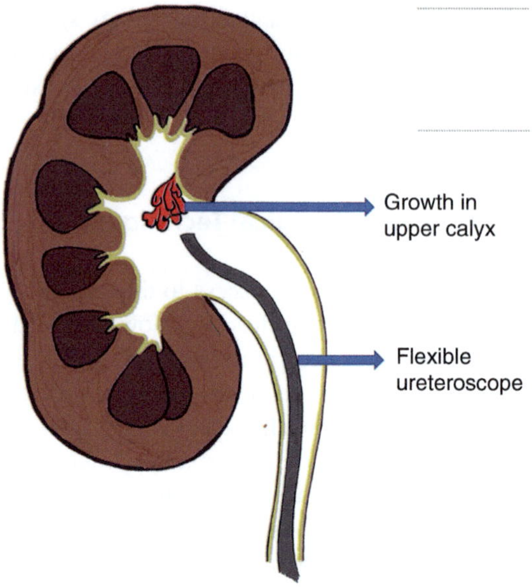

Fig. 8.2 Flexible ureteroscopy to resect tumour located in pelvis and upper calyx

ureteral access sheath is optional. In the following lines, we have described our technique of doing an ureteroscopic ablation of an UTUC of the renal pelvis/upper ureter. We start by doing a thorough cystoscopic examination with the patient under general anaesthesia. Both ureteric orifices are visualized, and a 0.035 inch nitinol guidewire with hydrophilic coating is passed into the ureteric orifice and coiled in the PCS under fluoroscopic guidance. Then a rigid ureteroscope is used to inspect the intramural, lower and middle ureters. Then we removed the rigid ureteroscope and introduce a ureteral access sheath over the guidewire under fluoroscopic guidance and insert a 7.5 Fr flexible ureteroscope after removing the guidewire. The ureteral access sheath helps by creating a low-pressure system and also allows for repeated and faster access to the ureter. As soon as the tumour is visualised, we take washings of the area with normal saline and send the collected fluid for cytology. Then the tumour is sampled or removed completely using flexible ureteroscopic biopsy forceps. Sometimes nitinol baskets are used to remove pedunculated tumours. Base of the tumour is then fulgurated using Holmium YAG laser at low energy and frequency settings. Sometimes a pedunculated tumour is removed completely by resecting the base with a laser fibre. A 6 Fr double J stent is placed in the ureter. The retrieved specimens are sent for histologic examination.

The advantages of using a laser are that the relative safety and less chances of ureteric perforation due to the low depth of penetration of energy [25]. Other described techniques include use of an ureteric resectoscope using a Bugbee electrode and Nd:YAG laser [67]. There are no randomized controlled trials between ureteroscopic management and RNU, and most of the available literature is from case series [68, 69]. Cutress et al. reported overall recurrence rate of 53% for the upper tracts and 34% for the bladder, with a progression rate of 15% following ureteroscopic management for UTUC [68]. The recurrence rates and disease-free survival rates were worse for higher grade tumours. Daneshmand et al. reported an overall ipsilateral recurrence rate of 90% [70]. Therefore, every patient undergoing ureteroscopic management should be strictly counselled about the need for early second-look ureteroscopy and lifelong surveillance and follow-up, the need for subsequent RNU and the distinct possibility of tumour progression [71, 72]. Accuracy of ureteroscopic biopsies and limitations of the number of biopsies are two major concerns of the ureteroscopic approach. However, multiple reports have shown that the accuracy of ureteroscopic biopsy in matching the pathological grade after open surgery ranges from 70 to 92% [45]. This supports the notion that in UTUC, grade is the most important prognostic factor and although there may be some limitations in assessment of stage, lower grade tumours usually have non-invasive disease. There have also been concerns about seeding of the tumour to other urothelial surfaces after ureteroscopy. However, this has not been reliably demonstrated across multiple reports.

8.7.1.2 Percutaneous Access and Antegrade Ureterorenoscopy

This modality can be offered for patients with low-risk UTUCs of the renal pelvis, which are too large to be dealt with by flexible ureteros-

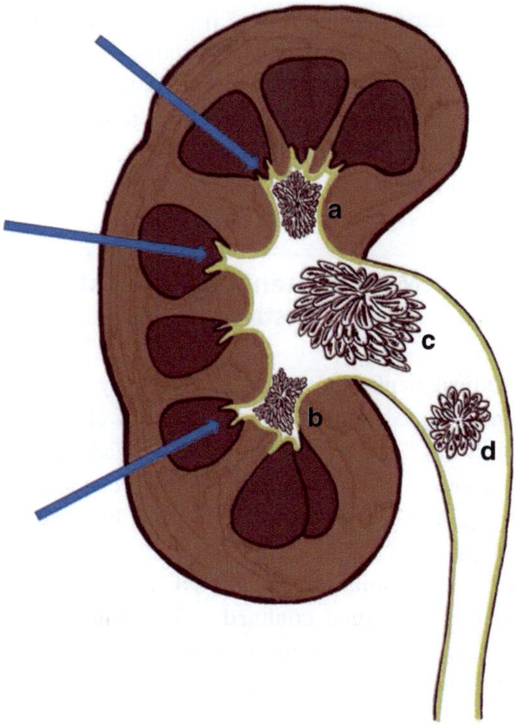

Fig. 8.3 Each tumour location needs a specific and precise puncture of the peripheral calyx. Tumours located in the upper and lower calyx (**a, b**) can be approached through puncture of the upper and lower calyces. Dealing with pelvic (**c**) and upper ureteric (**d**) tumours requires a middle or upper calyceal puncture

copy or for tumours of the lower calyx (Fig. 8.3) [68]. While the EAU recommends against using endoscopic means for tumours larger than 1 cm, there are multiple reports of successful nephroscopic treatment of larger tumours [68]. Another proposed advantage of nephroscopic approach is the ability to do topical chemotherapeutic agent instillation into the pelvicalyceal system and repeated nephroscopies through the sane tract. Disadvantages include potential tumour seeding outside the urinary tract by exposing non-urothelial surfaces to tumour cells [73]. Creating a nephrostomy tract also carries along with it the inherent risks of puncturing the kidney such as bleeding and complications of resection like systemic absorption of hypo-osmotic irrigating fluid and secondary ureteropelvic junction obstruction. Similar to ureteroscopic management, there are no randomised trials comparing this modality to radical nephroureterectomy. But literature review has shown that disease progression after nephroscopic management occurred in 17% with 6% progressing to metastases [68]. In all published reports comparing results of various modalities, low-grade tumours did well irrespective of modality used. Hence, we can assume that percutaneous management of UTUC can be offered to patients with low-grade disease amenable to resection by endoscopic means irrespective of the status of the contralateral kidney.

8.7.1.3 Upper Tract Instillation of Topical Chemotherapeutic Agents

Over the years, there have been multiple studies evaluating topical instillation of chemotherapeutic agents like mitomycin C, thiotepa and gemcitabine into the upper tracts after kidney-sparing management of UTUC. BCG has also been evaluated in the treatment of carcinoma in situ (CIS) of the upper tracts [74, 75]. Both antegrade instillation through a nephrostomy tract, retrograde instillation using reflux due to a double J stent and direct instillation through an open-ended single J stet has been used. Retrograde methods are unreliable, and the delivery of drugs to the upper tracts is suboptimal. Most of the studies on this topic are retrospective in nature with small sample sizes and therefore the quality of evidence supporting their use is poor. A meta-analysis of these studies assessing upper tract instillation of topical chemotherapeutic agents in low-grade Ta/T1 UTUC and BCG instillation in CIS after kidney-sparing surgery found no difference in the oncological outcomes in terms of recurrence and survival rates between the treated group and those reported in literature in untreated patients [76]. The OLYMPUS trial was a single-arm Phase III RCT, which showed that the use of mitomycin-containing reverse thermal gel (Jelmyto™, formerly called Mitogel) in the form of retrograde instillations as the first treatment of biopsy proven low-grade UTUC less than 15 mm, was associated with a complete response rate of 59% [77]. This compound stays in the upper tract in a gel form and gradually dissolves in urine providing higher concentrations of mitomycin to the urothelial surfaces compared to single-time instillations. On the basis of this evidence, Jelmyto™ has recently been FDA approved as a first-line treatment for small, biopsy proven Ta/T1 low-grade UTUC. The most frequently reported adverse effects were ureteric stenosis (44%), urinary tract infections (32%), hematuria (31%) and flank pain (30%).

8.7.2 Open/Minimally Invasive Techniques

For all practical purposes, segmental ureterectomy denotes distal ureterectomy and ureteroneocystostomy done for low-grade tumours of the distal ureters not amenable to endoscopic management or for high-grade tumours of the distal ureters in solitary kidneys where preservation of the functioning renal unit is necessary. Segmental resection of the ureters with ureteroureterostomy or ileal ureteric replacement in case of long segment ureteral excision can also be done for tumours of the proximal and mid ureters which cannot be managed endoscopically and the affected renal unit needs to be preserved.

8.7.2.1 Distal Ureterectomy with Ureteroneocystostomy

Most cases can be done by laparoscopic or robotic platforms. The patients are placed in Trendelenburg position after in-field catheterisation of the bladder. Ureter is mobilised up to the ureterovesical junction. Proximal ureter is cut above the level of the tumour and distally cuff of bladder is also excised. The various techniques of getting an appropriate cuff of bladder will be described in subsequent sections. Cystotomy on the posterior bladder wall is closed in 2 layers using absorbable sutures. Ureter is mobilised so that the cut end reaches the bladder in a tension-free manner. Ureteric reimplant is done on the bladder using Lisch Gregoir technique if non-refluxing reimplant is planned. If continued endoscopic surveillance of the upper tract is anticipated, a refluxing anastomosis may provide easier access in the future. If a long segment of the distal ureter has been excised, a psoas hitch may be done to bridge a gap of upto 5 cm. For longer defects, it may be necessary to do a Boari flap ureteroneocystostomy for an additional 10–15 cm of length.

8.8 Management of High-Risk Non-Metastatic UTUC

Radical nephroureterectomy either by open or endoscopic means is the treatment of choice for high-risk non-metastatic UTUC. Bladder cuff excision is an essential part of this procedure, and a regional lymphadenectomy should be done for all patients. The EAU recommends against performing minimally invasive RNU for any tumour that is not organ confined (T3/T4 and/or N+) because such patients have worse oncological outcomes when compared with open surgery. In the only surgical randomized controlled trial comparing laparoscopic and open extirpative surgery, Simone et al. showed no difference in metastasis-free and cancer-specific survival in patients with organ-confined disease [78]. However, in this study, patients with high-grade disease or at least pT3 stage benefited from open nephroureterectomy. UTUC is an aggressive tumour, and there are reports of retroperitoneal metastatic dissemination and seeding of trocar tracts during manipulation while doing minimally invasive surgeries [79, 80]. Precautions to minimise tumour spillage have been enumerated below:

- Avoid entering the urinary tract
- Avoid direct contact between the tumour and the instruments
- Perform the procedure in a closed system, avoid use of a morcellator and extract specimen in an Endobag
- Remove the kidney and ureter en bloc along with the bladder cuff

For organ confined disease, laparoscopic RNU has equivalent oncological outcomes compared to open RNU [81, 82]. Recent data also shows that robot-assisted laparoscopic approach has similar oncological outcomes as other modalities for organ-confined disease [83].

8.8.1 Technique of Radical Nephroureterectomy

Open radical nephroureterectomy can be done with the patient in either supine or modified flank position with exposure through an either subcostal, midline or thoraco-abdominal incision depending upon the patient's body habitus, size of the mass, need for a lymphadenectomy and the surgeon's preference. If a midline incision is not used, then removal of the bladder cuff necessitates a separate Gibson's or Pfannenstiel incision for bladder cuff removal. The nephrectomy part of the procedure is done the same way as an open radical nephrectomy, and the difference being that the ureter is not divided and is mobilised distally up to the ureterovesical junction. Also, the adrenal gland, unless directly involved by the tumour, is typically spared. Laparoscopic radical nephroureterectomy is done in modified flank position. The patient is fixed to the table so that he/she can be placed in supine position after completion of the nephrectomy part to complete the bladder cuff excision either through an open surgical incision or laparoscopically by placing other ports. Alternately the entire procedure can be completed laparoscopically without changing the patient's position or placing more ports in the modified flank position depending upon the patient's body habitus and the surgeon's expertise and comfort. Robot-assisted laparoscopic radical nephroureterectomy is being increasingly used for dealing with UTUC. Post positions have to be modified depending upon the robotic platform available.

8.8.2 Management of the Distal Ureter and Bladder Cuff

Complete resection of the intramural ureter along with a cuff of the bladder is of paramount importance in achieving superior oncological outcomes because of the significant rate of recurrence in the ureteric stump following RNU [84]. Non-definitive management of the ureteral end and bladder cuff also translates into inferior disease specific and overall survival [85]. There are at least five described techniques of dealing with the bladder cuff, although none of the techniques have been found to be superior to complete bladder cuff excision [86].

8.8.2.1 Open Distal Ureterectomy and Bladder Cuff Excision

This can be done by either extravesical, transvesical or combined approach using either a Gibson's or Pfannenstiel incision. Uncontrolled entry into the urinary tract is to be avoided at all times. Dissection should be carried out to the level of the intramural ureter in case of extravesical approach and the lateral vascular pedicles of the bladder may need to be divided to get adequate access to that part of the ureter. Taking care to stay away from the contralateral ureteric orifice, a cuff of bladder is removed en bloc with the ureter by applying a clamp to the bladder wall. Alternately, using the transvesical approach, intravesical dissection of the ureter is done including a 1 cm mucosal cuff around the orifice through an anterior cystotomy. In case of a protruding tumour at the orifice, a wider margin should be taken and sometimes even a partial cystectomy may be done to ensure negative margins. Cystotomy defects are closed in two layers, with the first layer closing the mucosa and the second layer including the detrusor and the adventitia. A Foley catheter is placed and maintained for 5 to 7 days, and a suction drain is left in the perivesical space.

8.8.2.2 Transvesical Ligation and Detachement

Two trocars are placed into the bladder after filling the bladder cystoscopically. An Endoloop is positioned around the ureteral orifice and a ureteral catheter is passed into the orifice. The orifice is retracted into the bladder using instruments passed through the trocar and the bladder cuff around the ureter is incised using a Collins knife. The Endoloop is cinched around the ureter after the cuff has been freed from all sides closing off the distal open end of the ureter. Then the patient is repositioned for nephrectomy part of the procedure. This technique should not be applied in patients with distal ureteral tumours, bladder disease and prior pelvic irradiation.

8.8.2.3 Transurethral Resection of the Ureteric Orifice

This is also known as the "pluck" technique. The ureteric orifice and the surrounding bladder mucosa are aggressively resected cystoscopically up to the level of the preivesical fat so that the distal ureteral end can be "plucked" off the bladder during the nephrectomy part of the procedure. This process has been mostly abandoned due to risk of tumour seeding extravesically.

8.8.2.4 Intussusception or "Stripping" Technique

This technique is associated with high failure rates of up to 18.7% and is contraindicated in the presence of ureteral tumours [87]. A ureteral catheter is placed first and then the nephrectomy is done. The distal ureter is secured to the intraluminal catheter by placing a circumferential tie around it from the abdominal side. On completion of the nephrectomy the ureter is transected between ties, and the bladder cuff is incised cystoscopically using a Collins knife. Pulling on the ureteral catheter everts the distal ureter inside the bladder. The intussuscepted ureter is then removed by traction out of the urethra.

8.8.2.5 Total Laparoscopic Technique

This technique utilises an endovascular stapler to harvest a cuff of the bladder. Alternately experienced laparoscopic surgeons can replicate the steps of open ureterectomy and bladder cuff excision laparoscopically. The concerns with this technique include the potential for leaving ureter mucosa within the staple line and inability for the pathologist to evaluate the distal margin because of the presence of staples. Laparoscopic stapling has been associated with a higher risk of positive margins, which in this disease is associated with significantly reduced survival [88]. Contraindications include the presence of distal ureteral tumours.

8.8.3 Lymph Node Dissection

Regional template-based lymphadenectomy should accompany all cases of radical nephroureterectomy in the treatment of UTUC [89]. Following a fixed template is more important than harvesting, an absolute number of lymph nodes as it improves cancer-specific survival and reduces the risk of local recurrence even in clinically and pathologically node-negative disease [90, 91]. Even for patients with low-risk UTUC, schedule for lymphadenectomy, a template-based lymph node dissection should be offered because preoperative staging is often inaccurate [16]. The templates followed for regional lymph node dissection in left- and right-sided UTUC are depicted in Fig. 8.4. A right-sided template dissection for UTUC is shown in Fig. 8.5.

8.8.4 Use of Perioperative Chemotherapy in Management of High-Risk UTUC

The use of cisplatin-based chemotherapy, both in the neoadjuvant and adjuvant settings, has been explored in the management of high-risk UTUC. Though most of this data was from retrospective series or small samples, it showed promising rates of pathological downstaging and complete response rates. Because UTUC is a rare disease, good-quality prospective data has not been available until now, to guide the use of cisplatin-based chemotherapy in either the adjuvant or neoadjuvant setting as a standard of care. The rationale behind advocating neoadjuvant chemotherapy is that the high rates of decreased renal function present intrinsically in patients of UTUC, result in postoperative renal deterioration and ultimately makes the patients ineligible to receive full-dose cisplatin-based chemotherapy.

8.8.4.1 Neoadjuvant Chemotherapy

A retrospective study on 150 patients with high-risk UTUC, who were treated with a variety of cisplatin-based regimens prior to undergoing RNU, showed a significant incidence of pathological downstaging of tumours and a 14% complete response rate [92]. A survival update

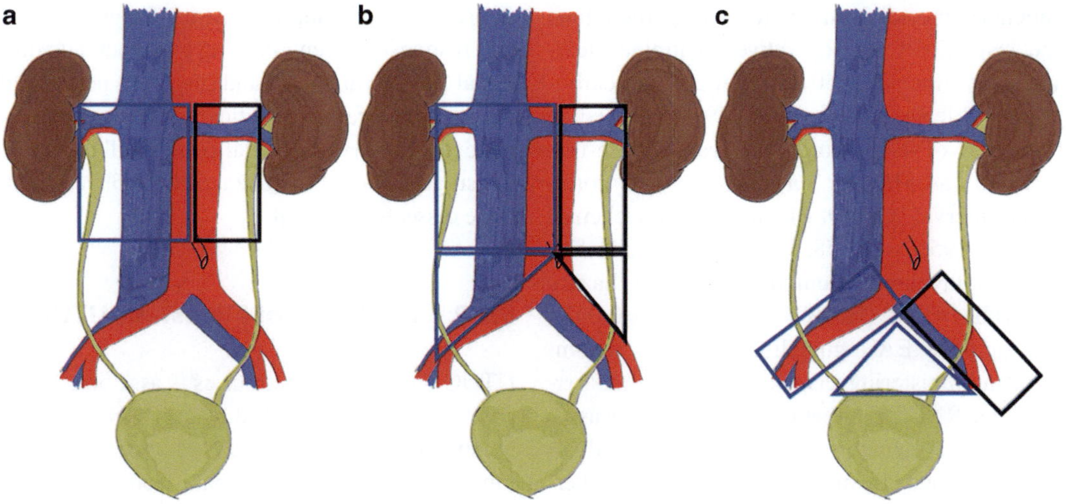

Fig. 8.4 (**a**) In addition to ipsilateral hilar nodes, the extended lymphadenectomy template for tumors of the renal pelvis includes paracaval, retrocaval, and interaortocaval lymph nodes for right-sided and para-aortic lymph nodes for left-sided tumours. The inferior mesenteric artery marks the inferior boundary of the template. (**b**) For tumours of the upper two-thirds of the ureter, this template is extended to the level of bifurcation of aorta. (**c**) The extended lymphadenectomy template for tumours in the distal ureter includes ipsilateral common, external and internal iliac, obturator and presacral nodes

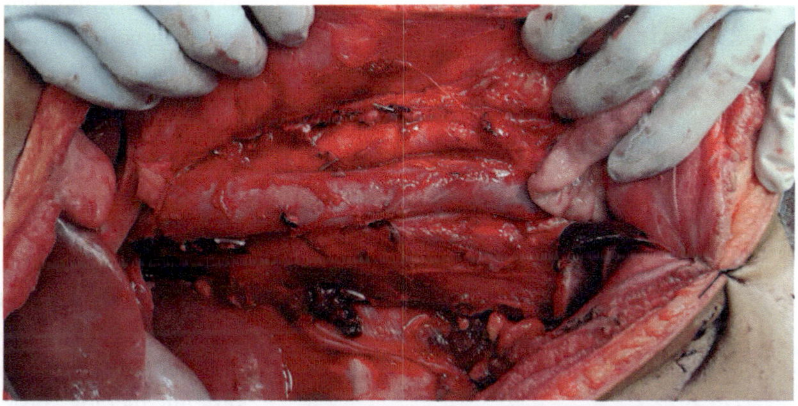

Fig. 8.5 Right-sided extended template dissection for UTUC showing removal of the paracaval, pre and retrocaval and inter-aortocaval lymph nodes

of these patients showed significant improvement in 5-year survival in those receiving neoadjuvant chemotherapy versus a matched historical cohort (94% vs. 58%, $p < 0.001$). The EA8141trial was the first prospective phase II trial which examined the use of cisplatin- and carboplatin-based chemotherapy in patients of high-risk UTUC, stratified as per their glomerular filtration rate [93]. This study met its predefined end points of 14% complete response and 60% downstaging to less than pT1N0 and thus confirms the efficacy of neoadjuvant chemotherapy in UTUC, especially in those patients expected to have renal deterioration after surgery. Based on this study, it is reasonable to consider neoadjuvant chemotherapy as the standard of care in patients of high-risk UTUC who are anticipated to have a creatinine clearance less than 50 postoperatively.

8.8.4.2 Adjuvant Chemotherapy

The phase III randomized controlled trial on Peri-Operative Chemotherapy Versus Surveillance in Upper Tract Urothelial Cancer (POUT) randomized patients having undergone nephroureterectomy with high risk of recurrence (pT2-4N0-3M0) to adjuvant chemotherapy (n = 125) versus surveillance (n = 123) [94].

Patients in the adjuvant arm received gemcitabine and cisplatin if post-operative creatinine clearance was more than 50 and gemcitabine carboplatin if clearance was 30 to 49. At a median follow-up of 17.6 months, 2-year disease-free survival was 51% for surveillance (95% confidence interval [CI] 39, 61) and 70% for chemotherapy (95% CI 58, 79). Progression-free survival favoured chemotherapy, with hazard ratio (HR) = 0.49 (95% CI 0.30, 0.79, $p = 0.003$). The updated EAU guidelines of 2021 recommend administering cisplatin-based chemotherapy after RNU in all patients of muscle-invasive UTUC. A systematic review and meta-analysis comparing neoadjuvant and adjuvant chemotherapy in high UTUC concluded that while both neoadjuvant and adjuvant chemotherapy were both beneficial compared to RNU alone, the level of evidence available for adjuvant chemotherapy was stronger compared to neoadjuvant therapy (positive Level I evidence versus Level II evidence at best) [95].

8.8.4.3 Postoperative Bladder Instillation of Single-Agent Chemotherapy

The rate of bladder recurrence after RNU, which ranges from 22 to 47%, can be decreased by a single-dose postoperative administration of mitomycin C within 2–10 days of surgery [96]. This benefit may even extend to patients undergoing kidney sparing surgery, but the evidence is still unexamined.

8.9 Management of Lymph Node Positive and Metastatic UTUC

8.9.1 Treatment of UTUC with Positive Regional Lymph Nodes without Distant Metastasis

Treatment of this stage of UTUC is similar to that of urothelial carcinoma of the bladder. When there is evidence of regional lymph node metastases, chemotherapy with cisplatin should be offered as a first-line treatment. If a good/maximal response is seen after 4 cycles, then an additional 2 cycles are given and surgery is performed only when there is a significant decrease or complete resolution of the nodal size. Needless to say, the surgery should include a full template lymph node dissection as well.

8.9.2 Treatment of Metastatic UTUC

UTUC with distant metastases is associated with poor overall survival. The role of RNU in such patients is limited to palliative surgery in symptomatic patients, although data from few observational studies show that there may be a survival benefit especially in patients fit to receive cisplatin-based chemotherapy and in those with only one distant metastatic site [97, 98]. These studies may have been subject to bias and no definite recommendation can be made based on these studies. Similarly, metastasectomy should be approached with caution although there are several reports documenting its benefit in terms of OS, especially in patients with a life expectancy of over 6 months [99]. This decision should be a shared decision and should be made on a case-to-case basis.

8.9.3 Systemic Therapy for Metastatic UTUC

The mainstay of treatment of metastatic UTUC is systemic therapy. Systemic therapy is either with platinum compound-based regimens or immunotherapy.

8.9.3.1 First-Line Setting

The MVAC regimen is associated with the highest response rates, even though complete and durable response beyond 12–24 months is rare and the toxicity is high. Dose dense MVAC wherein, all drugs are given at the same time with cell support has been shown to have lower toxicity and may show better response rates [100]. Carboplatin may be substituted for cisplatin in patients with decreased renal reserve, but response rates are inferior and so are survival rates [101]. A combination of gemcitabine, taxol and doxorubicin has been tried in certain patients and an improvement in renal function has been observed after a few weeks allowing these patients to switch to cisplatin-based regimens, but this needs to be investigated further [102]. Immunomodulation using immune checkpoint inhibitors appears to have the higher response rates in tumours showing high levels of microsatellite instability such as UTUCs. Most of the data on the use of immune checkpoint regulators is from trials on metastatic UTUCs in which majority of the patients have bladder cancer. Data from a phase III RCT showed that the use of avelumab maintenance therapy given after stable or good response after 4 to 6 cycles of gemcitabine plus cisplatin or carboplatin significantly prolonged OS as compared to best supportive care alone in those patients with advanced or metastatic urothelial carcinoma [103]. Atezolizumab was associated with an objective response rate of 39% in cisplatin-ineligible patients with metastatic UTUC (n = 119) [104]. Median OS in the overall cohort was 15.9 months and toxicity was acceptable. In a phase III RCT of 1213 patients with metastatic urothelial carcinoma, with 312 (26%) UTUC patients, the combination of atezolizumab with platinum-based chemotherapy was associated with limited PFS benefit as compared to platinum-based chemotherapy alone, and no significant impact was observed on OS. In a phase II trial (n = 370), pembrolizumab was associated with an objective response rate of 22% in cisplatin-ineligible patients with metastatic UTUC [105]. PD-L1 expression of 10% was associated with a greater response rate to pembrolizumab. In a phase III RCT of 351 patients with metastatic urothelial carcinoma, addition of pembrolizumab to platinum-based chemotherapy did not reach statistical significance for PFS and OS benefits as compared to platinum-based chemotherapy alone [106]. Another negative phase III RCT showed that durvalumab alone, or in combination with tremelimumab, did not prolong OS as compared to platinum-based chemotherapy for metastatic urothelial carcinoma but suggested that durvalumab alone may have better efficacy for these individuals as compared to those with bladder cancer [107]. Several trials are currently testing immunotherapy combinations with nivolumab (NCT03036098), pembrolizumab (NCT02178722) or durvalumab (NCT03682068) in patients with metastatic UC, including those with UTUC. Based on the above data, the EAU recommends offering pembrolizumab or atezolizumab as first-line therapy in cisplatin-ineligible patients depending on their PD L1 status [16]. If PD L1 status is negative, carboplatin is recommended as combination therapy.

8.9.3.2 Second-Line Setting

The treatment of metastatic UTUC progressing after first line systemic therapy remains challenging. Based on phase II trials, atezolizumab and nivolumab have been approved for use in patients progressing after first-line treatment with cisplatin-based regimens. Pembrolizumab has also been approved for this indication based on a phase III trial [108]. In a post-hoc subgroup analysis of locally advanced or metastatic UC, vinflunine was reported to be as effective in UTUC as for bladder cancer progressing after cisplatin-based chemotherapy. Erdafitinib, a tyrosine kinase inhibitor of FGFR1–4, showed a 43% response rate in patients of UTUC with visceral metastases who had progressed on first-line cisplatin-based therapy. Other drugs like durvalumab, avelumab and combination of nivolumab and ipilimumab need further studies. At present, the EAU recommends therapy with pembrolizumab, nivolumab or atezolizumab to patients progressing during or after cisplatin-based therapy. Vinflunine is to be offered as second-line treatment is immunotherapy or combination therapy is not feasible, and it can also be used as a third line or subsequent treatment [109].

8.10 Follow-Up

The follow-up of patients with UTUC post treatment has to be stringent to detect metachronous bladder tumours, distant and local recurrences. Bladder recurrence is not considered a distant recurrence. Cystoscopy, urine cytological exami-

Table 8.4 Recommendations for follow-up after treatment of UTUC

After radical nephroureterectomy	Low-risk tumours	Perform cystoscopy at 3 months. If negative, perform subsequent cystoscopy 9 months later and then yearly, for 5 years.
	High-risk tumours	Perform cystoscopy and urinary cytology at 3 months. If negative, repeat subsequent cystoscopy and cytology every 3 months for a period of 2 years, and every 6 months thereafter until 5 years, and then yearly.
		Perform computed tomography (CT) urography and chest CT every 6 months for 2 years, and then yearly.
After kidney-sparing surgery	Low-risk tumours	Perform cystoscopy and CT urography at 3 and 6 months and then yearly for 5 years.
		Perform ureteroscopy (URS) at 3 months.
	High-risk tumours	Perform cystoscopy, urinary cytology, CT urography and chest CT at 3 and 6 months, and then yearly.
		Perform URS and urinary cytology in situ at 3 and 6 months.

nation and cross-sectional imaging for the contralateral kidney form the mainstay of diagnostic modalities used in follow-up. It is important to note than follow-up should be more stringent after kidney-sparing surgery than after RNU. The follow-up recommendations have been adapted from the EAU guidelines and have been outlined in Table 8.4.

8.11 Points to Remember

- UTUC is a rare and aggressive disease with a tendency towards multifocality and repeated recurrences throughout the urothelium lined surfaces.
- Risk stratification of the UTUC and a risk-based approach towards treatment is of paramount importance to safeguard the renal reserve and proper oncological control.
- Low-risk UTUC should be offered kidney-sparing surgery whenever possible.
- High-risk UTUC should under RNU with bladder cuff excision.
- Adjuvant cisplatin-based chemotherapy and neoadjuvant cisplatin-based therapy, especially in those with anticipated fall in renal function postoperatively, have been associated with higher OS and cancer-specific survival.
- First-line and second-line treatment of metastatic UTUC is a challenging task and cisplatin-based therapy and immunotherapy with PD-1 and PD L-1 inhibitors are recommended.

References

1. Siegel RL, Miller KD, Fuchs HE, Jemal A. Cancer statistics, 2021. CA Cancer J Clin. 2021;71(1):7–33. https://doi.org/10.3322/caac.21654. Erratum in: CA Cancer J Clin. 2021 Jul;71(4):359.
2. Babjuk M, Burger M, Capoun O, Cohen D, Compérat EM, Escrig JL, Gontero P, Liedberg F, Masson-Lecomte A, Mostafid AH, Palou J. European association of urology guidelines on non–muscle-invasive bladder cancer (Ta, T1, and carcinoma in situ). Eur Urol. 2022;81(1):75–94.
3. Siegel R, Naishadham D, Jemal A. Global cancer statistics. CA Cancer J Clin. 2013;63(1):11–30.
4. Grollman AP. Aristolochic acid nephropathy: harbinger of a global iatrogenic disease. Environ Mol Mutagen. 2013;54(1):1–7.
5. Soria F, Moschini M, Haitel A, Wirth GJ, Karam JA, Wood CG, Rouprêt M, Margulis V, Karakiewicz PI, Briganti A, Raman JD. HER2 overexpression is associated with worse outcomes in patients with upper tract urothelial carcinoma (UTUC). World J Urol. 2017;35(2):251–9.
6. Cosentino M, Palou J, Gaya JM, Breda A, Rodriguez-Faba O, Villavicencio-Mavrich H. Upper urinary tract urothelial cell carcinoma: location as a predictive factor for concomitant bladder carcinoma. World J Urol. 2013;31(1):141–5.
7. Singla N, Fang D, Su X, Bao Z, Cao Z, Jafri SM, Xiong G, Zhang L, Hutchinson R, Sagalowsky A, Lotan Y. A multi-institutional comparison of clinicopathological characteristics and oncologic outcomes of upper tract urothelial carcinoma in China and the United States. J Urol. 2017;197(5):1208–13.
8. Nishiyama N, Hotta H, Takahashi A, Yanase M, Itoh N, Tachiki H, Miyao N, Matsukawa M, Kunishima Y, Taguchi K, Kitamura H. Upper tract urothelial carcinoma following intravesical bacillus Calmette-Guérin therapy for nonmuscle-invasive bladder cancer: results from a multi-institutional retrospective study. Urol Oncol. 2018;36(6):306–e9.

9. Sanderson KM, Rouprêt M. Upper urinary tract tumour after radical cystectomy for transitional cell carcinoma of the bladder: an update on the risk factors, surveillance regimens and treatments. BJU Int. 2007;100(1):11–6.
10. Ayyathurai R, Soloway MS. Monitoring of the upper urinary tract in patients with bladder cancer. Indian J Urol. 2011;27(2):238.
11. Xylinas E, Rink M, Margulis V, Karakiewicz P, Novara G, Shariat SF. Multifocal carcinoma in situ of the upper tract is associated with high risk of bladder cancer recurrence. Eur Urol. 2012;61(5):1069–70.
12. Li WM, Shen JT, Li CC, Ke HL, Wei YC, Wu WJ, Chou YH, Huang CH. Oncologic outcomes following three different approaches to the distal ureter and bladder cuff in nephroureterectomy for primary upper urinary tract urothelial carcinoma. Eur Urol. 2010;57(6):963–9.
13. Margulis V, Shariat SF, Matin SF, Kamat AM, Zigeuner R, Kikuchi E, Lotan Y, Weizer A, Raman JD, Wood CG. Upper tract Urothelial carcinoma collaboration. Outcomes of radical nephroureterectomy: a series from the upper tract Urothelial carcinoma collaboration. Cancer. 2009;115(6):1224–33.
14. Rouprêt M, Yates DR, Comperat E, Cussenot O. Upper urinary tract urothelial cell carcinomas and other urological malignancies involved in the hereditary nonpolyposis colorectal cancer (lynch syndrome) tumor spectrum. Eur Urol. 2008;54(6):1226–36.
15. Umar A, Boland CR, Terdiman JP, Syngal S, Chapelle AD, Rüschoff J, Fishel R, Lindor NM, Burgart LJ, Hamelin R, Hamilton SR. Revised Bethesda guidelines for hereditary nonpolyposis colorectal cancer (Lynch syndrome) and microsatellite instability. J Natl Cancer Inst. 2004;96(4):261–8.
16. EAU 2021 guidelines. https://uroweb.org/guidelines/upper-urinary-tract-urothelial-cell-carcinoma.
17. Dickman KG, Fritsche HM, Grollman AP, Thalmann GN, Catto J. Epidemiology and risk factors for upper urinary urothelial cancers. In: Xylinas E, Shariat SF, editors. Upper tract urothelial carcinoma. New York: Springer; 2015. p. 1–30.
18. Crivelli JJ, Xylinas E, Kluth LA, Rieken M, Rink M, Shariat SF. Effect of smoking on outcomes of urothelial carcinoma: a systematic review of the literature. Eur Urol. 2014;65(4):742–54.
19. McLaughlin JK, Silverman DT, Hsing AW, Ross RK, Schoenberg JB, Mimi CY, Stemhagen A, Lynch CF, Blot WJ, Fraumeni JF. Cigarette smoking and cancers of the renal pelvis and ureter. Cancer Res. 1992;52(2):254–7.
20. Jelaković B, Karanović S, Vuković-Lela I, Miller F, Edwards KL, Nikolić J, Tomić K, Slade N, Brdar B, Turesky RJ, Stipančić Ž. Aristolactam-DNA adducts are a biomarker of environmental exposure to aristolochic acid. Kidney Int. 2012;81(6):559–67.
21. Rosenquist TA, Grollman AP. Mutational signature of aristolochic acid: clue to the recognition of a global disease. DNA Repair. 2016;44:205–11.
22. Chen CH, Dickman KG, Moriya M, Zavadil J, Sidorenko VS, Edwards KL, Gnatenko DV, Wu L, Turesky RJ, Wu XR, Pu YS. Aristolochic acid-associated urothelial cancer in Taiwan. Proc Natl Acad Sci. 2012;109(21):8241–6.
23. Colin P, Koenig P, Ouzzane A, Berthon N, Villers A, Biserte J, Rouprêt M. Environmental factors involved in carcinogenesis of urothelial cell carcinomas of the upper urinary tract. BJU Int. 2009;104(10):1436–40.
24. Chen CJ, Chiou HY. Health hazards of environmental arsenic poisoning: from epidemic to pandemic. Singapore: World Scientific; 2011.
25. Matsuoka K, Lida S, Tomiyasu K, Inoue M, Noda S. Transurethral endoscopic treatment of upper urinary tract tumors using a holmium: YAG laser. Lasers Surg Med. 2003;32(5):336–40.
26. Asano K, Miki JU, Maeda S, Naruoka T, Takahashi H, Oishi Y. Clinical studies on inverted papilloma of the urinary tract: report of 48 cases and review of the literature. J Urol. 2003;170(4):1209–12.
27. McCarron JP, Mills C, Vaughn ED Jr. Tumors of the renal pelvis and ureter: current concepts and management. Semin Urol. 1983;1(1):75–81.
28. Rink M, Ehdaie B, Cha EK, Green DA, Karakiewicz PI, Babjuk M, Margulis V, Raman JD, Svatek RS, Fajkovic H, Lee RK. Stage-specific impact of tumor location on oncologic outcomes in patients with upper and lower tract urothelial carcinoma following radical surgery. Eur Urol. 2012;62(4):677–84.
29. Sung HH, Cho J, Kwon GY, Jeon HG, Jeong BC, Seo SI, Jeon SS, Choi HY, Lee HM. Clinical significance of micropapillary urothelial carcinoma of the upper urinary tract. J Clin Pathol. 2014;67(1):49–54.
30. Sakano S, Matsuyama H, Kamiryo Y, Hayashida S, Yamamoto N, Kaneda Y, Nasu T, Baba Y, Shimabukuro T, Suga A, Yamamoto M. Impact of variant histology on disease aggressiveness and outcome after nephroureterectomy in Japanese patients with upper tract urothelial carcinoma. Int J Clin Oncol. 2015;20(2):362–8.
31. Inman BA, Tran VT, Fradet Y, Lacombe L. Carcinoma of the upper urinary tract: predictors of survival and competing causes of mortality. Cancer. 2009;115(13):2853–62.
32. Cowan NC. CT urography for hematuria. Nat Rev Urol. 2012;9(4):218–26.
33. Raman JD, Shariat SF, Karakiewicz PI, Lotan Y, Sagalowsky AI, Roscigno M, Montorsi F, Bolenz C, Weizer AZ, Wheat JC, Ng CK. Does preoperative symptom classification impact prognosis in patients with clinically localized upper-tract urothelial carcinoma managed by radical nephroureterectomy? Urol Oncol. 2011;29(6):716–23.
34. Jena R, Sureka SK, Ruidas S, Lal H. Spontaneous renoalimentary fistula as a complication of upper tract urothelial carcinoma: unknown complication of a rare disease. BMJ Case Rep. 2019;12(10):e231720.

35. Cowan NC, et al. Multidetector computed tomography urography for diagnosing upper urinary tract urothelial tumour. BJU Int. 2007;99:1363.
36. Janisch F, Shariat SF, Baltzer P, Fajkovic H, Kimura S, Iwata T, Korn P, Yang L, Glybochko PV, Rink M, Abufaraj M. Diagnostic performance of multidetector computed tomographic (MDCTU) in upper tract urothelial carcinoma (UTUC): a systematic review and meta-analysis. World J Urol. 2020;38(5):1165–75.
37. Jena R, Sureka SK, Singh UP. Upper tract transitional cell carcinoma clinically mimicking inflammatory renal pathology: a report of three cases. Indian J Urol. 2021;37(2):169.
38. Takahashi N, Glockner JF, Hartman RP, King BF, Leibovich BC, Stanley DW, Fitz-Gibbon PD, Kawashima A. Gadolinium enhanced magnetic resonance urography for upper urinary tract malignancy. J Urol. 2010;183(4):1330–6.
39. NCCN guidelines version 2.2022. https://www.nccn.org/professionals/physician_gls/pdf/bladder.pdf.
40. Messer J, Shariat SF, Brien JC, Herman MP, Ng CK, Scherr DS, Scoll B, Uzzo RG, Wille M, Eggener SE, Steinberg G. Urinary cytology has a poor performance for predicting invasive or high-grade upper-tract urothelial carcinoma. BJU Int. 2011;108(5):701–5.
41. Malm C, Grahn A, Jaremko G, Tribukait B, Brehmer M. Diagnostic accuracy of upper tract urothelial carcinoma: how samples are collected matters. Scand J Urol. 2017;51(2):137–45.
42. McHale T, Ohori NP, Cieply KM, Sherer C, Bastacky SI. Comparison of urinary cytology and fluorescence in situ hybridization in the detection of urothelial neoplasia: an analysis of discordant results. Diagn Cytopathol. 2019;47(4):282–8.
43. Jin H, Lin T, Hao J, Qiu S, Xu H, Yu R, Sun S, Zhang P, Liu Z, Yang L, Liu L. A comprehensive comparison of fluorescence in situ hybridization and cytology for the detection of upper urinary tract urothelial carcinoma: a systematic review and meta-analysis. Medicine. 2018;97(52):e13859.
44. Rojas CP, Castle SM, Llanos CA, Cortes JA, Bird V, Rodriguez S, Reis IM, Zhao W, Gomez-Fernandez C, Leveillee RJ, Jorda M. Low biopsy volume in ureteroscopy does not affect tumor biopsy grading in upper tract urothelial carcinoma. Urol Oncol. 2013;31(8):1696–700.
45. Smith AK, Stephenson AJ, Lane BR, Larson BT, Thomas AA, Gong MC, Jones JS, Campbell SC, Hansel DE. Inadequacy of biopsy for diagnosis of upper tract urothelial carcinoma: implications for conservative management. Urology. 2011;78(1):82–6.
46. Bus MT, de Bruin DM, Faber DJ, Kamphuis GM, Zondervan PJ, Laguna Pes MP, de Reijke TM, Traxer O, van Leeuwen TG, de la Rosette JJ. Optical diagnostics for upper urinary tract urothelial cancer: technology, thresholds, and clinical applications. J Endourol. 2015;29(2):113–23.
47. Knoedler JJ, Raman JD. Advances in the management of upper tract urothelial carcinoma: improved endoscopic management through better diagnostics. Ther Adv Urol. 2018;10(12):421–9.
48. Breda A, Territo A, Guttilla A, Sanguedolce F, Manfredi M, Quaresima L, Gaya JM, Algaba F, Palou J, Villavicencio H. Correlation between confocal laser endomicroscopy (Cellvizio®) and histological grading of upper tract urothelial carcinoma: a step forward for a better selection of patients suitable for conservative management. Eur Urol Focus. 2018;4(6):954–9.
49. Bus MT, De Bruin DM, Faber DJ, Kamphuis GM, Zondervan PJ, Laguna-Pes MP, van Leeuwen TG, de Reijke TM, de la Rosette JJ. Optical coherence tomography as a tool for in vivo staging and grading of upper urinary tract urothelial carcinoma: a study of diagnostic accuracy. J Urol. 2016;196(6):1749–55.
50. Clements T, Messer JC, Terrell JD, Herman MP, Ng CK, Scherr DS, Scoll B, Boorjian SA, Uzzo RG, Wille M, Eggener SE. High-grade ureteroscopic biopsy is associated with advanced pathology of upper-tract urothelial carcinoma tumors at definitive surgical resection. J Endourol. 2012;26(4):398–402.
51. Brien JC, Shariat SF, Herman MP, Ng CK, Scherr DS, Scoll B, Uzzo RG, Wille M, Eggener SE, Terrell JD, Lucas SM. Preoperative hydronephrosis, ureteroscopic biopsy grade and urinary cytology can improve prediction of advanced upper tract urothelial carcinoma. J Urol. 2010;184(1):69–73.
52. Moch H, Cubilla AL, Humphrey PA, Reuter VE, Ulbright TM. The 2016 WHO classification of tumours of the urinary system and male genital organs—part a: renal, penile, and testicular tumours. Eur Urol. 2016;70(1):93–105.
53. Sauter G, Algaba F, Amin M, Busch C, Cheville J, Gasser T, Grignon DJ, Hofstadter F, Lopez-Beltran A, Epstein JI. Tumours of the urinary system: non-invasive urothelial neoplasias. In: Eble JN, Sauter G, JI E, Sesterhenn I, editors. WHO classification of classification of tumors of the urinary system and male genital organs. Lyon: IARCC Press; 2004. p. 29–34.
54. Brierley JD, et al. TNM classification of malignant tumours. 8th ed. Hoboken: Wiley-Blackwell; 2016.
55. Anderström C, Johansson SL, Pettersson S, Wahlqvist L. Carcinoma of the ureter: a clinicopathologic study of 49 cases. J Urol. 1989;142(2):280–3.
56. Kang CH, Yu TJ, Hsieh HH, Yang JW, Shu K, Huang CC, Chiang PH, Shiue YL. The development of bladder tumors and contralateral upper urinary tract tumors after primary transitional cell carcinoma of the upper urinary tract. Cancer. 2003;98(8):1620–6.
57. Williams AK, Kassouf W, Chin J, Rendon R, Jacobsen N, Fairey A, Kapoor A, Black P, Lacombe L, Tanguay S, So A. Multifocality rather than tumor location is a prognostic factor in upper tract urothelial carcinoma. Urol Oncol. 2013;31(7):1161–5.

58. Chromecki TF, Cha EK, Fajkovic H, Margulis V, Novara G, Scherr DS, Lotan Y, Raman JD, Kassouf W, Bensalah K, Weizer A. The impact of tumor multifocality on outcomes in patients treated with radical nephroureterectomy. Eur Urol. 2012;61(2):245–53.
59. Reddy M, Kader K. Follow-up management of cystectomy patients. Urol Clin. 2018;45(2):241–7.
60. Seisen T, Granger B, Colin P, Leon P, Utard G, Renard-Penna R, Comperat E, Mozer P, Cussenot O, Shariat SF, Roupret M. A systematic review and meta-analysis of clinicopathologic factors linked to intravesical recurrence after radical nephroureterectomy to treat upper tract urothelial carcinoma. Eur Urol. 2015;67(6):1122–33.
61. Rouprêt M, Babjuk M, Compérat E, Zigeuner R, Sylvester RJ, Burger M, Cowan NC, Gontero P, Van Rhijn BW, Mostafid AH, Palou J. European association of urology guidelines on upper urinary tract urothelial carcinoma: 2017 update. Eur Urol. 2018;73(1):111–22.
62. Hafner C, Knuechel R, Stoehr R, Hartmann A. Clonality of multifocal urothelial carcinomas: 10 years of molecular genetic studies. Int J Cancer. 2002;101(1):1–6.
63. Lughezzani G, Burger M, Margulis V, Matin SF, Novara G, Roupret M, Shariat SF, Wood CG, Zigeuner R. Prognostic factors in upper urinary tract urothelial carcinomas: a comprehensive review of the current literature. Eur Urol. 2012;62(1):100–14.
64. Chromecki TF, Ehdaie B, Novara G, Pummer K, Zigeuner R, Seitz C, Pycha A, Lee RK, Cha EK, Karakiewicz PI, Ng C. Chronological age is not an independent predictor of clinical outcomes after radical nephroureterectomy. World J Urol. 2011;29(4):473–80.
65. Xia L, Taylor BL, Pulido JE, Guzzo TJ. Impact of surgical waiting time on survival in patients with upper tract urothelial carcinoma: a national cancer database study. Urol Oncol. 2018;36(1):10–e15.
66. Seisen T, Peyronnet B, Dominguez-Escrig JL, Bruins HM, Yuan CY, Babjuk M, Böhle A, Burger M, Compérat EM, Cowan NC, Kaasinen E. Oncologic outcomes of kidney-sparing surgery versus radical nephroureterectomy for upper tract urothelial carcinoma: a systematic review by the EAU non-muscle invasive bladder cancer guidelines panel. Eur Urol. 2016;70(6):1052–68.
67. Carson CC. Endoscopic treatment of upper and lower urinary tract lesions using lasers. Semin Urol. 1991;9:185–91.
68. Cutress ML, Stewart GD, Zakikhani P, Phipps S, Thomas BG, Tolley DA. Ureteroscopic and percutaneous management of upper tract urothelial carcinoma (UTUC): systematic review. BJU Int. 2012;110(5):614–28.
69. Gadzinski AJ, Roberts WW, Faerber GJ, Wolf JS Jr. Long-term outcomes of nephroureterectomy versus endoscopic management for upper tract urothelial carcinoma. J Urol. 2010;183(6):2148–53.
70. Daneshmand S, Quek ML, Huffman JL. Endoscopic management of upper urinary tract transitional cell carcinoma: long-term experience. Cancer. 2003;98(1):55–60.
71. Villa L, Cloutier J, Letendre J, Ploumidis A, Salonia A, Cornu JN, Montorsi F, Traxer O. Early repeated ureteroscopy within 6–8 weeks after a primary endoscopic treatment in patients with upper tract urothelial cell carcinoma: preliminary findings. World J Urol. 2016;34(9):1201–6.
72. Vemana G, Kim EH, Bhayani SB, Vetter JM, Strope SA. Survival comparison between endoscopic and surgical management for patients with upper tract urothelial cancer: a matched propensity score analysis using surveillance, epidemiology and end results-medicare data. Urology. 2016;95:115–20.
73. Rouprêt M, Traxer O, Tligui M, Conort P, Chartier-Kastler E, Richard F, Cussenot O. Upper urinary tract transitional cell carcinoma: recurrence rate after percutaneous endoscopic resection. Eur Urol. 2007;51(3):709–14.
74. Redrow GP, Guo CC, Brausi MA, Coleman JA, Fernandez MI, Kassouf W, Keeley FX Jr, Margulis V, Raman JD, Roupret M, Shariat SF. Upper urinary tract carcinoma in situ: current knowledge, future direction. J Urol. 2017;197(2):287–95.
75. Giannarini G, Kessler TM, Birkhäuser FD, Thalmann GN, Studer UE. Antegrade perfusion with bacillus Calmette-Guérin in patients with non–muscle-invasive urothelial carcinoma of the upper urinary tract: who may benefit? Eur Urol. 2011;60(5):955–60.
76. Foerster B, D'Andrea D, Abufaraj M, Broenimann S, Karakiewicz PI, Rouprêt M, Gontero P, Lerner SP, Shariat SF, Soria F. Endocavitary treatment for upper tract urothelial carcinoma: a meta-analysis of the current literature. Urol Oncol. 2019;37(7):430–6.
77. Kleinmann N, Matin SF, Pierorazio PM, Gore JL, Shabsigh A, Hu B, Chamie K, Godoy G, Hubosky S, Rivera M, O'Donnell M. Primary chemoablation of low-grade upper tract urothelial carcinoma using UGN-101, a mitomycin-containing reverse thermal gel (OLYMPUS): an open-label, single-arm, phase 3 trial. Lancet Oncol. 2020;21(6):776–85.
78. Simone G, Papalia R, Guaglianone S, Ferriero M, Leonardo C, Forastiere E, Gallucci M. Laparoscopic versus open nephroureterectomy: perioperative and oncologic outcomes from a randomised prospective study. Eur Urol. 2009;56(3):520–6.
79. Rouprêt M, Smyth G, Irani J, Guy L, Davin JL, Saint F, Pfister C, Wallerand H, Rozet F. Oncological risk of laparoscopic surgery in urothelial carcinomas. World J Urol. 2009;27(1):81–8.
80. Ong AM, Bhayani SB, Pavlovich CP. Trocar site recurrence after laparoscopic nephroureterectomy. J Urol. 2003;170(4 Pt 1):1301.
81. Walton TJ, Novara G, Matsumoto K, Kassouf W, Fritsche HM, Artibani W, Bastian PJ, Martínez-Salamanca JI, Seitz C, Thomas SA, Ficarra V. Oncological outcomes after laparoscopic and

open radical nephroureterectomy: results from an international cohort. BJU Int. 2011;108(3):406–12.
82. Ni S, Tao W, Chen Q, Liu L, Jiang H, Hu H, Han R, Wang C. Laparoscopic versus open nephroureterectomy for the treatment of upper urinary tract urothelial carcinoma: a systematic review and cumulative analysis of comparative studies. Eur Urol. 2012;61(6):1142–53.
83. Clements MB, Krupski TL, Culp SH. Robotic-assisted surgery for upper tract urothelial carcinoma: a comparative survival analysis. Ann Surg Oncol. 2018;25(9):2550–62.
84. Xylinas E, Rink M, Cha EK, Clozel T, Lee RK, Fajkovic H, Comploj E, Novara G, Margulis V, Raman JD, Lotan Y. Impact of distal ureter management on oncologic outcomes following radical nephroureterectomy for upper tract urothelial carcinoma. Eur Urol. 2014;65(1):210–7.
85. Xylinas E, Kluth L, Passoni N, Trinh QD, Rieken M, Lee RK, Fajkovic H, Novara G, Margulis V, Raman JD, Lotan Y. Prediction of intravesical recurrence after radical nephroureterectomy: development of a clinical decision-making tool. Eur Urol. 2014;65(3):650–8.
86. Phé V, Cussenot O, Bitker MO, Rouprêt M. Does the surgical technique for management of the distal ureter influence the outcome after nephroureterectomy? BJU Int. 2010;108(1):130–8.
87. Giovansili B, Peyromaure M, Saïghi D, Dayma T, Zerbib M, Debré B. Stripping technique for endoscopic management of distal ureter during nephroureterectomy: experience of 32 procedures. Urology. 2004;64(3):448–52.
88. Matin SF, Gill IS. Recurrence and survival following laparoscopic radical nephroureterectomy with various forms of bladder cuff control. J Urol. 2005;173(2):395–400.
89. Dominguez-Escrig JL, Peyronnet B, Seisen T, Bruins HM, Yuan CY, Babjuk M, Böhle A, Burger M, Compérat EM, Gontero P, Lam T. Potential benefit of lymph node dissection during radical nephroureterectomy for upper tract urothelial carcinoma: a systematic review by the European Association of Urology guidelines panel on non–muscle-invasive bladder cancer. Eur Urol Focus. 2019;5(2):224–41.
90. Dong F, Xu T, Wang X, Shen Y, Zhang X, Chen S, Zhong S, Zhang M, Ding Q. Lymph node dissection could bring survival benefits to patients diagnosed with clinically node-negative upper urinary tract urothelial cancer: a population-based, propensity score-matched study. Int J Clin Oncol. 2019;24(3):296–305.
91. Lenis AT, Donin NM, Faiena I, Salmasi A, Johnson DC, Drakaki A, Gollapudi K, Blumberg J, Belldegrun A, Pantuck A, Chamie K. Role of surgical approach on lymph node dissection yield and survival in patients with upper tract urothelial carcinoma. Urol Oncol. 2018;36(1):9.e1.
92. Matin SF, Margulis V, Kamat A, Wood CG, Grossman HB, Brown GA, Dinney CP, Millikan R, Siefker-Radtke AO. Incidence of downstaging and complete remission after neoadjuvant chemotherapy for high-risk upper tract transitional cell carcinoma. Cancer. 2010;116(13):3127–34.
93. Margulis V, Puligandla M, Trabulsi EJ, Plimack ER, Kessler ER, Matin SF, Godoy G, Alva A, Hahn NM, Carducci MA, Hoffman-Censits J. Phase II trial of neoadjuvant systemic chemotherapy followed by extirpative surgery in patients with high grade upper tract urothelial carcinoma. J Urol. 2020;203(4):690–8.
94. Birtle AJ, Chester JD, Jones RJ, Johnson M, Hill M, Bryan RT, Catto J, Donovan J, French A, Harris C, Keeley F. Results of POUT: a phase III randomised trial of perioperative chemotherapy versus surveillance in upper tract urothelial cancer (UTUC). J Clin Oncol. 2018;36(6_Suppl):407.
95. Leow JJ, Chong YL, Chang SL, Valderrama BP, Powles T, Bellmunt J. Neoadjuvant and adjuvant chemotherapy for upper tract urothelial carcinoma: a 2020 systematic review and meta-analysis, and future perspectives on systemic therapy. Eur Urol. 2021;79(5):635–54.
96. Hwang EC, Sathianathen NJ, Jung JH, Kim MH, Dahm P, Risk MC. Single-dose intravesical chemotherapy after nephroureterectomy for upper tract urothelial carcinoma. Cochrane Database Syst Rev. 2019;5(5):CD013160.
97. Seisen T, Jindal T, Karabon P, Sood A, Bellmunt J, Rouprêt M, Leow JJ, Vetterlein MW, Sun M, Alanee S, Choueiri TK. Efficacy of systemic chemotherapy plus radical nephroureterectomy for metastatic upper tract urothelial carcinoma. Eur Urol. 2017;71(5):714–8.
98. Moschini M, Xylinas E, Zamboni S, Mattei A, Niegisch G, Evan YY, Bamias A, Agarwal N, Sridhar SS, Sternberg CN, Vaishampayan UN. Efficacy of surgery in the primary tumor site for metastatic urothelial cancer: analysis of an international, multicenter, multidisciplinary database. Eur Urol Oncol. 2020;3(1):94–101.
99. Faltas BM, Gennarelli RL, Elkin E, Nguyen DP, Hu J, Tagawa ST. Metastasectomy in older adults with urothelial carcinoma: population-based analysis of use and outcomes. Urol Oncol. 2018;36(1):9.e11.
100. Sternberg CN, De Mulder P, Schornagel JH, Theodore C, Fossa SD, Van Oosterom AT, Witjes JA, Spina M, Van Groeningen CJ, Duclos B, Roberts JT. Seven year update of an EORTC phase III trial of high-dose intensity M-VAC chemotherapy and G-CSF versus classic M-VAC in advanced urothelial tract tumours. Eur J Cancer. 2006;42(1):50–4.
101. Galsky MD, Chen GJ, Oh WK, Bellmunt J, Roth BJ, Petrioli R, Dogliotti L, Dreicer R, Sonpavde G. Comparative effectiveness of cisplatin-based and carboplatin-based chemotherapy for treatment of advanced urothelial carcinoma. Ann Oncol. 2012;23(2):406–10.

102. Campbell MT, Shah AY, Matin SF, et al. Optimizing management of upper tract urothelial carcinoma. Urol Oncol. 2017;35(7):492–8.
103. Powles T, Park SH, Voog E, Caserta C, Valderrama BP, Gurney H, Kalofonos H, Radulović S, Demey W, Ullén A, Loriot Y. Avelumab maintenance therapy for advanced or metastatic urothelial carcinoma. N Engl J Med. 2020;383(13):1218–30.
104. Balar AV, Galsky MD, Rosenberg JE, Powles T, Petrylak DP, Bellmunt J, Loriot Y, Necchi A, Hoffman-Censits J, Perez-Gracia JL, Dawson NA. Atezolizumab as first-line treatment in cisplatin-ineligible patients with locally advanced and metastatic urothelial carcinoma: a single-arm, multicentre, phase 2 trial. Lancet. 2017;389(10064):67–76.
105. Balar AV, Castellano D, O'Donnell PH, Grivas P, Vuky J, Powles T, Plimack ER, Hahn NM, de Wit R, Pang L, Savage MJ. First-line pembrolizumab in cisplatin-ineligible patients with locally advanced and unresectable or metastatic urothelial cancer (KEYNOTE-052): a multicentre, single-arm, phase 2 study. Lancet Oncol. 2017;18(11):1483–92.
106. Alva A, Csőszi T, Ozguroglu M, Matsubara N, Geczi L, Cheng SS, Fradet Y, Oudard S, Vulsteke C, Barrera RM, Fléchon A. LBA23 Pembrolizumab (P) combined with chemotherapy (C) vs. C alone as first-line (1L) therapy for advanced urothelial carcinoma (UC): KEYNOTE-361. Ann Oncol. 2020;31:S1155.
107. Powles T, van der Heijden MS, Castellano D, Galsky MD, Loriot Y, Petrylak DP, Ogawa O, Park SH, Lee JL, De Giorgi U, Bögemann M. Durvalumab alone and durvalumab plus tremelimumab versus chemotherapy in previously untreated patients with unresectable, locally advanced or metastatic urothelial carcinoma (DANUBE): a randomised, open-label, multicentre, phase 3 trial. Lancet Oncol. 2020;21(12):1574–88.
108. Bellmunt J, De Wit R, Vaughn DJ, Fradet Y, Lee JL, Fong L, Vogelzang NJ, Climent MA, Petrylak DP, Choueiri TK, Necchi A. Pembrolizumab as second-line therapy for advanced urothelial carcinoma. N Engl J Med. 2017;376(11):1015–26.
109. Heers H, De Geeter P, Goebell PJ, Matz U, De Schultz W, Edlich B, Retz M, Hegele A. Vinflunine in the treatment of upper tract Urothelial carcinoma–subgroup analysis of an observational study. Anticancer Res. 2017;37(11):6437–42.

Part III

Carcinoma Urinary Bladder

Diagnosis and Clinical Staging 9

Sammy Gharbieh, Kawa Omar,
Ramesh Thurairajah, Muhammed S. Khan,
and Rajesh Nair

9.1 Introduction

9.1.1 Epidemiology

Bladder cancer is the most common malignancy of the urinary tract, accounting for 3% of all new cancer diagnoses. It is a significant cause of cancer morbidity and mortality, with an estimated 555,000 people diagnosed with bladder cancer worldwide in 2018 [1]. In the United Kingdom, over 10,000 new cases and approximately 5500 deaths are reported annually [2]. The risk of bladder cancer is three times higher in men than in women, with 1 in 50 UK males and 1 in 133 UK females diagnosed with bladder cancer in their lifetime [2].

Bladder cancer is predominantly a disease of older adults, with over half of the cases in the United Kingdom occurring in those aged 75 years or over [2]. It largely appears to be a disease of the Western World, with the highest rates occurring in Europe and North America [1]. Bladder cancer incidence rates have decreased by 42% since the early 1990s and are projected to fall by 34% between 2014 and 2035 [2]. However, mortality rates have minimally changed, despite significant advances in diagnostic and therapeutic techniques. Bladder cancer remains the tenth most common cause of cancer deaths in the United Kingdom and the seventh most common cause of cancer deaths in males [2]. Currently, the 5- and 10-year survival rates for bladder cancer are 52.6% and 43.6%, respectively [2].

9.1.2 Aetiology and Risk Factors

Bladder cancer primarily affects the urothelium of the bladder. This specialised epithelial surface, also known as the transitional epithelium, extends to the rest of the urinary tract and lines the renal pelvis, ureters, bladder and proximal urethra. The single most important environmental risk factor for urothelial carcinoma is smoking, which is responsible for almost half of all bladder cancer cases in the UK [2]. Smokers have a threefold increased risk of the disease, as tobacco smoke contains known urothelial carcinogens which are metabolised and excreted by the kidneys. Due to their prolonged dwell time in the bladder, the risk of lower tract disease with smoking is higher than that of upper tract disease. The second most preventable risk factor for bladder cancer is occupational exposure to aromatic amines, which are often found in industries involving rubber, dyes, paint, petroleum and fungicides. As little as 2

S. Gharbieh · K. Omar · R. Thurairajah · M. S. Khan · R. Nair (✉)
Department of Urology, Guy's and St. Thomas' NHS Foundation Trust, Great Maze Pond, London, UK
e-mail: rajesh.nair1@gstt.nhs.uk

P. Singh et al. (eds.), *A Guide to Management of Urological Cancers*,
https://doi.org/10.1007/978-981-99-2341-0_9

years' exposure may be sufficient to increase this risk, but the latency period may be several decades, as is the case with tobacco smoke [3].

Therapeutic strategies for other pathologies may directly or indirectly predispose individuals to bladder cancer. Radiation therapy for pelvic malignancies, such as prostate, endometrial or rectal cancers, may directly increase the risk of second primary bladder tumours [4–6]. Other radiation-induced complications, such as haemorrhagic cystitis, ureteric and urethral strictures, may indirectly increase this risk by promoting chronic inflammation [7]. In addition, cytotoxic therapies for haematological malignancies, such as cyclophosphamide, may increase the risk of bladder cancer in a dose-dependent fashion, with higher doses leading to a 14.5-fold increased risk of disease [8].

A small proportion of bladder cancers (10%) are due to squamous cell carcinoma, adenocarcinoma and other rare forms such as small cell carcinoma and sarcoma. Squamous cell carcinoma of the bladder is most common in North and East Africa, where schistosomiasis is endemic [9]. In these regions, the mean age of bladder cancer incidence is 40–49 years, compared with over 70 years of age in the Western World. Schistosomal infection leads to chronic granulomatous inflammation of the mucosal and submucosal layers, directly leading to squamous metaplasia of the bladder urothelium. Granulomatous inflammation can also lead to bladder fibrosis, resulting in urinary stasis and bacterial superinfection. These bacteria generate N-nitrosamines, which themselves are carcinogenic and act on the metaplastic epithelium to promote progression to squamous cell carcinoma. Interestingly, the disease course is far more rapid than that of tobacco smoke or chemical exposure [10].

9.2 Classification and Grading

The TNM (tumour, node and metastasis) classification is the most widely used system for the staging of bladder cancer (Fig. 9.1a–c). Bladder cancers originate from the urothelium and spread through direct invasion into the submucosa, lamina propria, muscularis layers and serosa. Invasion of adjacent pelvic structures can also occur (i.e., prostate, urethra, vagina and uterus), as well as extension to local abdominal viscera. Lymphatic spread occurs via the internal iliac, obturator, external iliac and pre-sacral nodes. Distant metastases occur via haematogenous spread to the liver, lungs, bones and adrenal glands.

Approximately 75% of bladder cancer cases are non-muscle invasive (NMIBC), confined to the mucosa (Ta, Tis) or submucosa (T1) [11]. The remaining 25% of cases invade the muscularis propria (T2) and are termed muscle-invasive bladder cancers (MIBC). While MIBCs are high-grade cancers by definition, NMIBCs may be further classified into low- or high-grade tumours as per the WHO grading system. The WHO grading system provides a scale of tumour aggressiveness based on histological appearances: urethral carcinoma in situ, urothelial papilloma, papillary urothelial neoplasm of low malignant potential (PUNLMP), low-grade papillary urothelial carcinoma and high-grade papillary urothelial carcinoma (Table 9.1). The latest edition recognises two additional groups: urothelial proliferation of uncertain malignant potential, which refers to a 'thickened, hyperplastic urothelium with no atypical features', and urothelial dysplasia, which refers to a 'lesion with structural abnormalities believed to be preneoplastic but does not constitute carcinoma *in situ* (CIS)'.

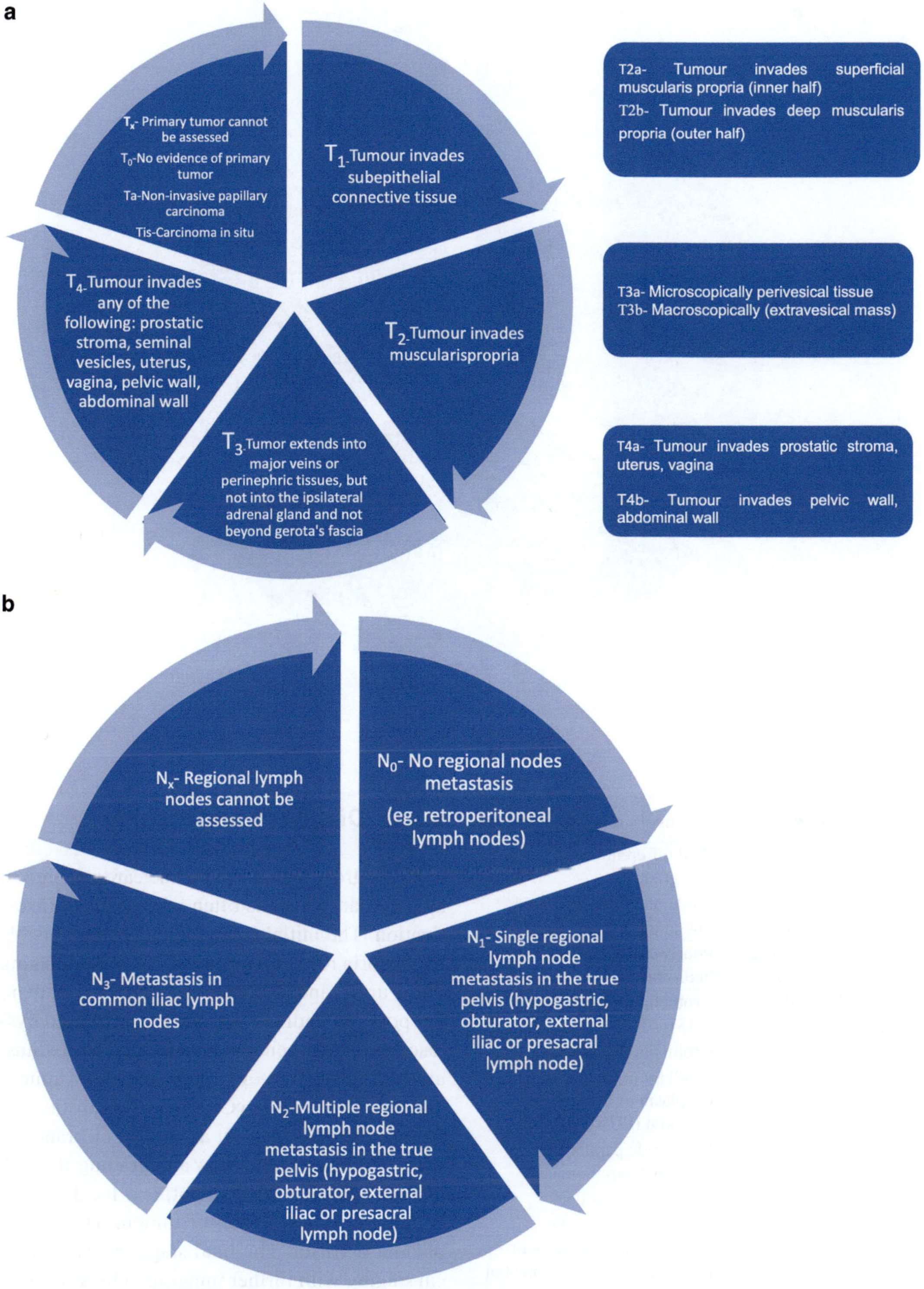

Fig. 9.1 (**a**) T staging; (**b**) nodal staging and (**c**) M staging

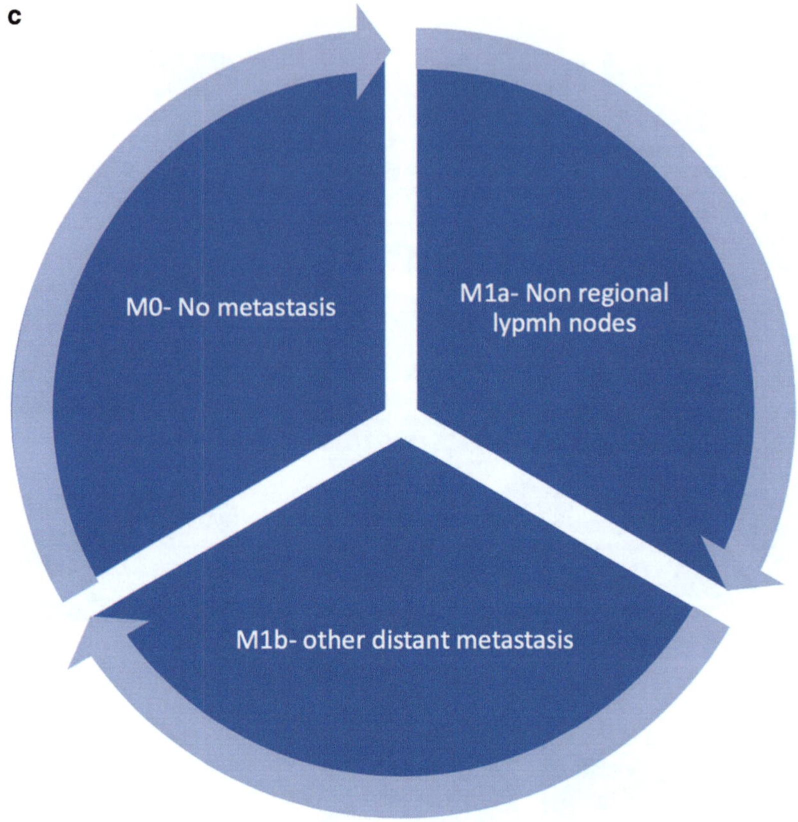

Fig. 9.1 (continued)

Table 9.1 WHO grading system of urothelial carcinoma

1973 WHO grading [12]	Grade 1 (G1)	Well differentiated, low-grade
	Grade 2 (G2)	Moderately differentiated, low-grade
	Grade 3 (G3)	Poorly differentiated, high-grade
2004 WHO grading [13]		Urothelial carcinoma in situ (CIS)
		Urothelial papilloma
		Papillary urothelial neoplasm of low malignant potential (PUNLMP)
		Low-grade papillary urothelial carcinoma
		High-grade papillary urothelial carcinoma
2016 edition [14]		Urothelial proliferation of uncertain malignant potential
		Urothelial dysplasia

9.3 Diagnosis and Staging

Painless gross haematuria is the cardinal sign of bladder cancer and is often what leads to investigation. The initial evaluation of patient visible haematuria relies on urine cytology and imaging of the upper and lower urinary tract [15]. If there are positive findings, the next step is rigid cystoscopy under general anaesthetic with transurethral resection of the bladder tumour (TURBT). TURBT is both a diagnostic and therapeutic procedure; it allows for clearance of visible tumours, diagnosis and grading through histopathological assessment, and local staging by determining whether the tumour has invaded bladder detrusor. The final stage involves clinical staging with further imaging to look for metastatic spread.

9.3.1 Cystoscopy

Cystoscopy is the gold standard investigation performed in the diagnostic work-up for bladder cancer, as it allows for direct visualisation of the urethra, urethral sphincter, prostate, bladder and ureteric orifices. The goal of cystoscopy is to identify all visible tumours to facilitate accurate staging and therefore treatment. The standard approach is white light cystoscopy (WLC), which, over the decades, has undergone significant technological advances associated with improved image quality. Despite this, its use remains operator dependent and false-negative rates of up to 20% have been reported, particularly with flat lesions such as CIS [16]. Tumour recurrence is remarkably common, with almost one-third of patients having disease identified at their first screening cystoscopy at 3 months, and half of patients demonstrating disease recurrence within their first year [17, 18]. Thus, complementary endoscopic technologies have been developed to improve lesion visualisation, detection and resection rates.

Photodynamic diagnosis (PDD), also known as blue-light cystoscopy, uses intravesical photosensitising agents to enable fluorescent imaging of the bladder wall. Prodrugs, 5-aminolevulinic acid (5-ALA) and hexaminolevulinate (Hexvix ®) are taken up by the urothelium, which results in the intracellular accumulation of photoactive porphyrines. Upon exposure to blue light (380–480 nm), abnormal cells emit a characteristic red fluorescence that is easily distinguishable from the blue background of healthy urothelium [19]. Numerous systematic reviews and meta-analyses have demonstrated the superiority of PDD over traditional WLC [20–25]. Bladder cancer detection rates are approximately 30% higher under PDD guidance, which may translate into more complete tumour resections, reduced risk of progression and prevention of cancer recurrence. One caveat is that PDD can be associated with false-positive results following intravesical treatment with Bacillus Calmette-Guerin (BCG), hence a delay in investigation is recommended for 9–12 weeks. Currently, PDD is the only approach other than traditional WLC that is approved for routine use, although numerous other technologies are underway [26, 27].

Narrow-band imaging (NBI) is another high-resolution technique that improves bladder cancer detection, without the need for intravesical contrast agents. It is a modification to traditional WLC, where only blue (415 nm) and green (540 nm) light bands are used as opposed to the entire visible light spectrum. Because these two light bands are strongly absorbed by haemoglobin, flat lesions such as CIS, which have dense capillaries, can easily be distinguishable from normal mucosa. This technology has been integrated into standard flexible and rigid cystoscopes and is associated with improved bladder cancer detection rates compared with WLC. NBI may even outperform PDD in term of diagnostic accuracy; however, there is inconclusive data on rates of disease recurrence and progression [21, 22, 28].

The Storz Professional Image Enhancement System (IMAGE 1S)®, previously known as SPIES, uses five different image enhancement modalities to improve tumour diagnosis. In addition to standard white light, it uses Spectra A, Spectra B, Chroma and Clara. Spectra A and B serve to increase colour contrast, Chroma improves the sharpness of images and Clara alters brightness to improve the visibility of dark spots. This image enhancement system is currently being investigated in a large international trial [29]. Other methods are also being developed, such as optical coherence tomography, confocal laser endomicroscopy and ultraviolet autofluorescence [19]. Whilst these new systems show promising results so far, they do not yet have routine clinical application.

9.3.1.1 TURBT: Resection Techniques

TURBT using a loop resectoscope has long been the standard method of endoscopic resection of NMIBC. Using a wire loop diathermy, resection is carried out in a piecemeal fashion otherwise known as the 'incise and scattering' technique. However, this technique contradicts the basic principles of oncological surgery, which is to remove the entire lesion to avoid seeding of tumour tissue. Other drawbacks include a relatively high rate of incomplete resections, thermal damage and cautery artefacts, which may prevent accurate histopathological assessment from the initial resection specimen [30, 31].

A significant advancement to the traditional TURBT is the en-bloc resection technique (ERBT), which aims to remove the entire tumour as a single specimen rather than in systematic fractions. It can be performed using different energy sources including electrical (monopolar or bipolar) cautery, laser (holmium/thulium) cautery and more recently water-jet resection. ERBT may improve resection quality and decrease recurrence rates, as there is a higher chance of obtaining detrusor muscle in the initial specimen whilst also minimising the risk of tumour scattering and fragmentation [32, 33]. The choice between conventional and en-bloc resection is based largely on the surgeon's preference in relation to the size and location of the lesion, as European guidelines currently do not specify which technique should be used [34]. Such modifications in resection techniques, combined with enhanced cystoscopy, show great promise to address some of the inherent shortcomings associated with conventional TURBT. However, large randomised multicentre trials are needed to further clarify outcomes and standardise procedures.

9.3.2 Urinary Biomarkers

Urine cytology is the most widely used non-invasive tool for detecting malignant urothelial cells. Whilst it has high diagnostic accuracy for high-grade tumours and CIS (sensitivity 80–90%, specificity 100%), it exhibits extremely low sensitivity for low-grade tumours (4–31%) [35]. Thus, the application of urine cytology is limited, and a negative sample does not exclude the presence of bladder cancer. Moreover, false positives can occur due to other inflammatory conditions or can result from chemo- or radiation therapy. In an attempt to overcome these limitations, several urinary biomarkers have been approved by the United States Food and Drug Administration (FDA) to use alongside cystoscopy. These include BTA stat (Polymedco), BTA TRAK (Polymedco), NMP22 enzyme-linked immune-sorbent assay (ELISA) (Matritech), NMP22 BladderChek Test (Alere), uCyt (Scimedx) and UroVysion (Abbott Molecular) [36]. Overall, these urinary biomarkers appear more sensitive than traditional cytology but are more costly and less specific in comparison.

The UK National Health Service (NHS) recently approved the use of two biomarkers to assist with the diagnosis and surveillance of bladder cancer. The first, ADXBLADDER-MCM5, is twice as sensitive as urine cytology and is not influenced by infection or inflammation. This test has an excellent negative predictive value up to 99% and has the advantage of providing rapid turnaround times using standard laboratory assays. However, overall performance is low, with a sensitivity of 51.9% and a specificity of 66.4% [37]. The second approved biomarker, URO17, is an immunocytochemistry-based test, which detects the oncoprotein Keratin 17 (K17). This test has shown 100% sensitivity in the detection of both recurrent and new cases of bladder cancer and a specificity of 96% and 92.6%, respectively [38, 39]. Thus, URO17 may be a sensitive and specific test for PUNLMP and other low-grade tumours that would otherwise be missed with conventional urine cytology.

The ideal biomarker for bladder cancer would reduce the need for serial cystoscopies, confidently exclude disease recurrence and detect progression toward invasive disease. Advancements in laboratory techniques have allowed the development of various biomarkers, including circulating cell-free tumour DNA (ctDNA), ctRNA, proteins, peptides and metabolites [32]. Whilst these may be key in the future of precision of medicine, large prospective multi-centre studies are still required to evaluate their performance compared to routine cystoscopy and urine cytology.

9.3.3 Imaging

9.3.3.1 Ultrasound

Imaging plays a pivotal role in the management of bladder cancer. Multiple imaging modalities may be used for diagnosis, locoregional staging and evaluation of distant metastases. Ultrasound is low-cost, widely available and a useful screening tool in the initial investigation of haematuria. Common sites for bladder tumours involve the posterior and lateral walls, which can be detected by ultrasound with approximately 95% accuracy [40]. Doppler ultrasound has the additional benefit of being able to distinguish a tumour from a blood clot. However, small tumours <0.5 cm or tumours at the bladder neck are difficult to delineate. Developments in contrast-enhanced sonography and three-dimensional ultrasound overcome some of the limitations in tumour characterisation with conventional ultrasound, but they are not in widespread use [41]. Although ultrasound cannot be used to exclude a diagnosis of bladder cancer, it offers additional benefits in the clinic setting by allowing the identification of renal lesions and evaluation of hydronephrosis.

9.3.3.2 Computed Tomography

Computed tomography (CT) is crucial in the assessment of visible haematuria. CT urography in particular is the most commonly used imaging modality to diagnose and stage urothelial malignancies [42]. CT urography is comparable to cystoscopy in terms of sensitivity and specificity but can miss very small or flat lesions that are more easily identified on endoscopic examination [43]. Despite this, CT urography is essential in the workup of bladder cancer due to the increased incidence of isolated or concurrent upper tract tumours [44]. One area where CT urography outperforms cystoscopy is with tumours arising within a bladder diverticulum (~1.5% of all bladder tumours), as endoscopic visualisation and tissue sampling are technically difficult [45].

CT urography is typically performed as a three-phase exam, comprising a noncontrast, contrast-enhanced nephrographic and delayed (excretory) phase. In the noncontrast phase, bladder cancer appears as a localised wall thickening, nodular mass or intraluminal polypoidal lesion. At the nephrographic phase, the bladder mass exhibits variable degrees of post-contrast enhancement. In the delayed phase, the tumour is seen as a soft tissue filling defect amidst a hyperattenuating lumen. However, CT urography cannot accurately assess the degree of bladder tumour invasiveness and is not ideal for differentiating NMBICs (≤T1) from MIBCs (≥T2). Tumours staged up to T3a can be reliably differentiated from the higher staged T3b and T4 tumours [46, 47].

CT is also essential in determining lymph node involvement. Lymph nodes are considered significant if the short axis is >10 mm in the abdomen and >8 mm in the pelvis [48]. However, these size criterions can produce false positives in the setting of reactive lymph nodes, leading to over-staging in up to 30% of cases. Conversely, metastases in lymph nodes with the short axis less <8 mm may be missed [49].

9.3.3.3 Magnetic Resonance Imaging

Magnetic resonance imaging (MRI) is considered superior to CT for local staging because of its high soft tissue contrast resolution and multiplanar imaging capabilities. Differentiation of normal bladder wall from bladder tumour can accurately be assessed on anatomic T2-weighted images; however, functional imaging techniques can provide more detail on the depth of tumour invasion as well as tumour grade [50, 51]. This has led to the development of multiparametric MRI, which uses anatomic and functional sequences in combination. These include T2-weighted imaging (T2WI), diffusion-weighted imaging (DWI) and dynamic contrast-enhanced (DCE) imaging [52, 53].

On T2WI, NMIBCs display intermediate-to-high signal intensity with an intact hypointense muscle wall, while MIBCs interrupt the hypointense line of the detrusor muscle. DWI captures the Brownian movement of water molecules; malignant tissues have a higher cellular density, leading to restriction of this movement and resulting in high-signal intensity. Hypervascular malignant tumours show early contrast enhancement, which can be captured on DCE-imaging, providing a scale on tumour aggressiveness [54].

The Vesical Imaging-Reporting and Data System (VI-RADS) was developed in recent years to standardise the interpretation and reporting of bladder cancer staging [55]. This

Table 9.2 VI-RADS scoring system [56]

VI-RADS category	T2WI (SC)	DCE-MRI (CE)	DWI (DW)
1	Uninterrupted low SI line representing the muscularis propria	No early enhancement of muscularis propria	Intact intermediate SI muscularis propria
	Lesion <1 cm		Lesion <1 cm
2	As above (SC 1), but with lesion >1 cm	As above (CE 1), but with early enhancement of inner layer	As above (DW 1), but with lesion >1 cm
3	Lack of SC 2 findings, with no clear disruption of low SI muscular propria	Lack of CE 2 findings, with no clear disruption of muscularis propria	Lack of DW 2 findings, with no clear disruption of muscularis propria
	Associated presence of exophytic tumour without stalk or sessile tumour without high SI thickened inner layer		
4	Intermediate SI tumour interrupts low SI line (muscularis propria)	Early enhancing tumour extends into muscularis propria	High SI tumour on DWI and low SI tumour on ADC extends into muscularis propria
5	Intermediate SI tumour extends into extravesical fat	Early enhancing tumour extends to entire bladder wall and to extravesical fat	High SI tumour on DWI and low SI tumour on ADC extending to the entire bladder wall and extra vesical fat
Final score			
VI-RADS 1		Muscle invasion highly unlikely	
		SC 1, CE 1, and DW 1	
VI-RADS 2		Muscle invasion unlikely	
		SC 2 + CE 2 and DW 2	
		SC 3 + CE 2 and DW 2	
VI-RADS 3		Muscle invasion equivocal	
		SC 3 + CE 3 and/or DW 3 (or below)	
VI-RADS 4		Muscle invasion likely	
		SC 4 + CE 4 and/or DW 4 (or below)	
		SC 5 + CE 4 and/or DW 4 (or below)	
VI-RADS 5		SC 4 + CE 5 and/or DW 5	
		SC 5 + CE 5 and/or DW 5	

ADC apparent diffusion coefficient, *DCE* dynamic contrast enhanced, *DWI* diffusion-weighted imaging, *SC* structural category, *SI* signal intensity, *T2WI* T2 weighted imaging

system incorporates tumour appearance on T2WI, DWI and DCE imaging to judge the risk of tumour invasion and produce an overall score of 1 to 5. VI-RADS 1 and 2 indicate an intact muscularis propria and no tumour invasion, VI-RADS 3 is equivocal for muscle invasion and VI-RADS 4 and 5 highly suggest muscle invasion with possible extra-vesical extension (see Table 9.2 for detail). The final overall score is based on the three categories and, if there is discrepancy between the structural T2WI and DCE imaging score, the findings on DWI predominate [55, 57].

Clinical Applications of MRI

Diagnostic pathways for bladder cancer have remained largely unchanged over the decades, with histopathologic confirmation via TURBT the reference standard for diagnosis and staging. Whilst TURBT is therapeutic for NMIBC, and its role in MIBC is predominantly diagnostic. The reliance on TURBT for bladder cancer staging not only has cost implications but also may increase the risk of complications and delay appropriate treatment. In these scenarios, multiparametric MRI can serve as a reliable, non-invasive tool to accurately stage and assess the disease.

Multiparametric MRI may be particularly useful in the pre-TURBT setting to help identify tumours that need a more radical approach [55]. For patients diagnosed with high-risk NMIBC at first TURBT, the VI-RADS score could be used to differentiate those who may be spared from secondary tumour resection from those who require it [58]. In MIBC, the VI-RADS score may recognise tumours likely to benefit from neoadjuvant therapy, identify those suited for bladder-sparing surgery and help plan a surgically feasible TURBT [53, 59, 60]. Whilst histopathological confirmation remains the cornerstone of bladder cancer diagnosis, the application of multiparametric MRI might enhance diagnostic and therapeutic pathways in a way that improves overall disease management.

9.4 Surveillance and Management

The European Association of Urology (EAU) has clear guidelines on the management of NMIBCs (Table 9.3) [34]. After initial TURBT, patients with NMIBC are stratified into low-, intermediate- and high-risk groups based on the probability of tumour recurrence and progression. All patients with NMIBC undergo strict follow-up, with repeat cystoscopy and urine cytology at regular intervals depending on the initial staging and grading of disease (Table 9.4) [61]. In higher-risk groups, surveillance imaging of the upper tract with CT urography is also undertaken. In the highest-risk groups, referral to specialist multidisciplinary team discussion is pertinent, as some

Table 9.3 EAU treatment recommendations for NMIBC according to risk stratification [61]

Risk category	Definition	Treatment recommendation
Low-risk	Primary, solitary, ta, G1 (PUNLMP, low-grade), <3 cm, no CIS	One immediate instillation of chemotherapy post-TURBT
Intermediate-risk	All tumours not defined in the two adjacent categories	One immediate instillation of chemotherapy followed by further instillations, with chemotherapy for a maximum of 1 year or 1 year full-dose BCG
High-risk	T1 tumours, G3 (high-grade) CIS, multiple and recurrent and large (>3 cm) ta G1/2 tumours	Intravesical full-dose BCG instillations for 1–3 years or cystectomy (in highest-risk tumours)
Subgroup of highest risk tumours	G3T1 associated with concurrent CIS; multiple and/or large G3T1 and/or recurrent G3T1; G3T1 with CIS in prostatic urethra/ unusual histology of urothelial carcinoma/ lympho-vascular invasion; BCG-failures	Radical cystectomy (RC) should be considered for all patients; for patients who refuse or are unsuitable for RC, intravesical full-dose BCG instillations for 1–3 years; RC is recommended for BCG failures

Table 9.4 Summary of risk-based guidelines from the EAU for the follow-up of patients after TURBT for NMIBC [61]

Years after diagnosis					
Risk category	1	2	3	4	5
Low-risk	Cystoscopy at 3 months and 12 months	Once-yearly for 5 years, discharge if disease-free at 5 years			
No upper tract imaging					
Intermediate-risk	Cystoscopy and cytology every 3–6 months		Cystoscopy and cytology every 6–12 months		Lifelong cystoscopy and cytology every 12 months
Upper tract imaging every 1–2 years					
High-risk	Cystoscopy and cytology every 3 months		Cystoscopy and cytology every 6 months		Cystoscopy and cytology every 6 months, and every 12 months thereafter
Upper tract imaging every 1–2 years					

will inevitably need to be considered for upfront radical cystectomy.

Radical cystectomy, pelvic lymph node dissection and urinary diversion is the standard therapy for MIBC and NMIBC that is not responsive to BCG [61]. Patients with decent performance status may receive neo-adjuvant chemotherapy in attempt to downstage the malignancy and facilitate micrometastatic control. Radical radiotherapy after neoadjuvant chemotherapy or on its own with radiosensitisers can be an alternative for patients who decline surgery or not suitable for major operation. Radiation therapy and/or chemotherapy may also be used for palliative purposes.

All patients with MIBC should receive a staging CT thorax-abdomen and pelvis to look for metastases. PET-CT or PET-MRI scans may be used to help troubleshoot equivocal lymph nodes or lesions suspicious for metastatic disease. Other specialist investigations, such as technetium-labelled radioisotope bone scans, may be performed in those with suspected bone metastases (bone pain and increased alkaline phosphatase). Ideally, imaging should be performed 6 weeks before radical surgery, as the rate of disease progression may be rapid. The overall 5-year survival rate for localised bladder tumours exceeds 90%, while that of metastatic disease is around 5% [62]. Thus, the importance of precise bladder cancer staging cannot be overemphasised.

References

1. Wong MCS, Fung FDH, Leung C, Cheung WWL, Goggins WB, Ng CF. The global epidemiology of bladder cancer: a joinpoint regression analysis of its incidence and mortality trends and projection. Sci Rep. 2018;8(1):1–2.
2. Cancer Research UK. Bladder cancer incidence statistics. https://www.cancerresearchuk.org/health-professional/cancer-statistics/statistics-by-cancer-type/bladder-cancer/incidence.
3. Saginala K, Barsouk A, Aluru JS, Rawla P, Padala SA, Barsouk A. Epidemiology of bladder cancer. Med Sci. 2020;8(1):15.
4. Moschini M, Zaffuto E, Karakiewicz PI, Andrea DD, Foerster B, Abufaraj M, et al. External beam radiotherapy increases the risk of bladder cancer when compared with radical prostatectomy in patients affected by prostate cancer: a population-based analysis. Eur Urol. 2019;75(2):319–28.
5. Wen L, Zhong G, Ren M. Increased risk of secondary bladder cancer after radiation therapy for endometrial cancer. Sci Rep. 2022;12(1):1032.
6. Guan X, Wei R, Yang R, Lu Z, Liu E, Zhao Z, et al. Risk and prognosis of secondary bladder cancer after radiation therapy for rectal cancer: a large population-based cohort study. Front Oncol. 2021;10:3158.
7. Chorbińska J, Krajewski W, Zdrojowy R. Urological complications after radiation therapy—nothing ventured, nothing gained: a narrative review. Transl Cancer Res. 2021;10(2):1096–118.
8. Travis LB, Curtis RE, Glimelius B, Holowaty EJ, Van Leeuwen FE, Lynch CF, et al. Bladder and kidney cancer following cyclophosphamide therapy for non-Hodgkin's lymphoma. J Natl Cancer Inst. 1995;87(7):524–31.
9. Mostafa MH, Sheweita SA, O'Connor PJ. Relationship between schistosomiasis and bladder cancer. Clin Microbiol Rev. 1999;12(1):97–111.
10. Zaghloul MS. Bladder cancer and schistosomiasis. J Egypt Natl Canc Inst. 2012;24(4):151–9.
11. Shen P, Lin M, Hong Y, He X. Bladder preservation approach versus radical cystectomy for high-grade non-muscle-invasive bladder cancer: a meta-analysis of cohort studies. World J Surg Oncol. 2018;16(1):197.
12. Mostofi FK, Sobin LH, Torloni H. Histological typing of urinary bladder tumours. International Classification of Tumours, No. 10. Geneva: World Health Organisation; 1973. p. 21–31.
13. Eble J, Sauter G, Epstein J, et al. Pathology and genetics of tumours of the urinary system and male genital organs. Lyon: IARC Press; 2004.
14. Humphrey PA, Moch H, Cubilla AL, Ulbright TM, Reuter VE. The 2016 WHO classification of tumours of the urinary system and male genital organs—part B: prostate and bladder tumours. Eur Urol. 2016;70(1):106–19.
15. Dulku G, Shivananda A, Chakera A, et al. Painless visible haematuria in adults: an algorithmic approach guiding management. Cureus. 2019;11(11):e6140.
16. Lotan Y, Bivalacqua TJ, Downs T, Huang W, Jones J, Kamat AM, et al. Blue light flexible cystoscopy with hexaminolevulinate in non-muscle-invasive bladder cancer: review of the clinical evidence and consensus statement on optimal use in the USA—update 2018. Nat Rev Urol. 2019;16(6):377–86.
17. Schwaibold HE, Sivalingam S, May F, Hartung R. The value of a second transurethral resection for T1 bladder cancer. BJU Int. 2006;97(6):1199–201.
18. Sylvester RJ, van der Meijden APM, Oosterlinck W, Witjes JA, Bouffioux C, Denis L, et al. Predicting recurrence and progression in individual patients with stage ta T1 bladder cancer using EORTC risk tables: a combined analysis of 2596 patients from seven EORTC trials. Eur Urol. 2006;49(3):466–77.
19. Schubert T, Rausch S, Fahmy O, Gakis G, Stenzl A. Optical improvements in the diagnosis of bladder

cancer: implications for clinical practice. Ther Adv Urol. 2017;9(11):251–60.
20. Rink M, Babjuk M, Catto JWF, Jichlinski P, Shariat SF, Stenzl A, et al. Hexyl Aminolevulinate–guided fluorescence cystoscopy in the diagnosis and follow-up of patients with non–muscle-invasive bladder Cancer: a critical review of the current literature. Eur Urol. 2013;64(4):624–38.
21. Burger M, Grossman HB, Droller M, Schmidbauer J, Hermann G, Drăgoescu O, et al. Photodynamic diagnosis of non–muscle-invasive bladder cancer with hexaminolevulinate cystoscopy: a meta-analysis of detection and recurrence based on raw data. Eur Urol. 2013;64(5):846–54.
22. Witjes JA, Babjuk M, Gontero P, Jacqmin D, Karl A, Kruck S, et al. Clinical and cost effectiveness of hexaminolevulinate-guided blue-light cystoscopy: evidence review and updated expert recommendations. Eur Urol. 2014;66(5):863–71.
23. Konecki T, Kutwin P, Łowicki R, Juszczak AB, Jabłonowski Z. Hexaminolevulinate in the management of nonmuscle invasive bladder cancer: a meta-analysis. Photobiomodul Photomed Laser Surg. 2019;37(9):551–8.
24. Chen C, Huang H, Zhao Y, Liu H, Luo Y, Sylvester RJ, et al. Diagnostic accuracy of photodynamic diagnosis with 5-aminolevulinic acid, hexaminolevulinate and narrow band imaging for non-muscle invasive bladder cancer. J Cancer. 2020;11(5):1082–93.
25. Russo GI, Sholklapper TN, Cocci A, Broggi G, Caltabiano R, Smith AB, et al. Performance of narrow band imaging (NBI) and photodynamic diagnosis (PDD) fluorescence imaging compared to white light cystoscopy (WLC) in detecting non-muscle invasive bladder Cancer: a systematic review and lesion-level diagnostic meta-analysis. Cancers. 2021;13(17):4378.
26. Babjuk M, Burger M, Capoun O, Cohen D, Compérat EM, Dominguez Escrig JL, et al. European Association of Urology guidelines on non–muscle-invasive bladder cancer (Ta, T1, and carcinoma in situ). Eur Urol. 2022;81(1):75–94.
27. Chang SS, Boorjian SA, Chou R, Clark PE, Daneshmand S, Konety BR, et al. Diagnosis and treatment of non-muscle invasive bladder cancer: AUA/SUO guideline. J Urol. 2016;196(4):1021–9.
28. Chen C, Huang H, Zhao Y, Liu H, Sylvester R, Lin T, et al. Diagnostic performance of image technique based transurethral resection for non-muscle invasive bladder cancer: systematic review and diagnostic meta-analysis. BMJ Open. 2019;9(10):e028173.
29. Gravas S, Stenzl A. The Storz Professional Image Enhancement System (SPIES) nonmuscle-invasive bladder cancer study: a multicenter international randomized controlled study. J Endourol. 2014;28:1254–5.
30. Kim LHC, Patel MI. Transurethral resection of bladder tumour (TURBT). Transl Androl Urol. 2020;9(6):3056–72.
31. Truong M, Liang L, Kukreja J, O'Brien J, Jean-Gilles J, Messing E. Cautery artifact understages urothelial cancer at initial transurethral resection of large bladder tumours. Can Urol Assoc J. 2017;11(5):203.
32. Zhang D, Yao L, Yu S, Cheng Y, Jiang J, Ma Q, et al. Safety and efficacy of en bloc transurethral resection versus conventional transurethral resection for primary nonmuscle-invasive bladder cancer: a meta-analysis. World J Surg Oncol. 2020;18(1):1–2.
33. van Putten K, Vernooij RW, Meijer RP, Zhu X. En-bloc resection versus conventional transurethral resection for patients with non-muscle-invasive bladder cancer. Cochrane Database Syst Rev. 2019;2019(11):CD013473.
34. Babjuk M, Böhle A, Burger M, Capoun O, Cohen D, Compérat EM, et al. EAU guidelines on non–muscle-invasive urothelial carcinoma of the bladder: update 2016. Eur Urol. 2017;71(3):447–61.
35. de Oliveira MC, Caires HR, Oliveira MJ, Fraga A, Vasconcelos MH, Ribeiro R. Urinary biomarkers in bladder Cancer: where do we stand and potential role of extracellular vesicles. Cancers. 2020;12(6):1400.
36. Sugeeta SS, Sharma A, Ng K, Nayak A, Vasdev N. Biomarkers in bladder cancer surveillance. Front Surg. 2021;8:735868.
37. Gontero P, Montanari E, Roupret M, Longo F, Stockley J, Kennedy A, et al. Comparison of the performances of the ADXBLADDER test and urinary cytology in the follow-up of non-muscle-invasive bladder cancer: a blinded prospective multicentric study. BJU Int. 2021;127(2):198–204.
38. Babu S, Mockler DC, Roa-Peña L, Szygalowicz A, Kim NW, Jahanfard S, et al. Keratin 17 is a sensitive and specific biomarker of urothelial neoplasia. Mod Pathol. 2019;32(5):717–24.
39. Vasdev N, Hampson A, Agarwal S, Swamy R, Chilvers M, Hampson A, et al. The role of URO17™ biomarker to enhance diagnosis of urothelial cancer in new hematuria patients—first European data. BJUI Compass. 2021;2(1):46–52.
40. Zhang J, Gerst S, Lefkowitz RA, Bach A. Imaging of bladder cancer. Radiol Clin N Am. 2007;45(1):183–205.
41. Abouelkheir RT, Abdelhamid A, Abou El-Ghar M, El-Diasty T. Imaging of bladder cancer: standard applications and future trends. Medicina. 2021;57(3):220.
42. Wong VK, Ganeshan D, Jensen CT, Devine CE. Imaging and management of bladder cancer. Cancers. 2021;13(6):1396.
43. Helenius M, Brekkan E, Dahlman P, Lönnemark M, Magnusson A. Bladder cancer detection in patients with gross haematuria: computed tomography urography with enhancement-triggered scan versus flexible cystoscopy. Scand J Urol. 2015;49(5):377–81.
44. Browne RFJ, Meehan CP, Colville J, Power R, Torreggiani WC. Transitional cell carcinoma of the upper urinary tract: spectrum of imaging findings. Radiographics. 2005;25(6):1609–27.
45. Di Paolo PL, Vargas HA, Karlo CA, Lakhman Y, Zheng J, Moskowitz CS, et al. Intradiverticular bladder can-

cer: CT imaging features and their association with clinical outcomes. Clin Imaging. 2015;39(1):94–8.
46. Lee CH, Tan CH, Faria S d C, Kundra V. Role of imaging in the local staging of urothelial carcinoma of the bladder. Am J Roentgenol. 2017;208(6):1193–205.
47. Mossanen M, Chang SL, Kimm S, Sonpavde GP, Kibel AS. Current staging strategies for muscle-invasive bladder cancer and upper tract urothelial cell carcinoma. Urol Clin N Am. 2018;45(2):143–54.
48. Pichler R, De Zordo T, Fritz J, Kroiss A, Aigner F, Heidegger I, et al. Pelvic lymph node staging by combined 18 F-FDG-PET/CT imaging in bladder cancer prior to radical cystectomy. Clin Genitourin Cancer. 2017;15(3):e387–95.
49. Thoeny HC, Froehlich JM, Triantafyllou M, Huesler J, Bains LJ, Vermathen P, et al. Metastases in Normal-sized pelvic lymph nodes: detection with diffusion-weighted MR imaging. Radiology. 2014;273(1):125–35.
50. Xu X, Zhang X, Tian Q, Zhang G, Liu Y, Cui G, et al. Three-dimensional texture features from intensity and high-order derivative maps for the discrimination between bladder tumors and wall tissues via MRI. Int J Comput Assist Radiol Surg. 2017;12(4):645–56.
51. Zhang X, Xu X, Tian Q, Li B, Wu Y, Yang Z, et al. Radiomics assessment of bladder cancer grade using texture features from diffusion-weighted imaging. J Magn Reson Imaging. 2017;46(5):1281–8.
52. de Haas RJ, Steyvers MJ, Fütterer JJ. Multiparametric MRI of the bladder: ready for clinical routine? Am J Roentgenol. 2014;202(6):1187–95.
53. Mirmomen SM, Shinagare AB, Williams KE, Silverman SG, Malayeri AA. Preoperative imaging for locoregional staging of bladder cancer. Abdom Radiol. 2019;44(12):3843–57.
54. Galgano SJ, Porter KK, Burgan C, Rais-Bahrami S. The role of imaging in bladder cancer diagnosis and staging. Diagnostics. 2020;10(9):703.
55. Pecoraro M, Takeuchi M, Vargas HA, Muglia VF, Cipollari S, Catalano C, et al. Overview of VI-RADS in bladder cancer. Am J Roentgenol. 2020;214(6):1259–68.
56. Makboul M, Farghaly S, Abdelkawi IF. Multiparametric MRI in differentiation between muscle invasive and non-muscle invasive urinary bladder cancer with vesical imaging reporting and data system (VI-RADS) application. Br J Radiol. 2019;92(1104):20190401.
57. Panebianco V, Narumi Y, Altun E, Bochner BH, Efstathiou JA, Hafeez S, et al. Multiparametric magnetic resonance imaging for bladder cancer: development of VI-RADS (vesical imaging-reporting and data system). Eur Urol. 2018;74(3):294–306.
58. Del Giudice F, De Berardinis E, Pecoraro M, Barchetti G, Campa R, Leonardo C, et al. Clinical implications of vesical imaging-reporting and data system (VI-RADS) on management of high-risk non-muscle invasive bladder cancers (HR-NMIBCs) candidate for repeated transurethral resection (re-TURBT): a single-center prospective analysis. Eur Urol Open Sci. 2020;19:e1014.
59. Griffiths G, Hall R, Sylvester R, Raghavan D, Parmar MK, the International Collaboration of Trialists, the Medical Research Council Advanced Bladder Cancer Working Party (now the National Cancer Research Institute Bladder Cancer Clinical Studies Group), the European Organisation for Research and Treatment of Cancer Genito-Urinary Tract Cancer Group, the Australian Bladder Cancer Study Group, the National Cancer Institute of Canada Clinical Trials Group, the Finnbladder, the Norwegian Bladder Cancer Study Group, the Club Urologico Espanol de Tratamiento Oncologico Group. International phase III trial assessing neoadjuvant cisplatin, methotrexate, and vinblastine chemotherapy for muscle-invasive bladder cancer: long-term results of the BA06 30894 trial. J Clin Oncol. 2011;29(16):2171–7.
60. Seisen T, Sun M, Lipsitz SR, Abdollah F, Leow JJ, Menon M, et al. Comparative effectiveness of trimodal therapy versus radical cystectomy for localized muscle-invasive urothelial carcinoma of the bladder. Eur Urol. 2017;72(4):483–7.
61. Witjes JA, Bruins HM, Cathomas R, Compérat EM, Cowan NC, Gakis G, et al. European Association of Urology guidelines on muscle-invasive and metastatic bladder cancer: summary of the 2020 guidelines. Eur Urol. 2021;79(1):82–104.
62. American Cancer Society. Cancer facts & figures 2022. https://www.cancer.net/cancer-types/bladder-cancer/statistics.

10 Pathology and Staging

Gauri Deshpande, Santosh Menon,
and Sangeeta Desai

10.1 Introduction

Urinary bladder carcinoma accounts for approximately 3% of the cancers worldwide and is the fourth most common cancer in men [1, 2]. In the United States, in the year 2021, the estimated number of new cases and the estimated deaths attributed to this cancer were 83,730 and 17,200, respectively [1]. The incidence of bladder cancers is increasing, more so in developed countries. The incidence of new bladder cases in India was 25,873 in the year 2020 and is projected to rise to 29,308 in 2025, as per the National Cancer Registry Programme [3]. Also, the incidence is markedly common in males and older age groups [4]. The most common histology is urothelial carcinoma (UC), seen in more than 90% of cases, while the remaining comprises of squamous cell carcinoma, adenocarcinoma, small cell carcinoma, etc. Bladder cancer is a heterogeneous disease, thus translating into multimodal treatment approaches [4, 5].

G. Deshpande · S. Menon (✉) · S. Desai
Department of Pathology, Tata Memorial Centre, Mumbai, India

10.2 Etiology and Risk Factors for Bladder Cancer

Tobacco smoking has been reported to be the one of the most important risk factors, which is associated with approximately 50% of new cases. It has been shown to increase the risk of bladder cancer 3–4 times. It is attributed to the carcinogens present in tobacco smoke namely beta-naphthylamine and polycyclic aromatic hydrocarbons [6]. The second most common risk factor is environmental and occupational exposure to carcinogens, prevalent in dye, paint, and rubber industries [7]. Urinary calculi have been shown to be associated with an increased risk of cancer in some studies [8]. Other less common risk factors include alcohol, red meat, obesity, radiation, and pathogenic infections, most commonly schistosomiasis, which is associated with squamous carcinoma of urinary bladder [2].

10.3 Pathology of Urothelial Carcinoma

Urothelial neoplasms comprise of a spectrum of tumors with different clinical and biological behaviors. This spectrum is translated from the heterogeneous morphological and genetic signatures of these neoplasms.

A common feature of urothelial carcinomas (UC) is the development of synchronous or

P. Singh et al. (eds.), *A Guide to Management of Urological Cancers*,
https://doi.org/10.1007/978-981-99-2341-0_10

metachronous multifocal tumors. Two theories have been proposed for this phenomenon: monoclonal theory and field cancerization effect [9–12]. The monoclonal theory suggests the role of a single transformed clone, which spreads by intraluminal/intraepithelial migration. The field cancerization theory emphasizes the independent mutational events, which can be simultaneous or sequential, at different sites. Various studies have suggested either monoclonal or field cancerization theories, while some studies have suggested coexistence of both [9, 13–16].

Urothelial neoplasms are classified primarily on the basis of the tumor architecture and cytologic atypia. Owing to continuing revelations in the molecular biology and clinical manifestations of these neoplasms, various nomenclatures and grading systems have been published. The ones most frequently used include the WHO 1973 classification, which was modified in the years 2004 and 2016. These classifications along with the recently published updates are elaborated below.

10.3.1 Grading of Urothelial Carcinoma

The grading of UC has always been a challenge, and various grading systems have been proposed. UC is morphologically a heterogeneous cancer with a varied spectrum, leading to considerable inter and intra-observer variability. The most frequently used grading systems in clinical practice include the 3-tier grading of the World Health Organization (WHO) put forth in 1973, and the WHO/ISUP 1998 grading system which was further endorsed in the year 2004 and 2016. The 2016 grading system is widely used at present; however, as most of the clinical data are based on the 1973 system, it retains its importance and many urologists still advocate use of the same [17–20].

10.3.1.1 The WHO 1973 Grading System

This grading system was proposed by Mostofi et al. [17] The UCs are graded based on the degree of cytological and architectural atypia, into three grades: G1, G2, and G3 (Table 10.1).

The major advantage of this system is the availability of long-term follow-up data, thus allowing comparison between different centers. The major disadvantage of this system is the vague and imprecise definition of G2 category, which leads to intra and interobserver variability and reproducibility [21, 22]. As a consequence, pathologists in several cases, resorted to subclassifying G2 into G1/2, for a tumor that was closer to G1 and G2/3, for a tumor which appeared morphologically closer to G3. These issues complicated the clinical decision-making [23].

10.3.1.2 The WHO/International Society of Urological Pathology (ISUP) 1998 Classification System

In 1998, a group comprising of Uropathologists representing the International Society of Urological Pathology, convened in Boston and developed a consensus grading system with a universally acceptable classification system for bladder tumors [24].

10.3.1.3 The WHO 2016 Grading System

The WHO 2016 classification (Table 10.2) essentially adopts the 1998/2004 classifications with

Table 10.1 The WHO 1973 grading system

	Architecture	Cytology
G1	Well organized slender papillae	No nuclear pleomorphism, regular chromatin distribution, no mitosis or necrosis
G2	Increased urothelial layers	Nuclear atypia between G1 and G3
G3	Marked loss of polarity	Marked nuclear pleomorphism, irregular nuclear membranes, coarse chromatin, high mitotic activity, necrosis

Table 10.2 WHO 2016 classification [25]

Non-invasive urothelial neoplasms	
Urothelial carcinoma in situ	Flat urothelial lesion with loss of polarity, large irregular hyperchromatic nuclei, mitoses reaching up to upper portion of urothelium; full thickness dysplasia is not required for the diagnosis; precursor for invasive carcinoma
Non-invasive papillary urothelial carcinoma, low grade	Papillary urothelial neoplasm with recognizable variation in architecture and cytology; moderate variation in nuclear size and shape; mitotic activity mainly in the lower half, scattered mitoses in upper half
Non-invasive papillary urothelial carcinoma, high grade	Papillary urothelial neoplasm with marked architectural and cytological atypia, hyperchromatic pleomorphic nuclei, and frequent mitotic figures
Papillary urothelial neoplasm of low malignant potential	Papillary urothelial neoplasm with increased thickness, minimal architectural, and cytological atypia (nuclear enlargement without pleomorphism)
Urothelial papilloma	Exophytic papillary growth of architecturally and cytologically normal urothelium with presence of fibrovascular core
Inverted urothelial papilloma	Inverted growth pattern comprising of trabeculae and anastomosing islands of cytologically normal urothelium, invaginating into lamina propria, but not muscularis propria
Urothelial proliferation of uncertain malignant potential	Increased thickness of urothelium with no cytological atypia and absence of papillary fronds; seen in treated cases of carcinoma or adjacent to carcinoma
Urothelial dysplasia	Flat urothelial lesion with cytological and architectural atypia falling short of CIS
Infiltrating urothelial carcinoma, including divergent differentiation (see Table 10.3)	

few refinements. This revision proposed a uniform terminology, eliminated the ambiguity in the 1973 grading system and redefined a high-grade UC category associated with high risk of progression [25] (Fig. 10.1).

This classification introduced the term papillary urothelial neoplasm of low malignant potential or PUNLMP, for a tumor characterized by very low risk of progression to a muscle invasive disease during its natural history [25]. This category, in most cases, corresponded to the grade 1 tumors of 1973 classification, which was shown by Jordan et al. [36] to have a survival curve similar to age matched noncancer controls. They suggested the term "papilloma" for these tumors; however, due to the genetic evidence of papilloma being a distinct entity and also a small chance of recurrences in these tumors, PUNLMP terminology was introduced [24]. Several studies further reconfirmed the fact that PUNLMP tumors have a low, but definite risk of recurrence as compared to low- and high-grade UCs, and hence, these need to be differentiated from papillomas [37–40]. Few experts have suggested merging PUNLMP and low-grade carcinomas into one category. However, others believe that PUNLMP genuinely exists, and it connotes an extremely low risk (<5%) of progression to invasive cancer in contrast to some low-grade UCs, which are associated with invasive disease. More evidence-based classification systems need to be introduced to deal with the grading of UCs.

10.3.1.4 Comparison of 1973 and 2016 WHO Classification of Urothelial Neoplasms

Currently, world over, the grading system used most frequently by pathologists is the WHO/ISUP 2016 grading system. However, in the European nations, urologists and pathologists favor the usage of WHO 1973 grading/classification in combination with 2016 WHO classification [41]. In a head to head comparison of the two grading system, Ruvolo et al. [42] studied a large cohort 35,986 patients graded according to both 1973 and 2016 classifications in stage Ta bladder cancers. Their study could not demonstrate the superiority of the three-tier grading system of WHO 1973 and found that the grade G2 was not an independent prognostic indicator [43]. Soukup et al. [21] in their study concluded that 2004/2016 WHO classification predicts recurrence and progression better than

1973 system; however, it cannot prognosticate the T1 subgroup. It is well established that the categories of WHO 1973 and WHO 2016 are not completely interchangeable, i.e., G1 does not equate to PUNLMP; G2 with low-grade urothelial carcinoma and G3 with the high-grade category when the two grading systems are compared. The major advantage of the WHO 2016 classification lies in the fact that it places some urothelial cancers of the grade G2 category (3-tier) into the high-grade category (as per the 2-tier grading), which ensures optimal and timely intravesical BCG therapy in such patients and also permits their close surveillance for detecting early recurrences [25].

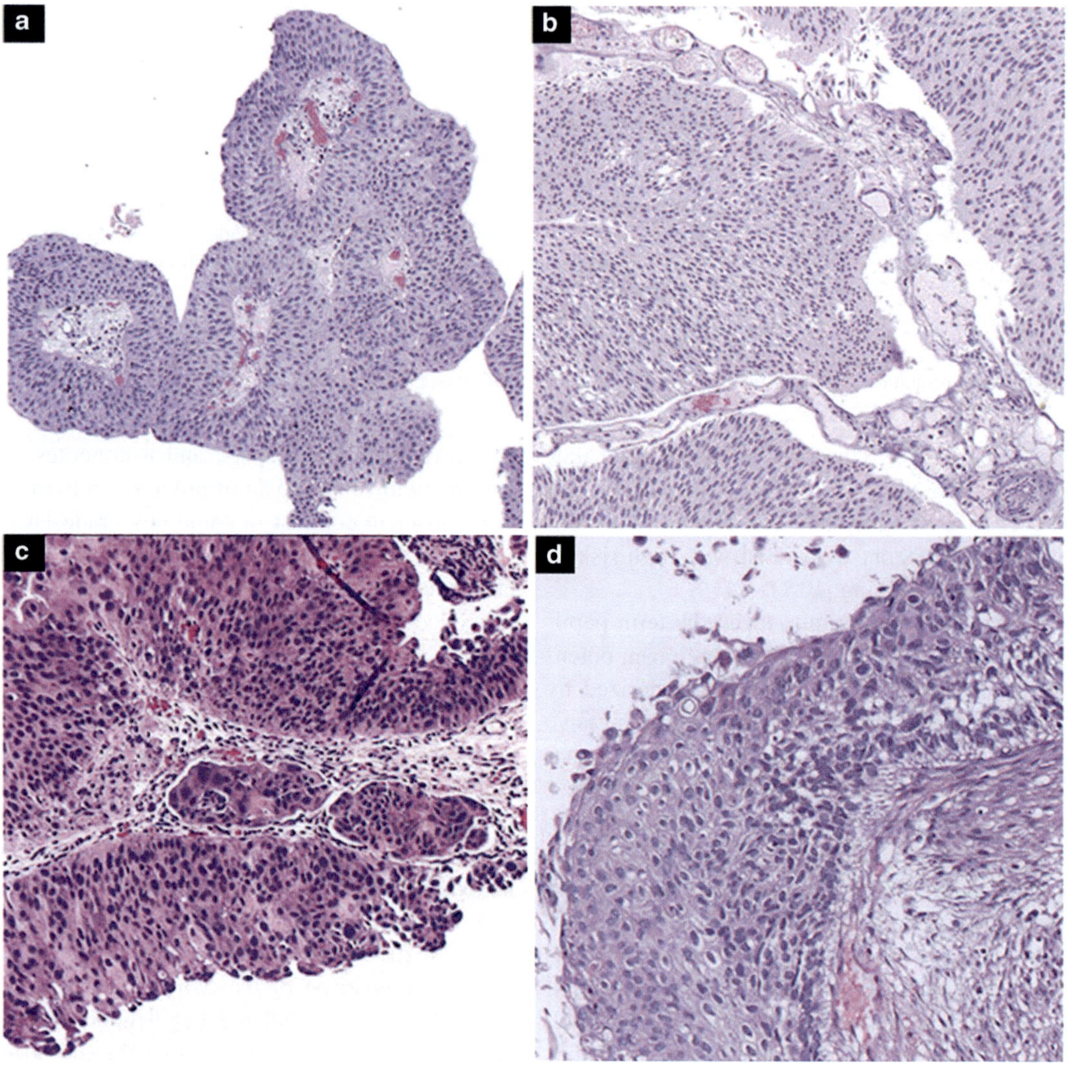

Fig. 10.1 Histopathology of urothelial carcinoma. (**a**) Papillary urothelial neoplasm of uncertain malignant potential; the papillae are lined by multilayered urothelium with preserved cell polarity and minimal to absent atypia (H & E, 100×). (**b**) Low-grade papillary urothelial carcinoma; the urothelium shows recognizable variation in architecture and cytology with mild-to-moderate nuclear atypia (H & E, 100×). (**c**) Lamina propria invasion; small nests of tumor cells seen within the lamina propria with surrounding retraction artefacts (H & E, 200×). (**d**) Urothelial carcinoma in situ; flat urothelial neoplasm with loss of polarity, irregular nuclei and mitosis reaching upto the upper urothelium (H & E, 200×). (**e**) Detrusor muscle invasion by high-grade urothelial carcinoma (H & E, 200×). (**f**) Squamous cell carcinoma (H & E, 200×)

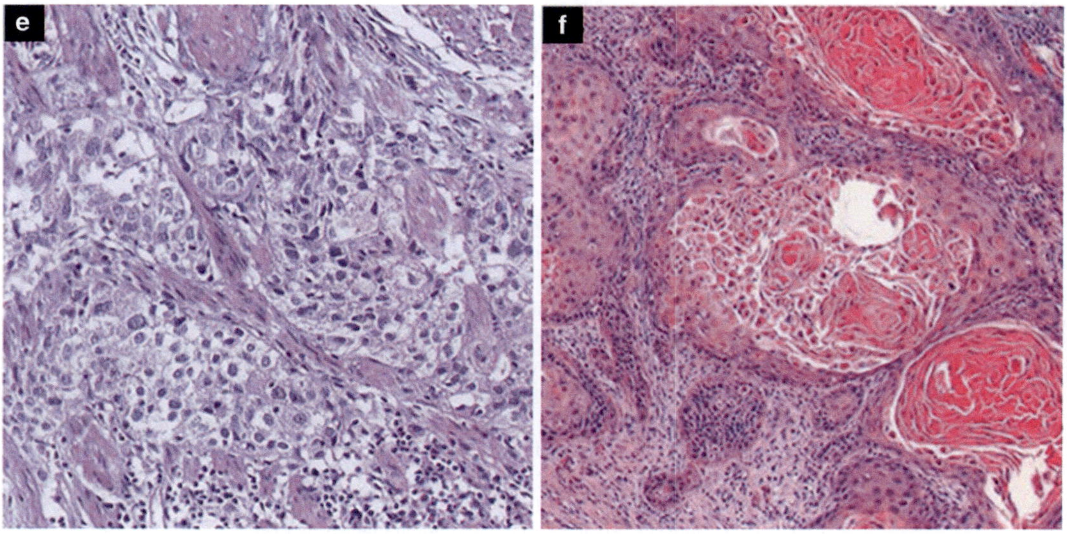

Fig. 10.1 (continued)

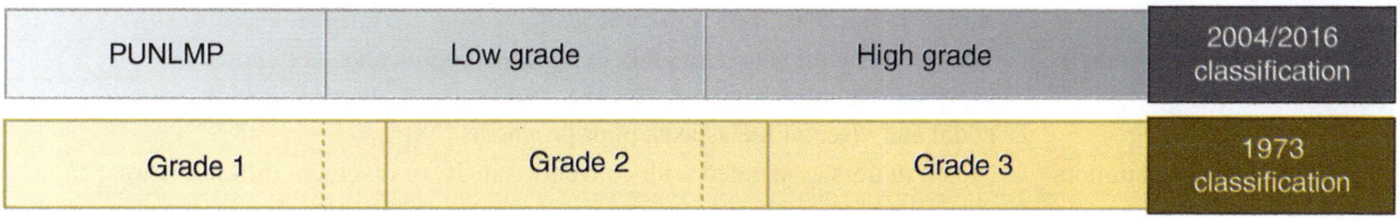

Fig. 10.2 Comparison of the 1973 and 2004/2016 WHO grading systems for urothelial carcinomas. The majority of 1973 grade 1 urothelial carcinomas are grouped into PUNLMP and some into low grade. The grade 2 predominantly comprises of low grade and the lower end of high-grade spectrum. The grade 3 is entirely grouped into high-grade urothelial carcinomas

The two major challenges in the grading systems include tumor heterogeneity and grading spectrum. UC is morphologically and genetically heterogeneous tumor. A single UC can show areas of low grade with intermixed high-grade morphology. The experts recommend the use of a cutoff of 5% high-grade areas to classify a heterogenous urothelial carcinoma as high grade [44]. Further, several experts believe that a tumor can be at the higher end spectrum of a low-grade carcinoma or at the lower end of a high-grade carcinoma. These cases within the continuous spectrum are the most difficult to grade and the WHO 1973 as well as the 2004/2016 have failed to some extent to provide a solution for these. As of now, the approach, as advocated by European Association of Urology (EAU), is to use both the systems simultaneously, which will help in reducing heterogeneity within subcategories and provide an accurate idea of the grade [41] (Fig. 10.2).

10.3.2 Urothelial Carcinoma with Divergent Differentiation and Variants

In the last decade or so, it has been increasingly recognized that there are a few subtypes/variants/divergent differentiations in the high-grade UC category, which may have distinct histomorphology, clinical presentation, behavior, and outcomes. These subtypes are summarized in Table 10.3.

Table 10.3 The histopathological features of UC with divergent differentiation

Squamous differentiation	Presence of intercellular bridges or keratinization; seen in 20% of UC; aggressive biological course and node-positive disease; less responsive to chemotherapy [26, 27]
Glandular differentiation	True glands (tubular, enteric type, mucinous pattern, or signet ring cells); seen in 6% of UC; aggressive disease, less responsive to chemotherapy [28]
Trophoblastic differentiation	Syncytiotrophoblast-like giant cells; β-HCG levels may be elevated and can be used for monitoring; usually high grade and stage [28]
Nested UC	Deceptively bland appearing disorderly arranged nests of urothelial cells; atypia may be present in deeper layers; present at higher stages [29]
Microcystic UC	Bland-looking tumor arranged in micro and macrocysts; no survival difference between conventional and microcystic UC [30]
Micropapillary UC	Small nests and clusters without vascular cores, surrounded by lacunae; associated with UC in 80% cases; aggressive clinical course [31]
Lymphoepithelioma like UC	Nests and sheets of large epithelial cells with prominent nucleoli admixed within prominent lymphoid infiltrate; favorable outcome, respond well to chemotherapy [32]
Plasmacytoid UC	Monomorphic tumor cells with eosinophilic cytoplasm and eccentric nuclei; loss of E-cadherin; advanced stage and nodal metastasis [28]
Giant cell UC	Large bizarre pleomorphic giant cells in sheets and nests; advanced stage and nodal metastasis [33]
Lipid rich UC	Sheets of large cells with eccentrically placed nuclei and vacuolated cytoplasm similar to lipoblast; poor outcome [34]
Clear cell (glycogen rich) UC	Tumor cells with abundant clear cytoplasm; significance not known [35]
Sarcomatoid UC	Morphologically resembles sarcoma; heterologous elements may be present; nodal and visceral metastasis; poor prognosis [28]
Poorly differentiated tumors	Mixed tumors associated with conventional UC or divergent differentiation [28]

10.3.3 Updates by Genitourinary Pathology Society (GUPS), 2021

Recently, the members of GUPS reviewed the nomenclatures of flat and papillary urothelial lesions and considering the diagnostic dilemmas in routine reporting, recommended few new terminologies, which have been tabulated below (Table 10.4) [45]. These may be particularly useful in defining atypical lesions which are often encountered following intravesical BCG therapy, although long-term evidence on the utility, inter and intra-observer variability, and reproducibility in usage of these terms needs to be determined.

The GUPS updates also recommend reporting of noninvasive low-grade papillary urothelial carcinoma with <10% noninvasive high-grade component with a disclaimer regarding lack of sufficient data and studies suggesting their behavior as low-grade tumors. The utility and feasibility of application of these terminologies in routine pathology, especially in the clinical context with outcome data will be determined in future studies [45].

Table 10.4 GUPS recommendations for classification of flat and papillary urothelial neoplasms [45]

"Flat" urothelial lesions	
Atypical urothelial proliferation, flat	Thickened urothelium, no cytologic atypia; absence of true papillae; in isolation, is not associated with urothelial neoplasia
Urothelial dysplasia	Loss of polarity, nuclear enlargement, and chromatin irregularity, falling short of CIS; should be diagnosed with caution
Urothelial carcinoma in situ (CIS)	2016 WHO definition retained
Flat squamous lesions	Focal vs. extensive keratinizing squamous metaplasia or dysplasia; associated with increased risk of progression
Flat glandular lesions	Represent divergent differentiation in urothelial CIS or glandular dysplasia in the background of cystitis glandularis
Papillary urothelial lesions	
Atypical urothelial proliferation, tented	Narrow-based folds of urothelium with thickened layers, lacking fibrovascular cores, complex arborizations, and detached papillae; associated with low-grade papillary urothelial neoplasms
Papillary urothelial neoplasm of low malignant potential	2016 WHO definition retained
Low-grade papillary urothelial carcinoma	2016 WHO definition retained
High-grade papillary urothelial carcinoma	2016 WHO definition retained
Mixed (flat and papillary) and early papillary lesions with cytologic atypia	
Early low-grade papillary urothelial carcinoma	Undulating folds, ill-formed papillae (no definite fibrovascular core), thickened urothelium; low-grade cytological atypia
CIS with early papillary formations	Undulating folds, ill-formed papillae (no definite fibrovascular core), thickened urothelium, high-grade cytological atypia
Tumors with inverted patterns	Inverted PUNLMP, inverted non-invasive papillary urothelial carcinoma, low grade and high grade

10.4 Molecular Pathogenesis of Bladder Cancer

Traditionally, two pathways have been described for the development of bladder cancer: papillary and non-papillary pathways. The low-grade non-muscle invasive bladder cancers (NMIBC) arise through urothelial hyperplasia in the papillary pathway and are associated with frequent recurrences, but less tendency of progression. The high-grade muscle invasive bladder cancers (MIBC) arise through urothelial dysplasia and carcinoma in situ (non-papillary pathway) and are associated with poor prognosis [46] (Fig. 10.3).

Few common molecular alterations in bladder cancers have been elaborated below:

10.4.1 Molecular Alterations in Papillary Pathway (NMIBC)

Activation of RTK/RAS/RAF/MAPK pathway can result from activating mutations in *FGFR3* or *RAS*; hence, these two mutations are reported to be mutually exclusive. *FGFR3* activating mutations are reported in ~80% of low-grade NMIBC, 30% of high grade NMIBC and 10% of MIBC [47, 48]. These mutations have shown significant association with lower recurrence rate and favorable prognosis.

Other common alterations include mutations in PI3K/AKT/mTOR pathway and *TERT* promoter pathway along with copy number alterations in 9p and 9q loci, harboring the *CDKN2A* and *CDKN2B* genes [47, 49–51].

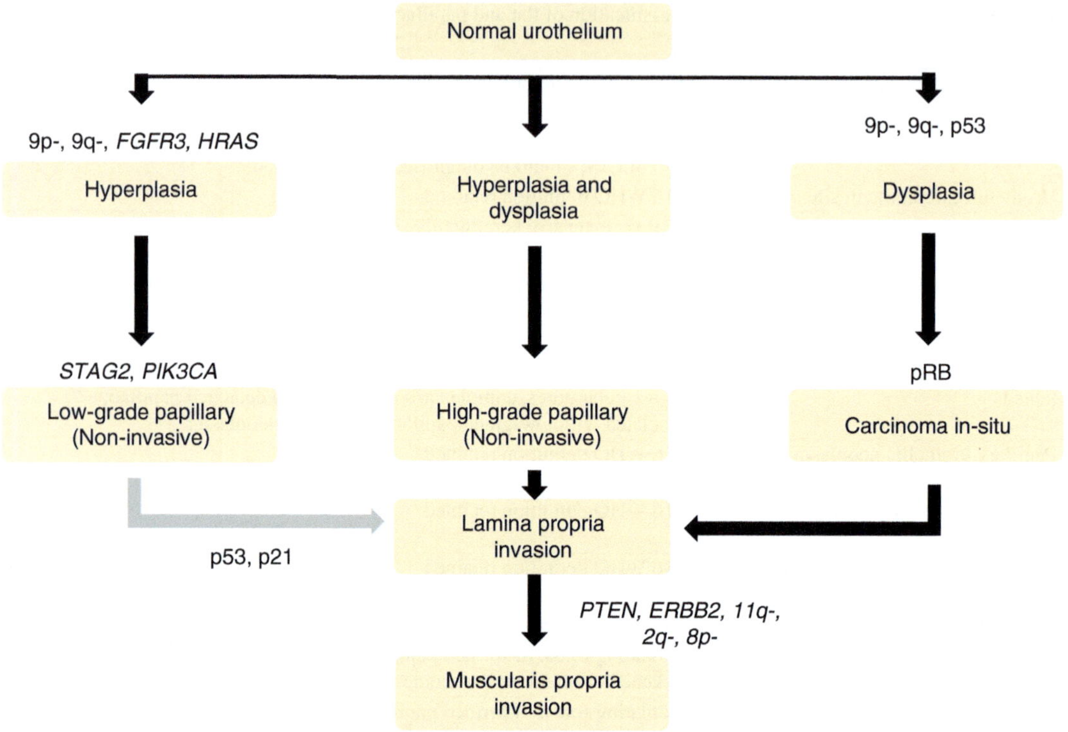

Fig. 10.3 Schematic diagram to show molecular pathways involved in urothelial carcinogenesis

10.4.2 Molecular Alterations in Non-papillary Pathway (MIBC)

TP53 mutations are the most frequently observed alterations in MIBC, present in up to 50%. These have been associated with higher stage and poor prognosis. Similarly, *RB1* inactivation has been associated with higher grade and aggressive clinical course [4, 47, 52, 53].

Defects in DNA repair genes (30% of MIBC) include *ERCC2* as the most commonly altered gene, activating mutations in *EGFR*, amplification of *HER2* are some of the other alterations reported [47, 50].

The Cancer Genome Atlas (TCGA) in the year 2014 identified UC as having extremely high number of alterations, second only to lung cancers. These alterations included 302 mutations, 204 segmental copy number alterations, and 22 rearrangements [47]. In addition, individual researchers have attempted subclassification of bladder cancers on the basis of molecular alterations. Hedegaard et al. [48] classified NMIBC into three classes depending on gene expression studies. Robertson et al. [54] classified T1 high-grade tumors into five molecular subtypes by transcriptomic profiling with significant therapeutic relevance. Robertson et al. [53] also classified MIBC into five molecular subgroups with significantly different survival rates, on transcriptomic profiling. Choi et al. [55], using mRNA expression profiling, proposed a clinically relevant classification system. MIBCs were divided into basal and luminal subtypes akin to breast carcinomas. The basal subgroup, although associated with worse survival, showed excellent response to neoadjuvant chemotherapy, while luminal subgroup is relatively resistant to chemotherapy. A third group comprising of a luminal like tumor was noted with an activated wild-type p53 signature, which was also resistant to neoadjuvant chemotherapy [55]. In an attempt to make this classification affordable, Choi et al. [55] and Rebola et al. [56] proposed the use of immunohistochemistry as a surrogate for molecular classification. In the year 2020, Kamoun et al. [52]

Table 10.5 Consensus molecular classification of MIBC [52]

	Proportion (%)	Immunohistochemistry	Mutations	Potential therapy
Luminal-Papillary (LumP)	24	GATA3, FOXA1 FGFR3, CK20, Uroplakin 2	*FGFR3, KDM6A*	FGFR3 inhibitors, low response to neoadjuvant chemotherapy
Luminal non-specified (LumNS)	8	GATA3, FOXA1 FGFR3, CK20, Uroplakin 2	*ELF3*	Immunotherapy, low response to neoadjuvant chemotherapy
Luminal unstable (LumU)	15	GATA3, FOXA1 FGFR3, CK20, Uroplakin 2	*TP53, ERCC2*	Immunotherapy, neoadjuvant chemotherapy
Stroma rich	15	Vimentin, Desmin, SMA	Not known	Not known
Basal squamous (Ba/sq)	35	CK14, CK5/6, STAT3, Desmoglein	*TP53, RB1*	Immunotherapy, EGFR inhibitors, neoadjuvant chemotherapy
Neuroendocrine like (NE-like)	3	Synaptophysin, chromogranin, INSM1, CD56	*TP53, RB1*	Immunotherapy, combined chemotherapy

derived and developed a consensus molecular classification for bladder cancer based on comprehensive integrative analysis of various other available molecular subgroups and classifications. The various genetic aberrations and the potential targeted therapeutic pathways of these molecular subgroups have been elaborated in Table 10.5.

10.4.3 Utility of Immunohistochemistry (IHC)

Many studies have shown limited utility of IHC in borderline cases. Positivity for CK20 and loss of CD44 have been associated with higher grade tumors [57]. In flat urothelial lesions, diffuse and strong nuclear staining for p53 and full thickness expression of CK20 is diagnostic of carcinoma in situ [58]. Rebola et al. [56] and Choi et al. [55] suggested the use of a 2-marker panel (CK20 and CK5/6) as surrogate for the molecular subtypes of bladder cancer [55, 56]. Ki67, which is a proliferative index marker, has been shown to be useful in diagnosis as well as prognosis in bladder cancers. The most important indication of Ki67 was described by Mallofre et al. [59] in distinguishing reactive urothelial atypia from carcinoma in situ, wherein the latter shows high proliferative index. In grading of UCs, although a steady rise in the percentage of Ki67-positive cells has been reported in PUNLMP, low-grade and high-grade papillary UCs respectively, no standard cutoff values are established, and hence routine use as a stand-alone marker is not recommended. Various studies have studied the prognostic role of Ki67 wherein higher levels of expression in nonmuscle-invasive bladder cancers have been associated with poor prognosis, shorter recurrence rates, and higher chances of progression to muscle-invasive bladder cancers [60–63].

10.5 Staging of Urothelial Neoplasms

Pathological staging is one of the most important prognostic factors in assessment of bladder cancers and aids in the clinical decision making. The staging is based on the extent of tumor invasion into the bladder wall. The staging of bladder cancers follows the American Joint Committee on Cancer (AJCC) 8th edition (TNM 8th) Staging system (Fig. 10.4).

10.5.1 T Stage

10.5.1.1 Stage pT0 Tumors

pT0 stage is designated for no residual viable tumors, post cystectomy, when the biopsy or transurethral resection (TUR) shows muscle

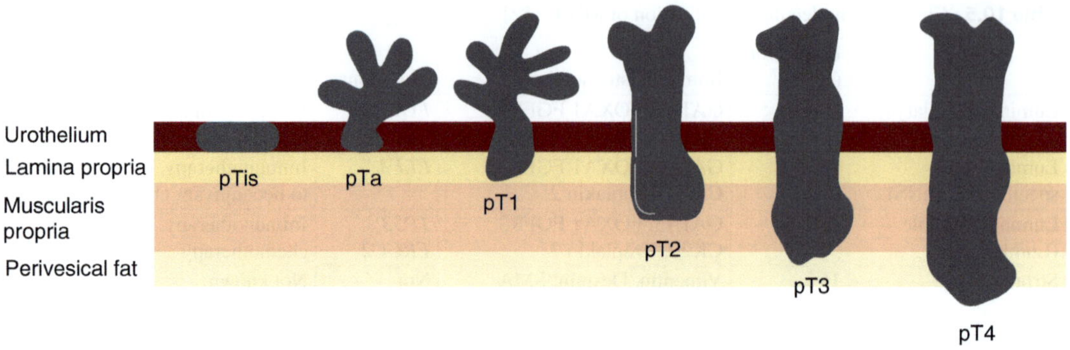

Fig. 10.4 Schematic diagram to show the depth of invasion

invasive bladder cancer. With the increasing use of neoadjuvant chemotherapy (NACT), the incidence of pT0 tumors is steadily rising (~30%). Also, it has been reported in meta-analyses that the patients who achieved complete response post NACT, had better overall and recurrence-free survival than those who did not achieve complete response [64, 65]. Pokuri et al. [66] studied the predictors of response to NACT and concluded that as compared to variant histologies, pure urothelial carcinomas were associated with significantly higher chances of pT0 [66]. In another study, the presence of lymphovascular emboli (LVE) and CIS was significantly associated with reduced overall survival [67].

10.5.1.2 Stage pTa Tumors

For pTa (noninvasive papillary urothelial carcinomas), the histological grade is the most important prognostic factor [68]. In addition, the presence of CIS should also be documented, as it carries a poor prognosis.

10.5.1.3 Stage pTis Tumors

Urothelial CIS is a flat urothelial lesion with urothelial cells showing significant nuclear pleomorphism, hyperchromasia, and increased mitotic activity [25]. It can be present alone or in association with invasive carcinomas, and it carries a poor prognosis in both the scenarios [41]. In a TURBT, presence of extensive CIS in addition to a high-grade papillary urothelial carcinoma may aid in deciding an early cystectomy [5, 41]. Certain features for the diagnosis of CIS in this case include presence of normal urothelium between the CIS and papillary neoplasm, CIS present in an entirely different fragment or CIS being histologically different from papillary tumor [69].

10.5.1.4 Stage pT1 Tumors

Lamina propria (LP) invasion without invasion of muscularis propria (MP) is considered as pT1. The identification of LP invasion has its own challenges. Pseudo invasion can be due tangential sectioning of tissue, thermal artefacts, inflammation induced by the tumor, or involvement of von Brunn nests. On the contrary, invasion can be misinterpreted with certain variants (nested or microcystic variant), wherein the cytology is deceptively bland [69]. Further, various studies have shown significant interobserver variability in diagnosis of LP invasion with complete agreement in 47–80% of cases [70, 71]. A few morphological features that may aid in the diagnosis of LP invasion include [72]:

- Single-cell infiltration or irregular nests
- Disrupted basement membrane contour
- Finger-like extensions from the base of the tumor
- Presence of retraction artefacts around clusters of tumors (these should be differentiated from LVE)
- Paradoxical maturation (the invasive cells contain more eosinophilic cytoplasm or squamoid appearance)
- Stromal response (if present)

In pT1 tumors, the histological grade is a strong prognostic factor; however, studies aimed at analyzing the association of grade and recurrence in pT1 tumors have reported contradicting results [18, 73, 74]. In recent years, the consensus has been to label almost all LP invasive UCs as high grade by default. This is based on the observation that low-grade UC, very rarely, if at all, are invasive in nature.

Since the stage pT1 is heterogeneous encompassing varied histological features, multiple attempts have been made to substage pT1. These mainly fall under two categories: histo-anatomical substaging (invasion above or below muscularis mucosae) or linear depth based substaging (depth of invasion cutoff 3 mm). Both the systems have their own pros and cons including difficulty in assessment of true muscularis mucosae in the former and the agreement on a true cutoff in the latter) [69]. Hence, at present, the AJCC 8th edition does not recommend substaging of pT1 tumors. Although not yet a standard, some experts document the presence of microinvasive carcinoma (depth < 2 mm) [75], particularly in cases with CIS, as it is associated with significant increase in lymph nodal metastasis and poor prognosis.

10.5.1.5 Stage pT2 Tumors

pT2 is characterized by tumor invading the muscularis propria. The identification of MP and its distinction from muscularis mucosae can be an extremely difficult task in TUR specimens. Beukers et al. [76] reported a 26% rate of downstaging of tumor in cystectomy because of misinterpretation of MP invasion. Hyperplastic muscularis mucosae can simulate MP. The distinction between the two can be made:

- Morphologically: Muscularis mucosae is thin wispy muscle fibers in lamina propria associated with thick-walled vessels and MP include large smooth muscle bundles with rounded contours.
- Immunohistochemistry: Smoothelin can help in distinguishing between the two, as MP shows staining for the marker [77].

The AJCC 8th edition has further divided pT2 into pT2a (invasion of superficial MP) and pT2b (invasion of deep MP). Various studies assessing the survival advantage of this subdivision have yielded contradictory results [78–86].

10.5.1.6 Stage pT3 Tumors

pT3 tumors are defined as invasion into the perivesical soft tissue beyond MP. The assessment of this feature is extremely unreliable in biopsy or TUR specimens, as adipose tissue can be present in the LP as well as in the MP [69]. In cystectomy specimens also, the arrangement of MP can be irregular and in cases with NACT, complicated by diffuse therapy-related changes.

The subdivision of pT3 into pT3a and pT3b has been controversial in the literature with studies showing no definite survival benefit and vice versa [87–94]. The assessment of macroscopic tumor extension is highly dependent on the awareness of the grossing personnel. In addition, the gross assessment can be particular difficult in cases with NACT [69].

10.5.1.7 Stage pT4 Tumors

pT4 tumors include extension beyond the perivesical fat into adjacent organs (pT4a) or the pelvic/abdominal wall (pT4b).

Prostatic invasion by UC is seen in 7–38% of radical cystoprostatectomy specimens [69]. Prostatic invasion has been defined in three ways:

- Intraurethral: Spread along the prostatic urethra, further invading into prostatic stroma
- Extravesical: Invasion into the extravesical fat, back into prostate
- Bladder neck: Through the bladder neck into prostate

The AJCC 8th edition considers the latter two conditions as pT4a. For intraurethral spread of tumor, the AJCC recommends a two-stage system for the bladder tumor and the prostatic urethral tumor [69]. It is important to differentiate these spreads, as direct invasion of prostate has been shown to confer worse prognosis than a prostatic urethral tumor invading the prostate [95–99]. Similarly, seminal vesical invasion has been reported to confer a poor prognosis after radical cystoprostatectomy [100].

Direct tumor extension into the vagina or uterus is rare and is reported in 3–6% of radical cystectomies [69]. This finding has been shown to be associated with worse prognosis [101].

Invasion of the pelvic/abdominal wall is rare, seen in 2% of all resections [69]. As expected, pT4b stage is associated with extremely worse prognosis [102].

10.5.2 N Stage

- Regional lymph nodes: Perivesical, iliac (internal and external), obturator, common iliac, and sacral.
- Extranodal extension should be documented.
- No definite criteria on minimum number of lymph nodes to be dissected, with different studies using different cutoffs [103–105]

10.5.3 M Stage

M1 is subdivided into M1a (lymph nodes beyond common iliac) and M1b (non-nodal metastasis) as the latter is associated with relatively worser outcomes than the former [106].

10.6 Conclusion

Urothelial neoplasms are extremely heterogeneous in both histomorphology and at the molecular level. Accurate pathological grading and staging are necessary for optimal patient management. The grading systems will continue to evolve, as the molecular pathways of these neoplasms are unraveled.

References

1. Siegel RL, Miller KD, Fuchs HE, Jemal A. Cancer statistics, 2021. CA Cancer J Clin. 2021;71:7–33.
2. Saginala K, Barsouk A, Aluru JS, Rawla P, Padala SA, Barsouk A. Epidemiology of bladder cancer. Med Sci (Basel). 2020;8:15.
3. Indian Council of Medical Research. Projection of cancer cases in India. New Delhi: Indian Council of Medical Research; 2020.
4. Grignon DJAF, Epstein J. Urothelial tumours. In: Holger M, Humphrey PA, Ulbright TM, Reuter VE, editors. Tumours of the urinary tract. 4th ed. Lyon: IARC; 2016.
5. Flaig TW, Spiess PE, Agarwal N, Bangs R, Boorjian SA, Buyyounouski MK, et al. Bladder cancer, version 3.2020, NCCN clinical practice guidelines in oncology. J Natl Compr Canc Netw. 2020;18:329–54.
6. Freedman ND, Silverman DT, Hollenbeck AR, Schatzkin A, Abnet CC. Association between smoking and risk of bladder cancer among men and women. JAMA. 2011;306:737–45.
7. Golka K, Wiese A, Assennato G, Bolt HM. Occupational exposure and urological cancer. World J Urol. 2004;21:382–91.
8. Shih C-J, Chen Y-T, Ou S-M, Yang W-C, Chen T-J, Tarng D-C. Urinary calculi and risk of cancer: a nationwide population-based study. Medicine (Baltimore). 2014;93:e342.
9. Jones TD, Wang M, Eble JN, MacLennan GT, Lopez-Beltran A, Zhang S, et al. Molecular evidence supporting field effect in urothelial carcinogenesis. Clin Cancer Res. 2005;11:6512–9.
10. Cheng L, Davidson DD, Maclennan GT, Williamson SR, Zhang S, Koch MO, et al. The origins of urothelial carcinoma. Expert Rev Anticancer Ther. 2010;10:865–80.
11. Cheng L, Zhang S, MacLennan GT, Williamson SR, Lopez-Beltran A, Montironi R. Bladder cancer: translating molecular genetic insights into clinical practice. Hum Pathol. 2011;42:455–81.
12. Koss LG, Tiamson EM, Robbins MA. Mapping cancerous and precancerous bladder changes. A study of the urothelium in ten surgically removed bladders. JAMA. 1974;227:281–6.
13. Sidransky D, Frost P, Von Eschenbach A, Oyasu R, Preisinger AC, Vogelstein B. Clonal origin of bladder cancer. N Engl J Med. 1992;326:737–40.
14. Habuchi T, Takahashi R, Yamada H, Kakehi Y, Sugiyama T, Yoshida O. Metachronous multifocal development of urothelial cancers by intraluminal seeding. Lancet. 1993;342:1087–8.
15. Takahashi T, Habuchi T, Kakehi Y, Mitsumori K, Akao T, Terachi T, et al. Clonal and chronological genetic analysis of multifocal cancers of the bladder and upper urinary tract. Cancer Res. 1998;58:5835–41.
16. Fadl-Elmula I, Gorunova L, Mandahl N, Elfving P, Lundgren R, Mitelman F, et al. Cytogenetic monoclonality in multifocal uroepithelial carcinomas: evidence of intraluminal tumour seeding. Br J Cancer. 1999;81:6–12.
17. Mostofi FK. Histological typing of urinary bladder tumors, International histological classification of tumors, vol. 17. Geneva: WHO; 1973.
18. Otto W, Denzinger S, Fritsche HM, Burger M, Wieland WF, Hofstädter F, et al. The WHO classification of 1973 is more suitable than the WHO classification of 2004 for predicting survival in pT1 urothelial bladder cancer. BJU Int. 2011;107:404–8.
19. Chen Z, Ding W, Xu K, Tan J, Sun C, Gou Y, et al. The 1973 WHO classification is more suitable than the 2004 WHO classification for predicting prog-

nosis in non-muscle-invasive bladder cancer. PLoS One. 2012;7:e47199.
20. Compérat E, Burger M, Gontero P, Mostafid AH, Palou J, Rouprêt M, et al. Grading of urothelial carcinoma and the new "World Health Organisation classification of tumours of the urinary system and male genital organs 2016". Eur Urol Focus. 2019;5:457–66.
21. Soukup V, Čapoun O, Cohen D, Hernández V, Babjuk M, Burger M, et al. Prognostic performance and reproducibility of the 1973 and 2004/2016 World Health Organization grading classification Systems in non-muscle-invasive Bladder Cancer: a European Association of Urology non-muscle invasive bladder cancer guidelines panel systematic review. Eur Urol. 2017;72:801–13.
22. Bosschieter J, Hentschel A, Savci-Heijink CD, Patrick van der Voorn J, Rozendaal L, Vis AN, et al. Reproducibility and prognostic performance of the 1973 and 2004 World Health Organization classifications for grade in non-muscle-invasive bladder cancer: a multicenter study in 328 bladder tumors. Clin Genitourin Cancer. 2018;16:e985–e92.
23. Pauwels RP, Schapers RF, Smeets AW, Debruyne FM, Geraedts JP. Grading in superficial bladder cancer. (1). Morphological criteria. Br J Urol. 1988;61:129–34.
24. Epstein JI, Amin MB, Reuter VR, Mostofi FK, Committee TBCC. The World Health Organization/ International Society of Urological Pathology Consensus Classification of Urothelial (transitional cell) neoplasms of the urinary bladder. Am J Surg Pathol. 1998;22:1435–48.
25. Humphrey PA, Moch H, Cubilla AL, Ulbright TM, Reuter VE. The 2016 WHO classification of tumours of the urinary system and male genital organs-part B: prostate and bladder tumours. Eur Urol. 2016;70:106–19.
26. Roehrborn CG, Sagalowsky AI, Peters PC. Long-term patient survival after cystectomy for regional metastatic transitional cell carcinoma of the bladder. J Urol. 1991;146:36–9.
27. Pollack A, Zagars GK, Cole CJ, Dinney CP, Swanson DA, Grossman HB. The relationship of local control to distant metastasis in muscle invasive bladder cancer. J Urol. 1995;154:2059–64.
28. Lopez-Beltran A, Cheng L. Histologic variants of urothelial carcinoma: differential diagnosis and clinical implications. Hum Pathol. 2006;37:1371–88.
29. Drew PA, Furman J, Civantos F, Murphy WM. The nested variant of transitional cell carcinoma: an aggressive neoplasm with innocuous histology. Mod Pathol. 1996;9:989–94.
30. Lopez Beltran A, Montironi R, Cheng L. Microcystic urothelial carcinoma: morphology, immunohistochemistry and clinical behaviour. Histopathology. 2014;64:872–9.
31. Johansson SL, Borghede G, Holmäng S. Micropapillary bladder carcinoma: a clinicopathological study of 20 cases. J Urol. 1999;161:1798–802.
32. Williamson SR, Zhang S, Lopez-Beltran A, Shah RB, Montironi R, Tan PH, et al. Lymphoepithelioma-like carcinoma of the urinary bladder: clinicopathologic, immunohistochemical, and molecular features. Am J Surg Pathol. 2011;35:474–83.
33. Lopez-Beltran A, Blanca A, Montironi R, Cheng L, Regueiro JC. Pleomorphic giant cell carcinoma of the urinary bladder. Hum Pathol. 2009;40:1461–6.
34. Lopez-Beltran A, Amin MB, Oliveira PS, Montironi R, Algaba F, McKenney JK, et al. Urothelial carcinoma of the bladder, lipid cell variant: clinicopathologic findings and LOH analysis. Am J Surg Pathol. 2010;34:371–6.
35. Kotliar SN, Wood CG, Schaeffer AJ, Oyasu R. Transitional cell carcinoma exhibiting clear cell features. A differential diagnosis for clear cell adenocarcinoma of the urinary tract. Arch Pathol Lab Med. 1995;119:79–81.
36. Jordan AM, Weingarten J, Murphy WM. Transitional cell neoplasms of the urinary bladder. Can biologic potential be predicted from histologic grading? Cancer. 1987;60:2766–74.
37. Holmäng S, Hedelin H, Anderström C, Holmberg E, Busch C, Johansson SL. Recurrence and progression in low grade papillary urothelial tumors. J Urol. 1999;162:702–7.
38. Holmäng S, Andius P, Hedelin H, Wester K, Busch C, Johansson SL. Stage progression in ta papillary urothelial tumors: relationship to grade, immunohistochemical expression of tumor markers, mitotic frequency and DNA ploidy. J Urol. 2001;165:1124–8.
39. Pan CC, Chang YH, Chen KK, Yu HJ, Sun CH, Ho DM. Prognostic significance of the 2004 WHO/ ISUP classification for prediction of recurrence, progression, and cancer-specific mortality of non-muscle-invasive urothelial tumors of the urinary bladder: a clinicopathologic study of 1,515 cases. Am J Clin Pathol. 2010;133:788–95.
40. Maxwell JP, Wang C, Wiebe N, Yilmaz A, Trpkov K. Long-term outcome of primary papillary urothelial neoplasm of low malignant potential (PUNLMP) including PUNLMP with inverted growth. Diagn Pathol. 2015;10:3.
41. Babjuk M, Böhle A, Burger M, Capoun O, Cohen D, Compérat EM, et al. EAU guidelines on non–muscle-invasive urothelial carcinoma of the bladder: update 2016. Eur Urol. 2017;71:447–61.
42. Collà Ruvolo C, Würnschimmel C, Wenzel M, Nocera L, Califano G, Tian Z, et al. Comparison between 1973 and 2004/2016 WHO grading systems in patients with ta urothelial carcinoma of urinary bladder. J Clin Pathol. 2022;75:333–7.
43. Collà Ruvolo C, Würnschimmel C, Wenzel M, Nocera L, Celentano G, Mangiapia F, et al. Comparison between 1973 and 2004/2016 World Health Organization grading in upper tract urothelial carcinoma treated with radical nephroureterectomy. Int J Clin Oncol. 2021;26:1707–13.
44. Reis LO, Taheri D, Chaux A, Guner G, Mendoza Rodriguez MA, Bivalacqua TJ, et al. Significance of

a minor high-grade component in a low-grade non-invasive papillary urothelial carcinoma of bladder. Hum Pathol. 2016;47:20–5.
45. Amin MB, Comperat E, Epstein JI, True LD, Hansel D, Paner GP, et al. The genitourinary pathology society update on classification and grading of flat and papillary urothelial neoplasia with new reporting recommendations and approach to lesions with mixed and early patterns of neoplasia. Adv Anat Pathol. 2021;28:179–95.
46. Jones PA, Droller MJ. Pathways of development and progression in bladder cancer: new correlations between clinical observations and molecular mechanisms. Semin Urol. 1993;11:177–92.
47. The Cancer Genome Atlas Research Network. Comprehensive molecular characterization of urothelial bladder carcinoma. Nature. 2014;507:315–22.
48. Hedegaard J, Lamy P, Nordentoft I, Algaba F, Høyer S, Ulhøi BP, et al. Comprehensive transcriptional analysis of early-stage urothelial carcinoma. Cancer Cell. 2016;30:27–42.
49. Platt FM, Hurst CD, Taylor CF, Gregory WM, Harnden P, Knowles MA. Spectrum of phosphatidylinositol 3-kinase pathway gene alterations in bladder cancer. Clin Cancer Res. 2009;15:6008–17.
50. Minoli M, Kiener M, Thalmann GN, Kruithof-de Julio M, Seiler R. Evolution of urothelial bladder cancer in the context of molecular classifications. Int J Mol Sci. 2020;21:5670.
51. Meeks JJ, Carneiro BA, Pai SG, Oberlin DT, Rademaker A, Fedorchak K, et al. Genomic characterization of high-risk non-muscle invasive bladder cancer. Oncotarget. 2016;7:75176–84.
52. Kamoun A, de Reyniès A, Allory Y, Sjödahl G, Robertson AG, Seiler R, et al. A consensus molecular classification of muscle-invasive bladder cancer. Eur Urol. 2020;77:420–33.
53. Robertson AG, Kim J, Al-Ahmadie H, Bellmunt J, Guo G, Cherniack AD, et al. Comprehensive molecular characterization of muscle-invasive bladder cancer. Cell. 2017;171:540–56.e25.
54. Robertson AG, Groeneveld CS, Jordan B, Lin X, McLaughlin KA, Das A, et al. Identification of differential tumor subtypes of T1 bladder cancer. Eur Urol. 2020;78:533–7.
55. Choi W, Porten S, Kim S, Willis D, Plimack ER, Hoffman-Censits J, et al. Identification of distinct basal and luminal subtypes of muscle-invasive bladder cancer with different sensitivities to frontline chemotherapy. Cancer Cell. 2014;25:152–65.
56. Rebola J, Aguiar P, Blanca A, Montironi R, Cimadamore A, Cheng L, et al. Predicting outcomes in non-muscle invasive (ta/T1) bladder cancer: the role of molecular grade based on luminal/basal phenotype. Virchows Arch. 2019;475:445–55.
57. Desai S, Dug Lim S, Jimenez RE, Chun T, Keane TE, McKenney JK, et al. Relationship of cytokeratin 20 and CD44 protein expression with WHO/ISUP grade in pTa and pT1 papillary urothelial neoplasia. Mod Pathol. 2000;13:1315–23.
58. McKenney JK, Amin MB. The role of immunohistochemistry in the diagnosis of urinary bladder neoplasms. Semin Diagn Pathol. 2005;22:69–87.
59. Mallofré C, Castillo M, Morente V, Solé M. Immunohistochemical expression of CK20, p53, and Ki-67 as objective markers of urothelial dysplasia. Mod Pathol. 2003;16:187–91.
60. Compérat E, Camparo P, Haus R, Chartier-Kastler E, Radenen B, Richard F, et al. Aurora-a/STK-15 is a predictive factor for recurrent behaviour in non-invasive bladder carcinoma: a study of 128 cases of non-invasive neoplasms. Virchows Arch. 2007;450:419–24.
61. van Rhijn BWG, Zuiverloon TCM, Vis AN, Radvanyi F, van Leenders GJLH, Ooms BCM, et al. Molecular grade (FGFR3/MIB-1) and EORTC risk scores are predictive in primary non–muscle-invasive bladder cancer. Eur Urol. 2010;58(3):433–41.
62. Burger M, van der Aa MN, van Oers JM, Brinkmann A, van der Kwast TH, Steyerberg EC, et al. Prediction of progression of non-muscle-invasive bladder cancer by WHO 1973 and 2004 grading and by FGFR3 mutation status: a prospective study. Eur Urol. 2008;54:835–43.
63. Missaoui N, Bdioui A, Baccouche A, Belkacem O, Hmida W, Mokni M, et al. Significance of p53, p27, Ki-67, E-cadherin, and HER2 expression in upper urinary tract urothelial carcinoma. J Egypt Natl Canc Inst. 2020;32:36.
64. Petrelli F, Coinu A, Cabiddu M, Ghilardi M, Vavassori I, Barni S. Correlation of pathologic complete response with survival after neoadjuvant chemotherapy in bladder cancer treated with cystectomy: a meta-analysis. Eur Urol. 2014;65:350–7.
65. Lavery HJ, Stensland KD, Niegisch G, Albers P, Droller MJ. Pathological T0 following radical cystectomy with or without neoadjuvant chemotherapy: a useful surrogate. J Urol. 2014;191:898–906.
66. Pokuri VK, Syed JR, Yang Z, Field EP, Cyriac S, Pili R, et al. Predictors of complete pathologic response (pT0) to neoadjuvant chemotherapy in muscle-invasive bladder carcinoma. Clin Genitourin Cancer. 2016;14:e59–65.
67. Kassouf W, Spiess PE, Brown GA, Munsell MF, Grossman HB, Siefker-Radtke A, et al. P0 stage at radical cystectomy for bladder cancer is associated with improved outcome independent of traditional clinical risk factors. Eur Urol. 2007;52:769–74.
68. MacLennan GT, Kirkali Z, Cheng L. Histologic grading of noninvasive papillary urothelial neoplasms. Eur Urol. 2007;51:889–98.
69. Magers MJ, Lopez-Beltran A, Montironi R, Williamson SR, Kaimakliotis HZ, Cheng L. Staging of bladder cancer. Histopathology. 2019;74:112–34.
70. Tosoni I, Wagner U, Sauter G, Egloff M, Knönagel H, Alund G, et al. Clinical significance of interobserver differences in the staging and grading of superficial bladder cancer. BJU Int. 2000;85:48–53.
71. Bol MG, Baak JP, Buhr-Wildhagen S, Kruse AJ, Kjellevold KH, Janssen EA, et al. Reproducibility

and prognostic variability of grade and lamina propria invasion in stages ta, T1 urothelial carcinoma of the bladder. J Urol. 2003;169:1291–4.
72. Lopez-Beltran A, Cheng L. Stage pT1 bladder carcinoma: diagnostic criteria, pitfalls and prognostic significance. Pathology. 2003;35:484–91.
73. Cao D, Vollmer RT, Luly J, Jain S, Roytman TM, Ferris CW, et al. Comparison of 2004 and 1973 World Health Organization grading systems and their relationship to pathologic staging for predicting long-term prognosis in patients with urothelial carcinoma. Urology. 2010;76:593–9.
74. van Rhijn BW, van Leenders GJ, Ooms BC, Kirkels WJ, Zlotta AR, Boevé ER, et al. The pathologist's mean grade is constant and individualizes the prognostic value of bladder cancer grading. Eur Urol. 2010;57:1052–7.
75. McKenney JK, Gomez JA, Desai S, Lee MW, Amin MB. Morphologic expressions of urothelial carcinoma in situ: a detailed evaluation of its histologic patterns with emphasis on carcinoma in situ with microinvasion. Am J Surg Pathol. 2001;25:356–62.
76. Beukers W, Meijer T, Vissers CJ, Boormans JL, Zwarthoff EC, van Leenders GJLH. Down-staging (<pT2) of urothelial cancer at cystectomy after the diagnosis of detrusor muscle invasion (pT2) at diagnostic transurethral resection (TUR): is prediction possible? Virchows Arch. 2012;461:149–56.
77. Fernandez N, Zhai Q. The value of smoothelin to determine invasion depth of urothelial carcinoma by differentiating hyperplastic muscularis mucosa from muscularispropia. Am J Clin Pathol. 2012;138:A342.
78. Jewett HJ. Carcinoma of the bladder: influence of depth of infiltration on the 5-year results following complete extirpation of the primary growth. J Urol. 1952;67:672–80.
79. Herr HW. Staging invasive bladder tumors. J Surg Oncol. 1992;51:217–20.
80. Hall RR, Prout GR. Staging of bladder cancer: is the tumor, node, metastasis system adequate? Semin Oncol. 1990;17:517–23.
81. Skinner DG. Current state of classification and staging of bladder cancer. Cancer Res. 1977;37:2838–42.
82. Tokgoz H, Türkölmez K, Resorlu B, Kose K, Tulunay O, Beduk Y. Pathological staging of muscle invasive bladder cancer. Is substaging of pT2 tumors really necessary? Int Braz J Urol. 2007;33:777–83.
83. Boudreaux KJ Jr, Clark PE, Lowrance WT, Rumohr JA, Barocas DA, Cookson MS, et al. Comparison of american joint committee on cancer pathological stage T2a versus T2b urothelial carcinoma: analysis of patient outcomes in organ confined bladder cancer. J Urol. 2009;181:540–6.
84. Tilki D, Reich O, Karakiewicz PI, Novara G, Kassouf W, Ergün S, et al. Validation of the AJCC TNM substaging of pT2 bladder cancer: deep muscle invasion is associated with significantly worse outcome. Eur Urol. 2010;58:112–7.
85. Sonpavde G, Khan MM, Svatek RS, Lee R, Novara G, Tilki D, et al. Prognostic risk stratification of pathological stage T2N0 bladder cancer after radical cystectomy. BJU Int. 2011;108:687–92.
86. Gakis G, Schilling D, Renninger M, Seibold J, Sievert KD, Stenzl A. Comparison of the new American joint Committee on cancer substratification in node-negative pT2 urothelial carcinoma of the bladder: analysis of patient outcomes in a contemporary series. BJU Int. 2011;107:919–23.
87. Quek ML, Stein JP, Clark PE, Daneshmand S, Miranda G, Cai J, et al. Microscopic and gross extravesical extension in pathological staging of bladder cancer. J Urol. 2004;171:640–5.
88. Boudreaux KJ Jr, Chang SS, Lowrance WT, Rumohr JA, Barocas DA, Cookson MS, et al. Comparison of American joint Committee on cancer pathologic stage T3a versus T3b urothelial carcinoma: analysis of patient outcomes. Cancer. 2009;115:770–5.
89. Dincel C, Kara C, Balci U, Ozer K, Ozbir S, Sefik E, et al. Comparison of microscopic (pT3a) and gross extravesical extension (pT3b) in pathological staging of bladder cancer: analysis of patient outcomes. Int Urol Nephrol. 2013;45:387–93.
90. Scosyrev E, Yao J, Messing E. Microscopic invasion of perivesical fat by urothelial carcinoma: implications for prognosis and pathology practice. Urology. 2010;76:908–14.
91. Neuzillet Y, Lebret T, Molinie V, Yonneau L, Herve J-M, Theodore C, et al. Perivesical fat invasion in bladder cancer: implications for prognosis comparing pT2b, pT3a and pT3b stages and consequences for adjuvant chemotherapy indications. BJU Int. 2012;110:1736–41.
92. Bastian PJ, Hutterer GC, Shariat SF, Rogers CG, Palapattu GS, Lotan Y, et al. Macroscopic, but not microscopic, perivesical fat invasion at radical cystectomy is an adverse predictor of recurrence and survival. BJU Int. 2008;101:450–4.
93. Philip AT, Amin MB, Tamboli P, Lee TJ, Hill CE, Ro JY. Intravesical adipose tissue: a quantitative study of its presence and location with implications for therapy and prognosis. Am J Surg Pathol. 2000;24:1286–90.
94. Tilki D, Svatek RS, Karakiewicz PI, Novara G, Seitz M, Sonpavde G, et al. pT3 substaging is a prognostic indicator for lymph node negative urothelial carcinoma of the bladder. J Urol. 2010;184:470–4.
95. Esrig D, Freeman JA, Elmajian DA, Stein JP, Chen SC, Groshen S, et al. Transitional cell carcinoma involving the prostate with a proposed staging classification for stromal invasion. J Urol. 1996;156:1071–6.
96. Knoedler JJ, Boorjian SA, Tollefson MK, Cheville JC, Thapa P, Tarrell RF, et al. Urothelial carcinoma involving the prostate: the association of revised tumour stage and coexistent bladder cancer with survival after radical cystectomy. BJU Int. 2014;114:832–6.
97. NjinouNgninkeu B, Lorge F, Moulin P, Jamart J, Van Cangh PJ. Transitional cell carcinoma involving the

prostate: a clinicopathological retrospective study of 76 cases. J Urol. 2003;169:149–52.
98. Ayyathurai R, Gomez P, Luongo T, Soloway MS, Manoharan M. Prostatic involvement by urothelial carcinoma of the bladder: clinicopathological features and outcome after radical cystectomy. BJU Int. 2007;100:1021–5.
99. Vallo S, Gilfrich C, Burger M, Volkmer B, Boehm K, Rink M, et al. Comparative analysis of the effect of prostatic invasion patterns on cancer-specific mortality after radical cystectomy in pT4a urothelial carcinoma of the bladder. Urol Oncol. 2016;34:432.e1–8.
100. Daneshmand S, Stein JP, Lesser T, Quek ML, Nichols PW, Miranda G, et al. Prognosis of seminal vesicle involvement by transitional cell carcinoma of the bladder. J Urol. 2004;172:81–4.
101. May M, Bastian PJ, Brookman-May S, Fritsche HM, Tilki D, Otto W, et al. Gender-specific differences in cancer-specific survival after radical cystectomy for patients with urothelial carcinoma of the urinary bladder in pathologic tumor stage T4a. Urol Oncol. 2013;31:1141–7.
102. Liberman D, Alasker A, Sun M, Ismail S, Lughezzani G, Jeldres C, et al. Radical cystectomy for patients with pT4 urothelial carcinoma in a large population-based study. BJU Int. 2011;107:905–11.
103. Pedrosa JA, Koch MO, Cheng L. Lymph node-positive bladder cancer: surgical, pathologic, molecular and prognostic aspects. Expert Rev Anticancer Ther. 2013;13:1281–95.
104. Herr HW, Bochner BH, Dalbagni G, Donat SM, Reuter VE, Bajorin DF. Impact of the number of lymph nodes retrieved on outcome in patients with muscle invasive bladder cancer. J Urol. 2002;167:1295–8.
105. Wright JL, Lin DW, Porter MP. The association between extent of lymphadenectomy and survival among patients with lymph node metastases undergoing radical cystectomy. Cancer. 2008;112:2401–8.
106. Galsky MD, Moshier E, Krege S, Lin CC, Hahn N, Ecke T, et al. Nomogram for predicting survival in patients with unresectable and/or metastatic urothelial cancer who are treated with cisplatin-based chemotherapy. Cancer. 2013;119:3012–9.

Management of Non-Muscle Invasive Bladder Cancer

11

Subodh K. Regmi

11.1 Background

Bladder cancer is the ninth most common cancer in the world with almost 430,000 new cases seen in 2012 [1]. A strong male preponderance is seen worldwide and interestingly 60% of the cases and 50% of the deaths occur in less developed countries. Considering the fact that more than 75% of these are nonmuscle invasive bladder cancer (NMIBC) at presentation [2], bladder cancer does represent a significant burden in terms of the continuity of care that is required with respect to surveillance strategies and intravesical therapies.

It is important to realize that NMIBC is not a single entity and represents a clinically and pathologically variable spectrum of superficial bladder cancer. It is, therefore, our prerogative to highlight the unique pathological and clinical differences and focus on management strategies specific to the risk-based stratification of these unique entities.

Over the years, there have been several advancements in the surgical management, adjuvant/intravesical treatment, as well as surveillance strategies. The basic tenet of managing NMIBC is central to the guiding principle of prevention and early detection of muscle-invasive bladder cancer, which is associated with significant disease andtreatment-related adverse effects.

11.2 Initial Presentation and Management

Presentation of most bladder cancer whether superficial or deep is similar. Atypical presentation is sometimes seen, and a high index of suspicion is necessary to avoid a missed opportunity at early diagnosis and treatment.

11.2.1 Presentation

The most common presentation is with gross visible hematuria. Microscopic hematuria, irritative urinary symptoms, and incidental diagnosis at cross-sectional imaging or pelvic ultrasound are other less common presentations. About 12% of hematuria workups result in a diagnosis of bladder cancer with the incidence being higher for gross (18.9%) than microscopic hematuria (4.8%) [3].

11.2.2 Initial Workup

The initial workup of patients with gross hematuria is well defined: cross-sectional imaging with contrast for evaluation of the upper urinary tract, urine cytol-

S. K. Regmi (✉)
Department of Urology, University of Minnesota, Minneapolis, MN, USA
e-mail: regmi014@umn.edu

P. Singh et al. (eds.), *A Guide to Management of Urological Cancers*,
https://doi.org/10.1007/978-981-99-2341-0_11

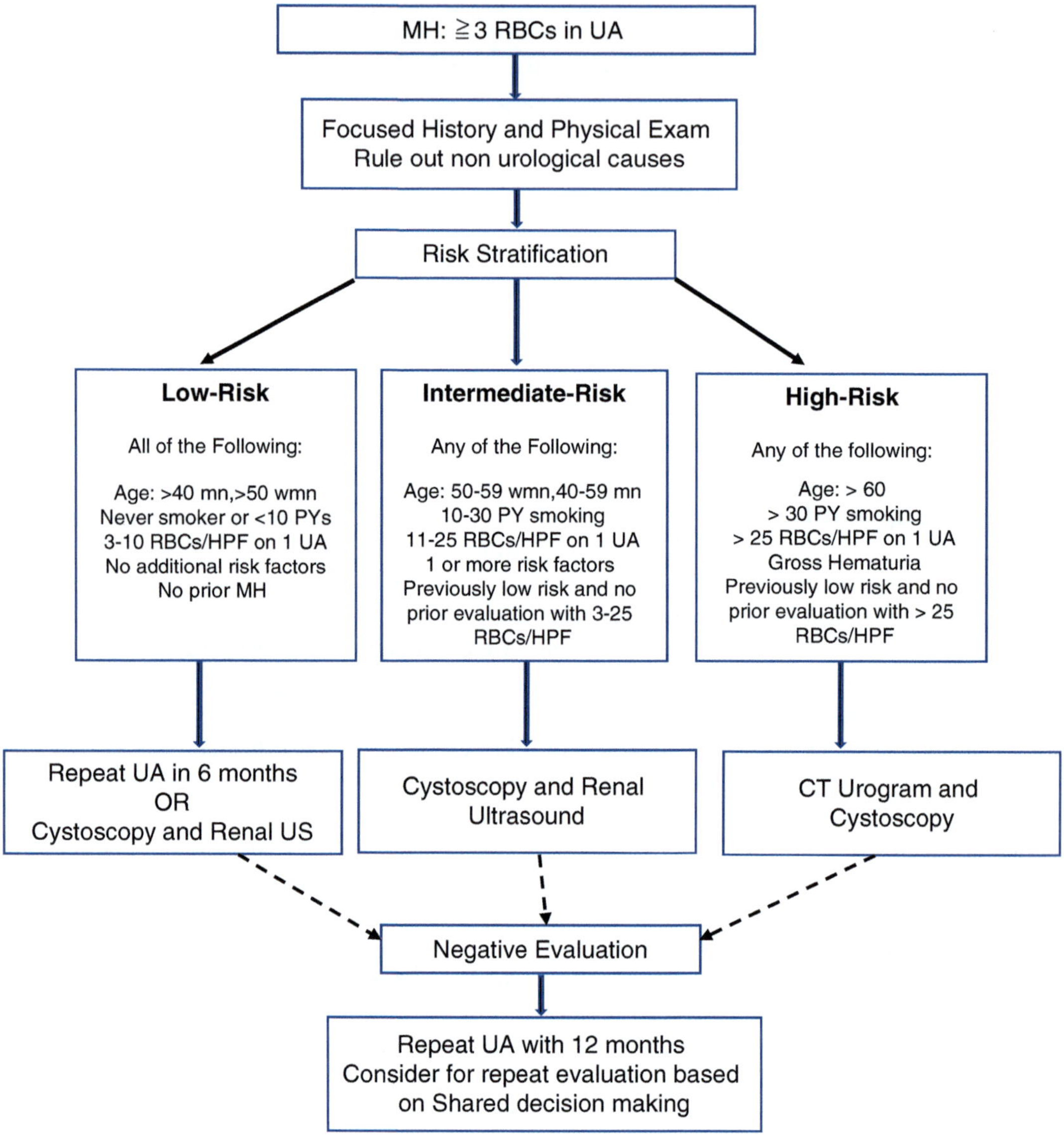

Fig. 11.1 Schematic Approach to Microscopic Hematuria Based on the AUA Recommendations [4]. MH, microscopic hematuria; RBCs, red blood cells; UA, urinalysis; mn, men; wmn, women; PYs, pack years; HPF, high-power field; US, ultrasound

ogy assessment, and office cystoscopy. CT urogram is the preferred approach for cross-sectional imaging, whereas MR urogram can serve as an alternate strategy in patients with contrast allergy.

The evaluation of patients with microscopic hematuria has shown several variations as well as deficiencies not only among the urologists but also among the referring providers. The AUA/SUFU guidelines for microscopic hematuria evaluation aim to not only address these deficiencies but also to focus on a risk-based assessment of microscopic hematuria with a shared decision-making model thus keeping the patient at the center of all the care [4]. The overall goal with this risk-based approach is to avoid unnecessary testing and at the same time, providing a framework for the referring physician as well as the evaluating urologist. A schematic approach to microscopic hematuria based on these recommendations is provided in Fig. 11.1.

11.2.3 Office Cystoscopy

The in-office cystoscopy is an important part of the initial workup for patients with gross hematuria and intermediate and high-risk microscopic hematuria according to the new AUA recommendations [4, 5]. Flexible cystoscopy is the most preferred option specially in men as it is better tolerated than rigid cystoscopy. The goal of this in-office evaluation is to identify and record the macroscopic features of the tumor including site, size, number, as well as locations along with the other mucosal abnormalities. A preferred approach is to use a bladder diagram to represent these findings [6]. The use of enhanced cystoscopy like blue light cystoscopy and narrow-band imaging (NBI) is an option in surveillance office cystoscopies and is discussed later.

11.2.4 Urine Cytology and Other Urinary Biomarkers

The sensitivity of urine cytology is high for high grade tumors (84%) and lower for low grade tumors (16%) [6].The sensitivity for CIS detection is variable (28–100%) [7]. In experienced hands the specificity, however, is high (>90%). This variation in the sensitivity across the spectrum of NMIBC highlights the inherent limitations of the urine cytology which can be further compounded by the problems of sample collection and issues like cellularity and urinary tract infection to name a few [6].

Therefore, there has always been a recurring interest in identifying potential urinary biomarkers that could supplant or even replace urine cytology in the initial diagnostic workup. There is also a recent push to identify reliable biomarkers, which could potentially rationalize the use of the office cystoscopy for initial diagnosis as well as surveillance in appropriate cases [7]. The most ideal scenario would be in the workup of microscopic hematuria where this could potentially avoid the need for further imaging as well as cystoscopy. For this to be a possibility, these biomarkers should have a high negative predictive value and a high specificity [8].

Among the classical biomarkers NMP 22, BTA, ImmunoCyt, and UroVysion need mentioning. UroVysion test, based on fluorescent in situ hybridization, is not affected by the degree of hematuria or inflammation and maintains its sensitivity even in the post Bacillus Calmette Guerin (BCG) treatment setting [9]. ImmunoCyt, which is now off the market in most countries, was useful even in the setting of low-grade pathology, but is affected by UTI, hematuria, BPH, and also required significant technical expertise along with other technical constraints [6, 7, 9].

There are several newer sets of biomarkers being investigated based on the epigenetic changes, DNA alterations as well as urinary mRNA assays which are now commercially available as multigene panels. The most popular of these is the Cx Bladder panel which are available as three separate tests that are catered to specific situations with relation to NMIBC. Cx Bladder Triage helps to rule out bladder cancer in low-risk patients with hematuria, Cx Bladder Detect complements cystoscopy in bladder cancer detection and Cx Bladder Monitor is helpful in bladder cancer surveillance along with cystoscopy. The Cx Bladder platform has a reasonable sensitivity (82%) and specificity (90%) [10].

11.2.5 Imaging in NMIBC

The AUA recommends performing upper tract imaging in newly diagnosed bladder cancer patients [5]. Interestingly, the likelihood of identifying concomitant upper tract disease in bladder cancer patients is only about 1.8%, which increases to 7.5% for those in the trigone [11]. This detection is also higher during follow-up for high grade and large tumors. Therefore, the EAU does not have a blanket recommendation for upper tract imaging in all patients of bladder cancer [6]. Whenever performed, CT urogram remains the preferred imaging modality, and MR urogram could be reserved for those with iodinated contrast allergies. Renal and bladder ultrasound is inferior to these modalities especially for hematuria workup [12].

Vesical image reporting and data system (VI-RADS) is a five-point system developed by multidisciplinary experts in 2018 [13] and since validated by other studies [14] for its ability to detect muscle-invasive disease using MRI of the bladder. VI-RADS Grades 1–2 represent very low and low likelihood of muscle invasiveness, grade 3 is equivocal, and grades 4–5 represent high and very high likelihood of muscle invasiveness [13]. It is not in widespread use yet but may have implications for usage in identifying muscle invasive disease, risk stratification, as well as surveillance in selected patients in the future.

11.3 Transurethral Resection

11.3.1 Initial Resection

The goal of transurethral resection in NMIBC is to ensure complete tumor resection of endoscopically evident tumors and to have a correct pathological diagnosis. The resection therefore should aim at either en-bloc or fractioned resection of all visible tumor with minimal use of coagulation to minimize cautery artefacts [6]. Recently, en-bloc resection has gained popularity, and in a recent meta-analysis, it was found to be comparable or even superior to the standard resection in most clinical outcomes [15]. Whatever the technique is employed, the surgeon should aim to perform a complete evaluation of the urethra as well as the bladder and a bimanual palpation or additional bladder biopsies wherever indicated. The use of enhanced cystoscopy techniques like photodynamic diagnosis (PDD) using blue light cystoscopy and narrow band imaging (NBI) can increase the detection of additional tumors and ensure a complete resection and can be included whenever available. A recently conducted Cochrane review found that blue light cystoscopy had a favorable outcome when compared to white light cystoscopy in terms of recurrence and progression of disease [16]. However, higher costs have limited the use of this technology to only specialized academic centers.

Collected specimens should be separately labeled if possible and a separate specimen for the tumor base/muscle should be taken so that the pathologist can easily identify detrusor muscle to comment on the tumor involvement of muscles. Adequate anesthesia should be used with provisions for muscle relaxation and/or obturator nerve block especially in tumors on the lateral bladder wall on prior assessments.

11.3.2 The Role of a Second Resection

There is a significant risk of residual disease in T1 bladder cancers reaching up to 51% and about 8% risk of under staging the disease [17].The AUA recommends that the repeat resection be performed within 6 weeks of initial resection in patients with Ta/T1 high-grade disease [5]. Repeat resection has also been associated with several treatment-related outcomes including improved recurrence-free survival, BCG response, as well as overall survival in select patients [6]. It has important implications in providing prognostic information with relation to disease upstaging of T1 disease even when there was detrusor muscle present muscle in the previously resected specimen [18].

11.4 Pathology of NMIBC

Correct pathological diagnosis is of the greatest importance in NMIBC for many reasons. The accuracy of grading as well as documentation of the depth of invasion along with the identification of in situ carcinoma (CIS) as well as Lymphovascular invasion has important implications. The identification of muscle in the initial TUR specimen is equally important and needs to be appropriately conveyed in the pathology reports. Pathologists and urologists should coordinate to ensure adequate reporting of prior intravesical therapy or radiation therapy [19]. In difficult situations, the opinion of an experienced genitourinary pathologist should be sought.

11.4.1 Pathological Classification

Noninvasive urothelial tumors are the most common variety of bladder cancer. It includes in situ carcinoma, high- and low-grade carcinoma (HG and LG) and papillary urothelial neoplasm of low malignant potential. 95% of all invasive cancers are high grade though some low-grade cancers can also show invasive features. CIS is a high-grade cancer, though it has noninvasive features. The World health organization in 2016 (Table 11.1) updated its classification of the invasive and noninvasive tumors with recognition of divergent differentiation in invasive urothelial tumors [20]. This update, however, still holds the 1997 proposed grading system for urothelial tumors by the International Society of Urologic Pathologists (ISUP).

Divergent tumors are those where the common type of urothelial tumor is seen along with variable percentages of other histological variants like glandular, squamous, small cell and trophoblastic. These are more commonly associated with locally advanced and invasive disease but are different from variants of urothelial cancers which lack the typical urothelial morphology and have an aggressive clinical course and their appropriate reporting is important as it directly impacts the approach to management [21]. Some divergent tumors can be more aggressive than the other variants, especially when they have nested, micropapillary or the small cell mixed histology.

Table 11.1 WHO 2016 classification of invasive and noninvasive urothelial tumors [20]

Non-invasive urothelial tumors	Invasive urothelial tumors
Urothelial carcinoma in situ	Infiltrating urothelial carcinoma with divergent differentiation
Papillary urothelial carcinoma, low grade	Nested, including large nested
Papillary urothelial carcinoma, high grade	Microcystic
Papillary urothelial neoplasm of low malignant potential	Micropapillary
Urothelial papilloma	Lymphoepithelioma-like
Inverted urothelial papilloma	Plasmacytoid/signet ring cell/diffuse
Urothelial proliferation of uncertain malignant potential (hyperplasia)	Sarcomatoid
Urothelial dysplasia	Giant cell
	Poorly differentiated
	Lipid rich
	Clear cell
	Tumours of Maüllerian type
	Tumors arising in a bladder diverticulum

11.4.2 Pathological Staging

Based on the 2017 TNM classification [22], NMIBC (T) categories include the following

1. Ta: Noninvasive papillary carcinoma.
2. CIS: carcinoma in-situ: flat tumor.
3. T1: Papillary carcinoma invasive to the sub-epithelial connective tissue.

CIS may be categorized as primary, secondary, or concomitant based on the clinical history and the presence of concomitant papillary histology. The WHO also finds benefits in further sub-classifying the T1 tumors based on the depth of the invasion as this has been shown to be of prognostic value [6].

11.4.3 Prognostication and Risk Stratification in NMIBC

Several agencies have actively been involved over the years in developing prognostication models for NMIBC. The risk calculator put forward by the European Organization for Research and Treatment of Cancer (EORTC) provides the risk of recurrence and progression at 1 and 5 years. Prior recurrence rate, number of tumors, and tumor size have been identified as important factor in prediction of recurrence, whereas T-stage, presence of CIS, and grade are predictive of disease progression based on this calculator [23]. Similarly, the Club Urologico Espanol de Tratamiento Oncologico (CUETO) model predicts the risks of recurrence and progression in patients who have been treated with 5–6 months of BCG [24].

There are several fallacies in each of the risk models, which may not have a significant influence in making clinical decisions. Therefore, there have been some recent changes especially in the EORTC model in 2016, which still fall short in terms of being a clinically valuable tool for making treatment-related decisions.

AUA and the EAU have both come up with their risk stratification tools to aid clinicians in making treatment-related decisions. The EAU 2021 NMIBC scoring model is based on the metanalysis of over 3000 patients who have had TURB and intravesical chemotherapy. This has identified tumor stage, WHO 1973 grade, WHO 2004/2016 grade, concomitant CIS, number of tumors, tumor size, and age as predictors of progression on multivariate analysis. Thereafter, the EAU 2021 scoring model stratifies patient into four distinct risk categories: low risk, intermediate risk, high risk, and very high risk [25]. An online calculator is available to aid clinicians in identifying the risk category and probability of progression for an individual patient [6].

The AUA NMIBC risk stratification is also based on the T stage, grade, number, size, presence of CIS but also uses LVI, variant histology, high-grade prostatic involvement along with incorporation of prior BCG therapies. It stratifies patients into low risk, intermediate risk, and high risk categories as shown in Table 11.2 [5] and has been validated by recent studies [26].

Table 11.2 Risk stratification based on the AUA guidelines 2016 [5]

Low risk	Intermediate risk	High risk
Solitary low grade ta ≤ 3 cm	Low grade: Ta Recurrence <1 year	High grade: Ta, recurrent
PUNLMP	Ta > 3 cm	Ta > 3 cm
	Ta multifocal	Any T1
	T1	Any: Carcinoma in situ
	High grade: Ta ≤ 3 cm	Lymphovascular invasion
		Variant histology
		BCG failure in high-grade case
		High-grade prostatic involvement

11.5 Intravesical Therapy in NMIBC

TURB in NMIBC can completely remove/resect the tumor. Nevertheless, adjuvant treatment is necessary based on risk stratification of an individual patient to decrease the risk of recurrence and progression to muscle invasive bladder cancer. Most of the approved and utilized therapies are in the form of intravesical therapies with one current exception, pembrolizumab.

11.5.1 Intravesical Chemotherapy

The primary use of intravesical chemotherapy is in low- and intermediate-risk disease and as a secondary option in high-risk disease. The common agents used for this are mitomycin c (MMC), anthracyclines (valrubicin, doxorubicin, and epirubicine) and Gemcitabine.

11.5.1.1 Intravesical Chemotherapy Indications

The most foremost indication for intravesical chemotherapy is in the immediate postoperative period. A single post/perioperative instillation of chemotherapeutic agent decreases in the recurrence risk by about 12% [27]. MMC, doxorubicin, and epirubicin have all shown benefits in this setting, and recently gemcitabine was also seen to be superior to placebo in reducing recurrence after resection [6]. It is contraindicated in the setting of bladder perforation or a suspicion of bladder perforation, as severe intrabdominal complications can arise.

Intravesical chemotherapy is also indicated as an adjuvant therapy in intermediate-risk disease though it is not as effective as BCG in preventing recurrences [28]. This schedule is not very well defined and usually involves an induction schedule of 6 weekly doses followed by either monthly or quarterly doses for a period not more than a year [6, 28]. A combination of intravesical chemotherapy and BCG has also been explored by some clinical trials and evaluated by a metanalysis which found a benefit in the recurrence-free survival without any changes in the progression-free survival. This metanalysis also did not find any significant difference in the toxicities between combination schedules and BCG alone [29]. Finally, intravesical chemotherapy as a salvage option can be explored in low-grade recurrences after BCG therapy for primarily intermediate-risk disease [6]. Valrubicin is an FDA-approved alternative in BCG refractory CIS; however, it has a very low response rate (21%) and is therefore not used very widely.

11.5.1.2 Improving the Delivery of Intravesical Chemotherapy

Several options have been explored to enhance the delivery of intravesical chemotherapy for increasing treatment efficacy. Adjusting the pH (MMC), increasing the dwell time (MMC), and increasing the concentration (Epirubicin) have been found to enhance the efficacy in separate studies [6]. Device-assisted delivery of MMC has been explored with microwave-assisted thermotherapy and electromotive drug administration (EMDA) have been proposed based on small studies but is not commonly practiced.

11.5.2 Intravesical BCG Immunotherapy

BCG is the cornerstone of adjuvant intravesical treatment in NMIBC for the past four decades or more based on the early works of Morales and Lamm. The mechanism of action of BCG is still under investigation but strongly implicates the active involvement of both urothelial cells as well as the immune cells. Bladder cells are responsible for attachment and internalization of the BCG and secreting cytokines and chemokines and finally presenting the cancer antigens along with BCG to the cells of the immune system. CD4+, CD8+ lymphocytes, natural killer cells, macrophages, dendritic cells, and granulocytes can then directly kill the cancer cells. BCG may also have some direct toxicity on the cancer cells [30].

The widespread use of BCG and the limited number of production facilities manufacturing it has led to variable periods of BCG shortage in the past 5–6 years. This along with the limited options available for patients with BCG failure/toxicity has led to the exploration of newer avenues of adjuvant therapy for NMIBC.

11.5.2.1 Efficacy of BCG

Overall reduction in recurrence rates has been seen up to 44–52% for all types of NMIBC. Similarly, the 10 year progression rate to MIBC in BCG-treated patients was 38% compared to 63% in TURB alone [31]. When used with a maintenance schedule, BCG had a 32% reduction in the risk of recurrence compared to MMC, whereas there was a 28% increase in recurrence for patients without BCG maintenance [6]. BCG-treatedd patients have an overall 9.8% progression rate compared to 13.8% in non-BCG-treated controls [6]. This efficacy generally extends to all superficial tumors (Ta, T1, and CIS). Additionally, this efficacy is seen across all strains of BCG used.

11.5.2.2 Side Effects with BCG

BCG is certainly associated with more side effects than intravesical chemotherapy. In a multicenter randomized study, it was found that 20% patients stopped BCG due to intolerable side effects, and local side effects were the most common. It was also seen that the incidence of serious side effects was less than 5%, and the maintenance schedule was not associated with an increase in incidence [32]. The frequency of BCG-associated infections was also rare [6]. Although there were initial concerns about the safety of BCG usage in elderly population, recent reports have shown that age is not an important factor in the incidence of treatment-related side effects in patients receiving BCG for intermediate- and high-risk diseases [33].

However, there are certain clear contraindications to BCG treatment, and these should be strictly followed. These are treatment within 2 weeks of the TURB, visible gross hematuria, traumatic catheterization, and patients with symptomatic UTI. Microscopic hematuria, pyuria, and asymptomatic bacteriuria are not contraindications for treatment nor do they require additional antibiotic usage prior to treatment [6]. It is reasonable to grade the severity of BCG-related toxicity based on the recommendations of the International Bladder Cancer Group (IBCG) [34].The IBCG classifies the BCG toxicity into four grades. It also recommends management strategies based on this grouping, including suspension of BCG treatments in grades 2 and 3 and complete cessation in grade 4 toxicity.

11.5.2.3 Optimizing BCG Schedules

The induction schedule of 6 weekly intravesical doses is based on the empirical dosing schedule proposed by Morales in 1976 [35]. Interestingly, subsequent studies that utilized less frequent dosing have not shown similar efficacy, and the original empirical schedule has prevailed [6]. A maintenance dosing is recommended is for optimal efficacy following the induction schedule. The proposed number of maintenance doses is variable and can be up to a maximum of 27 doses in a 3 year period based on the schedule proposed by Lamm et al. [36]. The single standard dose of BCG is 80/81 mg, whereas the original studies had used 60 mg, and there have been several studies that have looked at feasibilities for reduction of the standard dose to1/2 or 1/3 dose with variable results in terms of recurrence and no difference in the toxicities [6]. There are over 10 strains of BCG available, but no difference has been found in the efficacy between the individual strains [37].

Combination strategies of BCG with MMC and interferon (IFN) have not yielded favorable results and have resulted in worse side effects [37]. There are several ongoing trials looking at potential BCG combinations in BCG naïve as well as patients with BCG failure to further expand the horizon of BCG therapeutics in bladder cancer [38].

11.5.2.4 BCG Failures

BCG failure has been variably defined over the years, with focus on the recurrence and progression of disease. When CIS or HGT1 disease progresses, it results in muscle invasive disease, and there are no avenues for bladder preservation. Therefore, when defining BCG failures, disease recurrences at specific time frames are used. The EAU guidelines for bladder cancer have four categories of BCG failures defined: BCG refractory, BCG relapsing, BCG Unresponsive, and BCG intolerance. The definitions and proposed alternatives for management are highlighted in Table 11.3.

Table 11.3 Definitions and management of BCG failure based on EAU guidelines 2021 [6]

Category of BCG failure	Definition	Management
BCG refractory	T1 HG recurrence at 3 mo	Same a BCG unresponsive
	Ta HG recurrence after 3 mo and/or at 6 mo, after either reinduction or first course of maintenance	
	CIS (without ta/T1) present at 3 mo and persists at 6 mo after either reinduction or a first course of maintenance	
	HG recurrence during BCG maintenance	
BCG relapsing	HG recurrence after completion of BCG maintenance, despite an initial response	1. RC
		2. Repeat BCG induction
		3. Bladder preserving strategies
		4. LG recurrences for intravesical chemotherapy
BCG unresponsive	All BCG refractory tumors	1. RC
	T1/ta HG recurrence within 6 mo of adequate BCG exposure	2. Clinical trial enrollment
	CIS within 12 mo of completion of adequate BCG exposure	3. Bladder preserving strategies
		(a) MMC (microwave assisted)
		(b) Intravenous pembrolizumab
		(c) Nadofaragene firadenovac
BCG intolerant	Severe side effects prevent BCG completion	Limited evidence available to make recommendations

HG high grade, *mo* months, *LG* low grade

11.5.3 Risk-Based Intravesical Adjuvant Therapy Recommendations

AUA recommends intravesical therapy in the following scenarios [5]:

1. A single dose of intravesical chemotherapy (MMC or Epirubicin) is recommended in patients with suspected low- or intermediate-risk disease within 24 h of bladder tumor resection.
2. In patients with low-risk disease, further intravesical therapy is not indicated.
3. Patients with intermediate-risk disease, induction chemotherapy, or immunotherapy with BCG can be considered.
4. Intermediate-risk disease patients can be considered for maintenance therapy for 1 year with either BCG or chemotherapy if they respond to the initial induction schedule.
5. High-risk patients should receive 6 weekly doses of BCG induction and if they respond to this, a maximum of 3 years of maintenance BCG is recommended at 3, 6, 12, 18, 24, 30, and 36 months.

11.6 Newer Approaches to Adjuvant Treatment

The FDA in 2020 approved pembrolizumab for the treatment of patients with BCG-unresponsive, high-risk, NMIBC with carcinoma in situ (CIS) with or without papillary tumors. This approval was based on the single-arm Phase II study, which showed a 41% complete response at 3 months. The median duration of this complete response was for 16.2 months, and only 46% of the complete responders had a sustained response at 12 months. The scheduled dosing of the Pembrolizumab in this trial was for 200 mg intravenous every 3 months for a total duration of 24 months or until a confirmed disease recurrence was seen [39]. There has been significant criticism for this approval though as the evidence is nonrandomized with the potential of significant harm considering the possible adverse effects and the delay in consideration for cystectomy [40].

Nadofaragene firadenovac (rAd-IFNa/Syn3) is a recombinant adenovirus-mediated intravesical therapy that delivers interferon alfa-2b cDNA into the bladder epithelium and has been recently submitted to the FDA for approval in BCG-unresponsive NMIBC. This submission is based on a recently concluded Phase 3, multicenter, repeat dose open-label study. Patients on the trial received 75 mL of the drug (3×10^{11} viral particles per mL) as a single dose and repeat dosing was done at 3, 6, and 9 months. In total, 53.4% people showed an initial response at 3 months, and this was sustained in 45.5% at 12 months [41].

Currently, there are several clinical trials that are either completed or ongoing, which are looking at immune checkpoint inhibitors, targeted therapies, other chemotherapeutic agents, and viral or bacterial-based therapies along with those that are in combination with BCG. These agents are being explored in the realms of BCG naïve, BCG relapsing/recurrent disease, and BCG unresponsive/refractory disease. The need to investigate the alternatives in the BCG naïve population was probably also brought about by the recent issues with BCG scarcity [38].

11.7 Radical Cystectomy (RC) in NMIBC

The AUA guidelines are very clear and distinct on recommendations for radical cystectomy in NMIBC [5]. RC should not be offered to patients with Ta low- or intermediate-risk disease until bladder reserving therapies have completely failed. In a fit patient with persistent T1HG disease on repeat resection or those with associated CIS, LVI, and variant histology, we can consider offering initial RC. Additionally, in high-risk patients with persistent or recurrent disease within 1 year following two inductions cycles or BCG maintenance, RC should be offered.

11.8 Surveillance Strategies

In office, cystoscopy and urine cytology along with periodic upper tract imaging form the cornerstone of surveillance in NMIBC. Several newer urinary markers are being investigated as an alternative to the cystoscopy, however, based on the existing knowledge, cannot replace it. In patients with positive cytology and no detectable recurrences on cystoscopy, a mapping or PDD-guided biopsies and evaluation with CT urography and prostatic urethral biopsies is indicated. A simplified surveillance scheme as per the AUA recommendations in given in Table 11.4.

Table 11.4 Follow-up schema of surveillance for NMIBC as per AUA guidelines [5]

AUA risk category	Surveillance timing	Additional measures
Low risk	First cystoscopy at 3 months	Small ta recurrences can be fulgurated in the office
	Second 6–9 months later	
	Then annually for up to 5 years	
	Shared decision making for surveillance after 5 years	
Intermediate risk	First cystoscopy + cytology at 3 months	Consider surveillance upper tract imaging once a year
	Then 3–6 monthly for first 2 years	
	6 monthly for years 3 and 4	
	Yearly thereafter	
High risk	First cystoscopy + cytology at 3 months	
	Then 3–4 monthly for first 2 years	
	6 monthly for years 3 and 4	
	Yearly thereafter	

11.9 Conclusion

Management of NMIBC is based upon timely detection and accurate staging with TURB and repeat resection along with upper tract imaging whenever indicated. It is important to accurately identify the pathological grade and the presence of adverse pathological factors to follow a risk-based approach to NMIBC management. Adjuvant intravesical therapy is the cornerstone of management in preventing/limiting recurrences, and the option of radical cystectomy should be timely considered and discussed with eligible patients. The horizon for newer therapeutics in NMIBC looks very bright with the eagerly awaited results from several ongoing clinical trials.

References

1. Antoni S, Ferlay J, Soerjomataram I, Znaor A, Jemal A, Bray F. Bladder cancer incidence and mortality: a global overview and recent trends. Eur Urol. 2017;71(1):96–108. https://doi.org/10.1016/j.eururo.2016.06.010.
2. Burger M, Catto JWF, Dalbagni G, Grossman HB, Herr H, Karakiewicz P, et al. Platinum priority—review—bladder cancer epidemiology and risk factors of urothelial bladder cancer. Eur Urol. 2013;63:234–41.
3. Edwards TJ, Dickinson AJ, Natale S, Gosling J, McGrath JS. A prospective analysis of the diagnostic yield resulting from the attendance of 4020 patients at a protocol-driven haematuria clinic. BJU Int. 2006;97(2):301–5.
4. Barocas DA, Boorjian SA, Alvarez RD, Downs TM, Gross CP, Hamilton BD, et al. AUA microhematuria 2020. J Urol. 2020;204:778–86.
5. Chang SS, Boorjian SA, Chou R, Clark PE, Daneshmand S, Konety BR, et al. Diagnosis and treatment of non-muscle invasive bladder cancer: AUA/SUO guideline. J Urol. 2016;196(4):1021–9. https://doi.org/10.1016/j.juro.2016.06.049.
6. Babjuk M, Burger M, Capoun O, Cohen D, Compérat EM, Dominguez Escrig JL, et al. European Association of Urology guidelines on non–muscle-invasive bladder cancer (Ta, T1, and carcinoma in situ). Eur Urol. 2022;81(1):75–94.

7. Têtu B. Diagnosis of urothelial carcinoma from urine. Mod Pathol. 2009;22(2):S53–9. https://doi.org/10.1038/modpathol.2008.193.
8. Schmitz-Dräger BJ, Kuckuck EC, Zuiverloon TCM, Zwarthoff EC, Saltzman A, Srivastava A, et al. Microhematuria assessment an IBCN consensus—based upon a critical review of current guidelines. Urol Oncol. 2016;34(10):437–51.
9. Ng K, Stenzl A, Sharma A, Vasdev N. Urinary biomarkers in bladder cancer: a review of the current landscape and future directions. Urol Oncol. 2021;39(1):41–51.
10. O'Sullivan P, Sharples K, Dalphin M, Davidson P, Gilling P, Cambridge L, et al. A multigene urine test for the detection and stratification of bladder cancer in patients presenting with hematuria. J Urol. 2012;188(3):741–7.
11. Palou J, Rodríguez-Rubio F, Huguet J, Segarra J, Ribal MJ, Alcaraz A, et al. Multivariate analysis of clinical parameters of synchronous primary superficial bladder cancer and upper urinary tract tumor. J Urol. 2005;174(3):859–61.
12. Hilton S, Jones LP. Recent advances in imaging cancer of the kidney and urinary tract. Surg Oncol Clin N Am. 2014;23(4):863–910.
13. Panebianco V, Narumi Y, Altun E, Bochner BH, Efstathiou JA, Hafeez S, et al. Multiparametric magnetic resonance imaging for bladder cancer: development of VI-RADS (vesical imaging-reporting and data system). Eur Urol. 2018;74(3):294–306.
14. Panebianco V, Pecoraro M, Del Giudice F, Takeuchi M, Muglia VF, Messina E, et al. VI-RADS for bladder cancer: current applications and future developments. J Magn Reson Imaging. 2022;55(1):23–36. https://doi.org/10.1002/jmri.27361.
15. Teoh JY-C, MacLennan S, Chan VW-S, Miki J, Lee H-Y, Chiong E, et al. An international collaborative consensus statement on en bloc resection of bladder tumour incorporating two systematic reviews, a two-round delphi survey, and a consensus meeting. Eur Urol. 2020;78(4):546–69.
16. Maisch P, Koziarz A, Vajgrt J, Narayan V, Kim MH, Dahm P. Blue vs. white light for transurethral resection of non-muscle-invasive bladder cancer: an abridged cochrane review. BJU Int. 2022;130(6):730–40. https://doi.org/10.1111/bju.15723.
17. Cumberbatch MGK, Foerster B, Catto JWF, Kamat AM, Kassouf W, Jubber I, et al. Repeat transurethral resection in non–muscle-invasive bladder cancer: a systematic review. Eur Urol. 2018;73(6):925–33.
18. Naselli A, Hurle R, Paparella S, Buffi NM, Lughezzani G, Lista G, et al. Role of restaging transurethral resection for T1 non–muscle invasive bladder cancer: a systematic review and meta-analysis. Eur Urol Focus. 2018;4(4):558–67.
19. Babjuk M, Burger M, Compérat EM, Gontero P, Mostafid AH, Palou J, et al. European Association of Urology guidelines on non-muscle-invasive bladder cancer (TaT1 and carcinoma in situ)—2019 update. Eur Urol. 2019;76(5):639–57.
20. Humphrey PA, Moch H, Cubilla AL, Ulbright TM, Reuter VE. The 2016 WHO classification of tumours of the urinary system and male genital organs—part B: prostate and bladder tumours. Eur Urol. 2016;70(1):106–19.
21. Regmi SK, Konety BR. Variant histology: management pearls. In: Kamat AM, Black PC, editors. Bladder cancer: a practical guide. Cham: Springer International Publishing; 2021. p. 323–41. https://doi.org/10.1007/978-3-030-70646-3_27.
22. Brierley JD, Gospodarowicz MK, Wittekind C. TNM classification of malignant tumours. Oxford: John Wiley & Sons; 2017.
23. Sylvester RJ, van der Meijden APM, Oosterlinck W, Witjes JA, Bouffioux C, Denis L, et al. Predicting recurrence and progression in individual patients with stage ta T1 bladder cancer using EORTC risk tables: a combined analysis of 2596 patients from seven EORTC trials. Eur Urol. 2006;49(3):466–77.
24. Jesus F-G, Rosario M, Eduardo S, Miguel U, Luis M-P, Marcelino G, et al. Predicting nonmuscle invasive bladder cancer recurrence and progression in patients treated with Bacillus Calmette-Guerin: the CUETO scoring model. J Urol. 2009;182(5):2195–203. https://doi.org/10.1016/j.juro.2009.07.016.
25. Sylvester RJ, Rodríguez O, Hernández V, Turturica D, Bauerová L, Bruins HM, et al. European Association of Urology (EAU) prognostic factor risk groups for non–muscle-invasive bladder cancer (NMIBC) incorporating the WHO 2004/2016 and WHO 1973 classification systems for grade: an update from the EAU NMIBC guidelines panel. Eur Urol. 2021;79(4):480–8.
26. Ritch CR, Velasquez MC, Kwon D, Becerra MF, Soodana-Prakash N, Atluri VS, et al. Use and validation of the AUA/SUO risk grouping for nonmuscle invasive bladder cancer in a contemporary cohort. J Urol. 2020;203(3):505–11. https://doi.org/10.1097/JU.0000000000000593.
27. Sylvester RJ, Oosterlinck W, van der Meijden APM. A single immediate postoperative instillation of chemotherapy decreases the risk of recurrence in patients with stage Ta T1 bladder cancer: a meta-analysis of published results of randomized clinical trials. J Urol. 2004;171(6 Part 1):2186–90.
28. Porten SP, Leapman MS, Greene KL. Intravesical chemotherapy in non-muscle-invasive bladder cancer. Indian J Urol. 2015;31(4):297.
29. Huang D, Jin Y-H, Weng H, Huang Q, Zeng X-T, Wang X-H. Combination of intravesical Bacille Calmette-Guérin and chemotherapy vs. Bacille Calmette-Guérin alone in non-muscle invasive bladder cancer: a meta-analysis. Front Oncol. 2019;9:121. https://doi.org/10.3389/fonc.2019.00121.
30. Redelman-Sidi G, Glickman MS, Bochner BH. The mechanism of action of BCG therapy for bladder cancer—a current perspective. Nat Rev Urol. 2014;11(3):153–62. https://doi.org/10.1038/nrurol.2014.15.

31. Bassi P. BCG (Bacillus of Calmette Guerin) therapy of high-risk superficial bladder cancer. Surg Oncol. 2002;11(1):77–83.
32. van der Meijden APM, Sylvester RJ, Oosterlinck W, Hoeltl W, Bono AV. Maintenance Bacillus Calmette-Guerin for Ta T1 bladder tumors is not associated with increased toxicity: results from a European Organisation for Research and Treatment of Cancer Genito-Urinary Group Phase III Trial. Eur Urol. 2003;44(4):429–34.
33. Oddens JR, Sylvester RJ, Brausi MA, Kirkels WJ, van de Beek C, van Andel G, et al. Increasing age is not associated with toxicity leading to discontinuation of treatment in patients with urothelial non-muscle-invasive bladder cancer randomised to receive 3 years of maintenance bacille Calmette–Guérin: results from European Organisation for Research and Treatment of Cancer Genito-Urinary Group study 30911. BJU Int. 2016;118(3):423–8. https://doi.org/10.1111/bju.13474.
34. Witjes JA, Palou J, Soloway M, Lamm D, Brausi M, Spermon JR, et al. Clinical practice recommendations for the prevention and management of intravesical therapy–associated adverse events. Eur Urol Suppl. 2008;7(10):667–74.
35. Morales A, Eidinger D, Bruce A. Intracavitary Bacillus Calmette-Guerin in the treatment of superficial bladder tumors. J Urol. 1976;116(2):180–2. https://doi.org/10.1016/S0022-5347(17)58737-6.
36. Lamm DL, Blumenstein BA, Crissman JD, Montie JE, Gottesman JE, Lowe BA, et al. Maintenance Bacillus Calmette-Guerin immunotherapy for recurrent Ta, T1 and carcinoma in situ transitional cell carcinoma of the bladder: a randomized southwest oncology group study. J Urol. 2000;163(4):1124–9.
37. Boehm BE, Cornell JE, Wang H, Mukherjee N, Oppenheimer JS, Svatek RS. Efficacy of Bacillus Calmette-Guérin strains for treatment of nonmuscle invasive bladder cancer: a systematic review and network meta-analysis. J Urol. 2017;198(3):503–10.
38. Shore ND, Palou Redorta J, Robert G, Hutson TE, Cesari R, Hariharan S, et al. Non-muscle-invasive bladder cancer: an overview of potential new treatment options. Urol Oncol. 2021;39(10):642–63.
39. Balar AV, Kamat AM, Kulkarni GS, Uchio EM, Boormans JL, Roumiguié M, et al. Pembrolizumab monotherapy for the treatment of high-risk non-muscle-invasive bladder cancer unresponsive to BCG (KEYNOTE-057): an open-label, single-arm, multicentre, phase 2 study. Lancet Oncol. 2021;22(7):919–30.
40. Gill J, Prasad V. Pembrolizumab for non–muscle-invasive bladder cancer—a costly therapy in search of evidence. JAMA Oncol. 2021;7(4):501–2. https://doi.org/10.1001/jamaoncol.2020.6142.
41. Boorjian SA, Alemozaffar M, Konety BR, Shore ND, Gomella LG, Kamat AM, et al. Intravesical nadofaragene firadenovec gene therapy for BCG-unresponsive non-muscle-invasive bladder cancer: a single-arm, open-label, repeat-dose clinical trial. Lancet Oncol. 2021;22(1):107–17.

Management of MIBC

12

John Hayes, Saachi Chhaya, Harry Manning, Kenrick Ng, Anand Sharma, and Nikhil Vasdev

At presentation, approximately 25% of patients will have muscle-invasive bladder cancer (MIBC), and patients with non-MIBC may subsequently progress to MIBC. Prognosis is dependent on TNM stage (Table 12.1) and pelvic lymph node status. The disease requires a multidisciplinary approach, encompassing surgeon, oncologist, radiologist, pathologist and cancer specialist nurse.

Both CT and MRI imaging enable local assessment of tumour and lymphadenopathy. NICE and EAU Guidelines recommend CT imaging of the chest, abdomen and pelvis, with a urographic phase [1]. CT and MRI demonstrate similar accuracy when assessing for lymph node metastases. PET-CT can be considered to aid radical treatment decisions when there are equivocal findings.

The broad treatment options comprise radical cystectomy (RC), with urinary diversion, and radical radiotherapy (RRT) (Table 12.2). Both patient performance status and life expectancy influence the choice of modality. A Cochrane review demonstrated improved overall survival benefit at 5 years following RC (36% v. 20%) [2]. RRT is more likely given to patients with significant comorbidities, and non-randomised studies

Table 12.1 TMN classification of bladder cancer

T—primary tumour	
Tx	Primary tumour cannot be assessed
T0	No evidence of primary tumour
Ta	Non-invasive papillary carcinoma
Tis	Carcinoma in situ (CIS): "Flat tumour"
T1	Tumour invades subepithelial connective tissue
T2	Tumour invades muscle
T2a	Tumour invades superficial muscle (inner half)
T2b	Tumour invades deep muscle (outer half)
T3	Tumour invades peri-vesical tissue:
T3a	Microscopically
T3b	Macroscopically (extravesical mass)
T4	Tumour invades any of the following: Prostate stroma, seminal vesicles, uterus, vagina, pelvic wall, abdominal wall
T4a	Tumour invades prostate stroma, seminal vesicles, uterus or vagina
T4b	Tumour invades pelvic wall or abdominal wall
N—regional lymph nodes	
Nx	Regional lymph nodes cannot be assessed
N0	No regional lymph node metastasis
N1	Metastasis in a single lymph node in the true pelvis (hypogastric, obturator, external iliac or presacral)
N2	Metastasis in multiple regional lymph nodes in the true pelvis (hypogastric, obturator, external iliac or presacral)
N3	Metastasis in a common iliac lymph node(s)
M—distant metastasis	
M0	No distant metastasis
M1a	Non-regional lymph nodes
M1b	Other distant metastasis

J. Hayes (✉) · S. Chhaya · H. Manning · K. Ng · A. Sharma · N. Vasdev
Lister Hospital, Stevenage, UK
e-mail: john.hayes13@nhs.net

P. Singh et al. (eds.), *A Guide to Management of Urological Cancers*,
https://doi.org/10.1007/978-981-99-2341-0_12

Table 12.2 Radical cystectomy versus radical radiotherapy

	Radical cystectomy (RC)	Radical radiotherapy (RRT)
Benefits	Full staging with bladder and lymph node histology	Avoids major surgery
		Bladder preserving
Risks	Bleeding	Irritative LUTS
	Wound infection/chest infection/collection	Dysuria
	Deep venous thrombosis and pulmonary embolism	Small bladder capacity
	Anastomotic leak and stricture	Nausea
	Stomal stenosis	Proctitis
	Metabolic sequelae	Secondary malignancy

are subject to significant selection bias. No direct randomised comparisons have been undertaken between the two.

Relative indications for RC over RRT include the presence of CIS, upper urinary tract obstruction, severe storage LUTS, young patients and previous radiotherapy.

12.1 Radical Cystectomy: Removal of Tumour-Bearing Bladder

Radical cystectomy (RC), with urinary diversion, remains the standard treatment for localised MIBC (T2–T4a N0M0), in addition to recurrent high-risk NMIBC, BCG failure and extensive papillary disease. RC should be performed within 3 months, to reduce the risk of progression and disease-specific mortality [3]. The procedure should ideally be undertaken in high-volume centres (at least 10 and preferably >20 RCs per hospital/per year) in order to enhance both perioperative morbidity and mortality.

The EAU systematic review (2020) concluded that higher hospital volume was likely associated with lower in-hospital, 30- and 90-day mortality rates, in addition to lower positive surgical margins, and lower complication rates [4].

In men, standard RC includes removal of the bladder, prostate, seminal vesicles, distal ureters and regional lymph nodes (LN). In women, removal of the bladder, the entire urethra and adjacent vagina, uterus, distal ureters and LNs [5]. If a biopsy of the prostatic urethra has not been taken, a frozen section should be obtained peri-operatively, and the urethra should not be preserved if the margins are positive [1].

RC is known to result in impaired sexual and voiding dysfunction. Various nerve sparing approaches have been described to mitigate this. No consensus exists regarding which approach preserves function best. Concern remains regarding the impact of sparing techniques on oncological outcomes. Sexual preserving RC in men and women should not be offered as standard therapy, although they can be considered in well-motivated, highly selected individuals, with organ confined disease [6, 7].

Patients should be well counselled regarding surgery and the associated complications including bleeding, infection, rectal injury, impotency, incontinence, systemic complications (cardiovascular, venous thromboembolism and pulmonary embolism), specific urinary diversion complications and disease recurrence.

Patients should be commenced on pharmacological venous thromboembolism prophylaxis for a total of 4 weeks starting day 1 post-operatively [8].

12.2 Lymphadenectomy

Pelvic lymph node dissection (PLND) provides both accurate staging and confers a therapeutic effect. The presence of and number of positive lymph nodes is significantly associated with cancer-specific survival (5-year CSS 81% with N0 v. 40% with N+ve) [9].

Nodal spread from MIBC is predictable, comprising all LNs below the aortic bifurcation.

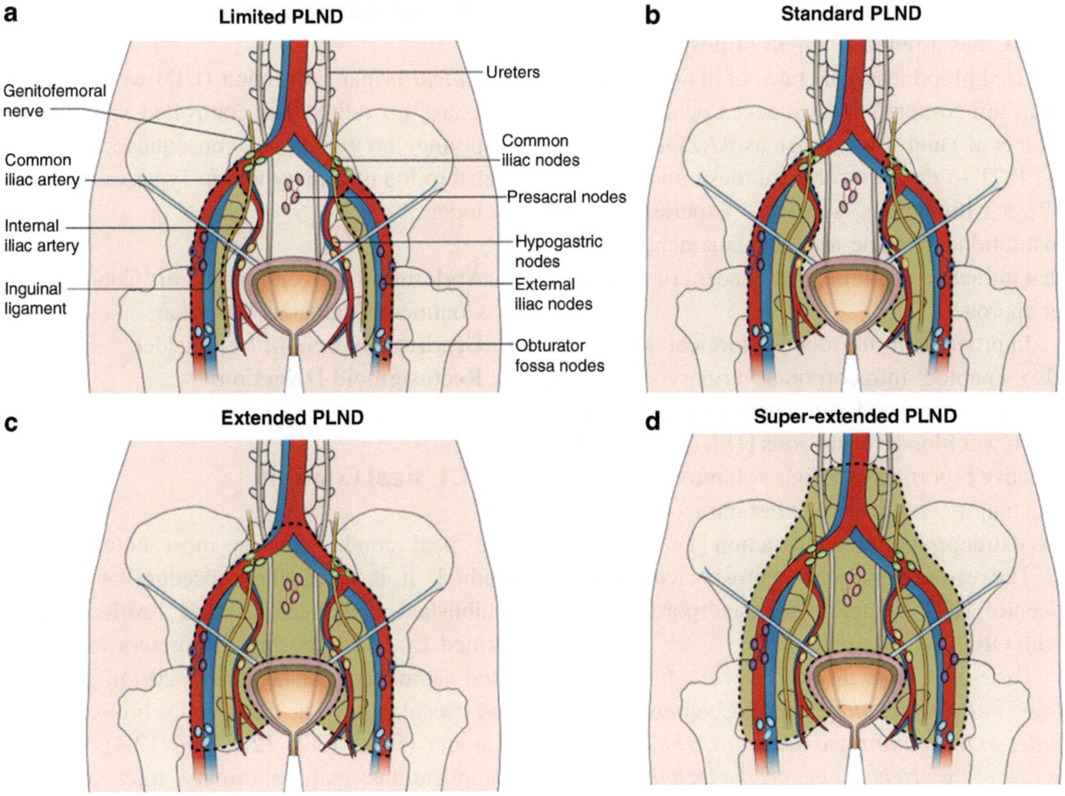

Fig. 12.1 Pelvic lymph node dissection. (**a**) Limited, (**b**) standard, (**c**) extended and (**d**) super-extended [11]

There are rarely nodes outside the pelvis if the pelvic nodes are negative [10]. The various extents of PLND (Fig. 12.1) include:

- **Limited PLND:** removal of nodal tissue from obturator fossae.
- **Standard PLND:** removal of nodal tissue cranially up to the common iliac bifurcation, with the ureter being the medial border, including the internal iliac, presacral, obturator fossa and external iliac nodes.
- **Extended PLND:** all LNs in the region of the aortic bifurcation, pre-sacral and common iliac vessels, medial to the ureters. Limits include genitofemoral nerve laterally, circumflex iliac vein, lacunar ligament and LN of Cloquet caudally.
- **Super-extended PLND:** to the level of inferior mesenteric artery.

A better oncological outcome is achieved with PLND. The evidence remains conflicting regarding whether the extent of dissection influences outcome, with several reporting benefits with (super)extended, in certain subsets of patients [12]. Cohort studies have suggested improved overall survival in the excision of >10 LNs [13]. There are presently two RCTs reviewing the effect of PLND extent (*SWOG 1011 and AUO*). EAU Guidelines state that *extended LND might have a therapeutic benefit compared to less extensive LND, but due to study bias no firm conclusions can be drawn* [1].

12.3 Robotic-Assisted Radical Cystectomy (RARC)

With the emergence of robotic technology, RARC offers enhanced surgical ergonomics, instrument dexterity and intra-operative visuals, albeit associated with significant cost and longer operative time. Oncological outcomes, including time to recurrence and positive surgical margin rates, are comparable with open RC (ORC). RARC has a reduced length of hospital stay and reduced blood loss. The rates of major complications are comparable. A recent Cochrane review (Rai et al.) and studies such as RAZOR, the largest RCT to date, corroborate these findings [14–17]. Ultimately, surgeon experience and institutional volume are the fundamental factors that influence outcome, independent of technique or approach.

Improvement in robotic surgical skills has also enabled intracorporeal urinary diversion, which is associated with shorter operative times and fewer blood transfusions [18]. A recent retrospective report, from a high-volume centre, found less major complications after intracorporeal versus extracorporeal reconstruction [19].

The results from *iROC*, a prospective UK multicentre RCT comparing intracorporeal RARC with ORC, are awaited.

Patients need to be made aware of the advantages and disadvantages of ORC versus *RARC in order to make informed decisions. The key factor is centre experience, not specific technique* [1].

12.4 Urinary Diversion

The *ideal* urinary diversion (UD) would be low pressure, no reflux, has controlled spontaneous emptying, no functional consequences and no reabsorption of urinary waste. Types of diversion include:

- **Abdominal Diversion**: Ileal Conduit and Continent Cutaneous Reservoir.
- **Urethral Diversion:** Neobladder.
- **Rectosigmoid Diversion.**

12.4.1 Ileal Conduit

The ileal conduit is the most common UD method. It is a reliable procedure, with well-established complications and results, and is formed by anastomosing the ureters to an isolated segment of distal ileum, 20 cm from the ileo-caecal valve. The distal end is brought out as a stoma (Figs. 12.2, 12.3, and 12.4). Specific complications include urinary tract infection,

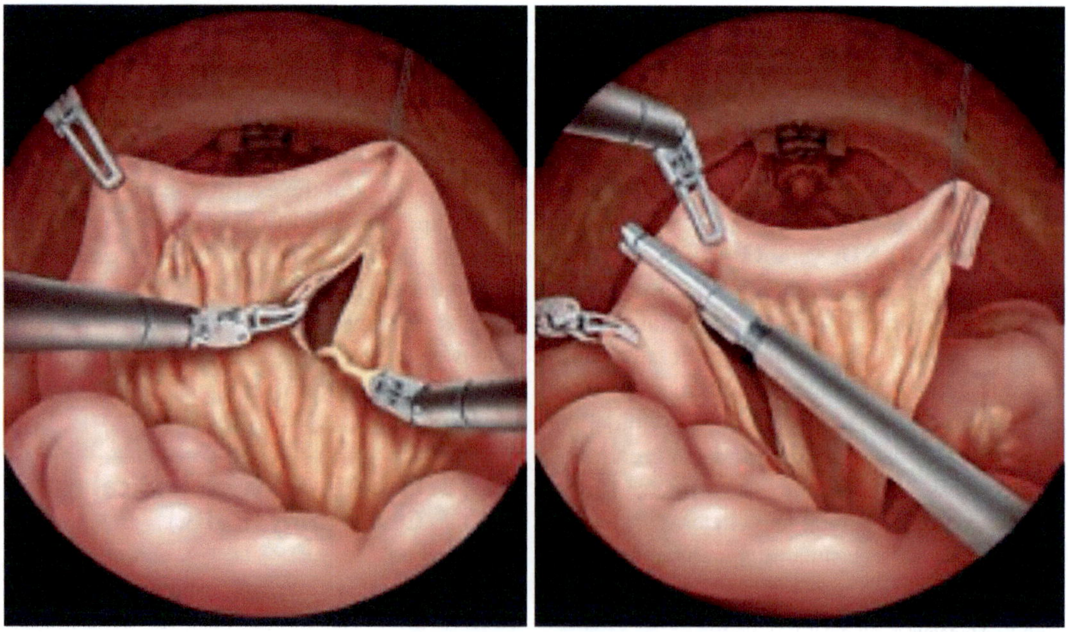

Fig. 12.2 Robotic-assisted intracorporeal ileal conduit "Marionette" Technique. Developing the mesenteric window and division of bowel segment (Reproduced from Guru K, Mansour A, Nyquist J. Robotic-assisted intracorporeal ileal conduit "Marionette" technique. *BJU Int.* 2010;106(9):1404–20)

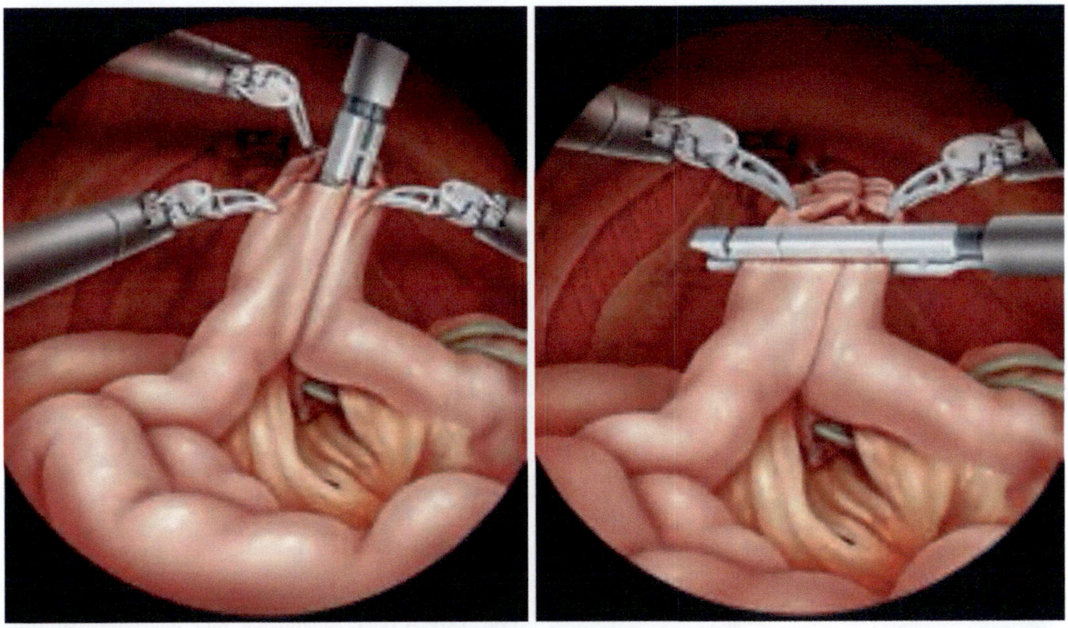

Fig. 12.3 Restoring bowel continuity with side-to-side anastomosis and closure of the end (Reproduced from Guru K, Mansour A, Nyquist J. Robotic-assisted intracorporeal ileal conduit "Marionette" technique. *BJU Int.* 2010;106(9):1404–20)

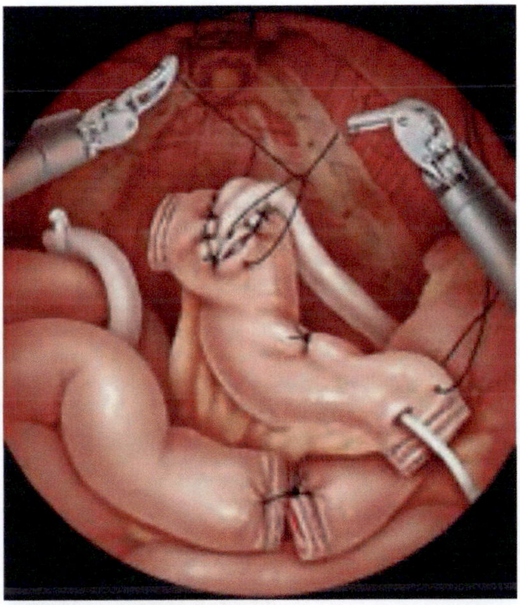

Fig. 12.4 "Bricker" ureteroenteric anastomosis with stent exiting distal end of the conduit via the same enterotomy used for washout of the conduit (Reproduced from Guru K, Mansour A, Nyquist J. Robotic-assisted intracorporeal ileal conduit "Marionette" technique. *BJU Int.* 2010;106(9):1404–20)

uretero-ileal leakage, ileo-ileal anastomotic leak, uretero-ileal anastomotic leak and stenosis, parastomal hernia and metabolic sequelae. Median length of postoperative hospital stay is considerably shorter compared to neobladder formation, and operative time is reduced [20].

Continent cutaneous diversion does not require an external collection device. The ureters drain into a low-pressure reservoir pouch, with an anti-reflux submucosal tunnel, which is drained by the patient via a catheterisable stoma (e.g., appendix—Mitrofanoff principle) brought out in the right iliac fossa.

12.4.2 Neobladder

This option of urinary diversion most resembles the native bladder. A reservoir is fashioned from bowel and the resultant pouch is anastomosed to the urethra. A number of techniques exist via both the open (Studer technique—Figs. 12.5, 12.6, 12.7, and 12.8) and robotic-assisted approaches (Figs. 12.9, 12.10, 12.11, and 12.12).

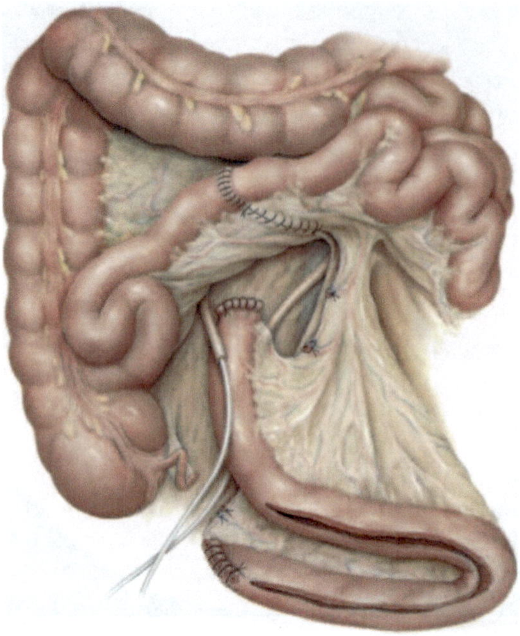

Fig. 12.5 Both ends of ileal segment closed and distal portion opened along anti-mesenteric border (Reproduced from Studer UE, Varol C, Danuser H. Orthotopic ileal neobladder. *BJU Int*. 2004;93(1):183–93. https://doi.org/10.1111/j.1464-410x.2004.04641.x)

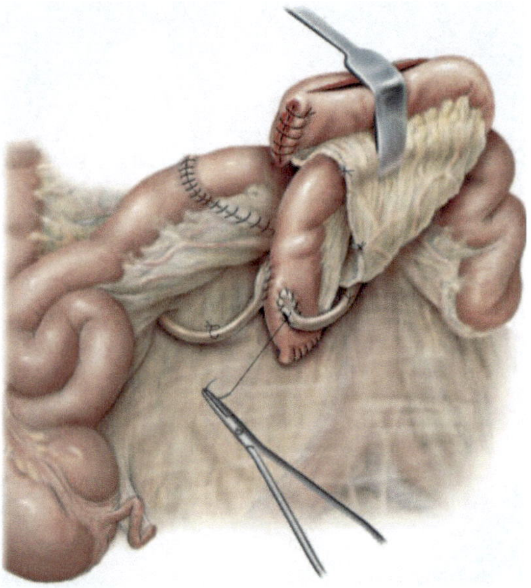

Fig. 12.6 Ureters spatulated and anastomosed using Nesbit technique (end-to-end anastomosis to longitudinal incisions along the antimesenteric border of afferent ileal segment (Reproduced from Studer UE, Varol C, Danuser H. Orthotopic ileal neobladder. *BJU Int*. 2004;93(1):183–93. https://doi.org/10.1111/j.1464-410x.2004.04641.x)

Increasingly being offered to patients, a neobladder negates the need for a stoma with reported daytime continence rates of up to 92% at 12 months [21]. A longer segment of ileum is required, increasing the risk of metabolic complications.

Absolute contraindications to neobladder formation include impaired renal function, severe hepatic dysfunction, compromised intestinal function and simultaneous urethrectomy or tumour infiltrating the prostate. Relative contraindications include bladder neck involvement, multifocal high-grade TCC in situ, positive lymph nodes, previous radiation, benign urethral pathology and obesity. Neobladder formation does not have an adverse impact on oncological outcomes when compared with ileal conduit [22]. No RCTs have been undertaken comparing the two approaches, or continent cutaneous diversion.

Regardless of UD technique, pre-operative patient counselling and education have been shown to improve quality of life measures [23].

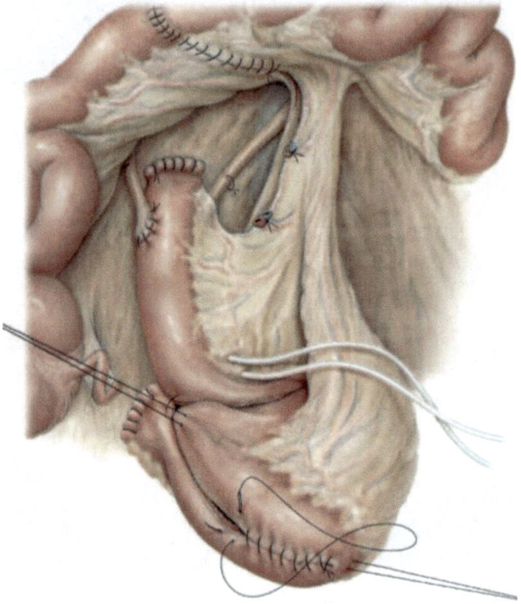

Fig. 12.7 Construction of the reservoir using opened U-shaped potion of distal ileal segment, with exteriorised ureteric catheters (Reproduced from Studer UE, Varol C, Danuser H. Orthotopic ileal neobladder. *BJU Int*. 2004;93(1):183–93. https://doi.org/10.1111/j.1464-410x.2004.04641.x)

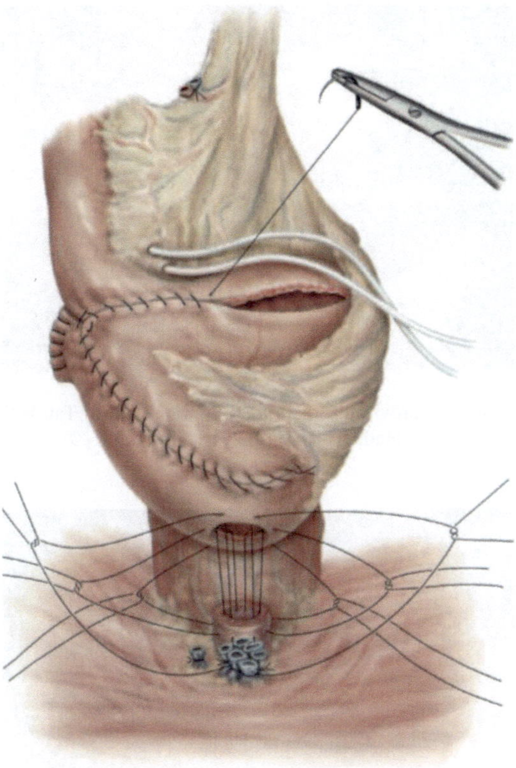

Fig. 12.8 Formation of urethra-enteric anastomosis (Reproduced from Studer UE, Varol C, Danuser H. Orthotopic ileal neobladder. *BJU Int*. 2004;93(1):183–93. https://doi.org/10.1111/j.1464-410x.2004.04641.x)

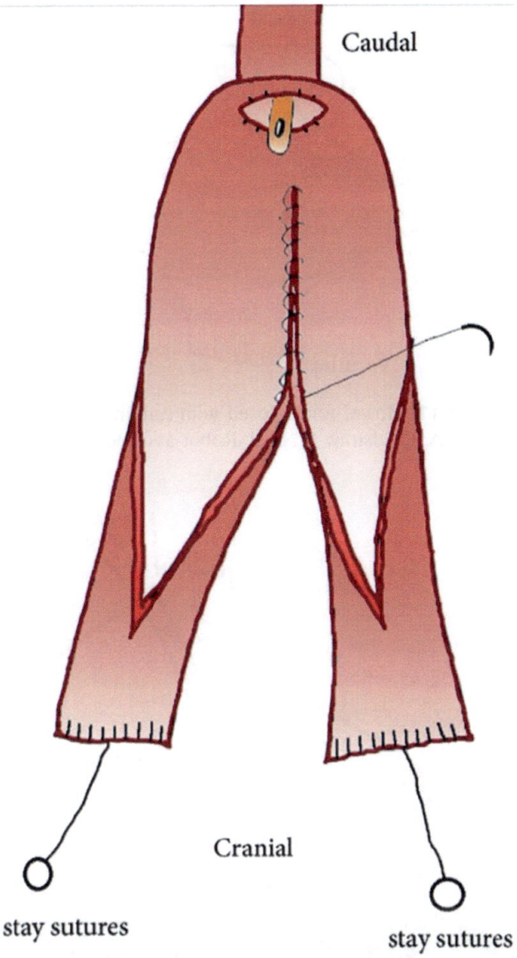

Fig. 12.9 Urethral-Ileal anastomosis and formation of posterior plate (Reproduced from Tan WS, Sridhar A, Goldstraw M, et al. Robot-assisted intracorporeal pyramid neobladder. *BJU Int*. 2015;116(5):771–9)

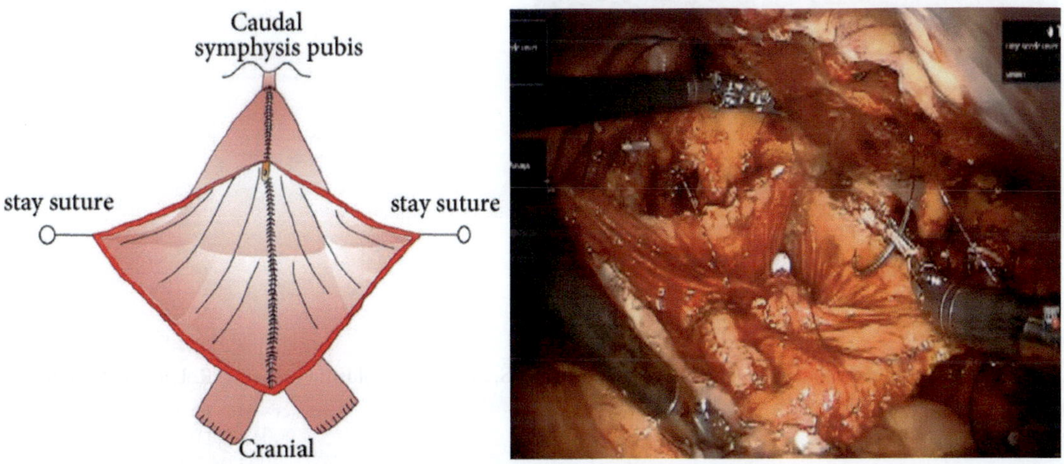

Fig. 12.10 Pyramid neobladder reconstruction (Reproduced from Tan WS, Sridhar A, Goldstraw M, et al. Robot-assisted intracorporeal pyramid neobladder. *BJU Int*. 2015;116(5):771–9)

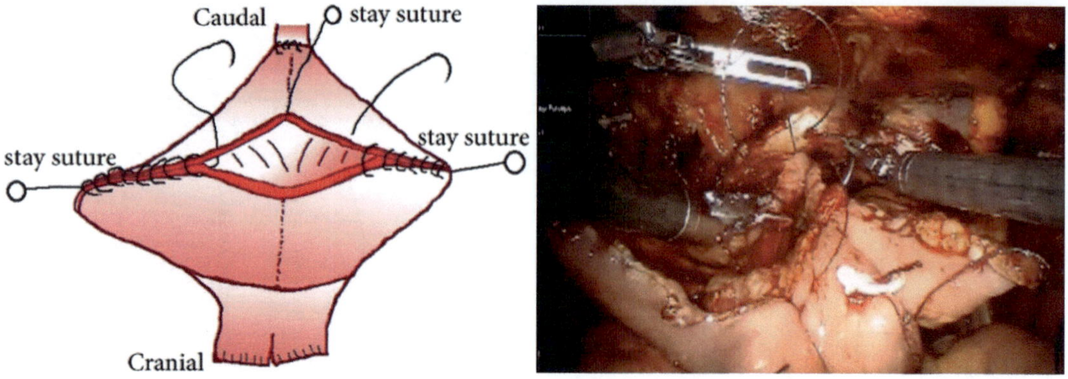

Fig. 12.11 Bowel folds closed with running 3-0 V-Loc. Stay sutures providing traction (Reproduced from Tan WS, Sridhar A, Goldstraw M, et al. Robot-assisted intracorporeal pyramid neobladder. *BJU Int*. 2015;116(5):771–9)

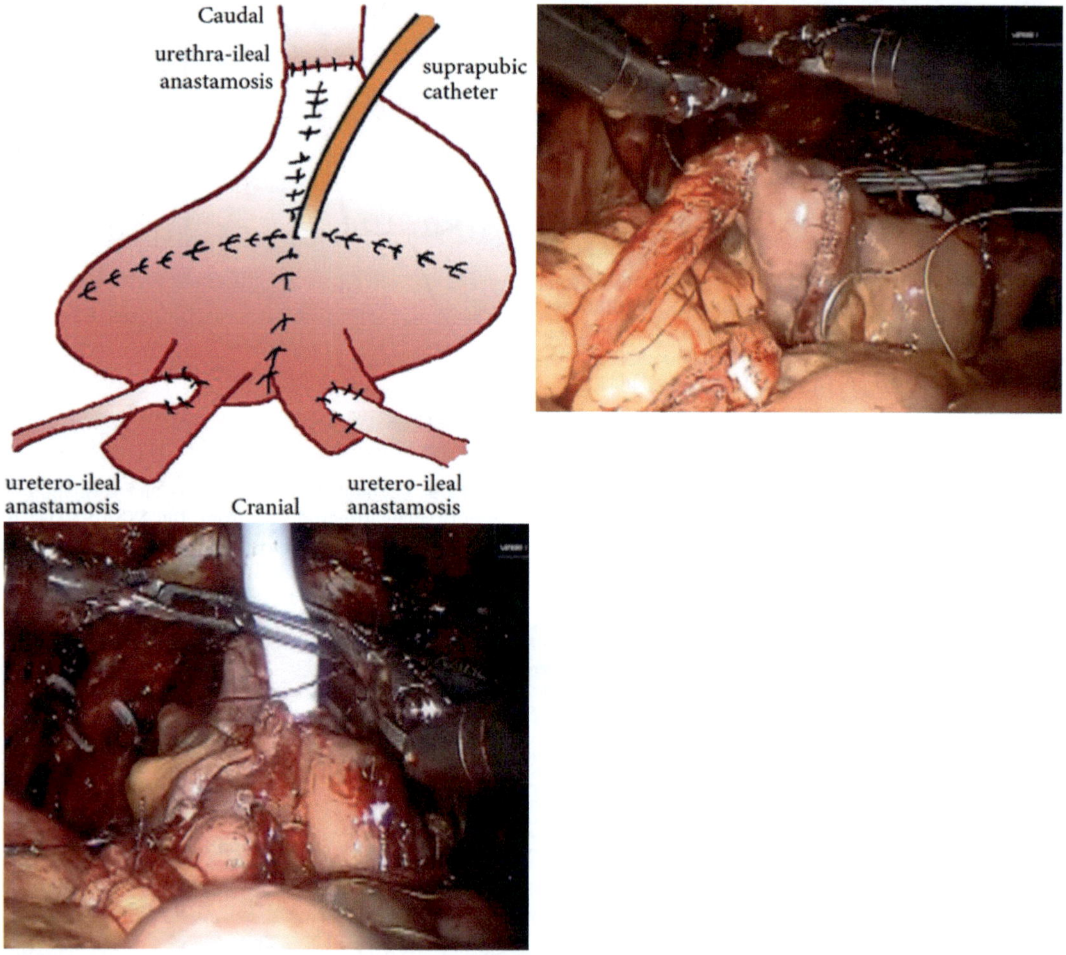

Fig. 12.12 Completed neobladder (Reproduced from Tan WS, Sridhar A, Goldstraw M, et al. Robot-assisted intracorporeal pyramid neobladder. *BJU Int*. 2015;116(5):771–9)

Neobladder formation is associated with improved psychological health, particularly in younger patients [24].

12.5 Bladder-Sparing Surgical Options

TURBT alone should only be considered as a therapeutic option for MIBC after radical TURBT, when the patient is not fit for RC, or declines surgery, or undergoes a multimodality bladder-preserving approach, comprising TURBT, systemic chemotherapy and radiotherapy, with ongoing cystoscopies to evaluate response.

The ideal patients for **partial cystectomy** have no hydronephrosis, a solitary tumour, within the bladder dome or anterior wall, which is amenable to resection with a 2cm surgical margin and no concomitant CIS.

Patients with MIBC who are medically fit and consent to radical cystectomy should not undergo partial cystectomy or maximal transurethral resection of bladder tumour as a primary curative therapy [1].

12.6 Salvage Cystectomy

Salvage cystectomy is indicated in non-responders to conservative treatment, recurrence after bladder-sparing treatment and non-urothelial cancer and is necessitated in approximately 10–15% of patients following multimodality therapy. Major late complications are a little higher when compared to primary RC [25, 26].

12.7 Post-Operative Surveillance

Following RC, patients remain at risk of tumour recurrence and appropriate surveillance is required (Table 12.3). Most recurrences occur 2 years post-operatively, occurring either locally within the pelvis, upper urinary tract and urethra or at distant anatomical sites. A recurrence rate of 48.6% has been reported after RC, following 20-year follow-up [27]. Recurrence is detected both symptomatically and on follow-up investigations, including cross-sectional imaging, laboratory testing and endoscopic examination of the urethral remnant.

Table 12.3 Various post-radical cystectomy (RC) follow-up protocols

	Post-radical cystectomy (RC)
NICE	• *Upper tract imaging* and *GFR*: At least annually
	• *CT-chest/abdomen/pelvis (CT-CAP)*: 6-, 12- and 24-months post-RC
	• Monitor for metabolic acidosis, B12 and folate deficiency, at least annually
	• Defunctioned urethra: Urethral washings for cytology
	• And/or urethroscopy annually for 5 years to detect urethral recurrence
EAU	• *Upper tract imaging*: 6 monthly for 3 years, then annually
	• Follow-up of urethra: Cytology and/or urethroscopy
	• Following neobladder: Regular measurements of pH and sodium bicarbonate substitution
	• Annual B12 levels
AUA	• *CT-CAP (or MRI)*: 6–12 month intervals for 2–3 years, then annually
	• *U&E and B12*: 3–6 month intervals for 2–3 years, then annually
	• Monitor urethral remnant for recurrence

12.7.1 Neoadjuvant Chemotherapy (NAC)

Neoadjuvant cisplatin-based chemotherapy is recommended in patients with T2–T4a cN0M0 bladder cancer [28, 29]. A 2003 meta-analysis of 11 randomised trials compared cisplatin-based neoadjuvant chemotherapy with local therapy against local therapy alone and demonstrated an improvement in overall survival by 5–8% and a lower risk of recurrence in the experimental arm [28].

However, the ideal neoadjuvant chemotherapy regimen has not yet been determined. Studies comparing various chemotherapy regimens show similar rates of pathologic complete response (pCR) for GC (gemcitabine and cisplatin) and MVAC (methotrexate, vinblastine, doxorubicin and cisplatin [30, 31]). MVAC could be the preferred option in young patients with a good performance status, affording a shortened time from diagnosis to surgery. For those unable to tolerate MVAC due to medical comorbidities, GC is an appropriate alternative. In a recently reported Phase III VESPER trial investigating the ideal perioperative treatment regimen, there was higher toxicity regarding asthenia and gastrointestinal side effects with dose-dense MVAC, accompanied by a better bladder control rate and 3-year progression-free survival compared with GC [32].

There has recently been increasing interest in the role of immunotherapy in the perioperative setting due to the potential of delivering durable response. At present, most studies using neoadjuvant immunotherapy have been performed in patients ineligible for cisplatin-based chemotherapy, and results from trials using neoadjuvant atezolizumab (ABACUS), pembrolizumab (PURE-01), combining durvalumab and tremelimumab (DUTRENEO) and nivolumab plus ipilimumab (NABUCCO) have reported response rates from 30% to 40% [33–36]. There have also been trials combining immunotherapy with chemotherapy such as BLASST-1 and HCRN gu14–188, which have also shown similar response rates, highlighting efficacy and tolerability of neoadjuvant immunotherapy use [37, 38]. However, further randomised controlled trials would be needed before neoadjuvant immunotherapy can be incorporated into standard practice. Neoaduvant radiotherapy is not recommended in routine practice, as studies show that neoadjuvant radiotherapy has no impact on survival when compared to cystectomy alone.

12.7.2 Adjuvant Therapy

Despite its proven benefits, there are concerns associated with the use of neoadjuvant chemotherapy. These include delays to surgery, toxicity, patient refusal and overtreatment of 10–15% of patients who have pT0 disease even without NAC. Clinicians and patients may decide to proceed with surgery without neoadjuvant treatment, reserving the option of adjuvant treatment at a later stage if they are deemed high risk for recurrence based on pathologic staging.

Adjuvant cisplatin-based combination chemotherapy may be offered to patients with pT3/4 and/or pN+disease, if no neoadjuvant chemotherapy has been delivered. While not as strongly recommended in international guidelines as neo-adjuvant treatment, meta-analyses have demonstrated evidence of overall survival and disease-free benefit in patients with MIBC receiving adjuvant cisplatin-based chemotherapy after RC [39]. However, caution should be exercised in adopting this as standard practice. Large retrospective studies have suggested superiority in survival for neoadjuvant versus adjuvant chemotherapy [40]. Furthermore, many meta-analyses for adjuvant chemotherapy are flawed by methodological limitations such as limited patient numbers and/or poor accrual.

Although adjuvant chemotherapy is widely used in clinical practice for the management of MIBC, a consensus has yet to be established on which regimen is most effective for improving overall survival. In a 2017 network meta-analysis, the only chemotherapy regimen associated with a significant improvement in both the PFS and OS was a combination involving gemcitabine/cisplatin/paclitaxel [41]. However, adjuvant chemotherapy may prolong disease-free survival among patients with locally advanced upper tract urothelial carcinoma, following the results of the Phase III POUT trial [42].

In 2021, the phase 3 CheckMate 274 trial was the first to demonstrate the role of adjuvant immunotherapy after RC. Disease-free survival was longer with adjuvant nivolumab than placebo, particularly in the PD-L1 biomarker-positive population where the risk of recurrence was reduced by 45% [43].

12.7.3 Bladder-Sparing Treatment

Removal of the bladder requires urinary diversions that can substantially impair quality of life post-surgery and cause concerns about postoperative impairment of renal function as previously reported in several studies [44, 45]. Another form of treatment offered to preserve the bladder is opting for trimodal therapy for bladder preservation (TMT), which incorporates maximal TURBT, radiation therapy and concurrent chemotherapy. This is an option for patients who are not candidates for cystectomy and for those who wish to preserve their bladder. This approach, however, requires careful surveillance for local recurrence or detection of new urothelial cancers. Most patients would prefer to keep their native bladder; however, the primary goal of treatment is to cure the cancer, with a view of preserving the bladder as a secondary goal.

Whilst bladder preservation seems like an ideal option, there remains a risk of recurrence in other parts of the bladder. The risk of recurrence is at least 50% or higher within 3 to 5 years of treatment amongst patients treated with the bladder sparing approach [46]. It is important that patients are given the relevant information about these risks, prior to making a treatment plan, whilst taking their own views, priorities and present quality of life, and general health into consideration. There are no select criteria for choosing patients who may undergo bladder preserving TMT approach of treatment; however, some important factors should be considered prior. These include:

- **Clinical T2 to T3a disease:** Increasing T stage is associated with decreased rates of complete response after chemoradiation, and it is noted that patients with clinical T2 to T3a disease may be favourable candidates for TMT. For patients with T3b or T4 disease, neoadjuvant chemotherapy followed by RC is preferred.
- **Absence of tumour-associated hydronephrosis:** It is also preferred to use TMT if there is absence of tumour-associated hydronephrosis, and adequate renal function is needed in order to receive cisplatin-based chemotherapy.
- **Urothelial histology:** Prospective studies exploring the use of TMT have focused on patients with urothelial histology. These findings cannot be generalised to less common histological subtypes which may respond more poorly to chemotherapy (e.g., squamous cell carcinoma, adenocarcinoma, and micropapillary).
- **Others:** Other factors that are beneficial in TMT are absence of extensive CIS, unifocal tumours <6 cm in diameter and good bladder function and capacity.

These patients can have long-term cancer-specific survival rates similar to those who undergo RC.

Radiation therapy can be offered in the forms of external beam radiotherapy and brachytherapy in selected patients. External beam radiotherapy can be recommended for frail, older patients or those with multiple comorbidities, who are unable to undergo other approaches, to palliate local symptoms. However, local recurrence with radiotherapy alone is reported in up to 70% of patients, and 5-year survival ranges from 20 to 40%, therefore radiotherapy alone is not a suitable treatment in healthy and fit patients. Brachytherapy is a form of radiation therapy in which a source of radiation (radioisotope) is sealed and placed inside or next to the tumour site. The radiation source is kept in a protective capsule or wire, allowing the radiation to destroy only surrounding tissue and prevents the charge of the radioisotope from escaping into body fluids. Brachytherapy can be used in patients with a small solitary muscle-invasive bladder tumour, and it can also be used in combination with external beam radiotherapy to maximise benefits of radiation. In patients receiving this type of treatment, outcomes appear similar to those opting for RC, although this has not been reported in studies [47, 48]. Therefore, the use of brachytherapy is not routinely offered to patients outside specialist centres.

Advanced techniques, such as intensity-modulated radiation therapy (IMRT), are now used when possible due to the more accurate delivery of high-dose radiation to the tumour and adjacent areas. There is no standardised dose, frequency or fields and restaging paradigms agreed, and there tend to be variations in between treatment centres. An adequate amount of radiation is needed to eradicate all tumour and to treat adjacent areas that are at high recurrence risk. A balance has to be made in also minimising the dose of radiation to adjacent normal tissues such as colon, rectum, small intestine, hips and normal bladder, in order to minimise any toxicity. Generally, 40–45 Gy is given to the bladder, prostatic or proximal urethra and the adjacent lymph node basin in the pelvis. A further dose of 10–15 Gy is given to the bladder and 10 Gy dose to the tumour. Salvage cystectomy can be done in patients who do not have complete response to this initial approach or develop invasive recurrence during follow-up.

Radiotherapy was used for decades as monotherapy for patients unfit to undergo cystectomy. However, recent evidence demonstrates that using sensitising chemotherapy in concordance with radiotherapy after maximal TURBT gives better outcomes than radiotherapy alone [49]. The perfect chemotherapy regimen has not been established; however, cisplatin-based chemotherapy is generally favoured, and 5-FU plus mitomycin in patients where cisplatin is contraindicated due to impaired kidney function or poor performance status, for example. Concurrent chemotherapy can sensitise tumour cells to the effects of radiation, and therefore able to improve outcomes. The addition of neoadjuvant and adjuvant chemotherapy to concurrent chemoradiation is intended to eradicate distant micro-metastases that are not treated by radiotherapy. It can be considered if it is a well-informed decision that accepts the uncertainty or benefit of neoadjuvant or adjuvant chemotherapy.

The risk of developing metastases is high in the first few years posttreatment, therefore, follow-up should include imaging of the chest, abdomen and pelvis and urine cytology for evidence of recurrence. The frequency of imaging depends on the individual risk of recurrence, but usually should be performed every 3 to 6 months for the first 2 years, then as clinically indicated. Those patients, who opted for TMT approach, should undergo routine endoscopic surveillance of the bladder and urethra due to the high risk of local recurrence.

12.7.4 Metastatic Disease

Approximately 5–10% of patients with MIBC present with de novo metastatic disease. Furthermore, approximately 50% of patients with MIBC who present as localised disease (T2–T4) will relapse after radical treatment. Lymph nodes, bones, lung, liver and peritoneum are the most common sites of metastasis.

In a similar fashion to neoadjuvant chemotherapy, cisplatin combination therapies remain the primary choice of treatment. There are multiple cisplatin-based combination regimens used including methotrexate, vinblastine, doxorubicin and cisplatin (MVAC), dose dense MVAC and gemcitabine plus cisplatin.

MVAC is a standard first-line option. Increasing the dose intensity of MVAC by administering the treatment every 2 weeks with G-CSF support has also been evaluated. There has not been a significant proven difference between dose-intense treatment in OS, but there is an association with a reduction in toxicity. Toxicity is a concern with MVAC therapy, such as myelosuppression, neutropenic fever, sepsis, mucositis and nausea and vomiting. Approximately 20% of patients treated with high-dose intensity MVAC have long-term survival. However, the use of hematopoietic growth factor support may benefit and ameliorate some toxicities such as myelosuppression [50].

The combination of gemcitabine plus cisplatin has similar efficacy to MVAC and less toxicity associated. MVAC versus GC has, in a phase III trial, displayed similar results in response rates (46% vs. 49%) and survival (14.8 vs. 13.8 months). In cisplatin-ineligible patients, gemcitabine and carboplatin can be used in combination—a common strategy prior to the introduction of immunotherapy.

In patients who are ineligible for first-line platinum-based chemotherapy, immunotherapy such as checkpoint inhibitor immunotherapy targeting programmed cell death-1 protein (PD-1) or its ligand (PD-L1) can be used. Atezolizumab is an option for initial therapy for metastatic disease patient. Immunotherapy is preferred in patients with indolent disease limited to lymph nodes and without autoimmune conditions [51]. Alternatively, the Phase II KEYNOTE-052 trial demonstrated that pembrolizumab was an appropriate option as initial therapy. The response rate was 29% for the cohort with a median overall survival of 11.3 months. The US approved pembrolizumab as initial therapy in patients who are not eligible for any platinum-containing chemotherapy. Atezolizumab has also gained approval by FDA as initial therapy for patients ineligible for platinum-based chemotherapy and for those who are cisplatin ineligible and their tumours express PD-L1.

Avelumab is used as maintenance therapy in those patients without disease progression on platinum-based chemotherapy, rather than supportive treatment alone, as this approach achieves improved overall survival (OS) and progression-free survival [52]. If the patients are not eligible for maintenance immunotherapy, they can be observed with supportive care. Avelumab can be continued until disease progression or toxicity development.

In patients with metastatic disease who have progressed during or after platinum-based chemotherapy, at least five PD-(L)1 inhibitors (three in Europe, pembrolizumab, atezolizumab and nivolumab) are approved so far. Pembrolizumab is the only one that demonstrated OS benefit in a phase III Trial (10.3 vs. 7.4 months in chemotherapy arm, which constituted an investigators' choice of docetaxel, paclitaxel or vinflunine) [53].

Targeted agents, such as Enfortumab vedotin, can be used when patients relapse following treatment with chemotherapy and immunotherapy. Enfortumab vedotin is an antibody targeting the cell adhesion molecule nectin-4 linked to a microtubule inhibitor conjugate; this antibody is reported to improve both OS and PFS over chemotherapy in trials [54]. This is the first example of a gene-targeted therapy that was approved for bladder cancer. Patients who are ineligible for or decline-targeted therapy may be offered single-agent chemotherapy, as an alternative; they can also be encouraged to enroll in clinical trials where available.

12.7.5 Palliative Treatment

Patients with locally advanced MIBC (T4b invading the pelvic or abdominal wall), with debilitating symptoms, such as bleeding, pain or urinary obstruction, may be candidates for palliative radiotherapy, or nephrostomy insertion for upper tract obstruction. Further adjuncts for haematuria treatment include intravesical rinsing with 1% silver nitrate or 1–2% alum, instillation of formalin or embolisation of pelvic arteries [55]. Palliative cystectomy with urinary diversion carries the greatest morbidity and should be considered only as a last resort (Fig. 12.14) [56].

References

1. Witjes JA, et al. European Association of Urology guidelines on muscle-invasive and metastatic bladder cancer: summary of the 2020 guidelines. Eur Urol. 2021;79(1):82–104.
2. Shelley MD, et al. Surgery versus radiotherapy for muscle invasive bladder cancer. Cochrane Database Syst Rev. 2002;1:CD002079.
3. Gore JL, et al. Mortality increases when radical cystectomy is delayed more than 12 weeks: results from a surveillance, epidemiology, and end results-Medicare analysis. Cancer. 2009;115:988.

4. Bruins HM, et al. The importance of hospital and surgeon volume as major determinants of morbidity and mortality after radical cystectomy for bladder cancer: a systematic review and recommendations by the European Association of Urology muscle-invasive and metastatic bladder cancer guideline panel. Eur Urol Oncol. 2020;3:131.
5. Stenzl A, et al. Cystectomy—technical considerations in male and female patients. EAU Updat Ser. 2005;3:138.
6. Hernandez V, et al. Oncological and functional outcomes of sexual function-preserving cystectomy compared with standard radical cystectomy in men: a systematic review. Urol Oncol. 2017;35:539.e17.
7. Veskimae E, et al. Systematic review of the oncological and functional outcomes of pelvic organ-preserving radical cystectomy (RC) compared with standard RC in women who undergo curative surgery and orthotopic neobladder substitution for bladder cancer. BJU Int. 2017;120:12.
8. Hammond J, et al. Rates of venous thromboembolism among patients with major surgery for cancer. Ann Surg Oncol. 2011;18:3240.
9. Tarin TV, et al. Lymph node-positive bladder cancer treated with radical cystectomy and lymphadenectomy: effect of the level of node positivity. Eur Urol. 2012;61(5):1025–30.
10. Dorin RP, et al. Lymph node dissection technique is more important than lymph node count in identifying nodal metastases in radical cystectomy patients: a comparative mapping study. Eur Urol. 2011;60:946.
11. Perera M, et al. Pelvic lymph node dissection during radical cystectomy for muscle-invasive bladder cancer. Nat Rev Urol. 2018;15(11):686–92.
12. Bruins HM, et al. The impact of the extent of lymphadenectomy on oncologic outcomes in patients undergoing radical cystectomy for bladder cancer: a systematic review. Eur Urol. 2014;66:1065.
13. Wright JL, et al. The association between extent of lymphadenectomy and survival among patients with lymph node metastases undergoing radical cystectomy. Cancer. 2008;112:2401.
14. Rai BP, et al. Robotic versus open radical cystectomy for bladder cancer in adults. Cochrane Database Syst Rev. 2019;4:CD011903.
15. Venkatramani V, et al. Predictors of recurrence, and progression-free and overall survival following open versus robotic radical cystectomy: analysis from the RAZOR trial with a 3-year followup. J Urol. 2020;203:522.
16. Parekh DJ, et al. Robot-assisted radical cystectomy versus open radical cystectomy in patients with bladder cancer (RAZOR): an open-label, randomised, phase 3, non-inferiority trial. Lancet. 2018;391:2525.
17. Rai BP, et al. Robot-assisted vs. open radical cystectomy for bladder cancer in adults. BJU Int. 2020;125(6):765–79.
18. Hussein AA, et al. Outcomes of intracorporeal urinary diversion after robot-assisted radical cystectomy: results from the International Robotic Cystectomy Consortium. J Urol. 2018;199:1302.
19. Zhang JH, et al. Large single institution comparison of perioperative outcomes and complications of open radical cystectomy, intracorporeal robot-assisted radical cystectomy and robotic extracorporeal approach. J Urol. 2020;203:512.
20. Novotny V, et al. Perioperative complications of radical cystectomy in a contemporary series. Eur Urol. 2007;51(2):397–401; discussion 401–2.
21. Hautmann RE, et al. Long-term results of standard procedures in urology: the ileal neobladder. World J Urol. 2006;24(3):305–14.
22. Yossepowitch O, et al. Orthotopic urinary diversion after cystectomy for bladder cancer: implications for cancer control and patterns of disease recurrence. J Urol. 2003;169:177.
23. Check DK, et al. Decision regret related to urinary diversion choice among patients treated with cystectomy. J Urol. 2020;203(1):159–63.
24. Yang LS, et al. A systematic review and meta-analysis of quality of life outcomes after radical cystectomy for bladder cancer. Surg Oncol. 2016;25(3):281–97.
25. Giacalone NJ, et al. Long-term outcomes after bladder-preserving tri-modality therapy for patients with muscle-invasive bladder cancer: an updated analysis of the Massachusetts General Hospital experience. Eur Urol. 2017;71:952.
26. Eswara JR, et al. Complications and long-term results of salvage cystectomy after failed bladder sparing therapy for muscle invasive bladder cancer. J Urol. 2012;187:463.
27. Volkmer BG, et al. Oncological follow up after radical cystectomy for bladder cancer-is there any benefit? J Urol. 2009;181(4):1587–93; discussion 1593.
28. Advanced Bladder Cancer Meta-analysis Collaboration. Neoadjuvant chemotherapy in invasive bladder cancer: a systematic review and meta-analysis. Lancet. 2003;361(9373):1927–34.
29. Meeks JJ, et al. A systematic review of neoadjuvant and adjuvant chemotherapy for muscle-invasive bladder cancer. Eur Urol. 2012;62(3):523–33.
30. Galsky MD, et al. Comparative effectiveness of gemcitabine plus cisplatin versus methotrexate, vinblastine, doxorubicin, plus cisplatin as neoadjuvant therapy for muscle-invasive bladder cancer. Cancer. 2015;121(15):2586–93.
31. Pfister C, et al. Randomized phase III trial of dose-dense methotrexate, vinblastine, doxorubicin, and cisplatin, or gemcitabine and cisplatin as perioperative chemotherapy for patients with muscle-invasive bladder cancer. Analysis of the GETUG/AFU V05 VESPER trial secondary endpoints: chemotherapy toxicity and pathological responses. Eur Urol. 2021;79(2):214–21.
32. Pfister C, et al. VESPER trial investigators. Randomized phase III trial of dose-dense methotrexate, vinblastine, doxorubicin, and Cisplatin, or gemcitabine and Cisplatin as perioperative chemotherapy for patients with muscle-invasive bladder cancer.

Analysis of the GETUG/AFU V05 VESPER trial secondary endpoints: chemotherapy toxicity and pathological responses. Eur Urol. 2021;79(2):214–21.
33. Powles T, et al. Clinical efficacy and biomarker analysis of neoadjuvant atezolizumab in operable urothelial carcinoma in the abacus trial. Nat Med. 2019;25:1706–14.
34. Necchi A, et al. Updated results of pure-01 with preliminary activity of neoadjuvant pembrolizumab in patients with muscle-invasive bladder carcinoma with variant histologies. Eur Urol. 2020;77:439–46.
35. Grande E, et al. Dutreneo trial: a randomized phase ii trial of durvalumab and tremelimumab versus chemotherapy as a neoadjuvant approach to muscle-invasive urothelial bladder cancer (MIBC) patients (PTS) prospectively selected by an interferon (inf)-gamma immune signature. J Clin Oncol. 2020;38:5012.
36. van Dijk N, et al. Preoperative ipilimumab plus nivolumab in locoregionally advanced urothelial cancer: the nabucco trial. Nat Med. 2020;26:1839–44.
37. Gupta S, et al. Results from blasst-1 (bladder cancer signal seeking trial) of nivolumab, gemcitabine, and cisplatin in muscle invasive bladder cancer (MIBC) undergoing cystectomy. J Clin Oncol. 2020;38:439.
38. Kaimakliotis HZ, et al. Phase II neoadjuvant (N-) gemcitabine (G) and pembrolizumab (P) for locally advanced Urothelial cancer (lauc): interim results from the cisplatin (c)-ineligible cohort of gu14-188. J Clin Oncol. 2020;38:5019.
39. Leow JJ, et al. Adjuvant chemotherapy for invasive bladder cancer: a 2013 updated systematic review and meta-analysis of randomized trials. Eur Urol. 2014;66(1):42–54.
40. Del Bene G, et al. Neoadjuvant vs. adjuvant chemotherapy in muscle invasive bladder cancer (MIBC): analysis from the RISC database. Front Oncol. 2018;8:463.
41. Kim HS, et al. Adjuvant chemotherapy for muscle-invasive bladder cancer: a systematic review and network meta-analysis of randomized clinical trials. Oncotarget. 2017;8(46):81204–14.
42. Birtle A, et al. Adjuvant chemotherapy in upper tract urothelial carcinoma (the POUT trial): a phase 3, open-label, randomised controlled trial. Lancet. 2020;395:1268–77.
43. Bajorin DF, et al. Adjuvant nivolumab versus placebo in muscle-invasive urothelial carcinoma. N Engl J Med. 2021;384(22):2102–14.
44. Nishikawa M, et al. Long-term changes in renal function outcomes following radical cystectomy and urinary diversion. Int J Clin Oncol. 2014;19:1105–11.
45. Isbarn H, et al. A population based assessment of perioperative mortality after cystectomy for bladder cancer. J Urol. 2009;182:70–7.
46. Tanaka H, Kijima T, Fujii Y. Bladder preservation therapy in muscle-invasive bladder cancer: current evidence and future perspectives. AME Med J. 2020;5:16.
47. van der Steen-Banasik E, et al. Brachytherapy versus cystectomy in solitary bladder cancer: a case control, multicentre, East-Netherlands study. Radiother Oncol. 2009;93(2):352–7.
48. Blank LE, et al. Results of bladder-conserving treatment, consisting of brachytherapy combined with limited surgery and external beam radiotherapy, for patients with solitary T1-T3 bladder tumors less than 5 cm in diameter. Int J Radiat Oncol Biol Phys. 2007;69(2):454–8.
49. James ND, et al. BC2001 investigators. Radiotherapy with or without chemotherapy in muscle-invasive bladder cancer. N Engl J Med. 2012;366(16):1477–88.
50. Gabrilove JL, et al. Effect of granulocyte colony-stimulating factor on neutropenia and associated morbidity due to chemotherapy for transitional-cell carcinoma of the urothelium. N Engl J Med. 1988;318(22):1414–22.
51. van der Heijden MS, et al. Atezolizumab versus chemotherapy in patients with platinum-treated locally advanced or metastatic urothelial carcinoma: a long-term overall survival and safety update from the phase 3 imvigor211 clinical trial. Eur Urol. 2021;80:7–11.
52. Powles T, et al. Avelumab maintenance therapy for advanced or metastatic Urothelial carcinoma. N Engl J Med. 2020;383(13):1218–30.
53. Fradet Y, et al. Randomized phase III KEYNOTE-045 trial of pembrolizumab versus paclitaxel, docetaxel, or vinflunine in recurrent advanced urothelial cancer: results of >2 years of follow-up. Ann Oncol. 2019;30(6):970–6.
54. Powles T, et al. Enfortumab vedotin in previously treated advanced urothelial carcinoma. N Engl J Med. 2021;384:1125–35.
55. Ghahestani SM, et al. Palliative treatment of intractable hematuria in context of advanced bladder cancer: a systematic review. Urol J. 2009;6:149.
56. Ok JH, et al. Medical and surgical palliative care of patients with urological malignancies. J Urol. 2005;174:1177.

13 Metastatic Carcinoma Urinary Bladder, Adjuvant Treatment and Follow-Up

Shuvadeep Ganguly, Sindhu Chitikela, and Atul Batra

13.1 Introduction

Bladder cancer is the second most common cancer of the genitourinary system after prostate cancer with a median age of presentation at 73 years [1]. As per GLOBOCAN 2020 data, cancer of urinary bladder is the tenth most common cancer worldwide and the 13th leading cause of cancer-related mortality [2]. Metastatic bladder cancer accounts for 5–10% of cases of bladder cancer during baseline presentation, but between 25 and 50% of patients with bladder cancer develop metastatic disease during their disease course [1, 3].

In India, cancer of urinary bladder is the 17th most common cancer overall and is the 21st leading cause of cancer-related deaths [4]. The sex-based difference in bladder cancer is more contrasting in India with male to female ratio of 8.9:1 as compared to what is seen in Western population (3:1 to 4:1) [5]. Similarly, there is a higher proportion of patients presenting with metastatic disease at baseline with 17.1% patients presenting with metastatic disease [6].

Neoadjuvant therapy is preferable for the management of localized muscle-invasive bladder carcinoma as nearly in a third of patients, adjuvant therapy is often delayed or not possible due to complications of radical cystectomy [7]. However, adjuvant therapy is recommended for patients who undergoes upfront radical cystectomy with high-risk features and with emerging data, immunotherapy is also being incorporated in adjuvant setting post neoadjuvant chemotherapy.

Palliative chemotherapy remains the cornerstone of the management of metastatic bladder cancer and was the only option available till a few years back. With newer therapies like immunotherapeutic drugs, antibody–drug conjugates and targeted therapies approved since 2016, the treatment landscape of metastatic bladder cancer has undergone a significant and exciting change over past 6 years [8]. In this chapter, we summarize currently available treatment options for first-line and subsequent-line management of metastatic bladder cancer as well as adjuvant therapy for muscle-invasive bladder cancer. Transitional cell carcinoma, which is derived from the pseudostratified epithelium of the urothelial tract, accounts for more than 90% of bladder cancer and is focused subsequently [3].

S. Ganguly · S. Chitikela · A. Batra (✉)
Department of Medical Oncology,
DR.B.R.A.I.R.C.H, All India Institute of Medical Sciences (AIIMS), New Delhi, India

P. Singh et al. (eds.), *A Guide to Management of Urological Cancers*,
https://doi.org/10.1007/978-981-99-2341-0_13

13.2 Workup and Prognosis in Metastatic Bladder Cancer

Organ involvement: Bladder cancer disseminates both via lymphatics as well as haematogenously. The most common pattern of organ involvement in case of metastatic bladder cancer includes nonregional lymph nodes, followed by bone, urinary tract, lung, and liver [9]. While ^{18}F-fluorodeoxyglucose positron emission computed tomography is not standard choice for evaluation of locally advanced bladder cancer, it is of significant utility for diagnosis of disseminated disease and monitoring response.

Outcome and prognostic factors: Metastatic bladder cancer has a significantly poor prognosis with 5-year survival of only 5% and median survival of around 12–15 months with standard-of-care chemotherapy [10]. It is, however, important to note that a significant proportion of patients at first-line setting remain ineligible for any therapy due to poor performance status; indeed in a real-world study in India, only 55.8% patients with metastatic bladder cancer received any chemotherapy [6].

Poor performance status (like Karnofsky performance status (KPS) <80) or presence of visceral metastases has been consistently shown to be poor prognostic factors (Bajorin risk factors) for outcome in urothelial malignancies [11, 12].

13.3 First-Line Management of Metastatic Bladder Cancer

The management algorithm for metastatic bladder cancer is summarized in Fig. 13.1.

13.3.1 Cisplatin-Based Chemotherapy

Cisplatin-based combination chemotherapy is the standard choice for the first-line chemotherapy for metastatic bladder cancer, for cisplatin-eligible patients. Defining cisplatin eligibility had initially been heterogenous across trials, and hence, subsequently, common criteria were proposed for defining cisplatin eligibility by Galsky et al. [13], which is mentioned in Table 13.1. It has been interestingly observed through a retrospective study that adherence to cisplatin eligibility is important and offering the option of cisplatin to eligible patients improves outcome [14].

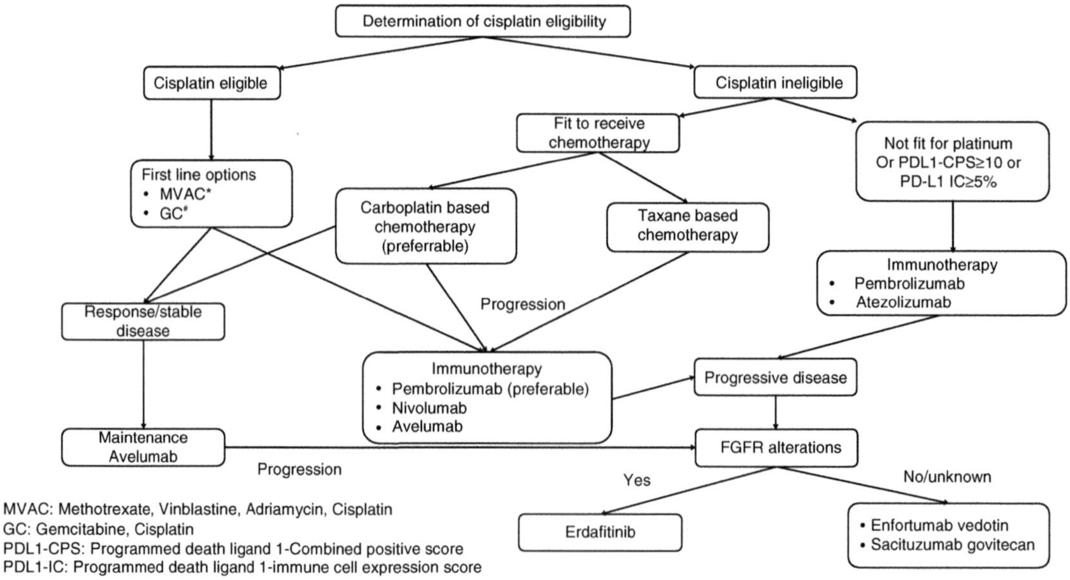

Fig. 13.1 Management algorithm of metastatic bladder cancer

Table 13.1 Criteria for cisplatin eligibility

Number	Parameter	Measurement
1	Performance status (PS)	Eastern Co-operative Oncology Group PS < 2
		Karnofsky performance status >60–70%
2	Creatinine clearance	>60 mL/min[a]
3	Pre-existing audiometric hearing loss	Not ≥Grade 2[b]
4	Pre-existing peripheral neuropathy	Not ≥Grade 2[b]
5	Heart failure	Not ≥New York Heart Association Grade III

[a]Preferably measured by urine creatinine clearance
[b]As per National Cancer Institute-common terminology criteria for adverse events

The common cisplatin-based combination chemotherapy regimens include MVAC (Methotrexate, Vinblastine, Adriamycin, and Cisplatin) and GC (Gemcitabine, Cisplatin), of which MVAC has been the historical standard for two decades. Other alternate regimens include CMV (Cisplatin, Methotrexate, and Vinblastine) and CISCA (Cisplatin, Cyclophosphamide, and Adriamycin).

MVAC regimen: It includes methotrexate 30 mg/m^2 on days 1, 15, and 22, vinblastine 3 mg/m^2 on days 2, 15, 22, adriamycin 30 mg/m^2 on day 2, and cisplatin 70 mg/m^2 on day 2 repeated every 28 days. It was prospectively evaluated in a randomized trial compared to single-agent cisplatin and demonstrated an improved response rate (39% vs. 12%) and overall survival (OS) (12.5 vs. 8.2 months). Even on long-term follow-up of 7 years, 3.7% patients in the MVAC group were survivors [12, 15]. MVAC had also demonstrated superior response and outcome over other cisplatin-based combination regimen like CISCA in randomized phase III study [16]. However, it is associated with significant toxicity like neutropenic sepsis (6–10%) and 4% treatment-related mortality [12, 15].

Dose-dense MVAC (ddMVAC) includes a modified regimen of MVAC, which omits day 15 and 22 doses of vinblastine and methotrexate and repeats cycle every 14 days along with primary growth factor support. ddMVAC was evaluated in comparison with classic MVAC regimen in a randomized trial, which demonstrated improvement in complete response rate (21% vs. 9%) and progression-free survival (PFS) (9.1 vs. 8.2 months), although it did not demonstrate improvement in OS [17]. Toxicity profile was similar. Although the improved response with ddMVAC may make it preferable for neoadjuvant setting, it may only be considered as an alternative option for metastatic disease.

GC regimen: Gemcitabine-cisplatin combination includes gemcitabine at 1000 mg/m^2 on days 1, 8, and 15 and cisplatin 70 mg/m^2 on day 2. In a phase III trial on 405 metastatic bladder patients, GC was compared with classic MVAC regimen, and it showed comparable survival outcomes (median PFS in the GC arm was 7.7 vs. 8.3 months in the MVAC arm). However, patients in the MVAC arm had higher incidence of neutropenic sepsis (12% vs. 1%) and mortality (3% vs. 1%) [18]. In view of better safety and tolerability profile, GC has emerged as the preferred first-line cisplatin-based combination therapy for metastatic bladder cancer.

13.3.2 Cisplatin-Ineligible Patients

Cisplatin ineligibility ranges anywhere between 30 and 60% of patients with upfront metastatic bladder cancer, especially due to advanced age and declining renal function [19]. For patients not eligible for cisplatin, carboplatin or taxane-based combination regimens are alternate options.

Carboplatin-based regimens: Carboplatin-based regimen was explored in a phase III randomized study EORTC trial 30986, which randomized 238 cisplatin-ineligible patients with upfront metastatic bladder cancer (ECOG PS ≥2 or creatinine clearance between 30 and 60 mL/

min) to gemcitabine-carboplatin and M-CAVI regimen (methotrexate, carboplatin, and vinblastine). There was no difference in PFS and OS in the two arms; however, gemcitabine-carboplatin had better toxicity profile (grade 3/4 toxicity of 21.2% vs. 9.3%), and hence it is considered as the preferred regimen for cisplatin-ineligible patients [20].

It is unclear whether carboplatin-based regimens are inferior to cisplatin as there is no randomized phase III study for comparison. A phase II randomized study in 110 patients compared gemcitabine-cisplatin and gemcitabine-carboplatin showed numerically higher objective response rate (49.1% vs. 40.0%) and median OS in the cisplatin arm (12.8 vs. 9.8 months) [21]. Splitting the dose of cisplatin over 2 days has also been explored as an alternative for cisplatin-ineligible patients and may provide an alternative to carboplatin-based regimen [22].

Taxane-based regimens: Taxanes, including paclitaxel and docetaxel, have modest single-agent activity in advanced bladder cancer and hence have been explored in combination for first-line management [23]. Combinations of gemcitabine and paclitaxel/docetaxel have been explored in several phase II trials, which demonstrated objective response rate between 33 and 70% and median OS between 13 and 16 months [24–27]. The above combinations are acceptable first-line alternatives for platinum-ineligible patients who are not eligible/affordable for immunotherapy.

13.3.3 Taxane-Platinum Combination

Due to activity of taxanes in advanced bladder malignancy, they have been explored in combination with platinum-based regimens, in doublet and triplet combinations. A phase III study compared the triplet combination of paclitaxel, gemcitabine and cisplatin (PGC) with gemcitabine, cisplatin regimen (GC) among 626 patients of advanced urothelial malignancy. PCG regimen showed improved objective response rate as compared to GC (55.5% vs. 43.6%) along with non-significant but numerically better OS (15.8 vs. 12.7 months), especially those in bladder primary. However, the triplet combination was associated with an increased incidence of febrile neutropenia (13.2% vs. 4.3%) [28]. However, it may be considered as an alternative for younger patients with good performance status.

The doublet combination regimens of platinum and taxane were also compared with classic MVAC in two randomized trials. In a phase III study, the combination of docetaxel and cisplatin showed inferior survival outcome as compared to MVAC arm (median OS 9.3 vs. 14.3 months in MVAC arm), while another phase III study comparing paclitaxel-carboplatin combination with MVAC showed similar survival outcomes (13.8 vs. 15.4 months in MVAC arm), although paclitaxel-carboplatin was better tolerated [29, 30]. Hence, platinum-taxane doublet combinations are not standard first-line choices for patients with advanced urothelial malignancy.

13.3.4 Immunotherapy in First Line

Immunotherapeutic drugs are preferred options for frontline management of patients with advanced urothelial malignancies who are ineligible for platinum-based chemotherapy (Table 13.2 and Fig. 13.1). Two agents, atezolizumab and pembrolizumab, have been approved in the United States for this indication.

Atezolizumab: Atezolizumab is a monoclonal antibody against programmed death-ligand 1 (PD-L1), which was evaluated in cohort 1 of phase II IMvigor210 study, which included chemotherapy naïve cisplatin-ineligible patients [33]. It demonstrated an objective response rate of 23%, median PFS of 2.7 months, and median OS of 15.9 months.

Based on this result, it was initially approved as first-line agent for cisplatin-ineligible patients on April 2017, however, based on interim efficacy analysis of atezolizumab monotherapy arm of phase III IMvigor130 study, currently, atezolizumab monotherapy is approved only for

Table 13.2 Currently approved indications for immunotherapeutic drugs in management of metastatic bladder cancer

Agent		Approved indication	Basis for approval
First line			
1	Pembrolizumab	Platinum-ineligible patients	Phase II KEYNOTE-052 study and phase III KEYNOTE-361 study [31, 32]
		Cisplatin-ineligible patients with PD-L1 CPS ≥ 10	
2.	Atezolizumab	Platinum-ineligible patients	Phase II IMvigor 210 study and phase III IMvigor 130 study [30, 33]
		Cisplatin-ineligible patients with PD-L1 IC expression ≥5%	
Second line			
1	Pembrolizumab	Progression on platinum-based chemotherapy or recurrence within 12 months of neoadjuvant/ adjuvant platinum therapy	Phase III KEYNOTE-045 study [34]
2	Nivolumab	Progression on platinum-based chemotherapy or recurrence within 12 months of neoadjuvant/ adjuvant platinum therapy	Phase II CheckMate 275 study [35][a]
3	Avelumab	Progression on platinum-based chemotherapy or recurrence within 12 months of neoadjuvant/ adjuvant platinum therapy	Expansion cohort of phase I JAVELIN Solid Tumor Trial [36][a]
Maintenance			
1	Avelumab	Patients who have not progressed after first-line treatment with platinum-based chemotherapy	Phase III JAVELIN bladder 100 trial [37]

PD-L1 CPS: Programmed death ligand 1 combined positive score
PD-L1 IC expression: Programmed death ligand 1 immune cell expression
[a]Approval subject to phase III data

patients ineligible for any platinum-based chemotherapy or cisplatin-ineligible patients with PD-L1 staining ≥5% in tumour-infiltrating immune cells [31, 38].

Pembrolizumab: Pembrolizumab is monoclonal antibody against programmed death-1 (PD-1), which was also evaluated in phase II KEYNOTE-052 study among cisplatin-ineligible patients. The study demonstrated an objective response rate of 28.6% with complete response 8.9% and a median OS of 8.9 months. The efficacy was enhanced in patients with PD-L1 combined positive score (CPS) of ≥10 (objective response rate of 47%) and those with lymph node only disease [32]. Based on this result, similar to atezolizumab, pembrolizumab also received accelerated approval for first-line management of cisplatin-ineligible patients. However, based on final results of phase III KEYNOTE-361 study, it is currently approved for patients who are not eligible for platinum-based chemotherapy or cisplatin-eligible patients with PD-L1 CPS ≥10 [31, 39].

Combination of chemo-immunotherapy in first line: The combination of immunotherapeutic drugs with chemotherapy in first line advanced urothelial malignancies have been investigated in two large-scale phase III randomized trials.

The phase III IMvigor130 study, which compared addition of atezolizumab with platinum-based chemotherapy in first-line metastatic urothelial cancer, demonstrated improvement in median PFS (8.2 vs. 6.3 months) on addition of atezolizumab but failed to show significant improvement in median OS (16 vs. 13.4 months) [38]. Similarly, in KEYNOTE-361 study, addition of pembrolizumab with platinum-based chemotherapy also did not show any improvement in median PFS (8.3 vs. 7.1 months) or OS (17 vs. 14.3 months) [39]. Hence, combination chemo-immunotherapy is not considered as a choice for frontline management of advanced bladder cancer for platinum-eligible patients.

Combination immunotherapy in first line: Combination of PD-1 inhibitor and cytotoxic T-lymphocyte antigen-4 (CTLA-4) inhibitor have demonstrated improved outcome in various tumour types. The phase III DANUBE trial explored durvalumab (PD-L1 inhibitor) alone or in combination with CTLA-4 inhibitor tremelimumab among treatment-naïve patients with advanced urothelial malignancy in comparison to chemotherapy. The study failed to show any improvement in OS with durvalumab monotherapy or combination with tremelimumab over standard platinum-based chemotherapy [40]. Combination of durvalumab with/without tremelimumab along with standard of care chemotherapy is being explored in NILE trial [41]. Pending results, incorporation of combination immunotherapy in first-line management of metastatic bladder cancer remains investigational.

13.3.5 Maintenance Therapy

Traditional first-line chemotherapy regimens rarely achieve any durable response in metastatic bladder cancer; hence, maintenance therapy has been explored to achieve improved outcome [37].

Avelumab: The phase III JAVELIN Bladder 100 trial investigated the role of maintenance avelumab compared to best-supportive care among patients who did not progress after 4–6 cycles of first-line gemcitabine-platinum chemotherapy regimen. The median OS with maintenance avelumab was 21.4 versus 14.3 months in best supportive care, and the improvement was more pronounced in PD-L1-positive subset and persisted even on extended follow-up [42, 43]. This trial established maintenance avelumab as standard of care after first-line platinum-based chemotherapy.

Other agents: Vinflunine maintenance has also been shown to improve PFS over best supportive care after nonprogression on first-line platinum-based chemotherapy in a phase II study; however, it failed to show any improvement in OS [44, 45]. Switch maintenance with pembrolizumab after platinum-based chemotherapy has also shown to improve PFS, but not OS in a phase II study [46]. Hence, vinflunine or pembrolizumab is not considered as standard choices for maintenance after platinum-based chemotherapy.

13.4 Second/Subsequent Line Management of Metastatic Bladder Cancer

13.4.1 Immunotherapy

Till 5 years back, there was no standard second-line choice for progressive urothelial malignancies. However, systemic immunotherapy with checkpoint inhibitors (PD-1 inhibitors and PD-L1 inhibitors) has emerged as the standard choice for second-line management of patients who have progressed beyond platinum-based chemotherapy (Table 13.2).

The accelerated approval of atezolizumab in second line in May 2016 based on exciting phase II study was quickly followed by further approval of four more immunotherapy agents, viz. pembrolizumab, nivolumab, avelumab, and durvalumab in platinum pretreated advanced urothelial malignancy [47]. However, durvalumab and atezolizumab failed to show meaningful survival benefit on subsequent phase III studies, following which their regulatory approvals have been withdrawn [34, 48].

Pembrolizumab: Pembrolizumab has been evaluated in a phase III open label KEYNOTE-045 study in comparison to physician choice chemotherapy (paclitaxel, docetaxel, and vinflunine) for patients with recurrent or progressive advanced urothelial malignancy after platinum-based chemotherapy. The study demonstrated improved median OS (10.3 vs. 7.4 months) with improved objective response rate (21.1% vs. 11.4%) and fewer adverse events (grade 3/4 adverse events of 15% vs. 49.4% in chemotherapy arm) [49]. The improved efficacy was consistent across the whole trial population irrespective of PD-L1 status. The benefit was durable even on long-term follow-up with median duration of response in pembrolizumab arm being 29.7 months compared to 4.4 months in chemotherapy arm [35]. The above results make pembrolizumab a standard second-line choice for recurrent/progressive metastatic urothelial malignancy.

Nivolumab: Nivolumab was evaluated in a single-arm phase II study in recurrent/progressive metastatic urothelial cancer among 270 patients. The study demonstrated an objective response rate of 19.6%, which was more so in patients with PD-L1 expression ≥1% (23.8%). The median survival of the whole cohort was 8.74 months and those with PD-L1 ≥ 1% was 11.3% [36]. Hence, nivolumab is an acceptable alternative in second-line setting with confirmatory phase III studies still awaited.

Avelumab: A pooled analysis of two expansion cohorts of phase I JAVELIN Solid Tumor study showed that avelumab demonstrated an objective response rate of 17% with 8% grade 3/4 adverse events. The median OS was 6.5 months which was enhanced in PD-L1 ≥ 5% population (8.2 months) [50]. Similar to nivolumab, avelumab is also an alternative in second-line management of advanced urothelial malignancy pending further confirmatory trials.

Durvalumab: While durvalumab was granted accelerated approval for second line advanced urothelial malignancy, the phase III DANUBE study failed to demonstrate any survival advantage of durvalumab with/without tremelimumab over platinum-based chemotherapy in first-line setting [40]. Following the results of DANUBE trial, the approval for durvalumab for second-line setting was withdrawn.

Atezolizumab: The phase III IMvigor 211 study also failed to show any benefit of atezolizumab over chemotherapy among 931 patients of platinum pretreated recurrent/progressive advanced urothelial malignancy. Hence, the approval of atezolizumab in second-line setting has been withdrawn [51].

Combination immunotherapy in second line: The combination of nivolumab and ipilimumab has been investigated in CheckMate-032 study. The cohort which received combination of nivolumab 1 mg/kg and ipilimumab 3 mg/kg showed an improved response rate of 38% and numerically higher PFS of 4.9 months and OS of 15.3 months [52]. These results make the combination an attractive option to be explored in further phase III studies.

13.4.2 Chemotherapy

There is no standard choice of second-line chemotherapy for metastatic urothelial malignancy, which have progressed beyond platinum-based chemotherapy. However, for patients ineligible for immunotherapy or progression following immunotherapy, single-agent chemotherapy remains the viable alternative in subsequent line. Several single-agent cytotoxic agents have activity in metastatic bladder cancer-like vinblastine, vinflunine, gemcitabine, paclitaxel, docetaxel, ifosfamide, methotrexate, pemetrexed and may be considered as second-line therapy if the agent was not exposed in first line [37].

Paclitaxel and docetaxel have objective response rate between 7 and 13% in various phase II studies for platinum-pretreated population of urothelial malignancy [23]. Nab-paclitaxel has similar response rate, median PFS, and OS as compared to paclitaxel [53]. They are commonly used in second-line setting, although there is lack of any randomized study showing the survival benefit with second-line taxane therapy. Pemetrexed has also been shown to have an objective response rate of 27.7% with median OS of 9.6 months in second-line setting and may be considered as an alternative [54].

Vinflunine: Vinflunine is the only chemotherapeutic agent, which has been evaluated in a randomized phase III study for second-line management of metastatic bladder cancer compared to best supportive care. Vinflunine demonstrated improved median OS (6.9 vs. 4.6 months) over best supportive care among 370 patients previously treated progressive urothelial malignancy [55]. The agent has been approved in Europe for second-line management of urothelial malignancies, although it is not available in India.

13.4.3 Targeted Therapy

Alterations in fibroblast growth factor receptor (*FGFR*) gene are seen in about 20% of advanced urothelial malignancies; the most common of which are activating missense mutations in *FGFR3* and in-frame *FGFR3-TACC3* fusions [56]. The presence of *FGFR* alterations is associated with lower grade for nonmuscle-invasive bladder cancer; however, in advanced disease, it is associated less durable response to chemotherapy or immunotherapy [57]. Erdafitinib, which is a small molecule tyrosine kinase inhibitor, specifically targeting *FGFR1–4*, has been the first targeted therapy approved for bladder cancer [58].

Erdafitinib: Erdafitinib was evaluated in a multicenter, open-label phase II study in patients with advanced urothelial malignancies with susceptible pathogenic *FGFR3* mutations or *FGFR3-FGFR2* fusions, which have progressed or relapsed within 12 months of adjuvant/neoadjuvant systemic chemotherapy or those ineligible for chemotherapy. The study included 99 patients, of which 22% received prior immunotherapy as well. Erdafitinib demonstrated an objective response rate of 40% with a median PFS of 5.5 months and OS of 13.8 months [59]. The most common side effect observed was hyperphosphatemia (78%), which is seen with *FGFR* inhibitors along with stomatitis and diarrhea. Detachment of retinal pigment epithelium is an important clinically concerning adverse effect, which led to discontinuation of the drug in 3% of patients. Based on this phase II study, it has been approved for progressive/recurrent advanced urothelial malignancies post systemic platinum chemotherapy or among those ineligible for chemotherapy and harboring susceptible pathogenic *FGFR3* mutations or *FGFR3-FGFR2* fusions.

Other *FGFR* inhibitors include infigratinib, rogaratinib, pemigatinib, which have also been evaluated in advanced urothelial malignancies. The FORT-1 study is ongoing which is evaluating rogaratinib versus chemotherapy post platinum-based chemotherapy. The objective response rate with rogaratinib was 19.5% (vs. 19.3% in chemotherapy); however, among patients with FGFR3 mutations, the objective response rate with rogaratinib was 52.4% [60, 61].

13.4.4 Antibody–Drug Conjugates

Two antibody–drug conjugates, enfortumab vedotin and sacituzumab govitecan have been evaluated and received approval for management of advanced urothelial malignancies on progression beyond chemotherapy and/or immunotherapy.

Enfortumab vedotin: Nectin-4 is a tumour-associated antigen, which is overexpressed in multiple malignancies including 97% of urothelial carcinomas. Enfortumab vedotin is an antibody drug conjugate that combines human nectin-4 antibody with monomethyl auristatin E, which is microtubule disruptive agent [62].

Enfortumab vedotin was compared with physician choice chemotherapy in phase III study among patients who had progression following systemic platinum-based chemotherapy as well as PD-1 or PD-L1 inhibitors. Among 608 patients, enfortumab vedotin showed improvement in median PFS (5.5 vs. 3.7 months) and median OS (12.8 vs. 8.9 months) as compared to chemotherapy. While treatment-related adverse events were similar in both arms and enfortumab vedotin was generally well tolerated, the clinically relevant adverse event observed with enfortumab vedotin arm included skin rash (43.9%), peripheral sensory neuropathy (46.3%), and treatment related hyperglycemia (6.4%).

The drug has also been evaluated in a phase II study among those patients who are cisplatin ineligible and had disease progression on immunotherapy. In this population, enfortumab vedotin demonstrated an objective response rate of 52% with a median PFS of 5.8 months and OS of 14.7 months [63]. Based on above two studies, enfortumab vedotin has been approved for cisplatin-ineligible patients after progression on immunotherapy and for patients after progression on systemic platinum-based chemotherapy as well as immunotherapy.

Sacituzumab govitecan: Sacituzumab govitecan is another antibody-drug conjugate that combines antibody against Trop2 along with SN-38, the active metabolite of irinotecan. In cohort 1 of TROPHY-U-01 study, the use of sacituzumab govitecan in platinum pretreated population showed an objective response rate of 27% with median PFS of 5.4 months and OS of 10.4 months [64]. Sacituzumab govitecan is also an acceptable alternative to enfortumab vedotin for patients with advanced urothelial malignancy, which have progressed following platinum-based chemotherapy and PD-1/PD-L1 inhibitors.

13.5 Local Management in Metastatic Bladder Cancer

While systemic chemotherapy is the mainstay of treatment of metastatic urothelial malignancy, incorporation of local treatment modalities like surgery or radiation therapy may be considered as a form of consolidation strategy or for palliation of symptoms.

Role of radiation: Radiation therapy may be utilized in metastatic urothelial carcinoma for multitude of purposes. It may be used for palliation of symptomatic bony metastases or pelvic obstructive symptoms or haematuria. It may also be utilized in elderly patients for palliation of symptoms who are not fit for surgery or any form of systemic therapy [65].

Radiation therapy may also be used as a consolidative intent after good response to chemotherapy in metastatic urothelial cancer. While the long-term prognosis is dismal in metastatic bladder cancer with systemic chemotherapy, few retrospective studies have shown that the use of additional consolidative radiation after good response to systemic chemotherapy resulted in improved survival outcomes in metastatic bladder cancer [66, 67].

Role of surgery: Based on a recent systematic review, which summarized the current role of surgery in metastatic bladder cancer, it is clear that offering consolidative surgery after good response to chemotherapy may offer a survival advantage [68]. Metastatectomy especially of limited pulmonary metastases or nodal metastases may be also considered in few cases. However, unlike renal cell carcinoma or ovarian carcinoma, there is no definite role of cytoreductive surgery in presence of overt metastatic disease. A retrospective review suggested that surgery helps in improvement in survival when the metastases are confined to one or two organs only [3].

Multidisciplinary approach is essential to select appropriate cases for the use of radiation therapy or surgical therapy as a consolidation approach following good response to chemotherapy.

13.6 Adjuvant Therapy in Muscle-Invasive Bladder Cancer

13.6.1 Benefit of Adjuvant Therapy and Patient Eligibility

The cornerstone of management of localized muscle-invasive bladder cancer is radical cystectomy; however, for locally advanced disease (pT3–T4) and node-positive disease, the 5-year recurrence-free survival is only between 35 and 40% with surgery alone [69].

Neoadjuvant cisplatin-based therapy has been demonstrated to have 5% overall survival advantage in locally advanced muscle-invasive bladder cancer; however, data for benefit of adjuvant chemotherapy specifically has been heterogenous due to small sample size of clinical trials and significant drop out [70]. A retrospective review which compared patients who received neoadjuvant versus adjuvant chemotherapy for muscle-invasive bladder cancer showed that patients who received neoadjuvant chemotherapy had improved disease-free survival but not overall survival or cancer-specific survival [71]. A meta-analysis that analysed individual patient data of 10 randomized trials comprising of 1183 patients demonstrated that adjuvant cisplatin-based chemotherapy improved overall survival with an absolute benefit of 6% at 5 years [72]. On the other hand, the EORTC-30994 open-label randomized trial that evaluated immediate adjuvant chemotherapy over deferred chemotherapy at relapse, did not demonstrate any overall survival advantage with immediate therapy although it significantly improved PFS [73]. This may be due to premature closure of the trial due to poor accrual. Even though the benefit of adjuvant chemotherapy post upfront radical cystectomy is not conclusively demonstrated, considering the survival advantage of neoadjuvant therapy and poor survival outcome with radical cystectomy alone, adjuvant chemotherapy should be considered uniformly for patients not receiving neoadjuvant chemotherapy.

Patients with muscle-invasive bladder cancer with pT2 disease have overall long-term cure rate of up to 80% with radical cystectomy alone; hence, adjuvant therapy is generally not recommended after patients who underwent upfront radical cystectomy. Adjuvant cisplatin-based chemotherapy is generally recommended for pT3–T4 and/or node-positive disease after upfront radical cystectomy [74].

With recent emerging evidence of benefit of adjuvant immunotherapy after neoadjuvant cisplatin-based chemotherapy, option of nivolumab as adjuvant therapy should also be gradually adopted into clinical practise [75].

13.6.2 Adjuvant Therapy for Patients Not Receiving Neoadjuvant Therapy

For patients who have not received any neoadjuvant therapy, adjuvant cisplatin-based chemotherapy should be considered for cisplatin-eligible patients. Cisplatin eligibility is defined as per uniform criteria as mentioned in Table 13.1 [13].

Cisplatin-eligible patients: There is no standard cisplatin-based adjuvant chemotherapy regimen of choice for adjuvant therapy. Three to four cycles of MVAC, dose dense MVAC or 4 cycles of gemcitabine-cisplatin (GC) are all acceptable alternatives [73]. These regimens have not compared head to head in adjuvant setting specifically. In the recently published GETUG-AFU V05 VESPER Trial, 6 cycles of dose dense MVAC every 2 weeks was compared with 4 cycles of GC every 3 weekly for both neoadjuvant and adjuvant setting, with 12% patients receiving therapy in adjuvant setting [76]. While the trial demonstrated improved PFS in dd-MVAC arm compared to GC arm in patients receiving neoadjuvant therapy, same could not be conclusively demonstrated in those receiving adjuvant therapy due to limited number of patients. However, GC regimen was better tolerated than dd-MVAC with only 60% patients completing planned 6 cycles of dd-MVAC. This suggests that the choice of regimen depends of age and general fitness of the patient.

Cisplatin-ineligible patients: For patients who are cisplatin ineligible, there is no regimen which has conclusively reported any survival advantage. Regimens incorporating taxane/carboplatin with gemcitabine/doxorubicin have been explored as adjuvant therapy in patients with renal failure in a nonrandomized study, with no benefit in disease-specific survival [77]. Hence, non-cisplatin-based regimens are not preferable as adjuvant therapy.

However, for cisplatin-ineligible patients, adjuvant immunotherapy with nivolumab is a better option for those with pT3–T4 or node-positive disease post radical cystectomy based on results obtained from CheckMate-274 trial, although benefit specifically in subgroup of cisplatin-ineligible patients was not demonstrated [75].

13.6.3 Adjuvant Therapy for Patients Receiving Neoadjuvant Therapy

Two trials have recently evaluated the use of immune checkpoint inhibitors post radical cystectomy for muscle-invasive bladder cancer. Both the trials included patients who have received neoadjuvant cisplatin-based chemotherapy and had ypT2–T4a or node-positive disease post-surgery or patients with upfront radical cystectomy but ineligible/declined cisplatin-based chemotherapy.

The IMvigor-010 study evaluated the use of adjuvant atezolizumab in the above setting among 804 patients and reported a median disease-free survival of 19.4 months in atezolizumab arm compared to 16.6 months in observation arm with no statistically significant difference [78]. On the other hand, in the CheckMate-274 trial, among 709 patients, use of adjuvant nivolumab for 1 year showed a median disease free survival of 20.8 months compared to 10.8 months in placebo arm, with a statistically significant difference [75]. Based on the above result, adjuvant nivolumab for 1 year is currently recommended as an adjuvant treatment for patients with muscle-invasive bladder cancer post radical cystectomy who had received neoadjuvant cisplatin-based chemotherapy and has ypT2–T4a or node-positive disease.

13.6.4 Surveillance in Localized Bladder Cancer Post Treatment

Long term follow-up is important to detect early recurrence in muscle-invasive bladder cancer following curative intent therapy. It remains unclear whether symptom guided follow-up is sufficient or image guided follow-up for detecting asymptomatic recurrence is important to detect recurrence, with one study which failed to show any benefit of asymptomatic imaging-based surveillance [79]. On the other hand, benefit of detecting asymptomatic early recurrence is demonstrated in a different study [80].

It is important to note that although recurrences are common within first 3 years, late recurrences are not negligible in proportion (post 5-year recurrence accounting for 12.2% of recurrences) and may be associated with a worse survival [81]. This suggests that a long-term follow-up beyond even 5 years is essential for bladder cancer.

However, consensus-based guidelines generally recommend imaging-based follow-up mainly incorporating contrast enhanced computed tomographic (CECT) scan of chest with abdomen and pelvis. A schedule suggested by European Association of Urology recommends a CECT scan every 6 monthly for 3 years followed by annually thereafter [82]. Similarly, National Comprehensive Cancer Network guidelines suggest CT or MR Urography including upper urinary tracts every 3–6 monthly for 2 years followed by annually till 5 years along with urine cytology. Renal ultrasonography annually is acceptable for 5–10 years post treatment [74].

13.7 Conclusion

Cisplatin-based systemic chemotherapy regimens (MVAC and GC) are the first-line management of metastatic bladder cancer. In real world, a significant proportion of patients are ineligible for cisplatin therapy, for which carboplatin or taxane-based regimens are alternate options. Systemic immunotherapy with PD-1 and PD-L1 inhibitors are preferred in second line management over chemotherapy or for patients not eligible for systemic chemotherapy. *FGFR* alterations are seen in 20% of advanced urothelial malignancies and for this subset, erdafitinib demonstrated improved survival compared to chemotherapy. Newer antibody–drug conjugates enfortumab vedotin and sacituzumab govitecan are options in later lines of therapy. For patients who undergo upfront radical cystectomy for muscle-invasive bladder cancer, patients with pT3–T4 or node-positive disease are eligible for adjuvant therapy. Cisplatin-based chemotherapy as used in metastatic settings are used for adjuvant treatment. For patients who has received neoadjuvant cisplatin-based chemotherapy and has ypT2–T4a or node-positive post therapy, or for cisplatin-ineligible patients without neoadjuvant therapy, adjuvant nivolumab for 1 year should be considered.

References

1. Saginala K, Barsouk A, Aluru JS, Rawla P, Padala SA, Barsouk A. Epidemiology of bladder cancer. Med Sci. 2020;8(1):15.
2. IARC, GLOBOCAN 2020: worldwide, both sexes, all ages. Bladder Cancer Fact Sheet. https://gco.iarc.fr/today/data/factsheets/cancers/30-Bladder-fact-sheet.pdf.
3. Wang P, Zang S, Li G, Qu W, Li S, Qiao Q, et al. The role of surgery on the primary tumor site in bladder cancer with distant metastasis: significance of

histology type and metastatic pattern. Cancer Med. 2020;9(24):9293–302.
4. IARC, GLOBOCAN 2020, both sexes, all ages. India Fact Sheet. https://gco.iarc.fr/today/data/factsheets/populations/356-india-fact-sheets.pdf.
5. Yuvaraja TB, Waigankar S, Bakshi G, Prakash G. Genitourinary cancers: summary of Indian data. South Asian J Cancer. 2016;5(3):122–4.
6. Prakash G, Pal M, Odaiyappan K, Shinde R, Mishra J, Jalde D, et al. Bladder cancer demographics and outcome data from 2013 at a tertiary cancer hospital in India. Indian J Cancer. 2019;56(1):54.
7. Donat SM, Shabsigh A, Savage C, Cronin AM, Bochner BH, Dalbagni G, et al. Potential impact of postoperative early complications on the timing of adjuvant chemotherapy in patients undergoing radical cystectomy: a high-volume tertiary cancer center experience. Eur Urol. 2009;55(1):177–86.
8. Osterman CK, Milowsky MI. New and emerging therapies in the management of bladder cancer. F1000Res. 2020;9:1146.
9. Bianchi M, Roghmann F, Becker A, Sukumar S, Briganti A, Menon M, et al. Age-stratified distribution of metastatic sites in bladder cancer: a population-based analysis. Can Urol Assoc J. 2014;8(3–4):148.
10. Flannery K, Boyd M, Black-Shinn J, Robert N, Kamat AM. Outcomes in patients with metastatic bladder cancer in the USA: a retrospective electronic medical record study. Future Oncol. 2019;15(12):1323–34.
11. Bajorin DF, Dodd PM, Mazumdar M, Fazzari M, McCaffrey JA, Scher HI, et al. Long-term survival in metastatic transitional-cell carcinoma and prognostic factors predicting outcome of therapy. J Clin Oncol. 1999;17(10):3173–81.
12. Saxman SB, Propert KJ, Einhorn LH, Crawford ED, Tannock I, Raghavan D, et al. Long-term follow-up of a phase III intergroup study of cisplatin alone or in combination with methotrexate, vinblastine, and doxorubicin in patients with metastatic urothelial carcinoma: a cooperative group study. J Clin Oncol. 1997;15(7):2564–9.
13. Galsky MD, Hahn NM, Rosenberg J, Sonpavde G, Hutson T, Oh WK, et al. Treatment of patients with metastatic urothelial cancer "unfit" for cisplatin-based chemotherapy. J Clin Oncol. 2011;29(17):2432–8.
14. Bamias A, Tzannis K, Harshman LC, Crabb SJ, Wong YN, Kumar Pal S, et al. Impact of contemporary patterns of chemotherapy utilization on survival in patients with advanced cancer of the urinary tract: a retrospective international study of invasive/advanced cancer of the Urothelium (RISC). Ann Oncol. 2018;29(2):361–9.
15. Loehrer PJ, Einhorn LH, Elson PJ, Crawford ED, Kuebler P, Tannock I, et al. A randomized comparison of cisplatin alone or in combination with methotrexate, vinblastine, and doxorubicin in patients with metastatic urothelial carcinoma: a cooperative group study. J Clin Oncol. 1992;10(7):1066–73.
16. Logothetis CJ, Dexeus FH, Finn L, Sella A, Amato RJ, Ayala AG, et al. A prospective randomized trial comparing MVAC and CISCA chemotherapy for patients with metastatic urothelial tumors. J Clin Oncol. 1990;8(6):1050–5.
17. Sternberg CN, de Mulder PH, Schornagel JH, Théodore C, Fossa SD, van Oosterom AT, et al. Randomized phase III trial of high-dose-intensity methotrexate, vinblastine, doxorubicin, and cisplatin (MVAC) chemotherapy and recombinant human granulocyte colony-stimulating factor versus classic MVAC in advanced urothelial tract tumors: European Organization for Research and Treatment of cancer protocol no. 30924. J Clin Oncol. 2001;19(10):2638–46.
18. von der Maase H, Hansen SW, Roberts JT, Dogliotti L, Oliver T, Moore MJ, et al. Gemcitabine and cisplatin versus methotrexate, vinblastine, doxorubicin, and cisplatin in advanced or metastatic bladder cancer: results of a large, randomized, multinational, multicenter, phase III study. J Clin Oncol. 2000;18(17):3068–77.
19. Dash A, Galsky MD, Vickers AJ, Serio AM, Koppie TM, Dalbagni G, et al. Impact of renal impairment on eligibility for adjuvant cisplatin-based chemotherapy in patients with urothelial carcinoma of the bladder. Cancer. 2006;107(3):506–13.
20. De Santis M, Bellmunt J, Mead G, Kerst JM, Leahy M, Maroto P, et al. Randomized phase II/III trial assessing gemcitabine/carboplatin and methotrexate/carboplatin/vinblastine in patients with advanced urothelial cancer who are unfit for cisplatin-based chemotherapy: EORTC study 30986. J Clin Oncol. 2012;30(2):191–9.
21. Dogliotti L, Cartenì G, Siena S, Bertetto O, Martoni A, Bono A, et al. Gemcitabine plus cisplatin versus gemcitabine plus carboplatin as first-line chemotherapy in advanced transitional cell carcinoma of the urothelium: results of a randomized phase 2 trial. Eur Urol. 2007;52(1):134–41.
22. Izumi K, Iwamoto H, Yaegashi H, Shigehara K, Nohara T, Kadono Y, et al. Gemcitabine plus cisplatin split *versus* gemcitabine plus carboplatin for advanced urothelial cancer with cisplatin-unfit renal function. In Vivo. 2019;33(1):167–72.
23. Galsky MD. The role of taxanes in the management of bladder cancer. Oncologist. 2005;10(10):792–8.
24. Gitlitz BJ, Baker C, Chapman Y, Allen HJ, Bosserman LD, Patel R, et al. A phase II study of gemcitabine and docetaxel therapy in patients with advanced urothelial carcinoma. Cancer. 2003;98(9):1863–9.
25. Ardavanis A, Tryfonopoulos D, Alexopoulos A, Kandylis C, Lainakis G, Rigatos G. Gemcitabine and docetaxel as first-line treatment for advanced urothelial carcinoma: a phase II study. Br J Cancer. 2005;92(4):645–50.
26. Meluch AA, Greco FA, Burris HA, O'Rourke T, Ortega G, Steis RG, et al. Paclitaxel and gemcitabine chemotherapy for advanced transitional-cell carcinoma of the Urothelial tract: a phase II trial of the Minnie pearl cancer research network. J Clin Oncol. 2001;19(12):3018–24.

27. Li J, Juliar B, Yiannoutsos C, Ansari R, Fox E, Fisch MJ, et al. Weekly paclitaxel and gemcitabine in advanced transitional-cell carcinoma of the Urothelium: a phase II Hoosier oncology group study. J Clin Oncol. 2005;23(6):1185–91.
28. Bellmunt J, von der Maase H, Mead GM, Skoneczna I, De Santis M, Daugaard G, et al. Randomized phase III study comparing paclitaxel/cisplatin/gemcitabine and gemcitabine/cisplatin in patients with locally advanced or metastatic urothelial cancer without prior systemic therapy: EORTC intergroup study 30987. J Clin Oncol. 2012;30(10):1107–13.
29. Bamias A, Aravantinos G, Deliveliotis C, Bafaloukos D, Kalofonos C, Xiros N, et al. Docetaxel and cisplatin with granulocyte colony-stimulating factor (G-CSF) versus MVAC with G-CSF in advanced urothelial carcinoma: a multicenter, randomized, phase III study from the Hellenic Cooperative Oncology Group. J Clin Oncol. 2004;22(2):220–8.
30. Dreicer R, Manola J, Roth BJ, See WA, Kuross S, Edelman MJ, et al. Phase III trial of methotrexate, vinblastine, doxorubicin, and cisplatin versus carboplatin and paclitaxel in patients with advanced carcinoma of the urothelium: a trial of the Eastern Cooperative Oncology Group. Cancer. 2004;100(8):1639–45.
31. Suzman DL, Agrawal S, Ning Y-M, Maher VE, Fernandes LL, Karuri S, et al. FDA approval summary: atezolizumab or pembrolizumab for the treatment of patients with advanced urothelial carcinoma ineligible for cisplatin-containing chemotherapy. Oncologist. 2019;24(4):563–9.
32. Vuky J, Balar AV, Castellano D, O'Donnell PH, Grivas P, Bellmunt J, et al. Long-term outcomes in KEYNOTE-052: phase II study investigating first-line pembrolizumab in cisplatin-ineligible patients with locally advanced or metastatic urothelial cancer. J Clin Oncol. 2020;38(23):2658–66.
33. Balar AV, Galsky MD, Rosenberg JE, Powles T, Petrylak DP, Bellmunt J, et al. Atezolizumab as first-line treatment in cisplatin-ineligible patients with locally advanced and metastatic urothelial carcinoma: a single-arm, multicentre, phase 2 trial. Lancet. 2017;389(10064):67–76.
34. Voluntary withdrawal Imfinzi US bladder indication. AstraZeneca. https://www.astrazeneca.com/media--centre/press-releases/2021/voluntary-withdrawal-imfinzi-us-bladder-indication.html.
35. Bellmunt J, Necchi A, De Wit R, Lee JL, Fong L, Vogelzang NJ, et al. Pembrolizumab (pembro) versus investigator's choice of paclitaxel, docetaxel, or vinflunine in recurrent, advanced urothelial cancer (UC): 5-year follow-up from the phase 3 KEYNOTE-045 trial. J Clin Oncol. 2021;39(15_Suppl):4532.
36. Sharma P, Retz M, Siefker-Radtke A, Baron A, Necchi A, Bedke J, et al. Nivolumab in metastatic urothelial carcinoma after platinum therapy (CheckMate 275): a multicentre, single-arm, phase 2 trial. Lancet Oncol. 2017;18(3):312–22.
37. Nadal R, Bellmunt J. Management of metastatic bladder cancer. Cancer Treat Rev. 2019;76:10–21.
38. Galsky MD, Arija JÁA, Bamias A, Davis ID, De Santis M, Kikuchi E, et al. Atezolizumab with or without chemotherapy in metastatic urothelial cancer (IMvigor130): a multicentre, randomised, placebo-controlled phase 3 trial. Lancet. 2020;395(10236):1547–57.
39. Powles T, Csőszi T, Özgüroğlu M, Matsubara N, Géczi L, Cheng SYS, et al. Pembrolizumab alone or combined with chemotherapy versus chemotherapy as first-line therapy for advanced urothelial carcinoma (KEYNOTE-361): a randomised, open-label, phase 3 trial. Lancet Oncol. 2021;22(7):931–45.
40. Powles T, van der Heijden MS, Castellano D, Galsky MD, Loriot Y, Petrylak DP, et al. Durvalumab alone and durvalumab plus tremelimumab versus chemotherapy in previously untreated patients with unresectable, locally advanced or metastatic urothelial carcinoma (DANUBE): a randomised, open-label, multicentre, phase 3 trial. Lancet Oncol. 2020;21(12):1574–88.
41. Galsky MD, Necchi A, Sridhar SS, Ogawa O, Angra N, Hois S, et al. A phase III, randomized, open-label, multicenter, global study of first-line durvalumab plus standard of care (SoC) chemotherapy and durvalumab plus tremelimumab, and SoC chemotherapy versus SoC chemotherapy alone in unresectable locally advanced or metastatic urothelial cancer (NILE). J Clin Oncol. 2021;39(6_Suppl):TPS504.
42. Powles T, Park SH, Voog E, Caserta C, Valderrama BP, Gurney H, et al. Avelumab maintenance therapy for advanced or metastatic urothelial carcinoma. N Engl J Med. 2020;383(13):1218–30.
43. Powles T, Park SH, Voog E, Caserta C, Pérez-Valderrama B, Gurney H, et al. Avelumab first-line (1L) maintenance for advanced urothelial carcinoma (UC): long-term follow-up results from the JAVELIN bladder 100 trial. J Clin Oncol. 2022;40(6_Suppl):487.
44. García-Donas J, Font A, Pérez-Valderrama B, Virizuela JA, Climent MÁ, Hernando-Polo S, et al. Maintenance therapy with vinflunine plus best supportive care versus best supportive care alone in patients with advanced urothelial carcinoma with a response after first-line chemotherapy (MAJA; SOGUG 2011/02): a multicentre, randomised, controlled, open-label, phase 2 trial. Lancet Oncol. 2017;18(5):672–681a.
45. Bellmunt Molins J, García-Donas Jiménez J, Valderrama BP, Virizuela Echaburu JA, Hernando-Polo S, Climent Durán MÁ, et al. Final overall survival analysis of the SOGUG phase 2 MAJA study: maintenance vinflunine versus best supportive care after first-line chemotherapy in advanced urothelial carcinoma. Clin Genitourin Cancer. 2020;18(6):452–60.
46. Galsky MD, Mortazavi A, Milowsky MI, George S, Gupta S, Fleming MT, et al. Randomized double-blind phase II study of maintenance pembrolizumab versus placebo after first-line chemotherapy in patients with metastatic urothelial cancer. J Clin Oncol. 2020;38(16):1797–806.
47. Konala VM, Adapa S, Aronow WS. Immunotherapy in bladder cancer. Am J Ther. 2022;29(3):e334–7.

48. Roche provides update on Tecentriq US indication in prior-platinum treated metastatic bladder cancer. https://www.roche.com/media/releases/med-cor-2021-03-08.
49. Bellmunt J, de Wit R, Vaughn DJ, Fradet Y, Lee JL, Fong L, et al. Pembrolizumab as second-line therapy for advanced urothelial carcinoma. N Engl J Med. 2017;376(11):1015–26.
50. Patel MR, Ellerton J, Infante JR, Agrawal M, Gordon M, Aljumaily R, et al. Avelumab in metastatic urothelial carcinoma after platinum failure (JAVELIN solid tumor): pooled results from two expansion cohorts of an open-label, phase 1 trial. Lancet Oncol. 2018;19(1):51–64.
51. Powles T, Durán I, van der Heijden MS, Loriot Y, Vogelzang NJ, De Giorgi U, et al. Atezolizumab versus chemotherapy in patients with platinum-treated locally advanced or metastatic urothelial carcinoma (IMvigor211): a multicentre, open-label, phase 3 randomised controlled trial. Lancet. 2018;391(10122):748–57.
52. Sharma P, Siefker-Radtke A, de Braud F, Basso U, Calvo E, Bono P, et al. Nivolumab alone and with ipilimumab in previously treated metastatic urothelial carcinoma: checkmate 032 nivolumab 1 mg/kg plus ipilimumab 3 mg/kg expansion cohort results. J Clin Oncol. 2019;37(19):1608–16.
53. Sridhar SS, Blais N, Tran B, Reaume MN, North SA, Stockler MR, et al. Efficacy and safety of nab-paclitaxel vs. paclitaxel on survival in patients with platinum-refractory metastatic urothelial cancer: the Canadian Cancer Trials Group BL.12 randomized clinical trial. JAMA Oncol. 2020;6(11):1751.
54. Sweeney CJ, Roth BJ, Kabbinavar FF, Vaughn DJ, Arning M, Curiel RE, et al. Phase II study of pemetrexed for second-line treatment of transitional cell cancer of the urothelium. J Clin Oncol. 2006;24(21):3451–7.
55. Bellmunt J, Théodore C, Demkov T, Komyakov B, Sengelov L, Daugaard G, et al. Phase III trial of vinflunine plus best supportive care compared with best supportive care alone after a platinum-containing regimen in patients with advanced transitional cell carcinoma of the urothelial tract. J Clin Oncol. 2009;27(27):4454–61.
56. Robertson AG, Kim J, Al-Ahmadie H, Bellmunt J, Guo G, Cherniack AD, et al. Comprehensive molecular characterization of muscle-invasive bladder cancer. Cell. 2017;171(3):540–556.e25.
57. Xiao JF, Caliri AW, Duex JE, Theodorescu D. Targetable pathways in advanced bladder cancer: FGFR signaling. Cancers. 2021;13(19):4891.
58. D'Angelo A, Bagby S, Galli IC, Bortoletti C, Roviello G. Overview of the clinical use of erdafitinib as a treatment option for the metastatic urothelial carcinoma: where do we stand. Expert Rev Clin Pharmacol. 2020;13(10):1139–46.
59. Loriot Y, Necchi A, Park SH, Garcia-Donas J, Huddart R, Burgess E, et al. Erdafitinib in locally advanced or metastatic Urothelial carcinoma. N Engl J Med. 2019;381(4):338–48.
60. Garje R, An J, Obeidat M, Kumar K, Yasin HA, Zakharia Y. Fibroblast growth factor receptor (FGFR) inhibitors in urothelial cancer. Oncologist. 2020;25(11):e1711–9.
61. Sternberg CN, Bellmunt J, Nishiyama H, Petrylak DP, Quinn DI, Nakajima K, et al. Phase II/III study of rogaratinib versus chemotherapy in patients with locally advanced or metastatic urothelial carcinoma selected based on FGFR1/3 mRNA expression. Ann Oncol. 2018;29:viii331.
62. Heath EI, Rosenberg JE. The biology and rationale of targeting nectin-4 in urothelial carcinoma. Nat Rev Urol. 2021;18(2):93–103.
63. Yu EY, Petrylak DP, O'Donnell PH, Lee JL, van der Heijden MS, Loriot Y, et al. Enfortumab vedotin after PD-1 or PD-L1 inhibitors in cisplatin-ineligible patients with advanced urothelial carcinoma (EV-201): a multicentre, single-arm, phase 2 trial. Lancet Oncol. 2021;22(6):872–82.
64. Tagawa ST, Balar AV, Petrylak DP, Kalebasty AR, Loriot Y, Fléchon A, et al. TROPHY-U-01: a phase II open-label study of sacituzumab govitecan in patients with metastatic urothelial carcinoma progressing after platinum-based chemotherapy and checkpoint inhibitors. J Clin Oncol. 2021;39(22):2474–85.
65. Fletcher A, Choudhury A, Alam N. Metastatic bladder cancer: a review of current management. ISRN Urol. 2011;2011:1–8.
66. Miranda AF, Howard JM, McLaughlin M, Meng X, Clinton T, Şanli Ö, et al. Metastasis-directed radiation therapy after radical cystectomy for bladder cancer. Urol Oncol. 2021;39(11):790.e1–7.
67. Abe T, Minami K, Harabayashi T, Sazawa A, Chiba H, Kikuchi H, et al. Prognostic impact of local radiotherapy on metastatic urothelial carcinoma patients receiving systemic chemotherapy. Jpn J Clin Oncol. 2020;50(2):206–13.
68. Abufaraj M, Dalbagni G, Daneshmand S, Horenblas S, Kamat AM, Kanzaki R, et al. The role of surgery in metastatic bladder cancer: a systematic review. Eur Urol. 2018;73(4):543–57.
69. Stein JP, Lieskovsky G, Cote R, Groshen S, Feng AC, Boyd S, et al. Radical cystectomy in the treatment of invasive bladder cancer: long-term results in 1,054 patients. J Clin Oncol. 2001;19(3):666–75.
70. Sternberg CN, Bellmunt J, Sonpavde G, Siefker-Radtke AO, Stadler WM, Bajorin DF, et al. ICUD-EAU international consultation on bladder cancer 2012: chemotherapy for urothelial carcinoma—neoadjuvant and adjuvant settings. Eur Urol. 2013;63(1):58–66.
71. Del Bene G, Calabrò F, Giannarelli D, Plimack ER, Harshman LC, Yu EY, et al. Neoadjuvant vs. adjuvant chemotherapy in muscle invasive bladder cancer (MIBC): analysis from the RISC database. Front Oncol. 2018;8:463.
72. Burdett S, Fisher DJ, Vale CL, Sternberg CN, Clarke NW, Parmar MKB, et al. Adjuvant chemotherapy for muscle-invasive bladder cancer: a systematic

review and meta-analysis of individual participant data from randomised controlled trials. Eur Urol. 2022;81(1):50–61.
73. Sternberg CN, Skoneczna I, Kerst JM, Albers P, Fossa SD, Agerbaek M, et al. Immediate versus deferred chemotherapy after radical cystectomy in patients with pT3–pT4 or N+ M0 urothelial carcinoma of the bladder (EORTC 30994): an intergroup, open-label, randomised phase 3 trial. Lancet Oncol. 2015;16(1):76–86.
74. Flaig TW, Spiess PE, Agarwal N, Bangs R, Boorjian SA, Buyyounouski MK, et al. Bladder cancer, version 3.2020, NCCN clinical practice guidelines in oncology. J Natl Compr Cancer Netw. 2020;18(3):329–54.
75. Bajorin DF, Witjes JA, Gschwend JE, Schenker M, Valderrama BP, Tomita Y, et al. Adjuvant nivolumab versus placebo in muscle-invasive urothelial carcinoma. N Engl J Med. 2021;384(22):2102–14.
76. Pfister C, Gravis G, Fléchon A, Chevreau C, Mahammedi H, Laguerre B, et al. Dose-dense methotrexate, vinblastine, doxorubicin, and cisplatin or gemcitabine and cisplatin as perioperative chemotherapy for patients with nonmetastatic muscle-invasive bladder cancer: results of the GETUG-AFU V05 VESPER trial. J Clin Oncol. 2022;40(18):2013–22.
77. Gallagher DJ, Milowsky MI, Iasonos A, Maluf FC, Russo P, Dalbagni G, et al. Sequential adjuvant chemotherapy after surgical resection of high-risk urothelial carcinoma. Cancer. 2009;115(22):5193–201.
78. Bellmunt J, Hussain M, Gschwend JE, Albers P, Oudard S, Castellano D, et al. Adjuvant atezolizumab versus observation in muscle-invasive urothelial carcinoma (IMvigor010): a multicentre, open-label, randomised, phase 3 trial. Lancet Oncol. 2021;22(4):525–37.
79. Volkmer BG, Kuefer R, Bartsch GC, Gust K, Hautmann RE. Oncological followup after radical cystectomy for bladder cancer—is there any benefit? J Urol. 2009;181(4):1587–93.
80. Boorjian SA, Tollefson MK, Cheville JC, Costello BA, Thapa P, Frank I. Detection of asymptomatic recurrence during routine oncological followup after radical cystectomy is associated with improved patient survival. J Urol. 2011;186(5):1796–802.
81. Soria F, Moschini M, Wirth GJ, Gust KM, Klatte T, Briganti A, et al. Characterization of late recurrence after radical cystectomy in a large multicenter cohort of bladder cancer patients. Urology. 2017;106:119–24.
82. EAU guidelines on MIBC: Introduction—Uroweb. Uroweb—European Association of Urology. https://uroweb.org/guidelines/muscle-invasive-and-metastatic-bladder-cancer.

Part IV

Prostate Cancer

Diagnosis and Clinical Staging 14

Harshit Garg, Dharam Kaushik, and Michael A. Liss

14.1 Screening

14.1.1 Screening: Basic Concept

Screening implies testing asymptomatic individuals to identify disease [1]. Population or mass screening implies systematic implementation of this screening in the entire population or sub-group of a population to reduce morbidity and mortality by early detection [2]. Prostate cancer screening using Prostate-Specific Antigen (PSA) remains one of the most controversial topics in urological literature and the decision of PSA testing in asymptomatic individuals is often complex.

14.1.2 Benefits of Prostate Cancer Screening with PSA Testing

The downward migration of prostate cancer stage at diagnosis, with the dramatic decrease in the incidence of metastatic disease at the time of presentation since 1988 is attributed in part to PSA screening [3]. PSA testing has also been shown to reduce prostate cancer mortality [4]. As per mathematical modeling estimates, PSA screening was responsible for a 45–70% reduction in prostate cancer mortality in the United States [5].

H. Garg (✉) · D. Kaushik · M. A. Liss
Department of Urology, University of Texas Health and Mays Cancer Centre, San Antonio, TX, USA

However, randomized trials comparing the disease-specific outcomes did not yield uniform results on PSA screening.

14.1.3 Potential Harms and Controversies with PSA Screening

Though prostate cancer is a major cause of death and disability, the benefits of early detection are, at best, moderate and often result in over-detection and hence, over-treatment of low-risk prostate cancer. Over-treatment refers to aggressive therapy leading to morbidity, with a low probability of clinical benefit. Furthermore, PSA testing often produces false-positive results leading to a negative prostate biopsy and unnecessarily causing patient anxiety, increased cost, and potential complications [6].

14.1.4 Evidence on PSA Screening

Various population-based screening studies including the European Randomized study of Screening for Prostate Cancer (ERSPC) trial [7, 8], Prostate Lung Colorectal and Ovarian (PLCO) cancer screening trial [9], Gotenburg trial [10, 11], and Cluster randomised triAl of PSA testing for Prostate cancer (CAP) [12] assessed the potential benefit of PSA screening and are sum-

P. Singh et al. (eds.), *A Guide to Management of Urological Cancers*,
https://doi.org/10.1007/978-981-99-2341-0_14

Table 14.1 Landmark trials in prostate cancer screening

Parameters	ERSPC trial [7, 8]	PLCO trial [9]	Gotenburg trial [10, 11]	CAP trial [12]
Participants	Asymptomatic men age 50–74 years [$n = 182{,}000$]	Asymptomatic men age 55–74 years [$n = 76{,}685$]	Asymptomatic men age 50–64 years [$n = 20{,}000$]	Asymptomatic men age 50–69 years [$n = 419{,}582$]
Intervention	PSA screening every 4 years	PSA screening annually for 6 years and DRE for 4 years	PSA screening every 2 years	Single PSA screening
Control	No screening	No screening	No screening	No PSA testing
Outcome	Prostate cancer mortality	Prostate cancer mortality	Prostate cancer mortality	Prostate cancer mortality
Study site	8 European countries	10 sites in USA	Sweden	United Kingdom
Duration	1994–2000	1993–2001	1994–2008	2001–2009
Median follow-up	11-year	13-year	14-year	10-year
Results	**11-year follow-up results:**	**13-year follow-up results:**	**14-year follow-up results:**	**10-year follow-up results:**
	Cumulative incidence of prostate cancer: 7.4% in screening group vs. 5.1% in control group	Cumulative incidence of prostate cancer: 108.4/10000 person-years (screening group) vs. 97.1/10000 person-years 9 control group)	Cumulative incidence of prostate cancer: 12.7% in screening group vs. 8.2% in control group ($p < 0.001$)	549 participants died of prostate cancer in intervention group compared to 647 in control group ($p = 0.50$)
	Rate ratio for death of prostate cancer was 0.79 for screening arm compared to control arm [95% CI, 0.69–0.91, $p = 0.001$]	12% relative increase of incidence in the intervention	Rate ratio for death of prostate cancer was 0.56 for screening arm compared to control arm [95% CI, 0.39–0.82, $p < 0.001$]	More low risk cancers diagnosed in intervention group
	21% reduction in prostate cancer mortality by PSA screening	No difference between disease specific mortality between two groups (RR = 1.09, 95% CI = 0.87–1.36)	44% reduction in prostate cancer mortality by PSA screening	No difference in all-cause mortality
	1055 individuals need to be screened and 37 additional need to be treated over 11 years to prevent one prostate cancer mortality	The results were similar after 15-year follow-up	293 individuals need to be screened and 12 additional need to be diagnosed over 14 years to prevent one prostate cancer mortality	
	Later, 13-year and 16-year follow-up data confirmed the mortality benefit and with 16-year follow-up, the number needed to screen, and the number needed to treat to prevent one prostate cancer death decreased to 570 and 18 respectively		Later, 18-year follow-up reported the reduction in absolute prostate-cancer specific mortality of 0.72 (95% CI, 0.5–0.94)	
			The number needed to screen and needed to diagnose decreased to 139 and 13 respectively	

(continued)

Table 14.1 (continued)

Parameters	ERSPC trial [7, 8]	PLCO trial [9]	Gotenburg trial [10, 11]	CAP trial [12]
Limitations	The ERSPC trial may have underestimated the benefit of PSA screening by using advanced age at first PSA testing (median > 60 years) and low intensity of screening (largely every 4 years)	Prescreening and high contamination of 40–52% per year in control arm [74% of participants in usual care arm were screened atleast once]	More than half of participants were also included in the main analysis of ERSPC trial, hence its independent role for interpretation is questionable	Single PSA testing
		Biopsy rate for those with elevated PSA was relatively lower as compared to European trials		Compliance for biopsy after raised PSA was only 40%
		In real sense compared 'fixed' screening vs. 'opportunistic' screening and did not truly test the hypothesis for value of PSA screening		

marized in Table 14.1. Each of these trials had certain limitations, with none of the trials addressing the potential benefit of screening in those with high-risk factors. For example, less than 5% of PLCO participants were African Americans and only 7% reported a family history of prostate cancer. In 2012, US Preventive Services Task Force (USPSTF) recommended against routine PSA testing [13]. This led to a decrease in screening and biopsy rates as well as diagnosis of localized prostate cancer, however, its effect on the diagnosis of metastatic prostate cancer remained unclear [14, 15]. A Cochrane review published in 2014 suggested that PSA screening is associated with increased diagnosis of prostate cancer and detection of more localized disease and less advanced disease. There was no disease-specific survival benefit nor overall survival benefit with PSA testing [16]. However, based on further evidence and systematic review [17], the USPSTF made a Grade C recommendation for periodic prostate cancer screening for men 55–69 years and recommended against screening for men with 70 years or older [18].

Both the European Association of Urology (EAU) [2] and the National Comprehensive Cancer Network (NCCN) [6] recommended guidelines for PSA screening (Table 14.2). The important considerations in PSA screening are the age of initiation of screening, frequency of PSA testing, and age of discontinuation of PSA testing.

14.1.5 Screening in High-Risk Population

14.1.5.1 Family History

Family history for high-risk of prostate cancer include [6].

- Having first degree relative with prostate cancer diagnosed before 60 years.
- Having one first or second degree relative with metastatic prostate cancer, ovarian cancer, pancreatic cancer, male breast cancer, female breast cancer ≤45 years, endometrial or colorectal cancer ≤50 years [19]..
- Having two or more first-or second-degree relatives with breast, prostate (but not localized grade group 1), colorectal or endometrial cancer at any age.

Though the risk of prostate cancer increases with the increased number of affected relatives, their cancer aggressiveness and outcomes appear similar between those with and without a family history [20, 21]. NCCN recommends shared decision-making about PSA screening at the age

Table 14.2 Screening recommendations of prostate cancer by European Association of Urology (EAU) and National Comprehensive Cancer Network (NCCN)

Guideline	EAU [2]	NCCN [6]
Age at onset	>50 years	>45 years
General population	>50 years: Annual PSA with DRE after shared decision making	45 years: PSA with DRE after shared decision making
	Risk adapted approach:	***Risk adapted approach:***
	If at risk initially, i.e., if PSA > 1 ng/mL in <40 years or PSA > 2 ng/mL in <60 years—repeat PSA every 2 years	If PSA < 1 ng/mL—every 2–4 years
	If not at risk: Postpone PSA for 8 years	PSA 1–3 ng/mL—every 1–2 years
Interruption	If LE < 15 years	Consider stopping:
		• If PSA < 1 ng/mL at age > 60 years
		• Age 75 years (especially if PSA < 3 ng/mL)
		• At age 75 years unless patient is very healthy with little/no comorbidities and especially if never have undergone PSA testing or have a rising PSA)
High risk population		
African descent	>45 years if African descent	>40 years in African American (annual screening preferable)
Positive family history	>45 years with family history	At age of onset 10 years prior to youngest family diagnosis
Genetic risk factor	>40 years with BRCA2+	>40 years in BRCA1/BRCA2+

DRE digital rectal examination, *PSA* prostate specific antigen, *LE* life expectancy

corresponding to 10 years before the age of the youngest family diagnosis [6].

14.1.5.2 Genetic Syndromes

Germline mutations in 16 DNA repair genes have been associated with prostate cancer-BRCA2 (5%), ATM (2%), CHEK2 (2%), BRCA1 (1%), RAD51D (0.4%), PALB2 (0.4%), ATR (0.3%) and NBN, PMS2, GEN1, MSH2, MSH6, RAD51C, MRE11A, BRIP1 or FAM175A [22]. Mutation carriers have an increased risk of prostate cancer before 65 years of age. Germline BRCA2 mutations are associated with a two- to sixfold increase in the risk of prostate cancer and association with BRCA1 is less consistent [23]. Moreover, prostate cancer with germline BRCA mutations appears to occur earlier, has a more aggressive phenotype, and has lower survival [24, 25]. The IMPACT study [26] evaluated prostate cancer screening using annual PSA testing in men aged 40–69 years with germline BRCA1/2 mutations. In their interim analysis, the overall incidence of prostate cancer and clinically significant prostate cancer was significantly higher in BRCA2 carriers but no difference BRCA1.

Another syndrome involving germline mutations in MLH1, MSH2, MSH6, PMS2, or EPCAM is Lynch Syndrome. It is associated with a 2 to 5.8-fold increase in the risk of prostate cancer [27].

The NCCN panel [6] recommends inquiring about personal or familial cancer germline mutations and referral for cancer genetics professional in case of positive history. Prostate cancer screening is recommended at age 40 years for BRCA2 carriers and other germline mutations and this screening should be done annually [6].

14.1.5.3 African Ancestry

Men with African ancestry have a 60% higher incidence of prostate cancer and a 36–39% increase in prostate cancer mortality in comparison with Caucasian men [28]. They are also at increased risk of aggressive prostate cancer and metastatic progression [29]. An analysis of SEER data from 2010 reported that non-Hispanic African Americans are diagnosed with prostate cancer 1.2 years earlier than non-Hispanic white men [30]. The probable reasons for this racial disparity include heritable genes linked to African ancestry and social determinants of health such as environmental exposures, patient and physician behaviors, delays in diagnosis, and suboptimal treatment [31, 32]. The NCCN panel recommends shared decision-making for annual PSA screening from age 40 years. However, there is no current evidence to suggest that testing at an earlier age would result in decreased morbidity and mortality compared to testing at 45 years of age [6].

14.2 Diagnosis of Prostate Cancer

Prostate cancer is often asymptomatic at an early stage and the presence of symptoms occur in locally advanced or metastatic disease. Locally advanced disease can present with obstructive lower urinary tract symptoms, pelvic pain, haematospermia, or decreased ejaculate volume and ureteral obstruction leading to renal failure. The metastatic disease can present with bony pain, pathological fractures, anemia, lower extremity edema, and rarely, paralysis. The diagnosis of prostate cancer involves digital rectal examination, biomarker testing including PSA, imaging including ultrasonography and multi-parametric Magnetic Resonance Imaging (mpMRI), and prostatic needle biopsy.

14.2.1 Digital Rectal Examination (DRE)

The early diagnosis of prostate cancer was primarily based on DRE before the availability of PSA testing. Though reproducibility of DRE findings is fair in experienced hands, the overall positive predictive value of DRE with normal PSA is poor. As per current NCCN guidelines [6], DRE alone should not be used as a standalone test without PSA testing and DRE is recommended as complementary testing with serum PSA in asymptomatic individuals. Furthermore, the greatest use of DRE is in those with elevated PSA as it aids in decisions regarding biopsy. In case of highly suspicious DRE, biopsy or further testing should be considered, irrespective of PSA value [6].

14.2.2 Biomarkers

Several biomarkers have been developed for the diagnosis and risk assessment of prostate cancer. PSA is the most common biomarker utilized in the diagnosis of prostate cancer. Various other biomarkers have been developed and become particularly important for patients with PSA levels between 3–10 ng/mL for selection of biopsy and for patients with prior negative biopsy to decide for repeat biopsy. Most of these biomarkers have been developed and validated independently. PSA is the most used biomarker [33] and various biomarkers related to PSA such as PSA velocity [34–36], PSA density [37, 38], free PSA (fPSA) [39] are commonly used. Newer biomarkers introduced include Prostate Cancer Antigen 3 (PCA3) [40, 41], Prostate Health Index (PHI) [42–44], 4 K score [45, 46], Confirm MDx [47], ExoDx Prostate (Intelliscore) [48], Select MDx [49, 50], Mi-Prostate Score (Mi-PS) [51–53] and Sentinel PCa [54] test. Table 14.3 describes the brief role of various biomarkers used in diagnosis of prostate cancer. Despite of availability of various novel biomarkers, no robust head-to-head comparisons exist at present, and no biomarker can be recommended over other at present time.

14.2.3 Imaging for Prostate Cancer

14.2.3.1 Ultrasonography

Transrectal high-frequency (5–10 Hz) ultrasonography can provide anatomic information about the prostate. On ultrasound, prostate cancer usually appears hypoechoic (60–70%) in the peripheral zone of the gland but can be hyperechoic or isoechoic (30–40%). Ultrasonography is also used in direct biopsies for suspicious lesions [55]. Further advances in ultrasound imaging appear promising to improve prostate cancer detection. Color ultrasonography with the incorporation of spectral waveform analysis of

Table 14.3 Various Biomarkers used in diagnosis of prostate cancer

S.No	Biomarker	Role in prostate cancer diagnosis
1	Prostate specific antigen (PSA)	PSA belongs to the human kallikrein gene family, located on chromosome 19, and is secreted in high concentrations (mg/mL) into seminal fluid. PSA circulates inbound (complexed) and unbound (free) forms. PSA has a half-life of 2–3 days [33] and serum levels of PSA serve as an initial assessment for diagnosis of prostate cancer. Serum PSA levels vary with age, race, prostate volume, urinary tract manipulation, and ejaculation. Androgens have a strong influence on PSA and 5-alpha reductase inhibitors used for the treatment of benign prostatic hyperplasia lower PSA levels.
2	PSA velocity (PSAV)	PSA velocity is the rate of change in PSA over time and determined by at least three separate PSA values calculated over at least 18 months. PSAV has been linked to PCSM and the relative risk of prostate cancer death is higher with PSAV>0.35 ng/mL/year [34]. Though the role of PSAV has been controversial with the risk of over-diagnosis and false-positive results, PSAV appeared to be an independent predictor of overall prostate cancer, intermediate and high-grade cancer in patients undergoing the second biopsy after initial negative biopsy [35, 36] as per current recommendations, PSAV has no role if PSA >10 ng/mL and PSAV (≥0.35 ng/mL) is only one criterion to consider while deciding to perform the biopsy in patients with low PSA, which should be seen in the light of other factors such as age, comorbidity, ancestry and family history [6].
3	PSA density (PSAD)	PSA density is defined as PSA value (in ng/mL) divided by prostate volume (in cc as measured on TRUS). PSAD potentially defines patients who do not have prostate cancer but have high PSA due to large prostate. Conventionally, a PSAD cutoff of 0.15 ng/mL was recommended earlier [37], which would spare up to 50% unnecessary biopsies, however, recent studies have challenged the sensitivity for this cutoff [38]. PSAD suffers from a lack of measurement of both PSA and prostate volume and thus, has limited acceptance. As per current guidelines, PSAD has not been incorporated into early detection guidelines for prostate cancer, but it could have some role in explaining elevated PSA after negative biopsies.

(continued)

Table 14.3 (continued)

S.No	Biomarker	Role in prostate cancer diagnosis
4	Percentage free PSA (%fPSA)	Unbound or fPSA is expressed as a ratio of total PSA and has the potential to improve early detection, staging, and monitoring of prostate cancer. The majority (60–90%) of circulating PSA is covalently bound to endogenous protease inhibitors- alpha-1 antichymotrypsin, alpha-1-antitrypsin, and protease C inhibitor. In addition, a large proportion of PSA is complexed with alpha-2-macroglobulin (AMG). Because of the shielding of PSA antigenic epitopes by AMG, this PSA-AMG cannot be measured using conventional assays. The unbound or free form of PSA is significantly lower in patients with prostate cancer. A 25% fPSA cutoff detected 95%of prostate cancers, thereby, avoiding 20% unnecessary prostate biopsies [39]. FDA approved the use of %fPSA for detection of prostate cancer in men with age $\geq$ 50 years with a non-suspicious DRE and PSA levels between 4–10 ng/mL.
5	Prostate cancer antigen 3 (PCA3)	PCA3 is a noncoding, prostate tissue-specific RNA that is overexpressed in prostate cancer. PCA3 over-expression in post DRE urine specimen is most useful to determine the need for repeat biopsy after prior negative biopsy. A PCA3 score cutoff of 25 is used and patients with a score $\geq$ 25 are 4.6 times more likely to have positive repeat biopsy than those with a score < 25 [40]. Similarly, the use of PCA3 in repeat biopsy would reduce the number of biopsies by almost half [41]. The FDA approved PCA3 for use in repeat biopsy setting in men age $\geq$ 50 years to decide for repeat biopsy, along with other factors.
6	Prostate health index (PHI)	PHI is a combination of tPSA, fPSA, and pro PSA tests. PHI has been approved by FDA for patients with PSA in the range of 4–10 ng/mL. In various studies, PHI correlated with cancer detection and had a good discriminative ability to predict cancer on biopsy [42, 43]. A PHI cutoff of 24 was shown to avoid 36% unnecessary biopsies while missing only 2.5% high-grade cancers [44].
7	4 K score	4 K score combines fPSA, tPSA, intact PSA, and human kallikrein 2 (hK2) and also includes age, DRE results, and prior biopsy status. 4 K score can be considered for patients before biopsy and for those with prior negative biopsy with risk of clinically significant prostate cancer. No optimal cutoff threshold exists for the 4 K score. However, a cutoff of >15% risk allowed for avoiding 58% unnecessary biopsies while 4.8% high-grade tumors were missed [45]. A meta-analysis involving 12 clinical validation studies reported pooled AURC for discrimination of grade group$\geq$2 prostate cancer of 0.81 (95% CI, 0.80–0.83) [46].

(continued)

Table 14.3 (continued)

S.No	Biomarker	Role in prostate cancer diagnosis
8	Confirm MDx	Confirm MDx is a tissue-based, multiplex epigenetic assay assessing hypermethylation of the promoter regions of GSTP1, APC, and RASSF1 in core biopsy tissue samples. This assay can be used before a repeat biopsy. The European MATLOC study [47] tested this assay in archived tissue from 498 patients with negative biopsies, who also had repeat biopsies within 30 months. They reported an NPV of 90% for this assay and the test was an independent predictor of patient outcome. Though not approved by FDA, confirm MDx can be considered as an option for individuals planning for repeat biopsy [6].
9	ExoDx prostate (IntelliScore)	Also known as EPI, this assay evaluates urine-based 3-gene exosome expression utilizing PCA3 and ERG (V-ETS erythroblastosis virus E26 oncogene homologs) RNA from urine, normalized to SPDEF (SAM pointed domain-containing ETS transcription factors). Its utility has been studied in biopsy-naïve men with age ≥ 50 years with PSA 2–10 ng/mL to discriminate GG ≥ 2 prostate cancer with GG1 cancer and benign pathology [48]. Waiting for FDA approval, the NCCN panel recommended that ExoDx can be considered as an option for patients with initial or repeat biopsies [6].
10	Select MDx	Select MDx is a gene expression assay to study DLX1 and HOXC6 expression against KLK3 as internal reference in a post DRE urine sample. DLX1 and HOXC6 have been associated with prostate cancer aggressiveness and this assay can be utilized to avoid unnecessary biopsies. Though not yet FDA approved, select MDx has been shown to have good predictive accuracy for GG ≥ 2 prostate cancer [49, 50] and can be potentially used in biopsy-naïve patients.
11	Mi-prostate score (mi-PS)	MiPS assay measures total serum PSA and post-DRE expression of PCA3 and the TMPRSS2:ERG fusion gene. The TMPRSS2:ERG fusion is an early event in prostate cancer and occurs at high frequency in prostate cancer [53]. Though few studies have shown its benefit to avoid unnecessary biopsies [51, 52], the NCCN panel [6] considers it an investigation at present, due to lack of validation, independent publications, and lack of clarity due to incremental value and cost-effectiveness and NCCN panel.
12	Sentinel PCa test	Recently introduced, this assay involves non-coding RNAs (sncRNA) isolated from urinary exosomes. Though this assay awaits further validation, it has been shown to differentiate prostate cancer from benign histopathology with high sensitivity and specificity [54].

the capsular and urethral arteries of the prostate using power Doppler can differentiate cancer from benign hypertrophy of the gland [56]. Further, the use of 3-D Doppler using microbubble contrast agents could also improve the detection of cancer [57]. Another ultrasound-based technique is HistoScanning (BK Medical, Peabody, MA). HistoScanning is a computer-aided ultrasound-based method that incorporates spectral analysis and pattern recognition to detect and characterize potentially suspicious lesions [58].

14.2.3.2 Magnetic Resonance Imaging (MRI)

For evaluation of the prostate, multiparametric (mp) MRI is used. mpMRI comprises dynamic contrast-enhanced (DCE) images and diffusion restriction imaging apart from anatomical T2-imaging. MRI has high soft tissue contrast and characterization, multiplanar imaging capability, and advanced computational methods to assess function. The resolution of MRI images in the pelvis can be augmented using an endorectal coil. The Prostate-Imaging Reporting and Data System (PIRADS) [59] is used to report findings of prostate MRI in a standardized manner and comprises of five-point scoring with PIRADS 1 and 2 indicating prostate cancer is highly unlikely and PIRADS 4 and 5 as prostate cancer is likely. As per recent PIRADSv2 [60], a PIRADS score of 3 or higher should be considered for biopsy.

14.2.4 Needle Biopsy of the Prostate

Tissue diagnosis of prostate cancer is mandatory for the diagnosis and definitive therapy. A needle biopsy is often used, and histological grade is the most important parameter on biopsy. The Gleason grading system is most used. Proposed in 1966 [61], the original Gleason grading comprised of pathological findings at low power magnification, and Gleason grade (1 to 5) is assigned to the predominant pattern (occupying the largest area of the specimen) and the second most common pattern. The sum of these patterns results in a score of 2–10. Later, it was shown that the tertiary Gleason pattern is an important prognostic marker, leading to modification in the Gleason grading system in 2005. Furthermore, the Gleason grading system was modified such that Gleason's total scores 2 to 5 were no longer assigned, and the lowest total score assigned was 6, even though the scale continued to range from 2–10. This resulted in further confusion with GS6, giving a false impression of a high score and presented as a barrier for active surveillance. Hence, the International Society of Urological Pathology (ISUP) proposed a new prostate cancer grading system in 2014 (Table 14.4) [62].

14.2.4.1 Use of Magnetic Resonance Imaging in Biopsy

Multi-parametric MRI can be used to select patients for prostate biopsy and to aid biopsy

Table 14.4 International Society of Urological Pathology (ISUP) 2014 Gleason grading of prostate cancer [61]

Gleason grade group	Gleason score	Pathological features	5 year biochemical recurrence free survival
1	≤6	Only individual discrete well-formed glands	96% (95% CI, 95–96%)
2	3 + 4 = 7	Predominantly well-formed glands with lesser component of poorly formed/fused/cribriform glands	88% (95% CI, 85–89%)
3	4 + 3 = 7	Predominantly poorly formed/fused/cribriform glands with lesser component of well-formed glands	63% (95% CI, 61–65%)
4	4 + 4 = 8	Only poorly formed/fused/cribriform glands	48% (95% CI, 44–52%)
	3 + 5 = 8	Predominantly well-formed glands with lesser component of lacking glands	
	5 + 3 = 8	Predominantly lacking glands and lesser component of well-formed glands	
5	9, 10	Lack gland formation (or with necrosis) with or without poorly formed fused/cribriform glands	26% (95% CI, 23–30%)

itself. Compared to TRUS biopsy, MRI-guided biopsy has a superior sensitivity for clinically significant prostate cancer [63]. Various clinical trials [64–69] have assessed the utility of MRI-targeted biopsy in prostate cancer (Box 14.1). Targeted biopsy techniques include cognitive or visual targeting (guiding with ultrasound, based on an MRI image), TRUS-MRI fusion platforms (merging stored MRI image with real-time ultrasound), or direct in-bore MR-guided biopsy (performed by intervention radiologist while the patient is in the scanner). A 2019 Cochrane systematic review [63] included 18 cross-sectional studies comparing template-guided biopsy with MRI only, MRI-targeted biopsy, MRI with or without MRI-targeted biopsy, and/or systematic biopsy for the detection of Grade Group ≥2 prostate cancer. Overall, MRI detected a greater number of significant prostate cancer, while detecting fewer insignificant prostate cancers. Another review showed that the use of MRI before biopsy for biopsy-naïve individuals would improve detection of clinically significant cancer, reduce the number of biopsy cores per procedure, reduce adverse effects and potentially reduce unnecessary biopsies [70]. As per current NCCN guidelines [6], MRI is recommended before biopsy, if available, and image-guided biopsy techniques should be employed routinely. As some significant cancers exist outside targets identified by MRI, a combined approach of targeted and systematic biopsy is advocated. In cases with prior one negative biopsy, the multiparametric MRI may help in the identification of missed cancer on prior biopsies and hence, should be done [6].

Box 14.1 Keypoints of landmark trials on utility of MRI-targeted biopsy in diagnosis of prostate cancer

PROMIS [prostate MR imaging study] study [63]
• Multicentre, paired cohort study
• 576 biopsy-naïve men with PSA < 15 ng/mL underwent multiparameteric MRI followed by TRUS biopsy and perineal template mapping biopsy
• Clinically significant prostate cancer was found in 40% of patients
• For detection of clinically significant prostate cancer, MRI was more sensitive and less specific [sensitivity = 93%, specificity = 41%] as compared to TRUS biopsy [sensitivity = 48%, specificity = 96%]
• If a normal MRI had been used to screen individuals for biopsy, 27% would have avoided biopsy
PRECISION [prostate evaluation for clinically important disease: Sampling using image-guidance or not] trial [64]
• Compared MRI-guided biopsy and conventional TRUS biopsy
• Randomized non-inferiority trial conducted in 25 centres across 11 countries
• 500 participants were randomized to MRI (with or without targeted biopsy) or 10–12 core TRUS biopsy
• MRI-guided biopsy had higher detection of clinically significant prostate cancer (38% in MRI group vs. 26% in standard TRUS biopsy) and lower detection of clinically insignificant prostate cancer (9% in MRI group vs. 22% in standard TRUS biopsy group)
MRI-FIRST trial [65]
• Compared MRI targeted biopsy and systematic TRUS biopsy
• Prospective multicentre paired diagnostic study conducted at 16 centres in France
• 251 men underwent pre-biopsy MRI, systematic biopsy and targeted biopsy (if MRI abnormal)
• 21% had normal MRI. Of these, 11% had clinically significant prostate cancer on systematic biopsy
• Clinically significant cancer was found in 29.9% on systematic biopsy, 32.3% on targeted biopsy and 37% using combined targeted and systematic biopsy
• There was no significant difference between targeted and systematic biopsy ($p = 0.38$). Omission of systematic biopsy and targeted biopsy would have missed 5.2% and 7.6% clinically significant prostate cancer
• Maximum detection of clinically significant prostate cancer required combination of targeted and systematic biopsy
4 M [met Prostaat MRI Meer mans (Dutch)] study [66]
• Prospective multicentre comparative study in four centres in Netherlands
• Compared in-bore MRI targeted biopsy with systematic biopsy

Box 14.1 (continued)

PROMIS [prostate MR imaging study] study [63]

- 626 biopsy naïve patients underwent pre-biopsy MRI followed by systematic biopsy and those with abnormal MRI also underwent in-bore MRI guided biopsy
- 49% of MRIs were normal
- Clinically significant prostate cancer was detected in 30% using combined approach, 25% using MRI-targeted approach and 23% using systematic approach
- No difference in clinically significant prostate cancer detection was seen between targeted and systematic biopsy
- Detection of clinically insignificant prostate cancer was lower using targeted approach
- In patients with abnormal MRI, 7% had cancer detected only on systematic biopsy while in patients with normal MRI, 4% had clinically significant cancer
- This trial represented best case scenario with experts interpreting MRI and performing targeted biopsy

Trio study [67]

- 2103 patients with abnormal MRI underwent both MRI-targeted and systematic biopsy
- Prostate cancer was diagnosed in 52.5% with systematic biopsy, 51.5% with MRI-targeted biopsy alone and 62.4% in combination of MRI-targeted and systematic biopsy
- The rate of detection of GG1 cancer was significantly lower while the rate of detection of GG $\geq$ 3 cancer was significantly higher with MRI-targeted biopsy as compared to systematic biopsy
- The combined approach resulted in additional 59 cancers diagnosis of GG $\geq$ 3 cancers that would have found by either method alone

PRECISE [PRostate evaluation for clinically important disease: MRI vs. standard evaluation procedures] trial [68]

- Canadian multicenter, randomized prospective trial
- 453 biopsy naïve patients with PSA $\leq$20 ng/mL
- Participants were randomized to undergo MRI followed by targeted biopsy only if PIRADS score $\geq$ 3 (MRI-TB group) or systematic TRUS biopsy
- The diagnosis of GG $\geq$ 2 cancer was similar in the two groups [35% in MRI-TB group vs. 30% in systematic biopsy group]
- MRI-TB group had lower rate of GG1 cancer (10%) as compared to systematic biopsy group (22%)
- 37% participants in MRI-TB group had negative MRI and avoided biopsy

14.2.4.2 Prostate Biopsy-Phase and Techniques

Initial Biopsy

Transrectal or transperineal systematic prostate biopsy under TRUS guidance with or without targeting of lesions seen on pre-biopsy MRI should be used for prostate biopsy. In the case of systematic biopsy, an extended pattern with at least 12-core biopsy should be preferred as compared to sextant biopsy [71, 72]. Both transperineal and transrectal appear reasonable options. The transperineal biopsy is associated with higher detection of clinically significant prostate cancer with lower risk of sepsis, however, extensive perineal template biopsy may lead to a higher rate of other complications such as urinary retention and definitive comparisons of more limited transperineal biopsy with conventional transrectal biopsy are lacking [6].

Repeat Biopsies

A negative prostate biopsy does not preclude prostate cancer and a repeat biopsy may be done in cases of high suspicion. The use of mpMRI followed by an appropriate targeted biopsy leads to a higher detection rate of clinically significant cancer than repeat systematic biopsy. The cancer detection rates by targeted fusion biopsies in individuals with prior negative biopsies range from 34–51% [73–75]. As per NCCN recommendations, targeted biopsy techniques help in the identification of regions of cancer missed on prior biopsies and should be considered strongly with a prior negative biopsy and persistent concern for cancer [6]. Additionally, biomarker testing can also be considered for informed decision-making.

Saturation Biopsy Techniques

Saturation biopsies involve the collection of cores systematically every few millimeters across the entire prostate to improve prostate cancer detection over standard 12-core biopsy. Saturation biopsies can be performed via transrectal or transperineal approaches with similar rates of cancer detection [76]. Transperineal prostate mapping biopsy is often used for saturation biopsy. The transperineal approach is associated with a lower risk of infection or sepsis, better saturation of gland, more accurate risk of assessment and is often more acceptable to patients as compared to the transrectal approach [77, 78] The transrectal approach can be performed routinely in the office while transperineal biopsy requires more extensive local or systemic analgesia. Though evidence is emerging in favor of saturation biopsy [79, 80], the NCCN panel does not recommend saturation biopsy strategy for all individuals with previous negative biopsies at this time, given the benefits seen for MRI and MRI-targeted biopsy in this patient population [6].

14.3 Staging of Prostate Cancer

The staging of prostate cancer involves the use of pretreatment parameters for predicting the extent and prognosis of the disease and helps in decision making for appropriate management. The most common parameters used for clinical staging include findings of digital rectal examination (determines the cT stage), PSA and its derivatives, prostate cancer features on biopsy, and radiological imaging. The pathological staging is determined after prostate removal and involves histological analysis of prostate, seminal vesicles, and pelvic lymph nodes if lymphadenectomy is performed.

The Whitmore and Jewett staging system of prostate cancer is of historical interest [81, 82] and current staging is based on tumor, node, and metastasis (TNM) classification system. First introduced in 1975 by American Joint Committee on Cancer (AJCC), this system has evolved, and the recent version (8th edition) was proposed in 2017 [83]. As per the latest version (Fig. 14.1a–c), the TNM stage is combined with the PSA level and Gleason grade group.

14.3.1 Risk Stratification and Nomograms

Risk assessment at the time of diagnosis of prostate cancers forms an integral component of prostate cancer management and assist in shared decision-making. Risk assessment indicates the likelihood of organ-confined disease and helps in management decisions such as the need for active surveillance or multimodal therapy.

Various nomograms and algorithms integrating multiple clinical parameters have been developed for improved staging and risk stratification of prostate cancer. These tools mostly incorporate DRE findings and radiographically determined clinical T stage, PSA, and histopathological grade on preoperative biopsy [84, 85].

D′ Amico et al. stratified prostate cancer into low-risk, intermediate-risk, and high-risk disease and demonstrated significant association with 10-year disease-free survival after radical prostatectomy with 83% for low risk, 46% for intermediate-risk, and 29% for high-risk disease [86]. Cancer of the Prostate Risk Assessment (CAPRA) score is another nomogram for pretreatment risk stratification. Both EAU [2] and NCCN [6] have incorporated risk stratification schemes and advocated treatment options based on their systems (Table 14.5).

Apart from risk stratification schemes, various nomograms have been proposed for predicting prognosis. The Partin tables were first to be commonly used for patient counseling in localized prostate cancer [87, 88]. These nomograms predict pathological stage based on preoperative features and can be used to inform treatment decision contemplating active surveillance [89, 90], radical prostatectomy [91, 92], neurovascular bundle

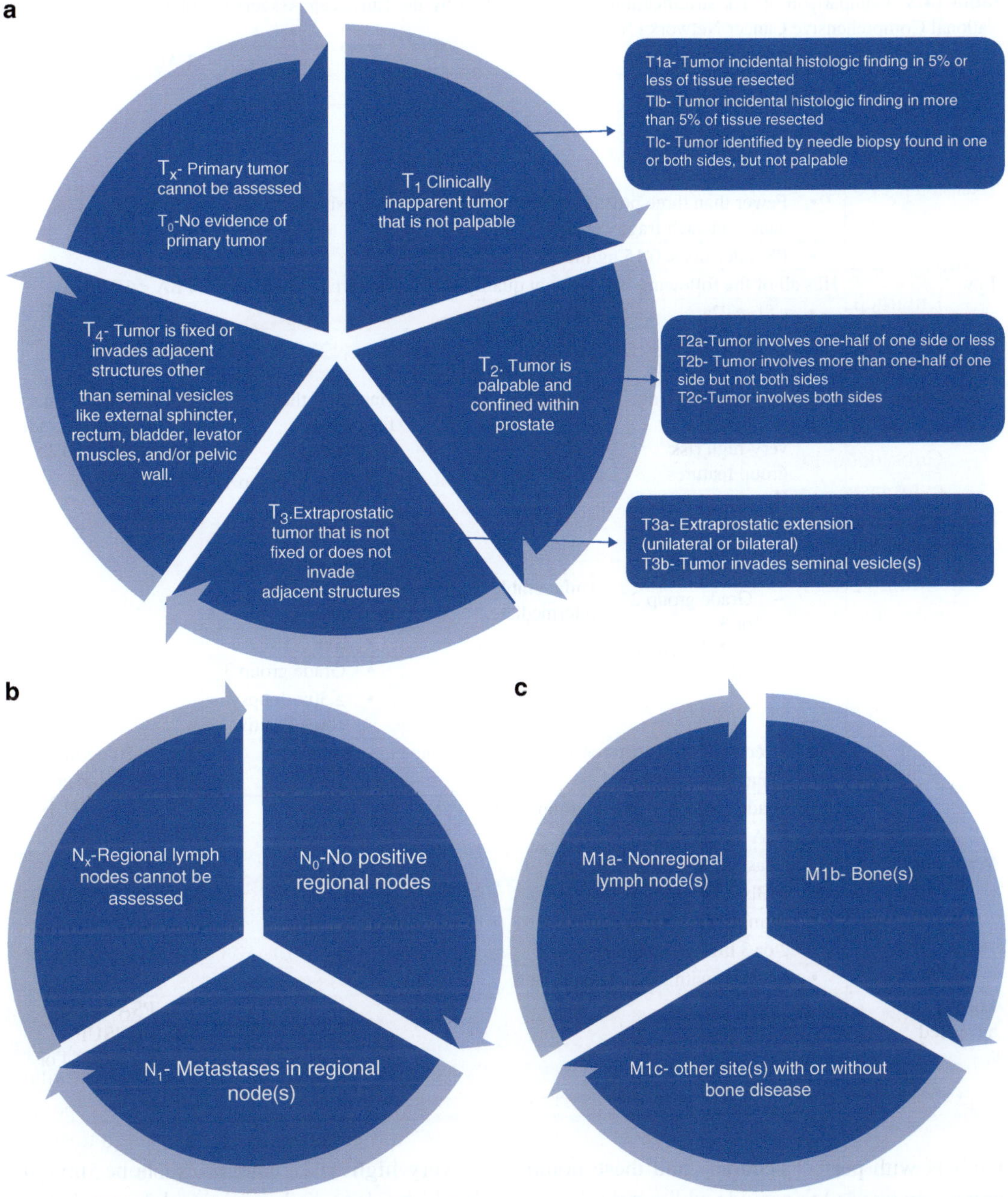

Fig. 14.1 (**a**) T staging, (**b**) N staging, (**c**) M staging

preservation [93, 94], or omission of pelvic lymph node dissection during radical prostatectomy [95, 96], brachytherapy [97, 98] or external beam radiotherapy [99]. The biochemical recurrence can be reassessed after definitive therapy using preoperative parameters, post-treatment PSA, and pathological grade and stage of the disease [100]. However, none of the current models

Table 14.5 Comparison of risk stratification system proposed by the European Association of Urology (EAU) and National Comprehensive Cancer Network (NCCN)

Risk group	NCCN [6]			EAU [2]
Very low	Has all of the following: • cT1c • Grade group 1 • PSA <10 ng/mL • Fewer than three prostate biopsy fragments/cores positive, ≤50% cancer in each fragment/core • PSA density < 0.15 ng/mL/g			
Low	Has all of the following but does not qualify for very low risk: • cT1–cT2a • Grade group 1 • PSA <10 ng/mL			PSA < 10 ng/mL and GS < 7 (ISUP grade 1) and cT1–2a
Intermediate	Has all of the following: • No high-risk or very-high risk group features • Has one or more intermediate risk factors (IRFs): – cT2b–cT2c – Grade group 2 or 3 PSA 10–20 ng/mL	Favorable intermediate	Has all of the following: • 1 IRF • Grade group 1 or 2 • <50% biopsy cores Positive	PSA 10–20 ng/mL or GS 7 (ISUP grade 2/grade 3) or cT2b
		Unfavorable intermediate	Has one or more of the following: • 2 or 3 IRFs • Grade group 3 • ≥ 50% biopsy cores Positive	
High	Has no very high-risk features and has exactly one high-risk feature • cT3a OR • Grade group 4 or grade group 5 OR • PSA >20 ng/mL			PSA > 20 ng/mL or GS > 7 (ISUP grade 4/grade 5) or cT2c
Very high	Has at least one of the following: • cT3b–cT4 • Primary Gleason pattern 5 • 2 or 3 high-risk features • >4 cores with grade group 4 or 5			
Locally advanced				Any PSA and any GS (any ISUP grade) cT3–cT4 or cN+

predicts with perfect accuracy and these nomograms can be used to provide additional information to NCCN or EAU risk groups.

14.3.2 Staging Evaluation

With a life expectancy of 5 years or less, asymptomatic patients with very low, low- and intermediate-risk prostate cancer need no further imaging until symptomatic. For high-risk or very-high risk categories, bone imaging should be done and pelvic ± abdominal imaging should be done if the nomogram predicts lymph node involvement, irrespective of life expectancy [6].

With life expectancy greater than 5 years and symptomatic, bone imaging is recommended in unfavorable intermediate risk, high or very high-risk disease. A conventional bone scan is an initial modality for bone imaging and CT, MRI or PET/CT or PET/MRI can be used in equivocal findings. Pelvic ± abdominal imaging is recommended for intermediate or higher risk disease when nomogram suggests a greater than 10% chance of lymph nodal involvement [6].

14.3.2.1 Imaging Techniques

Imaging is used for the detection and characterization of disease. Imaging could be anatomical (plain radiograph, CT, or MRI) or functional (radionuclide Bone scan, PET scan).

Plain Radiograph

It helps in the evaluation of symptomatic regions in the skeleton. However, a conventional plain radiograph will not detect bone lesions until nearly 50% of the mineral content of bone is lost or grained. CT or MRI is more useful to assess fracture risk as osteoblastic lesions may obscure cortical involvement on plain radiograph.

Bone Imaging

Bone scan refers to a conventional technetium-99m-MDP bone scan, wherein, Tc is taken up by bone with a fast turnover and imaged with gamma camera using planar imaging or 3D imaging with single-photon emission CT (SPECT). Sites of increased activity imply accelerated bone turnover and may indicate metastatic disease. A bone scan can also be used for monitoring prostate cancer during systemic therapy.

Computed Tomography (CT)

CT provides a high level of anatomic detail and may detect nodal or visceral metastatic disease or gross extracapsular spread. However, it is generally insufficient to evaluate the prostate gland. Whenever used, a CT scan should always be optimized for maximum diagnostic utility while minimizing radiation dose.

Magnetic Resonance Imaging (MRI)

Standard MRI can be used for examination of the pelvis and abdomen during initial staging and as a part of a workup for recurrence. MRI and CT scans are equivalent for pelvic lymph node evaluation.

Positron Emission Tomography (PET) Scan

F-18 fluoro-deoxyglucose (FDG)-PET is of limited use in the diagnosis of prostate cancer because of relatively low glucose metabolism in prostate cancer. However, other tracers are rapidly developing, and FDA-approved tracers include C-11 choline, F-18 sodium fluoride, and F-18 fluciclovine.

PET scan is not recommended for primary staging as earlier detection of bone metastatic disease may result in earlier use of newer and more expensive therapies, which might not improve oncologic outcomes or overall survival. Hence, a PET scan should be considered for further evaluation in primary staging of prostate cancer if the bone scan is equivocal for metastasis [6].

C-11 choline PET/CT and F-18 fluciclovine PET/CT can detect small volume disease in bone and soft tissue [101, 102]. These scans are recommended for use in patients with biochemical recurrence after primary treatment of prostate cancer for further soft tissue or bone evaluation. The FALCON trial [103] showed that the use of F-18 fluciclovine PET/CT resulted in the change of management in 64% of patients having biochemical recurrence after radical prostatectomy.

Gallium (Ga)-68 prostate-specific membrane antigen (PSMA) provides better detection of recurrences at lower PSA levels than FDA-approved agents and has comparable sensitivity (76–86%) and specificity (86–100%) [104, 105]. A comparative trial of PSMA PET/CT and F-18 fluciclovine PET/CT showed higher detection rates with PSMA in patients with biochemical recurrence [106]. A recent multicenter randomized trial, proPSMA study, investigated the role of PSMA-PET in patients with high-risk prostate cancer before definitive therapy and found PSMA PET/CT is more accurate than conventional imaging for the detection of positive pelvic nodes or distant metastatic disease [107].

Other investigational agents include F-18 fluorodihydrotestesterone (FDHT), which targets androgen receptor. It is ineffective in castration-naïve prostate cancer but has shown promising results in castration-resistant prostate cancer [108, 109]. C-11 acetate is another potential radiotracer that relies on increased levels of fatty acid synthesis. It performs similarly to C-11 choline but may have better specificity [110].

14.3.2.2 Germline Testing in Prostate Cancer

Germline testing is based on family history, histology, and risk groups.The NCCN panel [6] recommends germline genetic testing, with or without pre-test genetic counseling, for patients with prostate cancer and following:

1. A positive family history.
2. High-risk, very high risk, regional, or metastatic prostate cancer, regardless of family history.
3. Ashkenazi Jewish ancestry.
4. Intraductal/cribriform histology (associated with mismatch repair gene mutations and genomic instability).

Germline testing should include- MLH1, MSH2, MSH6, and PMS2 (for Lynch Syndrome) and the homologous recombination genes BRCA2, BRCA1, ATM, PALB2, and CHEK2.

Tumor testing recommendations include [6]:

1. Testing for somatic homologous recombination gene mutations (BRCA1, BRCA2, ATM, PALB2, FANCA, RAD51D, CHEK2, CDK12) is recommended for metastatic disease and can be considered for patients with regional (N1) prostate cancer.
2. Tumor testing for microsatellite instability or mismatch repair genes should be considered for patients with regional or metastatic castration-naïve prostate cancer and is recommended in metastatic castration resistant prostate cancer.
3. Multigene molecular testing can be considered for patients with low, intermediate, and high-risk prostate cancer and life expectancy ≥10 years.

If somatic mutations in BRCA2, BRCA1, ATM, CHEK2, or PALB2 are found, the patient should be referred for genetic counseling. Another type of genomic testing is to utilize the natural variation of single nucleotide polymorphisms (SNP) not based on mutational status. SNP's have been combined into polygenic hazard scores to guide level of risk of prostate cancer [111–114].

14.3.3 Molecular Staging of Prostate Cancer

Personalized or precision medicine is evolving in prostate cancer care. Molecular testing can provide insight into the biological behavior of cancer and aid in clinical decision-making.

One of the molecular assays involved the detection of circulating tumor cells (CTCs). The CTCs often referred to as liquid biopsy, are detected either through centrifugation/immunostaining methods or identification of the genetic material for prostate-specific biomarkers from circulating prostate cancer cells. They have been associated with pathological stage of prostate cancer and considerable investigation is underway to study their potential role in staging for early disease [115].

Several tissue-based molecular assays have been developed to improve prostate cancer risk stratification and help in decision-making for newly diagnosed men with prostate cancer. These assays could supplement current NCCN or EAU risk stratification and improve their prognostic ability. The Prolaris test (Myriad Genetics, Salt Lake City, UT) measures a panel of 31 cell cycle-related genes and 15 housekeeping controls involved in cancer proliferation [116]. The Oncotype Dx Prostate Cancer test (Genomic Health, Redwood City, CA) is a quantitative RT-PCR of 17 genes from five different pathways in prostate cancer [117]. The Decipher test uses the expression of 22 RNA biomarkers in various biological pathways of oncogenesis [118]. The ProMark assay a proteomic-based assay involving multiplex immunofluorescent staining of eight proteins, which correlate with prostate cancer aggressiveness [119]. Several other assays include ki-67 immunohistochemistry and PTEN fluorescence in situ hybridization or immunohistochemistry.

Several of the other assays are under development.

These molecular assays have been developed with extensive industry support, guidance, and involvement. These assays have been marketed under a less rigorous FDA regulatory pathway for biomarkers. Various studies have shown encouraging results [116, 119–123], though, a complete assessment of their clinical utility using prospective randomized clinical trials is lacking. The Molecular Diagnostic Service Program (MolDx) has approved four of these molecular assays-Decipher, Oncotype Dx Prostate, Prolaris, and ProMark. Following are the current recommendations of the NCCN panel [6] for use of these molecular assays:

- For men with low or favorable intermediate-risk cancer and life expectancy ≥10 years, use of Decipher, Oncotype Dx Prostate, Prolaris, or ProMark can be considered during initial risk stratification.
- For men with unfavorable intermediate- and high-risk prostate cancer and life expectancy ≥10 years, use of Decipher or Prolaris can be considered during initial risk stratification.
- Decipher may be considered to inform adjuvant treatment if adverse features are found on radical prostatectomy (pT2 disease with positive margins, any pT3 disease) or with PSA persistence or recurrence.

Conflict of Interest and Funding Dr. Michael A. Liss is supported through the DOD Prostate Cancer Research Program (PCRP) Physician Research Training Award. Opinions, interpretations, conclusions, and recommendations are those of the author and are not necessarily endorsed by the Department of Defense.

Dr. Dharam Kaushik is Stanley and Sandra Rosenberg Endowed Chair in Urologic Research. The funding sources had no role in opinions, interpretations, conclusions, and recommendations in this chapter.

References

1. Wald NJ. The definition of screening. J Med Screen. 2001;8(1):1. https://doi.org/10.1136/jms.8.1.1.
2. Mottet N, van den Bergh RCN, Briers E, et al. EAU-EANM-ESTRO-ESUR-SIOG guidelines on prostate cancer-2020 update. Part 1: screening, diagnosis, and local treatment with curative intent. Eur Urol. 2021;79(2):243–62. https://doi.org/10.1016/j.eururo.2020.09.042.
3. Paquette EL, Sun L, Paquette LR, Connelly R, McLeod DG, Moul JW. Improved prostate cancer-specific survival and other disease parameters: impact of prostate-specific antigen testing. Urology. 2002;60(5):756–9. https://doi.org/10.1016/s0090-4295(02)01960-x.
4. Schröder FH, Hugosson J, Carlsson S, et al. Screening for prostate cancer decreases the risk of developing metastatic disease: findings from the European Randomized Study of Screening for Prostate Cancer (ERSPC). Eur Urol. 2012;62(5):745–52. https://doi.org/10.1016/j.eururo.2012.05.068.
5. Etzioni R, Tsodikov A, Mariotto A, et al. Quantifying the role of PSA screening in the US prostate cancer mortality decline. Cancer Causes Control. 2008;19(2):175–81. https://doi.org/10.1007/s10552-007-9083-8.
6. Schaeffer E, Srinivas S, Antonarakis ES, et al. NCCN guidelines insights: prostate cancer, version 1.2021. J Natl Compr Cancer Netw. 2021;19(2):134–43. https://doi.org/10.6004/jnccn.2021.0008.
7. Schröder FH, Hugosson J, Roobol MJ, et al. Prostate-cancer mortality at 11 years of follow-up. N Engl J Med. 2012;366(11):981–90. https://doi.org/10.1056/NEJMoa1113135.
8. Hugosson J, Roobol MJ, Månsson M, et al. A 16-yr Follow-up of the European randomized study of screening for prostate cancer. Eur Urol. 2019;76(1):43–51. https://doi.org/10.1016/j.eururo.2019.02.009.
9. Andriole GL, Crawford ED, Grubb RL 3rd, et al. Prostate cancer screening in the randomized prostate, lung, colorectal, and ovarian cancer screening trial: mortality results after 13 years of follow-up. J Natl Cancer Inst. 2012;104(2):125–32. https://doi.org/10.1093/jnci/djr500.
10. Hugosson J, Carlsson S, Aus G, et al. Mortality results from the Göteborg randomised population-based prostate-cancer screening trial. Lancet Oncol. 2010;11(8):725–32. https://doi.org/10.1016/s1470-2045(10)70146-7.
11. Arnsrud Godtman R, Holmberg E, Lilja H, Stranne J, Hugosson J. Opportunistic testing versus organized prostate-specific antigen screening: outcome after 18 years in the Göteborg randomized population-based prostate cancer screening trial. Eur Urol. 2015;68(3):354–60. https://doi.org/10.1016/j.eururo.2014.12.006.

12. Martin RM, Donovan JL, Turner EL, et al. Effect of a low-intensity PSA-based screening intervention on prostate cancer mortality: the CAP randomized clinical trial. JAMA. 2018;319(9):883–95. https://doi.org/10.1001/jama.2018.0154.
13. Moyer VA. Screening for prostate cancer: U.S. Preventive Services Task Force recommendation statement. Ann Intern Med. 2012;157(2):120–34. https://doi.org/10.7326/0003-4819-157-2-201207170-00459.
14. Hu JC, Nguyen P, Mao J, et al. Increase in prostate cancer distant metastases at diagnosis in the United States. JAMA Oncol. 2017;3(5):705–7. https://doi.org/10.1001/jamaoncol.2016.5465.
15. Jemal A, Culp MB, Ma J, Islami F, Fedewa SA. Prostate cancer incidence 5 years after US Preventive Services Task Force recommendations against screening. J Natl Cancer Inst. 2021;113(1):64–71. https://doi.org/10.1093/jnci/djaa068.
16. Hayes JH, Barry MJ. Screening for prostate cancer with the prostate-specific antigen test: a review of current evidence. JAMA. 2014;311(11):1143–9. https://doi.org/10.1001/jama.2014.2085.
17. Fenton JJ, Weyrich MS, Durbin S, Liu Y, Bang H, Melnikow J. Prostate-specific antigen-based screening for prostate cancer: evidence report and systematic review for the US Preventive Services Task Force. JAMA. 2018;319(18):1914–31. https://doi.org/10.1001/jama.2018.3712.
18. Grossman DC, Curry SJ, Owens DK, et al. Screening for prostate cancer: US Preventive Services Task Force recommendation statement. JAMA. 2018;319(18):1901–13. https://doi.org/10.1001/jama.2018.3710.
19. Liss MA, Chen H, Hemal S, et al. Impact of family history on prostate cancer mortality in white men undergoing prostate specific antigen based screening. J Urol. 2015;193(1):75–9. https://doi.org/10.1016/j.juro.2014.07.085.
20. Bratt O, Drevin L, Akre O, Garmo H, Stattin P. Family history and probability of prostate cancer, differentiated by risk category: a nationwide population-based study. J Natl Cancer Inst. 2016;108(10):djw110. https://doi.org/10.1093/jnci/djw110.
21. Raheem OA, Cohen SA, Parsons JK, Palazzi KL, Kane CJ. A family history of lethal prostate cancer and risk of aggressive prostate cancer in patients undergoing radical prostatectomy. Sci Rep. 2015;5:10544. https://doi.org/10.1038/srep10544.
22. Pritchard CC, Mateo J, Walsh MF, et al. Inherited DNA-repair gene mutations in men with metastatic prostate cancer. N Engl J Med. 2016;375(5):443–53. https://doi.org/10.1056/NEJMoa1603144.
23. Agalliu I, Gern R, Leanza S, Burk RD. Associations of high-grade prostate cancer with BRCA1 and BRCA2 founder mutations. Clin Cancer Res. 2009;15(3):1112–20. https://doi.org/10.1158/1078-0432.Ccr-08-1822.
24. Mitra A, Fisher C, Foster CS, et al. Prostate cancer in male BRCA1 and BRCA2 mutation carriers has a more aggressive phenotype. Br J Cancer. 2008;98(2):502–7. https://doi.org/10.1038/sj.bjc.6604132.
25. Na R, Zheng SL, Han M, et al. Germline mutations in ATM and BRCA1/2 distinguish risk for lethal and indolent prostate cancer and are associated with early age at death. Eur Urol. 2017;71(5):740–7. https://doi.org/10.1016/j.eururo.2016.11.033.
26. Page EC, Bancroft EK, Brook MN, et al. Interim results from the IMPACT study: evidence for prostate-specific antigen screening in BRCA2 mutation carriers. Eur Urol. 2019;76(6):831–42. https://doi.org/10.1016/j.eururo.2019.08.019.
27. Ryan S, Jenkins MA, Win AK. Risk of prostate cancer in Lynch syndrome: a systematic review and meta-analysis. Cancer Epidemiol Biomark Prev. 2014;23(3):437–49. https://doi.org/10.1158/1055-9965.Epi-13-1165.
28. Odedina FT, Akinremi TO, Chinegwundoh F, et al. Prostate cancer disparities in Black men of African descent: a comparative literature review of prostate cancer burden among Black men in the United States, Caribbean, United Kingdom, and West Africa. Infect Agent Cancer. 2009;4(Suppl 1):S2. https://doi.org/10.1186/1750-9378-4-s1-s2.
29. Tsodikov A, Gulati R, de Carvalho TM, et al. Is prostate cancer different in black men? Answers from 3 natural history models. Cancer. 2017;123(12):2312–9. https://doi.org/10.1002/cncr.30687.
30. Robbins HA, Engels EA, Pfeiffer RM, Shiels MS. Age at cancer diagnosis for blacks compared with whites in the United States. J Natl Cancer Inst. 2015;107(3):dju489. https://doi.org/10.1093/jnci/dju489.
31. Han Y, Rand KA, Hazelett DJ, et al. Prostate cancer susceptibility in men of african ancestry at 8q24. J Natl Cancer Inst. 2016;108(7):djv431. https://doi.org/10.1093/jnci/djv431.
32. Mahal BA, Aizer AA, Ziehr DR, et al. Trends in disparate treatment of African American men with localized prostate cancer across National Comprehensive Cancer Network Risk Groups. Urology. 2014;84(2):386–92. https://doi.org/10.1016/j.urology.2014.05.009.
33. Stamey TA, Yang N, Hay AR, McNeal JE, Freiha FS, Redwine E. Prostate-specific antigen as a serum marker for adenocarcinoma of the prostate. N Engl J Med. 1987;317(15):909–16. https://doi.org/10.1056/nejm198710083171501.
34. Carter HB, Pearson JD, Metter EJ, et al. Longitudinal evaluation of prostate-specific antigen levels in men with and without prostate disease. JAMA. 1992;267(16):2215–20.
35. Vickers AJ, Till C, Tangen CM, Lilja H, Thompson IM. An empirical evaluation of guidelines on prostate-specific antigen velocity in prostate cancer detection. J Natl Cancer Inst. 2011;103(6):462–9. https://doi.org/10.1093/jnci/djr028.

36. Elshafei A, Li YH, Hatem A, et al. The utility of PSA velocity in prediction of prostate cancer and high grade cancer after an initially negative prostate biopsy. Prostate. 2013;73(16):1796–802. https://doi.org/10.1002/pros.22718.
37. Veneziano S, Pavlica P, Querzé R, Nanni G, Lalanne MG, Vecchi F. Correlation between prostate-specific antigen and prostate volume, evaluated by transrectal ultrasonography: usefulness in diagnosis of prostate cancer. Eur Urol. 1990;18(2):112–6. https://doi.org/10.1159/000463885.
38. Lujan M, Paez A, Llanes L, Miravalles E, Berenguer A. Prostate specific antigen density. Is there a role for this parameter when screening for prostate cancer? Prostate Cancer Prostatic Dis. 2001;4(3):146–9. https://doi.org/10.1038/sj.pcan.4500509.
39. Partin AW, Brawer MK, Subong EN, et al. Prospective evaluation of percent free-PSA and complexed-PSA for early detection of prostate cancer. Prostate Cancer Prostatic Dis. 1998;1(4):197–203. https://doi.org/10.1038/sj.pcan.4500232.
40. Gittelman MC, Hertzman B, Bailen J, et al. PCA3 molecular urine test as a predictor of repeat prostate biopsy outcome in men with previous negative biopsies: a prospective multicenter clinical study. J Urol. 2013;190(1):64–9. https://doi.org/10.1016/j.juro.2013.02.018.
41. Wei JT, Feng Z, Partin AW, et al. Can urinary PCA3 supplement PSA in the early detection of prostate cancer? J Clin Oncol. 2014;32(36):4066–72. https://doi.org/10.1200/jco.2013.52.8505.
42. Catalona WJ, Partin AW, Sanda MG, et al. A multicenter study of [−2]pro-prostate specific antigen combined with prostate specific antigen and free prostate specific antigen for prostate cancer detection in the 2.0 to 10.0 ng/mL prostate specific antigen range. J Urol. 2011;185(5):1650–5. https://doi.org/10.1016/j.juro.2010.12.032.
43. Loeb S, Shin SS, Broyles DL, et al. Prostate Health Index improves multivariable risk prediction of aggressive prostate cancer. BJU Int. 2017;120(1):61–8. https://doi.org/10.1111/bju.13676.
44. de la Calle C, Patil D, Wei JT, et al. Multicenter evaluation of the prostate health index to detect aggressive prostate cancer in biopsy naïve men. J Urol. 2015;194(1):65–72. https://doi.org/10.1016/j.juro.2015.01.091.
45. Parekh DJ, Punnen S, Sjoberg DD, et al. A multi-institutional prospective trial in the USA confirms that the 4Kscore accurately identifies men with high-grade prostate cancer. Eur Urol. 2015;68(3):464–70. https://doi.org/10.1016/j.eururo.2014.10.021.
46. Zappala SM, Scardino PT, Okrongly D, Linder V, Dong Y. Clinical performance of the 4K score test to predict high-grade prostate cancer at biopsy: a meta-analysis of us and European clinical validation study results. Rev Urol. 2017;19(3):149–55. https://doi.org/10.3909/riu0776.
47. Stewart GD, Van Neste L, Delvenne P, et al. Clinical utility of an epigenetic assay to detect occult prostate cancer in histopathologically negative biopsies: results of the MATLOC study. J Urol. 2013;189(3):1110–6. https://doi.org/10.1016/j.juro.2012.08.219.
48. McKiernan J, Donovan MJ, O'Neill V, et al. A novel urine exosome gene expression assay to predict high-grade prostate cancer at initial biopsy. JAMA Oncol. 2016;2(7):882–9. https://doi.org/10.1001/jamaoncol.2016.0097.
49. Haese A, Trooskens G, Steyaert S, et al. Multicenter optimization and validation of a 2-gene mRNA urine test for detection of clinically significant prostate cancer before initial prostate biopsy. J Urol. 2019;202(2):256–63. https://doi.org/10.1097/ju.0000000000000293.
50. Hendriks RJ, van der Leest MMG, Dijkstra S, et al. A urinary biomarker-based risk score correlates with multiparametric MRI for prostate cancer detection. Prostate. 2017;77(14):1401–7. https://doi.org/10.1002/pros.23401.
51. Tomlins SA, Day JR, Lonigro RJ, et al. Urine TMPRSS2:ERG plus PCA3 for individualized prostate cancer risk assessment. Eur Urol. 2016;70(1):45–53. https://doi.org/10.1016/j.eururo.2015.04.039.
52. Sanda MG, Feng Z, Howard DH, et al. Association between combined TMPRSS2:ERG and PCA3 RNA urinary testing and detection of aggressive prostate cancer. JAMA Oncol. 2017;3(8):1085–93. https://doi.org/10.1001/jamaoncol.2017.0177.
53. Perner S, Mosquera JM, Demichelis F, et al. TMPRSS2-ERG fusion prostate cancer: an early molecular event associated with invasion. Am J Surg Pathol. 2007;31(6):882–8. https://doi.org/10.1097/01.pas.0000213424.38503.aa.
54. Wang WW, Sorokin I, Aleksic I, et al. Expression of small noncoding RNAs in urinary exosomes classifies prostate cancer into indolent and aggressive disease. J Urol. 2020;204(3):466–75. https://doi.org/10.1097/ju.0000000000001020.
55. Harvey CJ, Pilcher J, Richenberg J, Patel U, Frauscher F. Applications of transrectal ultrasound in prostate cancer. Br J Radiol. 2012;85 Spec No 1(Spec Iss 1):S3–S17. https://doi.org/10.1259/bjr/56357549.
56. Turgut AT, Olçücüoglu E, Koşar P, Geyik PO, Koşar U, Dogra V. Power doppler ultrasonography of the feeding arteries of the prostate gland: a novel approach to the diagnosis of prostate cancer? J Ultrasound Med. 2007;26(7):875–83. https://doi.org/10.7863/jum.2007.26.7.875.
57. Unal D, Sedelaar JP, Aarnink RG, et al. Three-dimensional contrast-enhanced power doppler ultrasonography and conventional examination methods: the value of diagnostic predictors of prostate cancer. BJU Int. 2000;86(1):58–64. https://doi.org/10.1046/j.1464-410x.2000.00719.x.
58. Simmons LA, Autier P, Zát'ura F, et al. Detection, localisation and characterisation of prostate cancer by prostate HistoScanning™.

BJU Int. 2012;110(1):28–35. https://doi.org/10.1111/j.1464-410X.2011.10734.x.
59. Barentsz JO, Richenberg J, Clements R, et al. ESUR prostate MR guidelines 2012. Eur Radiol. 2012;22(4):746–57. https://doi.org/10.1007/s00330-011-2377-y.
60. Padhani AR, Weinreb J, Rosenkrantz AB, Villeirs G, Turkbey B, Barentsz J. Prostate imaging-reporting and data system steering committee: PI-RADS v2 status update and future directions. Eur Urol. 2019;75(3):385–96. https://doi.org/10.1016/j.eururo.2018.05.035.
61. Gleason DF. Classification of prostatic carcinomas. Cancer Chemother Rep. 1966;50(3):125–8.
62. Epstein JI, Egevad L, Amin MB, Delahunt B, Srigley JR, Humphrey PA. The 2014 International Society of Urological Pathology (ISUP) consensus conference on gleason grading of prostatic carcinoma: definition of grading patterns and proposal for a new grading system. Am J Surg Pathol. 2016;40(2):244–52. https://doi.org/10.1097/pas.0000000000000530.
63. Drost FH, Osses DF, Nieboer D, et al. Prostate MRI, with or without MRI-targeted biopsy, and systematic biopsy for detecting prostate cancer. Cochrane Database Syst Rev. 2019;4(4):CD012663. https://doi.org/10.1002/14651858.CD012663.pub2.
64. Ahmed HU, El-Shater Bosaily A, Brown LC, et al. Diagnostic accuracy of multi-parametric MRI and TRUS biopsy in prostate cancer (PROMIS): a paired validating confirmatory study. Lancet. 2017;389(10071):815–22. https://doi.org/10.1016/s0140-6736(16)32401-1.
65. Kasivisvanathan V, Rannikko AS, Borghi M, et al. MRI-targeted or standard biopsy for prostate-cancer diagnosis. N Engl J Med. 2018;378(19):1767–77. https://doi.org/10.1056/NEJMoa1801993.
66. Rouvière O, Puech P, Renard-Penna R, et al. Use of prostate systematic and targeted biopsy on the basis of multiparametric MRI in biopsy-naive patients (MRI-FIRST): a prospective, multicentre, paired diagnostic study. Lancet Oncol. 2019;20(1):100–9. https://doi.org/10.1016/s1470-2045(18)30569-2.
67. van der Leest M, Cornel E, Israël B, et al. Head-to-head comparison of transrectal ultrasound-guided prostate biopsy versus multiparametric prostate resonance imaging with subsequent magnetic resonance-guided biopsy in biopsy-naïve men with elevated prostate-specific antigen: a large prospective multicenter clinical study. Eur Urol. 2019;75(4):570–8. https://doi.org/10.1016/j.eururo.2018.11.023.
68. Ahdoot M, Wilbur AR, Reese SE, et al. MRI-targeted, systematic, and combined biopsy for prostate cancer diagnosis. N Engl J Med. 2020;382(10):917–28. https://doi.org/10.1056/NEJMoa1910038.
69. Klotz L, Chin J, Black PC, et al. Comparison of multiparametric magnetic resonance imaging–targeted biopsy with systematic transrectal ultrasonography biopsy for biopsy-naive men at risk for prostate cancer: a phase 3 randomized clinical trial. JAMA Oncol. 2021;7(4):534–42. https://doi.org/10.1001/jamaoncol.2020.7589.
70. Elwenspoek MMC, Sheppard AL, McInnes MDF, et al. Comparison of multiparametric magnetic resonance imaging and targeted biopsy with systematic biopsy alone for the diagnosis of prostate cancer: a systematic review and meta-analysis. JAMA Netw Open. 2019;2(8):e198427. https://doi.org/10.1001/jamanetworkopen.2019.8427.
71. Presti JC Jr, O'Dowd GJ, Miller MC, Mattu R, Veltri RW. Extended peripheral zone biopsy schemes increase cancer detection rates and minimize variance in prostate specific antigen and age related cancer rates: results of a community multi-practice study. J Urol. 2003;169(1):125–9. https://doi.org/10.1097/01.ju.0000036482.46710.7e.
72. Ukimura O, Coleman JA, de la Taille A, et al. Contemporary role of systematic prostate biopsies: indications, techniques, and implications for patient care. Eur Urol. 2013;63(2):214–30. https://doi.org/10.1016/j.eururo.2012.09.033.
73. Portalez D, Mozer P, Cornud F, et al. Validation of the European Society of Urogenital Radiology scoring system for prostate cancer diagnosis on multiparametric magnetic resonance imaging in a cohort of repeat biopsy patients. Eur Urol. 2012;62(6):986–96. https://doi.org/10.1016/j.eururo.2012.06.044.
74. Sonn GA, Chang E, Natarajan S, et al. Value of targeted prostate biopsy using magnetic resonance-ultrasound fusion in men with prior negative biopsy and elevated prostate-specific antigen. Eur Urol. 2014;65(4):809–15. https://doi.org/10.1016/j.eururo.2013.03.025.
75. Vourganti S, Rastinehad A, Yerram N, et al. Multiparametric magnetic resonance imaging and ultrasound fusion biopsy detect prostate cancer in patients with prior negative transrectal ultrasound biopsies. J Urol. 2012;188(6):2152–7. https://doi.org/10.1016/j.juro.2012.08.025.
76. Abdollah F, Novara G, Briganti A, et al. Transrectal versus trans-perineal saturation rebiopsy of the prostate: is there a difference in cancer detection rate? Urology. 2011;77(4):921–5. https://doi.org/10.1016/j.urology.2010.08.048.
77. Murphy DG, Weerakoon M, Grummet J. Is zero sepsis alone enough to justify transperineal prostate biopsy? BJU Int. 2014;114(1):3–4. https://doi.org/10.1111/bju.12390.
78. Grummet JP, Weerakoon M, Huang S, et al. Sepsis and 'superbugs': should we favour the transperineal over the transrectal approach for prostate biopsy? BJU Int. 2014;114(3):384–8. https://doi.org/10.1111/bju.12536.
79. Merrick GS, Gutman S, Andreini H, et al. Prostate cancer distribution in patients diagnosed by transperineal template-guided saturation biopsy. Eur Urol. 2007;52(3):715–23. https://doi.org/10.1016/j.eururo.2007.02.041.
80. Walz J, Graefen M, Chun FK, et al. High incidence of prostate cancer detected by saturation biopsy

after previous negative biopsy series. Eur Urol. 2006;50(3):498–505. https://doi.org/10.1016/j.eururo.2006.03.026.
81. Jewett HJ. The present status of radical prostatectomy for stages a and B prostatic cancer. Urol Clin North Am. 1975;2(1):105–24.
82. Whitmore WF Jr. Hormone therapy in prostatic cancer. Am J Med. 1956;21(5):697–713. https://doi.org/10.1016/0002-9343(56)90086-9.
83. Amin MB, Greene FL, Edge SB, et al. The eighth edition AJCC cancer staging manual: continuing to build a bridge from a population-based to a more "personalized" approach to cancer staging. CA Cancer J Clin. 2017;67(2):93–9. https://doi.org/10.3322/caac.21388.
84. Ankerst DP, Hoefler J, Bock S, et al. Prostate cancer prevention trial risk calculator 2.0 for the prediction of low- vs. high-grade prostate cancer. Urology. 2014;83(6):1362–7. https://doi.org/10.1016/j.urology.2014.02.035.
85. Ankerst DP, Straubinger J, Selig K, et al. A contemporary prostate biopsy risk calculator based on multiple heterogeneous cohorts. Eur Urol. 2018;74(2):197–203. https://doi.org/10.1016/j.eururo.2018.05.003.
86. D'Amico AV, Whittington R, Malkowicz SB, et al. Biochemical outcome after radical prostatectomy, external beam radiation therapy, or interstitial radiation therapy for clinically localized prostate cancer. JAMA. 1998;280(11):969–74. https://doi.org/10.1001/jama.280.11.969.
87. Makarov DV, Trock BJ, Humphreys EB, et al. Updated nomogram to predict pathologic stage of prostate cancer given prostate-specific antigen level, clinical stage, and biopsy Gleason score (Partin tables) based on cases from 2000 to 2005. Urology. 2007;69(6):1095–101. https://doi.org/10.1016/j.urology.2007.03.042.
88. Tosoian JJ, Chappidi M, Feng Z, et al. Prediction of pathological stage based on clinical stage, serum prostate-specific antigen, and biopsy Gleason score: partin tables in the contemporary era. BJU Int. 2017;119(5):676–83. https://doi.org/10.1111/bju.13573.
89. Kattan MW, Eastham JA, Wheeler TM, et al. Counseling men with prostate cancer: a nomogram for predicting the presence of small, moderately differentiated, confined tumors. J Urol. 2003;170(5):1792–7. https://doi.org/10.1097/01.ju.0000091806.70171.41.
90. Leyh-Bannurah SR, Dell'Oglio P, Tian Z, et al. A proposal of a new nomogram for predicting upstaging in contemporary D'Amico low-risk prostate cancer patients. World J Urol. 2017;35(2):189–97. https://doi.org/10.1007/s00345-016-1863-x.
91. Punnen S, Freedland SJ, Presti JC Jr, et al. Multi-institutional validation of the CAPRA-S score to predict disease recurrence and mortality after radical prostatectomy. Eur Urol. 2014;65(6):1171–7. https://doi.org/10.1016/j.eururo.2013.03.058.
92. Stephenson AJ, Scardino PT, Eastham JA, et al. Preoperative nomogram predicting the 10-year probability of prostate cancer recurrence after radical prostatectomy. J Natl Cancer Inst. 2006;98(10):715–7. https://doi.org/10.1093/jnci/djj190.
93. Graefen M, Haese A, Pichlmeier U, et al. A validated strategy for side specific prediction of organ confined prostate cancer: a tool to select for nerve sparing radical prostatectomy. J Urol. 2001;165(3):857–63.
94. Ohori M, Kattan MW, Koh H, et al. Predicting the presence and side of extracapsular extension: a nomogram for staging prostate cancer. J Urol. 2004;171(5):1844–9.; discussion 49. https://doi.org/10.1097/01.ju.0000121693.05077.3d.
95. Briganti A, Chun FK, Salonia A, et al. A nomogram for staging of exclusive nonobturator lymph node metastases in men with localized prostate cancer. Eur Urol. 2007;51(1):112–9.; discussion 19–20. https://doi.org/10.1016/j.eururo.2006.05.045.
96. Gandaglia G, Fossati N, Zaffuto E, et al. Development and internal validation of a novel model to identify the candidates for extended pelvic lymph node dissection in prostate cancer. Eur Urol. 2017;72(4):632–40. https://doi.org/10.1016/j.eururo.2017.03.049.
97. Potters L, Roach M 3rd, Davis BJ, et al. Postoperative nomogram predicting the 9-year probability of prostate cancer recurrence after permanent prostate brachytherapy using radiation dose as a prognostic variable. Int J Radiat Oncol Biol Phys. 2010;76(4):1061–5. https://doi.org/10.1016/j.ijrobp.2009.03.031.
98. Kattan MW, Potters L, Blasko JC, et al. Pretreatment nomogram for predicting freedom from recurrence after permanent prostate brachytherapy in prostate cancer. Urology. 2001;58(3):393–9. https://doi.org/10.1016/s0090-4295(01)01233-x.
99. Zelefsky MJ, Kattan MW, Fearn P, et al. Pretreatment nomogram predicting ten-year biochemical outcome of three-dimensional conformal radiotherapy and intensity-modulated radiotherapy for prostate cancer. Urology. 2007;70(2):283–7. https://doi.org/10.1016/j.urology.2007.03.060.
100. Kattan MW, Wheeler TM, Scardino PT. Postoperative nomogram for disease recurrence after radical prostatectomy for prostate cancer. J Clin Oncol. 1999;17(5):1499–507. https://doi.org/10.1200/jco.1999.17.5.1499.
101. Fuccio C, Castellucci P, Schiavina R, et al. Role of 11C-choline PET/CT in the re-staging of prostate cancer patients with biochemical relapse and negative results at bone scintigraphy. Eur J Radiol. 2012;81(8):e893–6. https://doi.org/10.1016/j.ejrad.2012.04.027.
102. Nanni C, Schiavina R, Brunocilla E, et al. 18F-fluciclovine PET/CT for the detection of prostate cancer relapse: a comparison to 11C-Choline PET/CT. Clin Nucl Med. 2015;40(8):e386–91. https://doi.org/10.1097/rlu.0000000000000849.

103. Scarsbrook AF, Bottomley D, Teoh EJ, et al. Effect of (18)F-fluciclovine positron emission tomography on the management of patients with recurrence of prostate cancer: results from the FALCON trial. Int J Radiat Oncol Biol Phys. 2020;107(2):316–24. https://doi.org/10.1016/j.ijrobp.2020.01.050.
104. Afshar-Oromieh A, Avtzi E, Giesel FL, et al. The diagnostic value of PET/CT imaging with the (68) Ga-labelled PSMA ligand HBED-CC in the diagnosis of recurrent prostate cancer. Eur J Nucl Med Mol Imaging. 2015;42(2):197–209. https://doi.org/10.1007/s00259-014-2949-6.
105. Perera M, Papa N, Christidis D, et al. Sensitivity, specificity, and predictors of positive (68) Ga-prostate-specific membrane antigen positron emission tomography in advanced prostate cancer: a systematic review and meta-analysis. Eur Urol. 2016;70(6):926–37. https://doi.org/10.1016/j.eururo.2016.06.021.
106. Calais J, Ceci F, Eiber M, et al. (18)F-fluciclovine PET-CT and (68)Ga-PSMA-11 PET-CT in patients with early biochemical recurrence after prostatectomy: a prospective, single-centre, single-arm, comparative imaging trial. Lancet Oncol. 2019;20(9):1286–94. https://doi.org/10.1016/s1470-2045(19)30415-2.
107. Hofman MS, Lawrentschuk N, Francis RJ, et al. Prostate-specific membrane antigen PET-CT in patients with high-risk prostate cancer before curative-intent surgery or radiotherapy (proPSMA): a prospective, randomised, multicentre study. Lancet. 2020;395(10231):1208–16. https://doi.org/10.1016/s0140-6736(20)30314-7.
108. Dehdashti F, Picus J, Michalski JM, et al. Positron tomographic assessment of androgen receptors in prostatic carcinoma. Eur J Nucl Med Mol Imaging. 2005;32(3):344–50. https://doi.org/10.1007/s00259-005-1764-5.
109. Larson SM, Morris M, Gunther I, et al. Tumor localization of 16beta-18F-fluoro-5alpha-dihydrotestosterone versus 18F-FDG in patients with progressive, metastatic prostate cancer. J Nucl Med. 2004;45(3):366–73.
110. Mohsen B, Giorgio T, Rasoul ZS, et al. Application of C-11-acetate positron-emission tomography (PET) imaging in prostate cancer: systematic review and meta-analysis of the literature. BJU Int. 2013;112(8):1062–72. https://doi.org/10.1111/bju.12279.
111. Kader AK, Liss MA, Trottier G, et al. Impact of prostate-specific antigen on a baseline prostate cancer risk assessment including genetic risk. Urology. 2015;85(1):165–70. https://doi.org/10.1016/j.urology.2014.07.081.
112. Liss MA, Xu J, Chen H, Kader AK. Prostate genetic score (PGS-33) is independently associated with risk of prostate cancer in the PLCO trial. Prostate. 2015;75(12):1322–8. https://doi.org/10.1002/pros.23012.
113. Huynh-Le MP, Fan CC, Karunamuni R, et al. Polygenic hazard score is associated with prostate cancer in multi-ethnic populations. Nat Commun. 2021;12(1):1236. https://doi.org/10.1038/s41467-021-21287-0.
114. Seibert TM, Fan CC, Wang Y, et al. Polygenic hazard score to guide screening for aggressive prostate cancer: development and validation in large scale cohorts. BMJ. 2018;360:j5757. https://doi.org/10.1136/bmj.j5757.
115. Galletti G, Portella L, Tagawa ST, Kirby BJ, Giannakakou P, Nanus DM. Circulating tumor cells in prostate cancer diagnosis and monitoring: an appraisal of clinical potential. Mol Diagn Ther. 2014;18(4):389–402. https://doi.org/10.1007/s40291-014-0101-8.
116. Cooperberg MR, Simko JP, Cowan JE, et al. Validation of a cell-cycle progression gene panel to improve risk stratification in a contemporary prostatectomy cohort. J Clin Oncol. 2013;31(11):1428–34. https://doi.org/10.1200/jco.2012.46.4396.
117. Knezevic D, Goddard AD, Natraj N, et al. Analytical validation of the oncotype DX prostate cancer assay—a clinical RT-PCR assay optimized for prostate needle biopsies. BMC Genomics. 2013;14:690. https://doi.org/10.1186/1471-2164-14-690.
118. Klein EA, Yousefi K, Haddad Z, et al. A genomic classifier improves prediction of metastatic disease within 5 years after surgery in node-negative high-risk prostate cancer patients managed by radical prostatectomy without adjuvant therapy. Eur Urol. 2015;67(4):778–86. https://doi.org/10.1016/j.eururo.2014.10.036.
119. Blume-Jensen P, Berman DM, Rimm DL, et al. Development and clinical validation of an in situ biopsy-based multimarker assay for risk stratification in prostate cancer. Clin Cancer Res. 2015;21(11):2591–600. https://doi.org/10.1158/1078-0432.Ccr-14-2603.
120. Hu JC, Tosoian JJ, Qi J, et al. Clinical utility of gene expression classifiers in men with newly diagnosed prostate cancer. JCO Precis Oncol. 2018;2:1–15. https://doi.org/10.1200/PO.18.00163.
121. Marascio J, Spratt DE, Zhang J, et al. Prospective study to define the clinical utility and benefit of decipher testing in men following prostatectomy. prostate Cancer Prostatic Dis. 2020;23(2):295–302. https://doi.org/10.1038/s41391-019-0185-7.
122. Cullen J, Rosner IL, Brand TC, et al. A biopsy-based 17-gene genomic prostate score predicts recurrence after radical prostatectomy and adverse surgical pathology in a racially diverse population of men with clinically low- and intermediate-risk prostate cancer. Eur Urol. 2015;68(1):123–31. https://doi.org/10.1016/j.eururo.2014.11.030.
123. Cuzick J, Stone S, Fisher G, et al. Validation of an RNA cell cycle progression score for predicting death from prostate cancer in a conservatively managed needle biopsy cohort. Br J Cancer. 2015;113(3):382–9. https://doi.org/10.1038/bjc.2015.223.

15 Pathology and Staging

Moushumi Suryavanshi and Garima Durga

Prostate cancer is the most common non-cutaneous malignancy worldwide. Recently in 2022, the World Health Organization (WHO) updated the histopathological classification of urinary and male genital tumours including prostate cancer (Table 15.1) in the fifth edition of their *Blue Book, wherein* they have revised the diagnostic terminology, epidemiology, pathogenesis, histopathology and diagnostic molecular pathology of genitourinary cancers.

Table 15.1 : WHO classification of prostate carcinoma (2022)

Acinar adenocarcinoma
Atrophic acinar adenocarcinoma
Pseudohyperplastic acinar adenocarcinoma
Microcystic acinar adenocarcinoma
Foamy gland acinar adenocarcinoma
Mucinous (colloid) acinar adenocarcinoma
Signet ring cell-like acinar adenocarcinoma
Pleomorphic giant cell acinar adenocarcinoma
Sarcomatoid acinar adenocarcinoma
Prostatic intraepithelial neoplasia-like carcinoma
Prostatic intraepithelial neoplasia
Intraductal carcinoma
Ductal adenocarcinoma
Urothelial carcinoma
Squamous neoplasms
Adenoid cystic (basal cell) carcinoma
Neuroendocrine tumours

M. Suryavanshi (✉)
Department of Molecular Biology, Amrita Medical Institute & Research Centre, Faridabad, India

G. Durga
Department of Molecular Biology, Amrita Medical Institute & Research Centre, Faridabad, India

Department of Lab services, Rajiv Gandhi Cancer Institute & Research Centre, Delhi, India

P. Singh et al. (eds.), *A Guide to Management of Urological Cancers*,
https://doi.org/10.1007/978-981-99-2341-0_15

15.1 Acinar Adenocarcinoma

It is an invasive epithelial malignancy of prostatic secretory cells. According to GLOBOCAN 2020 data, it is the second most common malignancy amongst males accounting for 1.4 million cases worldwide. Its highest incidence is in Europe (33.5%) and lowest incidence is in Asia (26.2%). There were an estimated 34,540 new cases of prostate cancer in India in 2020. Worldwide, prostate cancer is the fifth most common cause of death due to malignancy in men, with an estimated 375,304 deaths in 2020 [1]. Approximately, 75% of prostate cancer cases occur in males >65 years; incidence increases with age [2].

15.1.1 Aetiology

Risk factors [3] include the following:

1. Advancing age.
2. Lifestyle and food habits: heavy intake of red meat, animal fats, milk and dairy products.
3. Obesity.
4. Tobacco smoking: higher mortality.
5. Family history: positive family history leads to 1.5- to 2.5-fold increase in risk of prostate cancer.
6. Race: higher mortality rates in men of African-Caribbean and Middle and Southern African descent as compared to men in Eastern and South-central Asia.
7. Genetics: common molecular alterations include gene fusions involving ETS transcription factors, MYC overexpression, shortening of telomeres, inactivation of GSTP1, PTEN loss, TP53 inactivation and mutations in FLI1, SPOP, FOXA1, AR, IDH1 and DNA repair genes.

15.1.2 Localization

Majority of cancers (75–80%) are located in the peripheral zone and about 15–25% arise in the transition zone. The central zone is usually secondarily involved by cancers arising in other zones [3]. Most prostatic adenocarcinomas (85–90%) are multifocal, with an average of two to three separate tumours per gland [4].

15.1.3 Clinical Features

1. An elevated serum prostate-specific antigen (PSA) levels
2. An abnormal digital rectal examination
3. Urinary symptoms like frequency, retention and dysuria
4. Impotence, priapism and uraemia due to locally advanced disease
5. Bone pain/fractures, lower limb oedema and neurological symptoms due to metastatic disease (incidentally detected in the workup of unknown primary)
6. Anaemia and disseminated intravascular coagulation due to paraneoplastic syndromes

15.1.4 Imaging Features

1. *Transrectal ultrasound (TRUS)* of the prostate is the modality of choice for diagnosis in a clinically suspected case of prostate cancer, wherein systematic TRUS-guided needle core biopsy (NCB) has significantly improved the diagnostic rates [5]. Newer modalities in TRUS include three-dimensional ultrasound and contrast-enhanced ultrasound.
2. *Magnetic resonance imaging (MRI)* is a good modality to determine precise localization, size and extent of tumour. MRI-guided biopsy is conducted in suspected cases of prostate cancer with previous negative TRUS-guided NCB. Targeted fusion biopsy using pre-biopsy MRI with real-time TRUS significantly improves yield from suspicious lesions.

15.1.5 Tissue Sampling

1. Needle core biopsy (NCB):

   At least 12 systematic 18-gauge TRUS-guided core biopsies along with targeted cores from suspicious areas are obtained. Additional cores are taken from areas highlighted by MRI-USG fusion, if clinical suspicion of malignancy persists despite negative biopsy results. Single-core, site-specific, labelled submission is recommended for histopathological evaluation. Submission of more than two cores in a single container is associated with fragmentation.

All the containers are processed and reported individually.

2. Transurethral resection (TUR):

   Infrequently performed for benign prostatic hyperplasia (BPH). Tissue is submitted in entirety if specimen weighs <12 g. In specimens weighing >12 g, one additional cassette every 5 g of tissue is recommended. In case, an incidental small volume (<5%) carcinoma is detected, then entire remaining tissue should be evaluated. In our practice, we have opted to submit the entire tissue.

3. Radical prostatectomy (RP):

   Performed as an open, laparoscopic or robotic assisted procedure.

   The specimen is immersed adequately in 10% buffered neutral formalin. Thereafter, it is weighed, measured, inked, sliced and kept for fixation in formalin (at least 24 h). After optimum fixation, the prostate gland is grossed and representative sections are taken.

   Appropriate handling and systematic examination of a RP specimen is essential for the identification of histopathological tumour parameters such as grade, volume, stage, margins and extraprostatic extension (EPE) for optimizing patient treatment.

15.1.6 Gross Pathology

These tumours may or may not be apparent on gross examination. The ones which are recognizable are poorly delineated with firm, greyish yellow cut surface. The presence of largest nodule should be documented with location and size.

15.1.6.1 Microscopic Pathology

The histological diagnosis is based on a bunch of findings including architectural, nuclear, cytoplasmic and luminal features (Figs. 15.1 and 15.2; Table 15.2).

1. Architectural features:
   – Well-differentiated tumours comprise of loose or compact groups of well-formed glands with loss of basal cells around them.
   – Poorly differentiated tumours display ill-formed/fused glands, cribriform pattern, solid sheets or singly lying cells.
   – Neoplastic glands can be seen infiltrating in between benign glands. They have smaller calibre and sharp luminal borders as compared to benign glands.

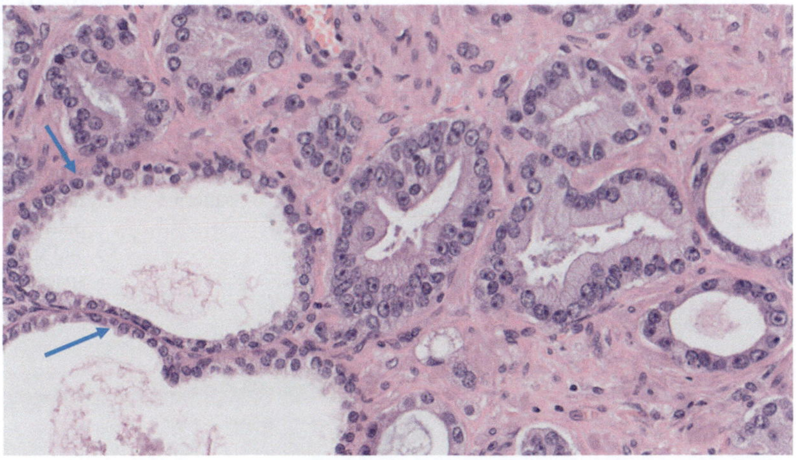

Fig. 15.1 Well-formed, discrete neoplastic glands lined by cells displaying nucleomegaly and prominent nucleoli. Benign glands are marked by arrow

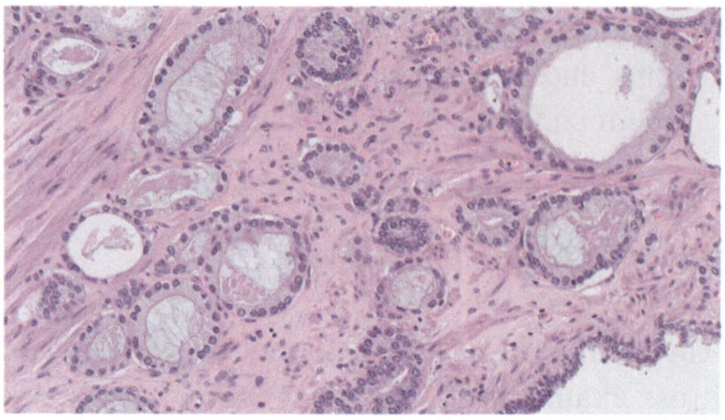

Fig. 15.2 Neoplastic glands show Wispy, blue-tinged mucin and granular eosinophilic material in the lumen

Table 15.2 Histopathological features pathognomonic of malignancy

Feature	Description
Mucinous fibroplasia (collagenous micronodules)	Hyalinized eosinophilic material often seen with intraluminal wispy blue mucin
Glomerulations	Cribriform cellular luminal proliferation adherent to one of the edges creating a crescentic space, resembling a renal glomerulus
Perineural/ intraneural invasion	Malignant glands around or within a nerve
Extraprostatic extension (EPE)	Growth of malignant glands in the extraprostatic fat

2. Nuclear features:
   - Enlarged, hyperchromatic nuclei with little or no pleomorphism
   - Prominent nucleoli
   - Mitoses and apoptosis rarely seen
3. Cytoplasmic features:
   - Cuboidal/columnar cells with amphophilic cytoplasm
4. Luminal features:
   - Wispy, blue-tinged intraluminal mucin
   - Granular eosinophilic luminal material
   - Crystalloids which are eosinophilic, rhomboid crystals with sharp edges
   - Comedonecrosis
   - Lack of corpora amylacea

Prostate Cancer Grading

Modified Gleason grading is recommended which utilizes the architecture of neoplastic cells. It is defined as the sum of the primary (most predominant in terms of surface area of involvement) grade and the secondary (second most predominant) grade and reported as the *Gleason score (GS)*. So the Gleason grade ranges from 1 (most well differentiated) to 5 (most poorly differentiated) and GS ranges from 2 to 10 (Table 15.3). If a tumour has only one histological pattern, then the primary and secondary patterns are assigned with the same number. GS should be assigned to the dominant nodule(s), if present.

In NCB, where more than two patterns are present and the worst grade is neither the primary nor the secondary grade, the predominant and

Table 15.3 Description of Gleason patterns

Gleason pattern 1	• Circumscribed nodule of closely packed, uniform, well-formed glands
	• Controversial and disregarded in current guidelines
Gleason pattern 2	• Nodule of loosely packed glands with minimal peripheral infiltration
	• Disregarded in current guidelines and grouped with Gleason pattern 3 according to 2014 International Society of Urological Pathology (ISUP) grading system under grade group 1
Gleason pattern 3	• Most common pattern; well-formed variably sized glands which infiltrate between benign ducts and acini (Fig. 15.3a, b)
Gleason pattern 4	• Poorly formed/fused glands, glomeruloid glands, cribriform structure and hypernephroid pattern (solid sheets of cells with clear cytoplasm) (Fig. 15.4)
Gleason pattern 5	• Solid sheets, cords or singly lying tumour cells, signet ring cells, any pattern with central comedonecrosis and solid nests with rosette-like spaces (Fig. 15.5a, b)

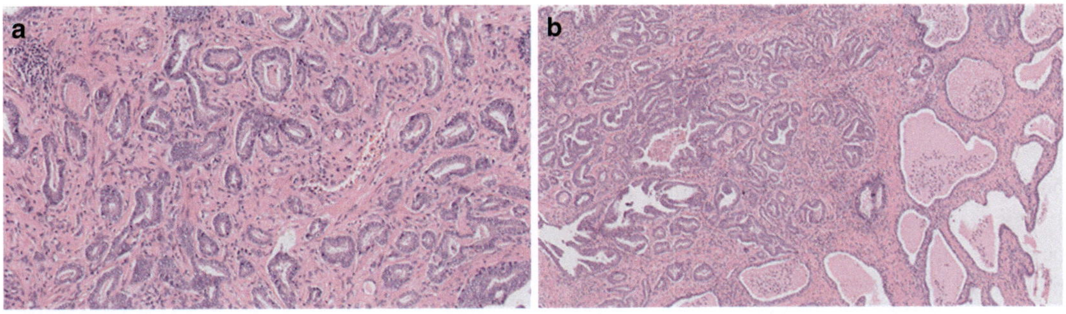

Fig. 15.3 (**a**) Acinar adenocarcinoma prostate showing well-formed and discrete glands corresponding to Gleason pattern 3. (**b**) Histomorphology showing well-formed and discrete neoplastic glands corresponding to Gleason pattern 3, adjacent to benign prostatic glands (on the right side)

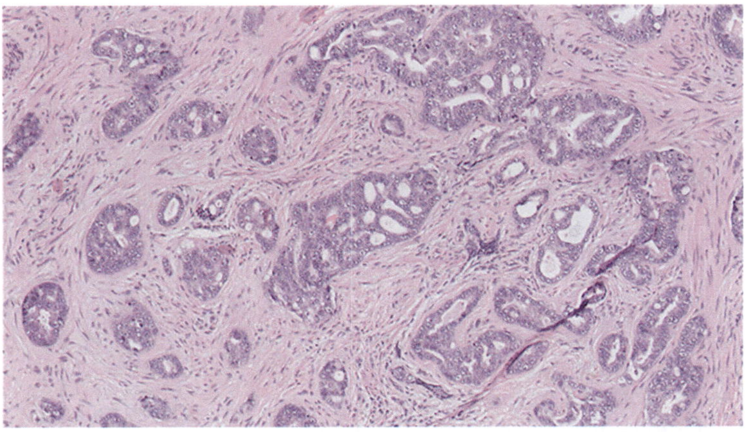

Fig. 15.4 Fused and cribriform glands in acinar adenocarcinoma corresponding to Gleason pattern 4

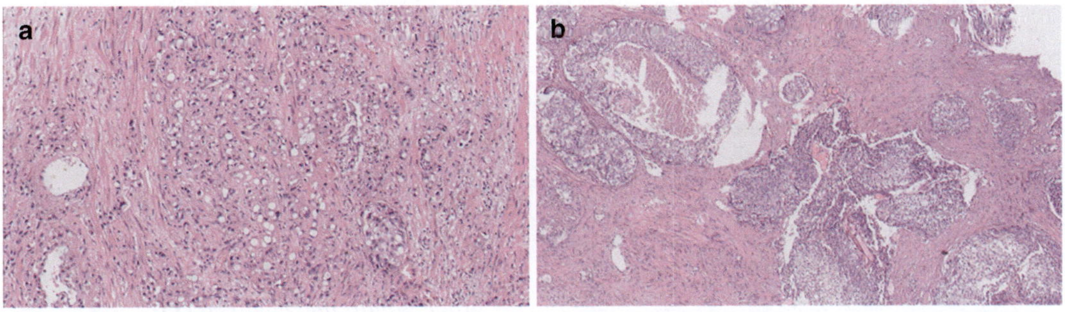

Fig. 15.5 (**a**) Neoplastic cells arranged in cords, nests, single cells and signet ring cells corresponding to Gleason pattern 5. (**b**) Tumour cells in solid nests and showing comedonecrosis (top-left corner), corresponding to Gleason pattern 5

highest grades are reported to arrive at a score. For example, 70% pattern 3, 25% pattern 4 and <5% pattern 5 is reported as GS 3 + 5 = 8. In NCB, percentage of pattern 4 should be reported in all GS 7 cases so as to stratify it further and choose patients who are eligible for active surveillance. Gleason grading is not done for cores showing tumour as micro focus or perineural invasion only.

The Tertiary Gleason pattern is defined as the third most common pattern in RP specimens. If it is Gleason pattern 5 and <5%, it should be reported as minor tertiary Gleason pattern 5. If it is ≥5%, it should be reported as the secondary pattern, rather than as the minor tertiary pattern.

It is recommended that the Gleason grading be performed using the ×4 and ×10 objective. It can be verified using the ×20 objective.

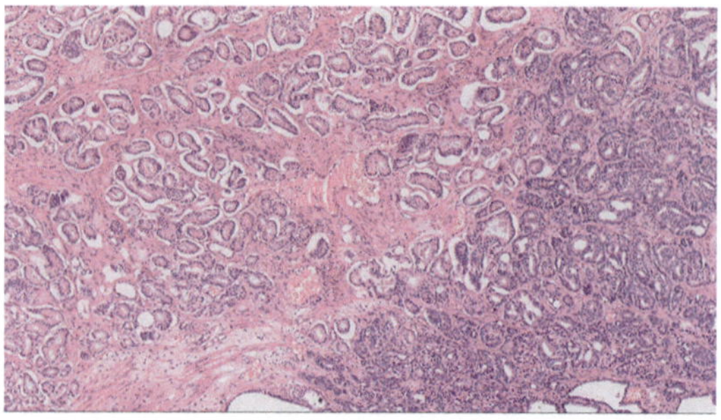

Fig. 15.6 Acinar adenocarcinoma with Gleason pattern 3 + 4. Note the well-formed and discrete glands (pattern 3) on the right and fused glands (pattern 4) on the left side

Grade Groups

Grade groups were Introduced in 2014 ISUP (International Society of Urological Pathology) conference to overcome the limitations of Gleason system.

These grade groups have been defined after a meta-analysis of 20,000 RP specimens such that each group is associated with a unique prognosis [6] (Table 15.4).

Merits of grade group system:

1. More accurate risk stratification. Gleason 3 + 4 = 7 and 4 + 3 = 7 form grade groups 2 and 3, reflective of their true prognostic differences.
2. More simplified categorization of 5 groups as opposed to 12 grades.
3. A more intuitive scale, starting at 1 as opposed to 6.

Current recommendation: to report both grade groups and modified GS

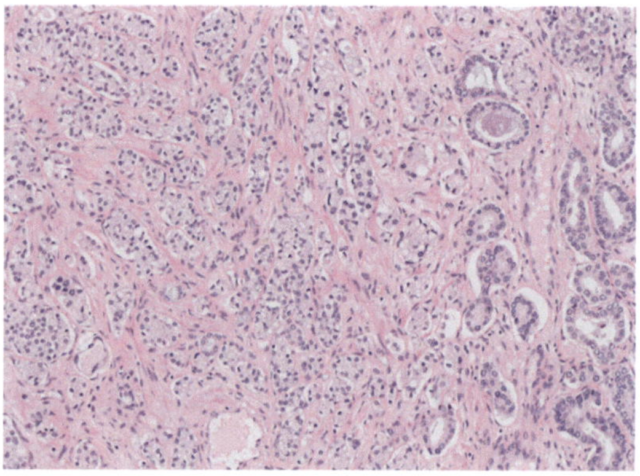

Fig. 15.7 Acinar adenocarcinoma with Gleason pattern 4 + 3. Note the well-formed and discrete neoplastic glands (pattern 3) on the left and fused glands (pattern 4) on the right side

Table 15.4 ISUP grade group system

ISUP grade	Definition	Gleason score
1	Only individual discrete well-formed glands	3 + 3 = 6
2	Predominantly well-formed glands with lesser component of poorly formed/fused/cribriform glands	3 + 4 = 7 (Fig. 15.6)
3	Predominantly poorly formed/fused/cribriform glands with lesser	4 + 3 = 7 (Fig. 15.7)
	Component of well-formed glands	
4	Only poorly formed/fused/cribriform glands or	4 + 4 = 8
	Predominantly well-formed glands and lesser component lacking glands	3 + 5 = 8
	Predominantly lacking glands and lesser component of well-formed glands	5 + 3 = 8
5	Lacks gland formation (or with necrosis) ± poorly formed/fused/cribriform glands	4 + 5 = 9
		5 + 4 = 9
		5 + 5 = 10

Immunohistochemistry (IHC) Studies

1. Basal cell markers: P63/P40 and CK34betaE12 display loss of basal cells around neoplastic glands (Fig. 15.8a, b).
2. AMACR: expressed in 80–100% of carcinomas (Fig. 15.8a, b)

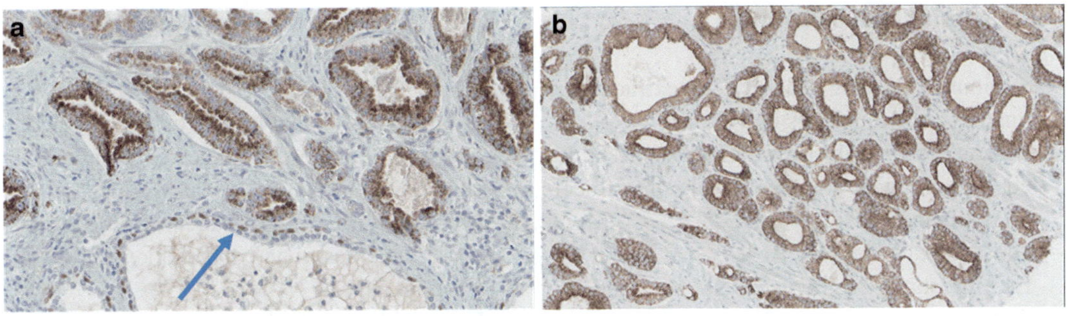

Fig. 15.8 (**a**) IHC shows absence of basal myoepithelial cell layer with negative p63, and positive AMACR in the neoplastic glands in contrast to the benign gland (arrow) which displays negative AMACR expression and p63 positive basal layer. (**b**) IHC performed with p63 + AMACR cocktail in acinar adenocarcinoma shows granular cytoplasmic AMACR expression and negative p63 highlighting loss of basal cells

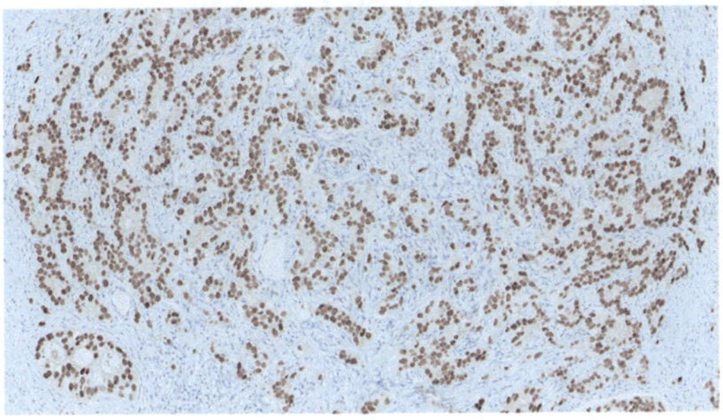

Fig. 15.9 NKX3.1 immunostain stains the prostatic carcinoma glands at the metastatic site

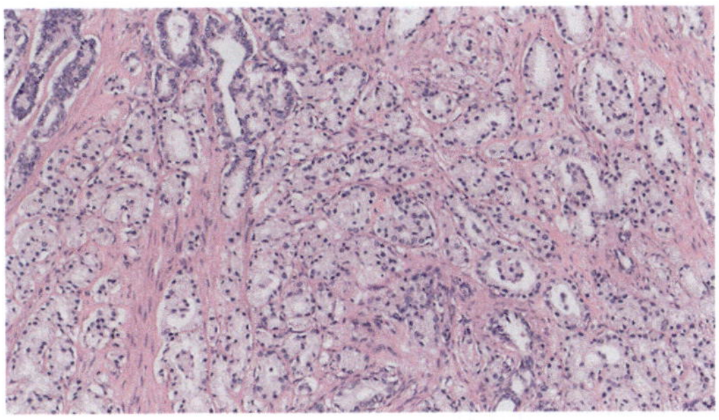

Fig. 15.10 Foamy gland carcinoma characterized by abundant xanthomatous cytoplasm. Note the presence of conventional acinar adenocarcinoma, at the top-left corner, within the same tumour

3. ERG-1: specific marker for neoplastic prostatic glands.
4. PTEN: prognostic and predictive biomarker; PTEN loss is associated with aggressive disease and poor response to androgen therapy.
5. NkX3.1: sensitive and specific marker for prostatic glands (Fig. 15.9).
6. Urothelial and colorectal markers: to rule out secondary involvement of the prostate.

15.2 Histological Patterns: No Prognostic Significance

15.2.1 Atrophic

- Flat atrophic glands with malignant nuclear features and infiltrative architecture
- Commonly seen as an after effect of hormone/radiation treatment
- Gleason pattern 3

15.2.2 Pseudohyperplastic

- Larger benign-appearing dilated branching glands with papillary in foldings lined by tall columnar cells with malignant nuclear features
- Gleason pattern 3

15.2.3 Microcystic

- Intermediate sized cystically dilated glands lined by flat cells
- Gleason pattern 3

15.2.4 Foamy Gland (Fig. 15.10)

- Glands/cribriform pattern/nests composed of cells with abundant foamy/xanthomatous cytoplasm
- Gleason pattern 3/pattern 4

15.2.5 Mucinous (Colloid)

- Tumour displaying at least 25% extracellular mucin pools (diagnosis on RP only).
- Discrete/fused/cribriform glands, nests or cords floating in abundant pools of extracellular mucin.
- Gleason pattern 3/pattern 4.
- Extraprostatic origin needs to be ruled out first.

15.3 Histological Subtypes: Prognostically Significant

15.3.1 Signet Ring-Like Cell (Plasmacytoid)

- Tumour displaying at least 25% signet ring-like cells (diagnosis possible on RP only) lying singly as well as in cords and sheets.
- Gleason pattern 4/pattern 5.
- Secondary involvement needs to be excluded.
- Poor prognosis.

15.3.2 Pleomorphic Giant Cell

- Tumour displaying markedly pleomorphic giant cells with anaplastic nuclei
- History of prior radiation and/or hormone therapy
- Poor prognosis

15.3.3 Sarcomatoid

- Biphasic tumour displaying varying admixture of malignant epithelial and mesenchymal components
- History of acinar adenocarcinoma treated with radiation and/or hormone therapy
- Poor prognosis

15.3.4 Prostatic Intraepithelial Neoplasia-Like

- Large glands displaying flat or tufted architecture and lined pseudostratified columnar or cuboidal epithelium
- Mimics HGPIN (high-grade prostatic intraepithelial neoplasia) and ductal adenocarcinoma
- Gleason pattern 3
- Favourable prognosis

15.4 Treatment Effects (Fig. 15.11)

15.4.1 To Radiation Therapy

- Atrophy/atypia of benign glands.
- Hyalinized, paucicellular stroma.
- Tumour cells arranged as poorly formed glands/singly with foamy, vacuolated cytoplasm, small pyknotic nuclei and inconspicuous nucleoli.
- Tumours with absent/minimal radiation effect associated with higher chance of recurrence.
- IHC with immunostains like CK, AMACR, p63 and ERG1 may be helpful.

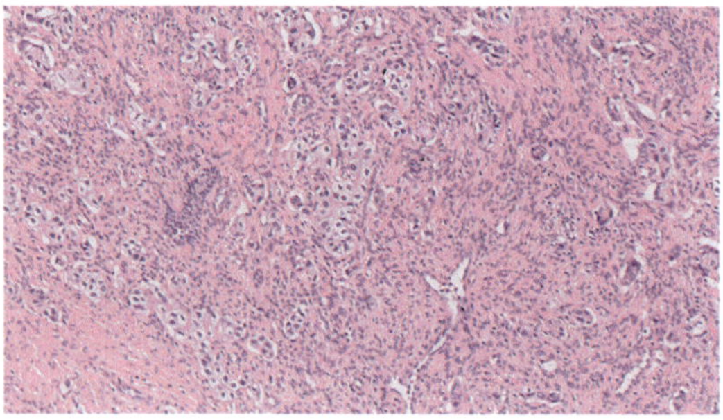

Fig. 15.11 Therapy effect seen as poorly formed glands with foamy, vacuolated cytoplasm, small pyknotic nuclei and inconspicuous nucleoli

15.4.2 To Hormonal Therapy

- Similar to effects of radiation treatment.
- In addition, squamous/urothelial metaplasia of benign glands may be seen.

Current guidelines: Report presence/absence of therapy effect. If present, comment on severity. Gleason grading is not applicable in presence of these changes.

15.5 Key Elements in Reports of Prostate Cancer

1. **Gleason grade, Gleason score and ISUP grade group:**
   - To be reported in NCB, TURP and RP.
   - In NCB, predict grade and stage in RP sample, tumour progression form a criterion for choosing active surveillance.
   - In TURP, it is a predictor of disease-specific survival.
   - *Current guidelines: report both GS and corresponding grade group.*
2. **Tumour quantity:**
   - To be reported in NCB, TURP and RP.
   - In NCB, shows correlation with RP stage, tumour volume, margin status, neurovascular bundle involvement and post treatment progression.
   - In TURP, it is essential to report as it is a required criterion for pTNM staging (T1).
   - In RP, show correlation with disease progression.
   - *Current guidelines: In NCB, report number of positive cores, proportion (percentage) and/or linear extent of tumour in millimetres. In TURP, report number of involved chips and ratio or percentage of involved to total chips. In RP, report percentage of tumour involvement by visual inspection.*
3. **Cribriform pattern:**
   - Defined as a proliferation with multiple punched-out lumina, without intervening stroma.
   - Associated with poorer outcome in GS 7 tumours.
   - *Current guidelines: report on the presence/absence of cribriform architecture in GS score 7 tumours.*
4. **Extraprostatic extension (EPE) (Fig. 15.12):**
   - Reported in ~36% of RP specimens, is an indicator of poor outcome.
   - If seen, it should be reported in CNB and TURP samples as well.
   - *Current guidelines: report location as well as extent (focal vs. non-focal) and status of margin at site of EPE.*
5. **Margin status (Fig. 15.13):**
   - Involvement of margin defined as tumour cells at the inked margin.
   - Classified as limited/non-limited.
   - Reported in 16–41% of RP; a predictor of biochemical recurrence.
   - *Current guidelines: report presence/absence, location and extent of positive margin in millimetres.*

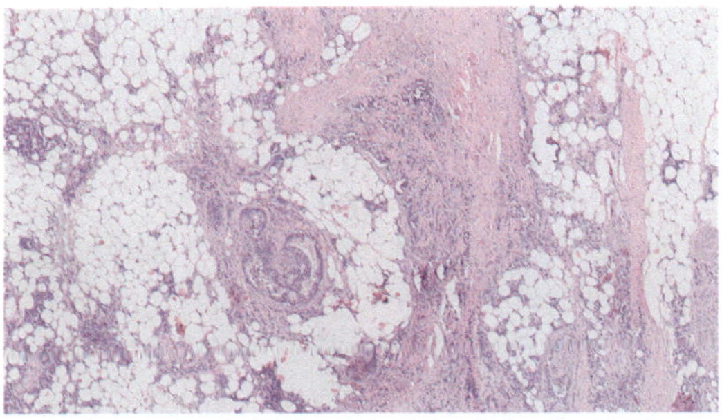

Fig. 15.12 EPE seen as presence of neoplastic cells into periprostatic adipose tissue

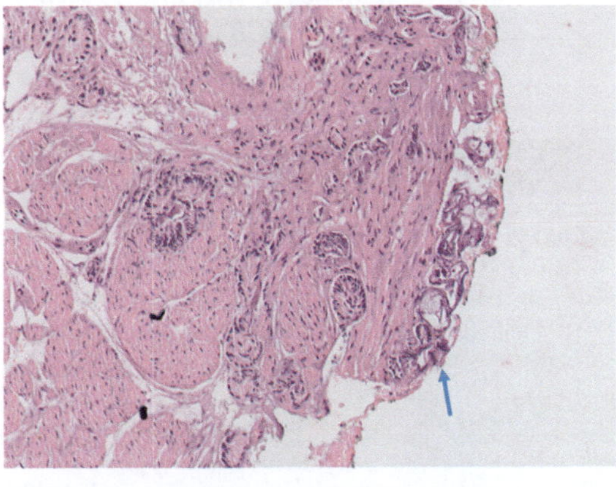

Fig. 15.13 Peripheral inked resected margin in RP specimen involved by neoplastic glands (marked by arrow)

6. **Perineural invasion (PNI) (Fig. 15.14):**
   - Defined as presence of prostate cancer along, around or within the nerve.
   - The presence of PNI in NCB is correlated with EPE on RP and with recurrence after radiation therapy.
   - *Current guidelines: report presence/absence of PNI.*
7. **Lymphovascular invasion (LVI):**
   - Defined as invasion of lymphatics/blood vessels by cancer cells.
   - Reported in up to 21.5% of RP specimens.
   - Associated with biochemical recurrence, disease progression and metastasis.
   - *Current guidelines: report presence/absence of LVI in RP.*
8. **Seminal vesicle (SV) invasion (Fig. 15.15):**
   - Defined as invasion of muscular wall of SV by cancer cells.
   - Associated with adverse prognosis.
   - *Current guidelines: report presence/absence of SV invasion (extraprostatic). If seen, it should be reported in NCB as well.*
9. **High-grade prostatic intraepithelial neoplasia (HGPIN) and atypical small acinar proliferation (ASAP):**
   - Correlates with presence of subsequent cancer in RP.
   - Optional to report in presence of invasive cancer.
10. **Intraductal carcinoma (IDC):**
    - Associated with higher GS, stage and lower progression-free survival.
    - *Current guidelines: Report presence/absence of IDC in NCB and RP.*
    - *Do not grade IDC without invasive cancer. Incorporate the grade of IDC into the GS when invasive cancer is present.*
11. **Treatment effect to prior hormonal or radiation therapy:**
    - Tumours with absent/minimal radiation effect associated with higher chance of recurrence.
    - Gleason grade assigned in prostate cancers lacking treatment effects.
    - *Current guidelines: Report presence/absence of therapy effect. If present, comment on severity. Gleason grading is not applicable in presence of these changes.*
12. **Nodal metastasis (Fig. 15.16):**
    - Presence/absence of tumour in the submitted nodes needs to be documented to determine the nodal stage.
    - Laterality does not affect the N stage.
    - Involvement of distant lymph nodes is classified as M1a.

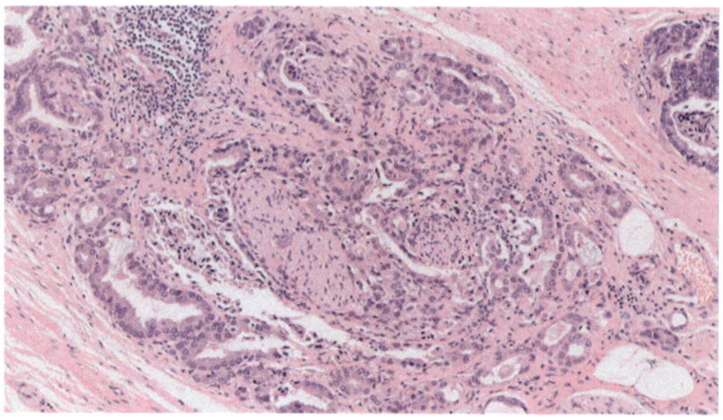

Fig. 15.14 PNI in a case of acinar adenocarcinoma

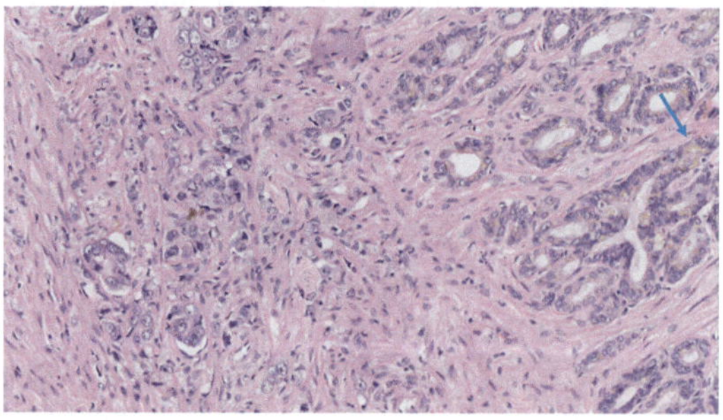

Fig. 15.15 Neoplastic cells invading into the SV. Note the golden yellow-brown lipofuscin pigment (arrow) in the cytoplasm of SV

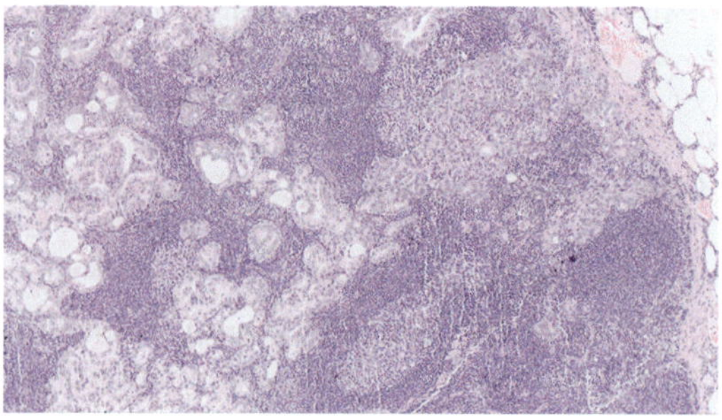

Fig. 15.16 Pelvic lymphnodal metastasis in a case of acinar adenocarcinoma of the prostate

13. **Pathological stage:**
    - Most important prognostic factor for recurrence and mortality.

Pathologic stage
1 pT category
pT1: There is no pathologic T1 classification
pT2: Organ confined
pT3: Extraprostatic extension
pT3a: Extraprostatic extension or microscopic invasion of the bladder neck
pT3b: Tumour invades seminal vesicle(s)
pT4: Tumour is fixed or invades adjacent structures other than seminal vesicles such as the external sphincter, rectum, bladder, levator muscles and/or pelvic wall
pN category
pN0: No positive regional nodes
pN1: Metastasis in regional nodes
pM category
pM1: Distant metastasis
pM1a: Nonregional lymph node(s)
pM1b: Bone(s)
pM1c: Other sites with or without bone disease

15.6 Prostatic Intraepithelial Neoplasia (PIN)

- Premalignant condition characterized by noninvasive proliferation of epithelial cells confined to pre-existing prostatic ducts and acini.
- Previously classified into low and high grade on the basis of degree of cytological atypia. Present guidelines however mandate reporting of only HGPIN which is characterized by severe atypia.
- Low-grade PIN is not to be reported due to poor interobserver reproducibility and a relatively low risk of cancer following re-biopsy [7, 8].

15.6.1 Epidemiology

Pure HGPIN is present in 5–6% of NCB and 1–5% of TUR specimens. In >80% cases, HGPIN coexists with adenocarcinoma. Its incidence increases with age, reaching up to 67% by eighth decade. It is seen more commonly and earlier in African Americans compared to Caucasians [9].

15.6.2 Localization

More commonly encountered in the peripheral zone of the prostate.

15.6.3 Clinical Presentation

Generally asymptomatic with or without raised serum PSA levels.

15.6.4 Genetic Profile

HGPIN shares similar genetic alterations with invasive cancer, including critical shortening of telomeres, MYC amplifications, TMPRSS2::ERG fusion, PTEN loss and loss of heterozygosity at chromosomes 6 and 8 and gain of chromosomes [10].

15.6.5 Microscopic Pathology

Architecturally benign prostatic acini and ducts are lined by cytologically atypical cells displaying severe atypia in the form of nuclear pseudostratification, overlapping, enlargement and prominent nucleoli. Basal layer may be preserved or fragmented (Fig. 15.17a).

Common histological patterns of HGPIN (without any clinical implications) are the following:

1. Tufting
2. Micropapillary
3. Cribriform
4. Flat

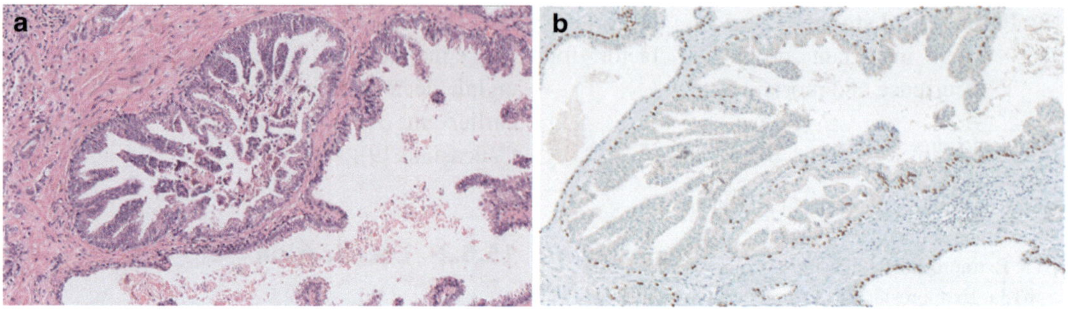

Fig. 15.17 (**a**) Microphotograph shows large prostatic ducts with luminal filiform structures exhibiting enlarged hyperchromatic nuclei forming a HGPIN. (**b**) p63 IHC shows intact basal myoepithelial cell layer around the duct of high-grade PIN

Uncommon patterns include signet ring cell, small cell, mucinous, foamy gland, inverted (hobnail) and PIN with squamous differentiation.

15.6.6 Ancillary Testing

1. Basal cell markers [p63, HMCK(34βE12)] highlight intact or fragmented (discontinuous) basal cell layer around the involved ducts (Fig. 15.17b).
2. AMACR and ERG1 staining in the lining acinar cells is variable.

15.6.7 Differential Diagnosis

1. Normal prostatic anatomical structures such as central zone glands or seminal vesicle/ejaculatory ducts.
2. Benign lesions such as prostatic glands with reactive atypia or cribriform hyperplasia or transitional metaplasia.
3. Malignant lesions such as acinar adenocarcinoma, IDC or ductal adenocarcinoma.

15.6.8 Prognosis

Median risk of cancer following diagnosis of HGPIN in NCB is ~21% (vs. 19% in benign cores).

Patients with multifocal (i.e. >3 cores), bilateral HGPIN are at higher risk of developing cancer and therefore should be more aggressively followed [9–11].

15.7 Intraductal Carcinoma of Prostate (IDC-P)

- Panluminal intra-acinar and/or intraductal proliferation of neoplastic epithelial cells with preservation of basal cells. The morphologic criteria of IDC-P exceed those seen in HGPIN either architecturally or cytologically [12].
- Categorized as a distinct entity by WHO in 2016; it is associated with high-grade, high-volume, high-stage prostate carcinoma [13].
- It mostly exists in the peripheral zone adjacent to high-grade carcinoma involving ducts in a retrograde manner ("regular IDC-P"). Rarely (0.06–0.26%), it may be as a de novo intraepithelial lesion unaccompanied by any lesion ("precursor IDC-P") [13, 14].
- Pure IDC-P in NCB mostly represents invasive tumour with an unsampled invasive component.

15.7.1 Epidemiology

Seen in 2.8% NCB and 20–40% RP specimens (with associated invasive carcinoma) [14]

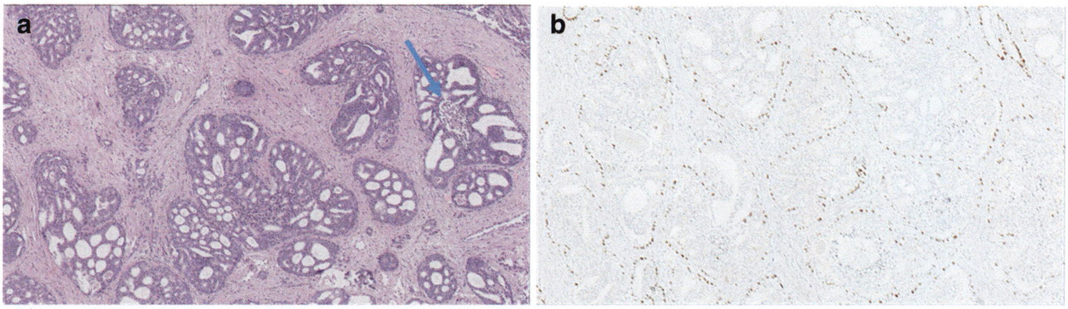

Fig. 15.18 (**a**) Microphotograph of IDC-P composed of large cribriform structure with preserved myoepithelial layer. Arrow shows a focus of comedonecrosis. (**b**) IHC in IDC-P shows intact myoepithelial layer with p63 expression

15.7.2 Microscopic Pathology

It is an expansile lesion of the prostatic ducts and acini, with the basal cell layer at least partially preserved. The normal architecture of the ducts and acini is preserved (Fig. 15.18a).

15.7.2.1 Histologic Criteria [12]

Malignant epithelium filling large acini or ducts with preservation of basal cells:

- Solid or dense cribriform pattern
- Loose cribriform or micropapillary pattern with either the following:
  - Marked nuclear atypia (nuclei 6× normal) or
  - Comedonecrosis

15.7.3 IHC Studies

The use of IHC to identify basal cells is optional, rather than mandatory, for the diagnosis of IDC-P:

1. Preserved or interrupted basal cells highlighted on staining with p63 or HMWK (Fig. 15.18b).
2. Neoplastic epithelial cells express AMACR/PSAP.
3. Loss of PTEN and positive ERG1 expression is seen in up to 80% of IDC-P while in HGPIN, PTEN expression is typically retained and ERG1 expression is uncommon (~18%).

15.7.3.1 Current Guidelines on Reporting IDC-P

1. Pure IDC should not be graded.
2. Incorporate IDC component of invasive prostate cancer in GS, for example, tumour with GS 4 + 3 and comedonecrosis IDC would be reported as GS 4 + 5 = 9.

15.7.4 Differential Diagnosis

1. Benign normal proliferations such as prostatic glands from central zone of the prostate/clear cell cribriform hyperplasia/basal cell hyperplasia
2. HGPIN
3. Invasive tumours such as acinar adenocarcinoma with cribriform architecture/ductal adenocarcinoma/urothelial carcinoma/metastatic adenocarcinoma

15.7.5 Prognosis

IDC on NCB is associated with poor prognostic features at RP such as higher GS (median score 8), high tumour volume, advanced stage and high rate of EPE and SV involvement. This is regardless of presence or absence of associated invasive carcinoma component in NCB [13].

A study by Porter et al. [15] suggested that IDC-P with concomitant invasive carcinoma is associated with higher rate of biochemical recurrence, metastasis and resistance to hormone and chemotherapy [15].

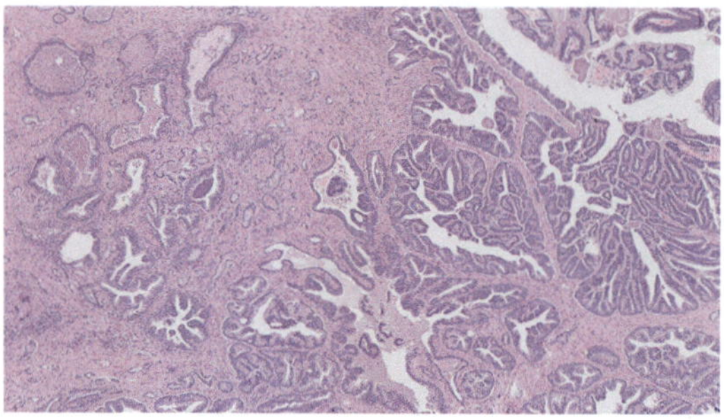

Fig. 15.19 Mixed acinar and ductal adenocarcinoma. Note the tall columnar pseudostratified lining of the ductal adenocarcinoma on the right side, in contrast to the acinar adenocarcinoma on the left

15.8 Ductal Adenocarcinoma

- It is a subtype of prostatic adenocarcinoma characterized by large glands lined by tall pseudostratified columnar cells.
- It mostly exists in combination with usual acinar adenocarcinoma. Rarely it may exist in pure form (0.2–0.4%) [16].
- It is located mostly in periurethral region but may exist in peripheral zone.
- It is composed of complex papillary and cribriform glands lined by columnar cells with abundant amphophilic cytoplasm, round-oval atypical nuclei, prominent nucleoli, coarse chromatin, frequent mitosis and intraluminal debris (Fig. 15.19).
- IHC findings are similar to usual acinar adenocarcinoma.
- Assigned Gleason pattern 4 to cribriform and papillary pattern and Gleason pattern 5 to comedonecrosis.
- More aggressive than the average acinar adenocarcinoma in terms of higher stage and increased mortality.

15.9 Urothelial Carcinoma (UC)

15.9.1 Classification

1. Primary: arises in prostatic urethra/prostatic glands (1–4% cases)
2. Secondary: arises in the urinary bladder and extends to involve prostate directly or through pagetoid spread (12–58% cases)

15.9.2 Microscopic Pathology

- Histopathological and IHC features similar to UC occurring anywhere in the genitourinary tract.
- Most pertinent IHC markers to distinguish UC from poorly differentiated prostatic adenocarcinoma are the urothelial markers GATA3, p63 and HMWCK and the prostatic markers PSAP and NKX3.1.

15.9.3 Prognosis

- Depends on extent, location and stage of disease.
- In primary cases, prostatic urethra staging is applied whereas in secondary cases, urinary bladder carcinoma staging is applied.

15.10 Squamous Neoplasms

- Include squamous cell carcinoma (SCC) and adenosquamous carcinoma.
- Rare entity (<0.6%); ~50% originate as a therapy effect of hormone or radiotherapy in prostate cancer cases.
- Microscopic features are similar to those of SCC of other origin. On IHC, the squamous component expresses HMWCK and is negative for PSAP, whereas the glandular component is positive for PSAP and negative for HMWCK.
- More aggressive and poor responder to treatment than usual prostate adenocarcinoma with median survival of 14–16 months.

15.11 Adenoid Cystic (Basal Cell) Carcinoma

- Malignant tumour composed of prostatic basal cells.
- Renamed so as to avoid confusion with the skin tumour.
- Very rare but aggressive neoplasm.
- Histologically composed of basaloid tumour cells with scant cytoplasm, high nuclear/cytoplasmic ratio, angulated nuclei and open chro-

matin arranged as nests with peripheral palisading in a desmoplastic stroma. It may also display adenoid cystic pattern. On IHC, it expresses CK7 (luminal), HMWCK (peripheral) and Bcl-2 and is negative for CK20.

15.12 Neuroendocrine Tumours

Classification:

- Adenocarcinoma with neuroendocrine differentiation
- Adenocarcinoma with Paneth cell-like neuroendocrine differentiation
- Well-differentiated neuroendocrine tumour
- Small cell neuroendocrine carcinoma
- Large cell neuroendocrine carcinoma

15.12.1 Adenocarcinoma with Neuroendocrine Differentiation

- Usual acinar/ductal adenocarcinoma with variable number of cells expressing neuroendocrine markers.
- Does not affect the outcome or treatment strategy.

15.12.2 Adenocarcinoma with Paneth Cell-Like Neuroendocrine Differentiation

- Usual acinar adenocarcinoma with variable number of cells with eosinophilic cytoplasmic granules reminiscent of paneth cells.
- Displays immunopositivity for neuroendocrine markers.

15.12.3 Well-Differentiated Neuroendocrine Tumour

- Very rare.
- Composed of round uniform cells in nests, acini with indistinct nucleoli, low mitosis and absent necrosis.

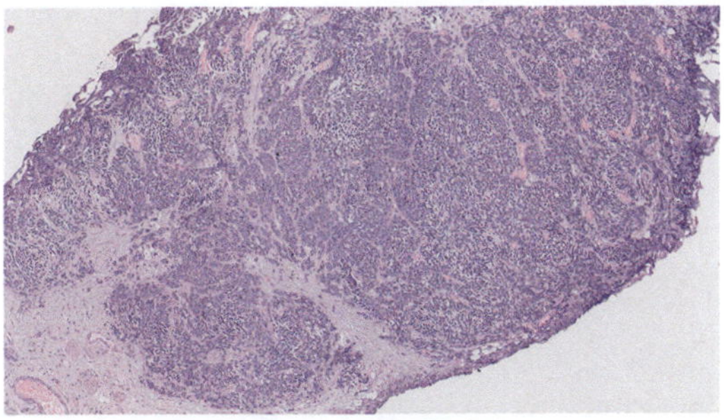

Fig. 15.20 Pure small cell carcinoma shows small round hyperchromatic cells lying in diffuse sheets, islands

- Displays positivity for neuroendocrine markers like synaptophysin/chromogranin/CD56/INSM1 and is negative for PSA.
- Advanced stage at presentation but good prognosis.

15.12.4 Small Cell Neuroendocrine Carcinoma (SmCC)

- Seen as pure (50–60%) or as admixed with usual acinar adenocarcinoma (40–50%) [17].
- Composed of cells lying in diffuse sheets, cords, rosettes or singly displaying nuclear moulding. The cells have high nuclear/cytoplasmic ratio, scant cytoplasm, fine chromatin, lack of nucleoli, high mitosis, apoptotic debris and geographic necrosis (Figs. 15.20 and 15.21a).
- Positive for neuroendocrine markers and p53. PSAP and NKX3.1 may be expressed focally in ~25% of cases. TTF1 expression is noted >50% cases. AR expression is lost (Fig. 15.21b–d).
- Not assigned any GS.
- 40–50% cases have past history of acinar adenocarcinoma, with time gap ranging from 1 to 300 months.
- Aggressive disease with advanced stage at presentation, poor prognosis and a median survival of <12 months.

15.12.5 Large Cell Neuroendocrine Carcinoma

- Very rare entity.
- Can be pure or as admixed with acinar adenocarcinoma or SmCC.

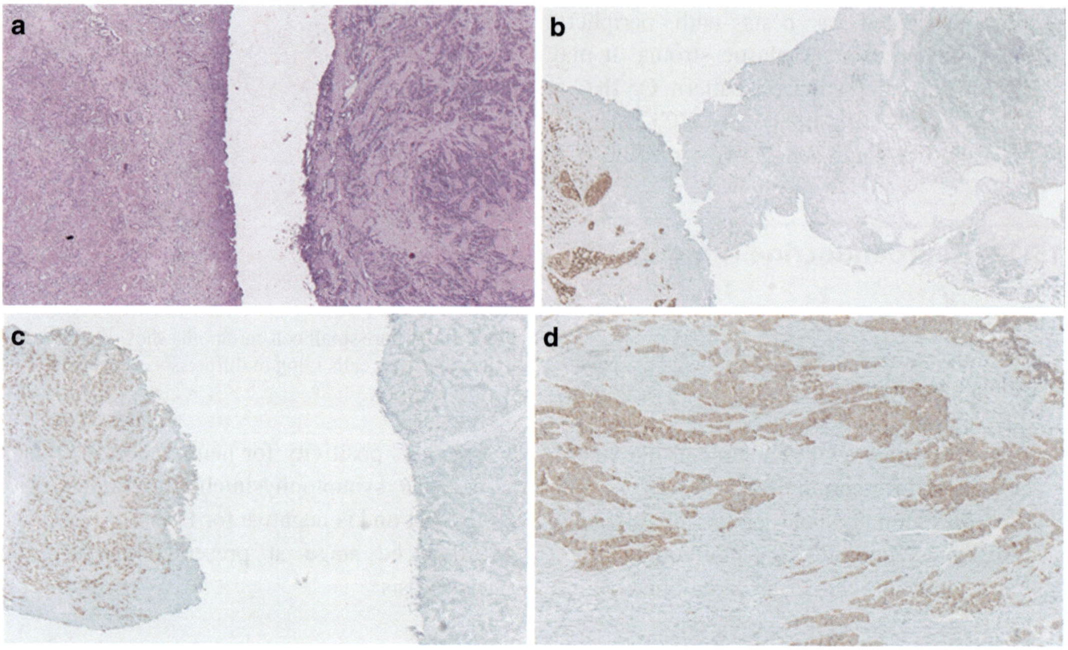

Fig. 15.21 (**a**) Mixed acinar (left side) and small cell carcinoma (right side). (**b, c**) IHC study shows positive expression of NKX3.1 and AR in acinar carcinoma (respectively), while being negative in small cell carcinoma component. (**d**) Diffuse synaptophysin positivity seen in small cell carcinoma.

- Composed of cells arranged as organoid nests with peripheral palisading and geographic necrosis. The cells have abundant cytoplasm, vesicular chromatin and nucleoli. IHC findings are similar to SmCCa.
- Poor prognosis.

15.12.6 Treatment-Related Neuroendocrine Prostatic Carcinoma (T-NEPCs) [17]

- Tumours demonstrating complete/partial neuroendocrine differentiation with adenocarcinoma after androgen deprivation therapy.
- Constitute 10–15% of prostatic adenocarcinomas.
- Originate due to transdifferentiation of castration-resistant prostate cancer on androgen deprivation therapy.
- Clinical and pathological features similar to usual small/large cell neuroendocrine carcinoma.
- Median survival is seven months.

15.13 Genomic Biomarkers in Prostate Cancer

Genomic biomarkers include different tools and technologies to predict, prognosticate and provide therapeutic options in prostate cancer patients. These markers can help screen patients with or without family history who are likely to develop cancer, predict likelihood of a positive biopsy, stratify low to intermediate-risk patients and predict response to molecular and immunotherapy. Each of these is discussed separately (Fig. 15.22).

Genetic susceptibility: Prostate cancer has a large amount of heritability. Around 85% cases are sporadic, 10–15% cases have prostate cancer in families and 3–5% is associated with high-risk genes [18]. Men with affected first-degree relatives are at much greater risk (1.5–2.5-fold) [19]. Familial prostate cancer is multifactorial and is affected by low- to moderate-risk variants, moderate- to high-risk genes and environmental insults along with aging. It is also known that men with family history are likely to have aggressive disease with an early age of onset by almost two years [20].

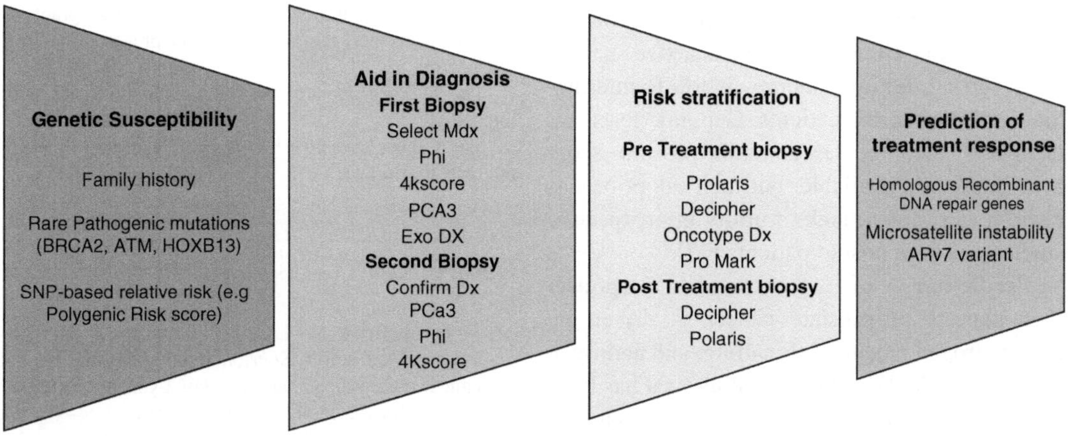

Fig. 15.22 Different roles of genomic biomarkers in prostate cancer

Genome-wide association studies (GWAS) have shown that cumulative effect of multiple single nucleotide polymorphisms (SNPs) significantly increases relative risk of prostate cancer in a person. SNPs are risk alleles occurring at >1% frequency in the normal population. More than 150 SNPs are known to be associated with prostate cancer, and these account for 38% familial risk in prostate cancer [21]. Polygenic risk scores (PRS) have been used in various studies based on the cumulative effect of the SNPs to identify the high-risk population [22] of prostate cancer.

DNA repair genes like BRCA1/BRCA2, ATM, CHEK2 and NBN are associated with 3–5% risk of prostate cancer [18]. Patients who carry germline variants like BRCA2 in a metastatic setting have been shown to respond to PARP (poly-ADP ribose polymerase) inhibitors and platinum-based chemotherapy [23]. A 3607 prostate cancer study conducted on unselected cases for familial history showed 17.2% pathogenic germline variants. Amongst these 30.7% were BRCA1/BRCA2, 4.5% were HOXB13, 14.1% were CHEK2 and 9.6% were ATM genes [24]. The Philadelphia Prostate Cancer Consensus group has provided a comprehensive consensus guideline for implementation of germline genetic testing in prostate cancer [25]. They recommended that all metastatic prostate cancers should be tested (both germline and somatic) for BRCA1/BRCA2, MMR (mismatch repair gene) and ATM genes. In men with first-degree relatives with prostate cancer especially with two or more male relatives with either prostate cancer in <60 years old, death from prostate cancer and metastatic prostate cancer should be considered. Patients with Ashkenazi Jewish lineage and intraductal histology and patients presenting at young age (40 years or 10 years prior to youngest prostate cancer in the family) should also be tested.

Aid in Diagnosis: Another important role of molecular diagnosis is in aiding diagnosis of prostate cancer. Prostate-specific antigen (PSA) is a commonly used biochemical marker. It is not a perfect marker and also can be elevated in benign conditions like benign prostatic hyperplasia or prostatitis. Tests like select MDx, PCA3 and Exodx performed on urine sample and biochemical tests like PHI®, 4k® and total/free PSA performed on blood may be helpful in solving the clinical dilemma of performing prostate biopsy in patients with mildly raised PSA. Clinically suspicious patients having suspicious/negative biopsy may be offered with tests like confirm MDx. This test is known to have a negative predictive value (NPV) of 88–90% compared to histopathology which has NPV of around 70%. Detailed information about these tests is beyond the scope of this chapter. Low-risk patients may be kept on surveillance, and patients selected as high risk are advised for guided prostatic biopsy [26]. The validity of these newer molecular tests has not been proven unequivocally due to multifocality, tumour heterogeneity, sampling bias and lack of validation across different populations in prostate cancer.

Risk stratification: After a positive biopsy report, another clinical dilemma is active surveillance versus additional therapy in low to intermediate prognostic risk patients. Genomic tests like decipher, Oncotype Dx genomic prostate score and Polaris are available, but their adoption has been modest due to lack of utility in prospective studies and high cost to patients [27].

Prediction of treatment response: Pathogenesis of prostate cancer is driven by AR (androgen receptor) signalling, and androgen receptor blockade/androgen withdrawal has been exploited therapeutically. AR splice variants are one of the mechanisms of resistance in CRPC (castration-resistant prostate cancer) patients. AR-V7 (splice variant) detected in circulating tumour cells predicts poor response to AR antagonists like enzalutamide or abiraterone [28]. Genomic landscape of metastatic prostate cancer has also shown that 23% of these tumours harbour germline or somatic mutations in genes involved in the DNA damage repair pathway. These patients are also good candidates for platinum-based chemotherapy or PARP inhibitor therapy based on PROFOUND and TOPARP trials [26]. It is recommended that these patients should be tested at least for DNA repair genes BRCA1/BRCA2 and preferably for other genes like ATM, BRIP1, BARD1, CDK12, CHEK1, CHEK2, FANCL, PALB2, RAD51B, RAD51C, RAD51D and RAD54L on germline/tissue/liquid biopsy to look for therapeutic options. 1–2% prostate cancer patients can also have microsatellite instability (MSI) which can be detected by MMR testing by IHC (immunohistochemistry) or MSI testing by PCR-based techniques [29, 30]. These patients are likely to respond well to immunotherapy.

Expanding genomic landscape of localized and metastatic prostate carcinoma with an increasing repertoire of targeted therapies and diagnostic tests for prognostic, predictive and therapeutic benefit to the patient is the way forward for personalized medicine.

Acknowledgments The authors wish to thank Dr. Meenakshi Kamboj, Dr. Divya Bansal and Dr. Ankur Kumar for their assistance in the preparation of this manuscript.

Declaration The authors declare that no funds, grants or other supports were received during the preparation of this manuscript.

The authors declare that they have no conflict of interest.

The authors have no relevant financial or non-financial interests to disclose.

References

1. Ferlay J, Ervik M, Lam F, Colombet M, Mery L, Piñeros M, Znaor A, Soerjomataram I, Bray F. Global cancer observatory: cancer today. Lyon: International Agency for Research on Cancer; 2020.
2. Smith SC. General concepts, prostate carcinoma. In: Amin MB, Tickoo SK, editors. Diagnostic pathology: genitourinary. 2nd ed. Salt Lake City, UT: Elsevier; 2016. p. 600–7.
3. Kench JG, Kristiansen G, Berney DM, et al. Acinar adenocarcinoma. In: WHO Classification of Tumours Editorial Board, editor. Urinary and male genital tumours, WHO classification of tumours series, vol. 8. 5th ed. Lyon: International Agency for Research on Cancer; 2022.
4. Andreoiu M, Cheng L. Multifocal prostate cancer: biologic, prognostic, and therapeutic implications. Hum Pathol. 2010;41(6):781–93. https://doi.org/10.1016/j.humpath.2010.02.011.
5. Rosoff JS, Prasad SM, Savage SJ. Ultrasonography in prostate cancer: current roles and potential applications in radiorecurrent disease. World J Urol. 2013;31(6):1353–9. https://doi.org/10.1007/s00345-013-1080-9.
6. Epstein JI, Egevad L, Amin MB, Delahunt B, Srigley JR, Humphrey PA, Grading Committee. The 2014 International Society of Urological Pathology (ISUP) consensus conference on Gleason grading of prostatic carcinoma: definition of grading patterns and proposal for a new grading system. Am J Surg Pathol. 2016;40(2):244–52. https://doi.org/10.1097/PAS.0000000000000530.
7. van Leenders GJLH, van der Kwast TH, Grignon DJ, Evans AJ, Kristiansen G, Kweldam CF, Litjens G, McKenney JK, Melamed J, Mottet N, Paner GP, Samaratunga H, Schoots IG, Simko JP, Tsuzuki T, Varma M, Warren AY, Wheeler TM, Williamson SR, Iczkowski KA, ISUP Grading Workshop Panel Members. The 2019 International Society of Urological Pathology (ISUP) consensus conference on grading of prostatic carcinoma. Am J Surg Pathol. 2020;44(8):e87–99. https://doi.org/10.1097/PAS.0000000000001497.
8. Epstein JI, Herawi M. Prostate needle biopsies containing prostatic intraepithelial neoplasia or atypical foci suspicious for carcinoma: implications for patient care. J Urol. 2006;175(3 Pt 1):820–34. https://doi.org/10.1016/S0022-5347(05)00337-X.
9. Al-Ahmadie H. Prostatic intraepithelial neoplasia. In: Amin MB, Tickoo SK, editors. Diagnostic pathology:

genitourinary. 2nd ed. Salt Lake City, UT: Elsevier; 2016. p. 590–9.
10. Netto GJ, Humphrey PA, Galluzzi CM. High-grade prostatic intraepithelial neoplasia. In: WHO Classification of Tumours Editorial Board, editor. Urinary and male genital tumours, WHO classification of tumours series, vol. 8. 5th ed. Lyon: International Agency for Research on Cancer; 2022.
11. Singh PB, Nicholson CM, Ragavan N, Blades RA, Martin FL, Matanhelia SS. Risk of prostate cancer after detection of isolated high-grade prostatic intraepithelial neoplasia (HGPIN) on extended core needle biopsy: a UK hospital experience. BMC Urol. 2009;9:3. https://doi.org/10.1186/1471-2490-9-3.
12. Guo CC, Epstein JI. Intraductal carcinoma of the prostate on needle biopsy: histologic features and clinical significance. Mod Pathol. 2006;19:1528–35.
13. Epstein JI, Oxley J, Ro JY, Van der Kwast T, Zhou M. lntraductal carcinoma. In: Moch H, Humphrey PA, Ulbright TM, Reuter VE, editors. WHO classification of tumours of the urinary system and male genital organs, 2016. 4th ed. Lyon: International Agency for Research on Cancer; 2016.
14. Wobker SE, Epstein JI. Differential diagnosis of Intraductal lesions of the prostate. Am J Surg Pathol. 2016;40(6):e67–82. https://doi.org/10.1097/PAS.0000000000000609.
15. Porter LH, Lawrence MG, Ilic D, Clouston D, Bolton DM, Frydenberg M, Murphy DG, Pezaro C, Risbridger GP, Taylor RA. Systematic review links the prevalence of Intraductal carcinoma of the prostate to prostate cancer risk categories. Eur Urol. 2017;72(4):492–5. https://doi.org/10.1016/j.eururo.2017.03.013.
16. Kwast THVD, Kristiansen G, McKenney JK. Ductal adenocarcinoma. In: WHO Classification of Tumours Editorial Board, editor. Urinary and male genital tumours, WHO classification of tumours series, vol. 8. 5th ed. Lyon: International Agency for Research on Cancer; 2022.
17. Rubin MA. Treatment-related neuroendocrine prostatic carcinoma. In: WHO Classification of Tumours Editorial Board, editor. Urinary and male genital tumours, WHO classification of tumours series, vol. 8. 5th ed. Lyon: International Agency for Research on Cancer; 2022.
18. Klein EA, Kupelian PA, Witte JS. Does a family history of prostate cancer result in more aggressive disease? Prostate Cancer Prostatic Dis. 1998;16:297–300.
19. Dias A, Kote-Jarai Z, Mikropoulos C, Eeles R. Prostate cancer Germline variations and implications for screening and treatment. Cold Spring Harb Perspect Med. 2018;8(9):a030379. https://doi.org/10.1101/cshperspect.a030379.
20. Gronberg H, Isaacs SD, Smith JR, Carpten JD, Bova GS, Freije D, Xu J, et al. Characteristics of prostate cancer in families potentially linked to the hereditary prostate cancer 1 (HPC1) locus. JAMA. 1997;27815:1251–5.
21. Ni Raghallaigh H, Eeles R. Genetic predisposition to prostate cancer: an update. Familial Cancer. 2022;21:101–14. https://doi.org/10.1007/s10689-021-00227-3.
22. Zheng SL, Sun J, Wiklund F, Smith S, Stattin P, Li G, Adami HO, et al. Cumulative association of five genetic variants with prostate cancer. N Engl J Med. 2008;3589:910–9.
23. Zafeiriou Z, Bianchini D, Chandler R, Rescigno P, Yuan W, Carreira S, Barrero M, et al. Genomic analysis of three metastatic prostate cancer patients with exceptional responses to carboplatin indicating different types of DNA repair deficiency. Eur Urol. 2019;751:184–92.
24. Nicolosi P, Ledet E, Yang S, Michalski S, Freschi B, O'Leary E, Esplin ED, et al. Prevalence of germline variants in prostate cancer and implications for current genetic testing guidelines. JAMA Oncol. 2019;54:523–8.
25. Giri VN, Knudsen KE, Kelly WK, Cheng HH, Cooney KA, Cookson MS, Dahut W, et al. Implementation of germline testing for prostate cancer: Philadelphia prostate cancer consensus conference 2019. J Clin Oncol. 2020;38:2798–811.
26. Cucchiara V, Cooperberg MR, Dall'Era M, et al. Genomic markers in prostate cancer decision making. Eur Urol. 2018;73(4):572–82. https://doi.org/10.1016/j.eururo.2017.10.036.
27. Mateo J, Carreira S, Sandhu S, et al. DNA-repair defects and olaparib in metastatic prostate cancer. N Engl J Med. 2015;373:1697–708.
28. Antonarakis ES, Lu C, Wang H, Luber B, Nakazawa M, Roeser JC, Chen Y, Mohammad TA, Chen Y, Fedor HL, Lotan TL, Zheng Q, De Marzo AM, Isaacs JT, Isaacs WB, Nadal R, Paller CJ, Denmeade SR, Carducci MA, Eisenberger MA, Luo J. AR-V7 and resistance to enzalutamide and abiraterone in prostate cancer. N Engl J Med. 2014;371(11):1028–38. https://doi.org/10.1056/NEJMoa1315815.
29. Hempelmann JA, Lockwood CM, Konnick EQ, et al. Microsatellite instability in prostate cancer by PCR or next-generation sequencing. J Immunother Cancer. 2018;6(1):29. https://doi.org/10.1186/s40425-018-0341-y.
30. Lotan TL, Tomlins SA, Bismar TA, Van der Kwast TH, Grignon D, Egevad L, Kristiansen G, Pritchard CC, Rubin MA, Bubendorf L. Report from the International Society of Urological Pathology (ISUP) consultation conference on molecular pathology of urogenital cancers. I. Molecular biomarkers in prostate cancer. Am J Surg Pathol. 2020;44(7):e15–29. https://doi.org/10.1097/PAS.0000000000001450.

Management of Localized and Locally Advanced Prostate Cancer

16

Siddharth Yadav and Anup Kumar

16.1 Introduction

Prostate cancer is the most common non-cutaneous malignancy, and roughly one in six American men will be diagnosed with prostate cancer throughout their lifetime [1]. In the developed world, the majority of the cancers (70%), at the time of the diagnosis, are localized to the prostate gland, whereas another 11% are locally advanced [2]. This can be attributed to the widespread practice of prostate-specific antigen (PSA)-based screening, whereas in the developing world, the percentage of metastatic disease is expected to be higher. Traditionally, the cancers localized to the prostate (stages T1 and T2) are called as localized prostate cancer, whereas stages T3 and T4 fall under the gamut of locally advanced disease. However, with a better understanding of the natural history of prostate cancer, various risk stratification methods, mostly by adding PSA levels and Gleason score (GS) to the clinical stage, have been proposed. Localized disease is usually subcategorized into low, intermediate, and high risk, and the locally advanced disease also falls under the high-risk prostate cancer. Such risk stratifications help to prognosticate the disease accurately, thereby assisting in the selection of appropriate treatment options.

S. Yadav · A. Kumar (✉)
Department of Urology, Robotics and Renal Transplant, SJH and VMMC, New Delhi, India

Patients with localized and locally advanced prostate cancers are usually offered treatment with a curative intent, provided they have a long life expectancy. If the life expectancy is short, that is less than 5–10 years, watchful waiting can be offered. However, those with a longer life expectancy need to weigh the benefits and the potential harms associated with active treatment and can be offered with active surveillance, curative radiotherapy, or radical prostatectomy. Besides these whole gland treatments, focal ablation modalities such as high intensity-focused ultrasonography and cryoablation have also been described. This review aims to discuss the various treatment options available to the patients with localized and locally advanced prostate cancer, the possible benefits and harms of each, and how to choose one over the other.

16.2 Localized Prostate Cancer

Men with localized prostate cancer have been shown to have long-term survival when treated expectantly, even in the absence of local treatment. The reported disease-specific survival rate in men diagnosed with localized prostate cancer, who did not receive local treatment, at 10, 15, and 20 years was 85%, 58%, and 32%, respectively, and the treatment-free survival rate at 10 years was 43% [3]. When stratified according to the degree of differentiation of the cancer, the

P. Singh et al. (eds.), *A Guide to Management of Urological Cancers*,
https://doi.org/10.1007/978-981-99-2341-0_16

10-year cancer-specific survival rate for men with well, moderately, and poorly differentiated tumors, who were initially untreated and managed conservatively, was 91%, 90%, and 74%, respectively [4]. The corresponding 10-year risk of dying of competing causes was 59%, 57%, and 56%, respectively [4]. Thus, besides the volume of the disease, the degree of differentiation of cancer, that is, the Gleason score, and the life expectancy plays an important role while planning local treatment in men with localized prostate cancer.

A life expectancy of at least 10 years is considered mandatory for contemplating local treatment in patients with localized disease. Besides age, the presence of comorbidities has been shown to increase the risk of death from non-prostate cancer causes. A 10-year competing risk analysis of men diagnosed with localized prostate cancer, who did not receive local treatment within the first 6 months, found that the majority of the deaths resulted from competing causes rather than the cancer [5]. The overall 5-year mortality rate in men 66–74 years of age with T1c disease and Gleason score 8–10 was 52% in those with ≥2 comorbidities of which only 9.6% died of the prostate cancer, whereas it was 26.4% in men without comorbidities and 13.6% of these had died of the cancer. The presence of comorbidities was shown to have a higher impact on the overall survival as compared to the age at diagnosis and the Gleason score [5]. Thus, men with localized prostate cancer and multiple comorbidities and shorter life expectancy can be spared from local treatment as they are unlikely to derive a survival benefit and can be advised watchful waiting.

Watchful waiting refers to conservative management where patients are just observed for the development of symptoms or imminent complications, when they are prescribed palliative treatment. The goal is to maintain the quality of life rather than actively treating the malignancy. The PIVOT (Prostate Intervention Versus Observation Trial) compared all-cause mortality in men with localized prostate cancer who underwent radical prostatectomy to men who were observed and found little to no benefit of radical prostatectomy (68% mortality in radical prostatectomy group vs. 73% in observation group [$p = 0.044$] at 22.1-year follow-up) with the surgery resulting in a gain of mean 1 year of life only [6]. Thus, in view of limited benefit in selected subgroup of patients, that too after a very long duration of follow-up, men with limited life expectancy and localized prostate cancer are best offered watchful waiting.

Risk stratification is commonly used to subclassify men with localized prostate cancer into low-risk (PSA <10 ng/mL, Gleason score < 7, and cT1–T2a), intermediate-risk (PSA 10–20 ng/mL, Gleason score 7, and cT2b), and high-risk (PSA > 20 ng/mL, Gleason score > 7, and cT2c) disease. Grouping patients with similar expected disease behavior eases the decision-making process and helps in making an informed decision.

16.2.1 Low-Risk Localized Prostate Cancer

Men with low-risk localized prostate cancer have an overall low risk of dying from the disease. The 10-year cancer-specific mortality rate of men 66–74 years of age with T1c and Gleason score 7 or less was found to be 4.8%, in men without comorbidities [5]. Men with long expected survival have the option to undergo curative treatment either in the form of radical prostatectomy or radiotherapy or can opt for active surveillance. The only randomized trial comparing active treatment (radical prostatectomy or radiotherapy) to active surveillance, the prostate testing for cancer and treatment (ProtecT) study, randomized 1643 patients into active monitoring (545), to surgery (553), and to radiotherapy (545) [7]. Fifty-six percent of the patients had low-risk disease, with 90% having PSA <10 ng/mL; 77% had Gleason score of 6 and 76% had T1c disease. The 10-year cancer-specific mortality and the overall mortality rates were similar between the groups, whereas the rates of disease progression and metastasis (6% in the active monitoring group vs. 2.6% in the active treatment group) were higher in the active monitoring group. Thus, in men with localized prostate cancer, deferred treatment in the form of active surveillance has similar oncologic outcomes, and the main concern in men with low-risk localized disease is overtreatment- and treatment-related adverse effects.

16.2.1.1 Active Surveillance

Majority of the men with long expected survival and low-risk prostate cancer, on one hand, are unlikely to derive large survival benefit from curative treatment; however, on the other hand, they have the most to lose if the disease progresses out of the curative window. Active surveillance aims to avoid overtreatment in men with localized prostate cancer by keeping them under close surveillance and offers treatment with a curative intent at progression. This strategy avoids overtreatment- and treatment-related adverse events in those who are unlikely to have survival benefit from upfront treatment, while at the same time aims to provide timely curative intervention to those with progressive disease, without compromising long-term survival.

Although the ProtecT study showed a higher rate of metastasis in men undergoing active monitoring, the major shortcoming of the ProtecT trial was the active monitoring protocol, which was significantly less stringent than the contemporary active surveillance protocols in the terms of clinical follow up, imaging, and repeat biopsies. Multiparametric magnetic resonance imaging and protocol mandated repeat biopsies were not utilized, and the follow-up was based on PSA measurement alone [7]. Nevertheless, even with less strict monitoring, ProtecT trial reinforces the importance of deferred active treatment in men with low-risk localized prostate cancer. A recent prospective study enrolled 1818 men with low-risk prostate cancer to active surveillance (6 monthly PSA, 12 monthly rectal exam, and multiparametric magnetic resonance imaging) and reported cumulative cancer-specific mortality and metastasis rate of 0.1% at 10 and 15 years [8]. The authors concluded that in men with Gleason grade group 1 cancer, the risk of metastasis or death was <1%, and the cumulative incidence of biopsy grade reclassification was 32% at 15 years. In men with favorable risk prostate cancer, the reported 10- and 15-year overall, cancer-specific, and metastasis survival rates are 93%, 99.9%, and 99.4% and 69%, 99.9%, and 99.4%, respectively, and the cumulative incidence of curative intervention is 50% at 10 years and 57% at 15 years and the median treatment-free survival is 8.5 years [9].

All men diagnosed with low-risk prostate cancer (PSA 10 ng/mL, cT1–T2a, and Gleason score < 7) can be offered with active surveillance. In patients where a MRI was not performed prior to enrolment into active surveillance, a MRI along with a combined systematic and guided biopsy should be performed at confirmatory biopsy; however, if MRI and a combined systematic and guided biopsy were performed prior to enrolment into active surveillance, a confirmatory biopsy may be omitted [10, 11]. Adding MRI-guided biopsy to systematic biopsy at the confirmatory biopsy upgrades cancer in an additional 7% of the patients [10]. There is still a lack of evidence and consensus on the follow-up protocol and the triggers to change the treatment. The follow-up protocol is usually based on 6 monthly PSA, yearly rectal examination, and repeated biopsy, usually at predefined intervals. Radiological progression on MRI can suggest cancer upgradation, with 39% of the patients having a pathological progression if there was radiological progression; however, 21% with stable MRI findings were also found to have pathological progression [12]. Others have also reported that pathological progression can be found in 30–50% of the patients without radiological progression [13, 14]. Triggered repeat biopsies should be performed if there is a change in PSA, rectal exam findings, or mpMRI findings; however, there is lack of consensus on the frequency and the duration of untriggered protocol-mandated repeat biopsies and repeat MRI. The most commonly used criteria to define progression are a change in Gleason score, change in the T stage, PSA doubling time < 3 years, more than two-thirds core positive or >50% core involvement; however, a consensus has not been reached [15].

16.2.1.2 Radical Prostatectomy

Radical surgery can be offered as a curative option to patients with low-risk localized cancer prostate, provided they have a long expected survival and are ready to accept the adverse effect profile for the prevention of disease progression. Radical prostatectomy can be performed by open, laparoscopic, or robotic approaches. The most recent review comparing the outcomes of robotic versus laparoscopic versus open radical prostatectomy found no significant differences in the oncologic, urinary, and sexual outcomes; however, both the robotic and the laparoscopic radical prostatectomies were associated with shorter hospital stay and lower blood loss as compared to the open approach [16]. Radical prostatectomy is typically performed by the anterior approach, by dropping the bladder and exposing the space of Retzius. A Retzius-sparing posterior approach has been described which preserves the anterior supporting structures of the prostate and thus can conceptually result in better continence outcomes. A recent review comparing Retzius-sparing radical prostatectomy to the conventional radical prostatectomy showed improved continence rates at 1 and 3 months but similar rates at 12 months of follow up; however, the chances of positive surgical margins were higher with the Retzius-sparing approach [17]. Sparing the neurovascular bundles during the radical prostatectomy improves the postoperative erectile function, which also depends on the age and the preoperative erectile function. Nerve sparing also results in better continence rates without adversely affecting the oncologic outcomes; thus, a nerve-sparing approach can be offered to patients interested in maintaining the sexual functions. An extended pelvic lymph node dissection, including the obturator, internal iliac, and the external iliac nodes is performed along with radical prostatectomy in patients at high risk of nodal metastasis as calculated by either the Briganti nomogram, Roach formula, Partin's tables, or MSKCC (Memorial Sloan Kettering Cancer Center) nomogram [18]. The addition and the extent of pelvic lymph node dissection does not seem to improve the oncologic outcomes but are important for staging and prognosis [19].

As compared to the active surveillance, in patients with low-risk disease, radical prostatectomy results in lower chances of metastasis and progression, but similar cancer-specific survival and the magnitude of difference may be even lower with the contemporary surveillance methods [7]. The LAPPRO (Laparoscopic Prostatectomy Robot Open) trial reported the oncologic and functional outcomes in 338 men with low-risk prostate cancer at 12 months of follow-up [20]. The positive surgical margin rate was 16.4%, the 12-month biochemical relapse rate was 2.4%, and 34.5% had an upgradation to either T3 or Gleason score ≥ 7 on the final histopathology report. The urinary continence rate, defined as less than 1 pad per day, was 84%, and the erectile function, defined as erections hard enough to penetrate more than half of the times, was 50% [20]. The 10-year cancer-specific survival was 99% [7]. The patients who shift from active surveillance to radical prostatectomy, either for personal reasons or for the increase in the tumor volume or Gleason score, also have similar oncologic outcomes as compared to those who chose upfront radical prostatectomy [21].

16.2.1.3 Radiotherapy

External beam radiotherapy is an alternative curative option for patients with low-risk localized prostate cancer with long expected survival desiring curative treatment. Intensity-modulated external beam radiotherapy (IMRT) has been shown to be superior to three-dimensional conformal radiotherapy (3D CRT) and is the current standard of care. IMRT uses a sophisticated computer program and inverse planning so that delivered radiation conforms to the area of interest, thus reducing the amount of radiation delivered to the surrounding structures. An image guiding system is also used to detect organ movement and correct the radiation path in the real time. The IMRT results in lower acute and late gastrointestinal toxicity and has similar or slightly higher genitourinary toxicity and similar oncologic outcomes [22]. Dose escalation has shown to improve survival in patients receiving radiotherapy, and a dose of 74–80 Gy is currently recommended. Moderate hypo-fractionation,

2.5–3.4 Gy per fraction, can reduce the number of sessions of radiotherapy making it convenient and cost effective for the patient and has similar oncologic outcomes and adverse event profile [23]. Ultra-hypofractionation, >3.4 Gy per fraction, with stereotactic body radiotherapy has also been shown to be equally effective, although long-term data is still awaited and some studies report slightly higher incidence of adverse events [24].

Men with low-risk prostate cancer can be offered with 74–80 Gy of IMRT with image-guided radiotherapy without adjuvant androgen deprivation therapy as a curative option. Radiotherapy is equally effective to radical prostatectomy in terms of cancer-specific survival and progression- and metastasis-free survival [7]. The 10-year biochemical disease-free survival, distant metastasis-free survival, and cancer-specific survival for low-risk disease after IMRT were 81%, 100%, and 100%, respectively [25]. The 10-year likelihood of developing grade 2 and 3 genitourinary toxicity was 11% and 5%, whereas the same for gastrointestinal toxicity was 2% and 1%, respectively [25]. Prior history of transurethral resection of prostate or severe lower urinary tract symptoms may be relative contraindications to radiation therapy due to the increased risk of urethral stricture or acute urinary retention.

Radiotherapy can also be delivered as brachytherapy, either as permanently implanted seeds or as a temporarily introduced radioactive source. Low-dose rate (LDR) brachytherapy uses permanently implanted radioactive seeds into the prostate and has been used for the treatment of low-risk prostate cancer in men without the history of transurethral resection of the prostate or outflow obstruction, either alone or in combination with external beam radiotherapy. The reported biochemical disease-free survival of LDR brachytherapy in men with low-risk prostate cancer is 89% at 12-year of follow-up [26]. High-dose rate (HDR) brachytherapy uses radioactive needles or catheters to deliver the desired radiation dose to the prostate within minutes, which are then removed. HDR brachytherapy is usually delivered in combination with external beam radiotherapy although some centers have utilized HDR brachytherapy as monotherapy in men with low- and intermediate-risk prostate cancer. The local control, distant metastasis-free survival, and cause-specific survival were 99.7%, 98.9%, and 99.1%, respectively [27]. There were no late grade 3–4 rectal toxicities developed and late grade 3–4 genitourinary toxicity reported in 4.9% (grade 3 in 4.7%) [27].

16.2.2 Intermediate-Risk Localized Prostate Cancer

Men with clinical stage T2 prostate cancer and a Gleason score of 5–7 without co-morbidities have a 9.5% chance of dying from the disease, whereas those with ≥2 comorbidities have a 1% chance [5]. Men with limited life expectancy can be safely observed, whereas those with a life expectancy of >10 years can be offered curative treatment in the form of radical prostatectomy or radiation therapy, and a selected few can be offered active surveillance as well.

16.2.2.1 Active Surveillance

Patients with Gleason pattern 4 on the needle biopsy have a threefold increased risk of metastasis as compared to those with Gleason score 6 [28]. The estimated 15 year metastasis-free survival of patients with Gleason 6 or less with PSA <10 ng/mL was 94%, Gleason 6 or less with PSA 10 to 20 ng/mL was 94%, Gleason 3 + 4 with PSA <20 ng/mL was 84%, and Gleason 4 + 3 with PSA < 20 ng/mL was 63% [28]. Thus, patients categorized into the intermediate-risk group because of PSA between 10 and 20 ng/mL can be safely offered with active surveillance; however, caution needs to be exercised for patients with Gleason score 7. Those with low-volume Gleason pattern 4 can be offered active surveillance, where those with large number of positive cores or Gleason score 4 + 3 are best treated upfront. The DETECTIVE group also recommends active surveillance in patients with Gleason grade group 2 disease with PSA <10 ng/mL and clinical stage cT2a with low core positivity [15]. Multiparametric MRI may also help in the detection and accurate biopsy of small foci of Gleason pattern 4 disease which might be missed on the systematic biopsy. The 10-year metastasis-free survival, cancer-specific survival, and overall survival in men with intermediate-risk prostate cancer were 91%, 97%, and 67%, respectively, which are inferior as compared to those with low-risk disease, especially in men with Gleason pattern 4 [28].

16.2.2.2 Radical Prostatectomy

Men with intermediate-risk prostate cancer and long expected survival can be offered with radical prostatectomy as a curative treatment option. Radical prostatectomy offers similar survival outcomes as compared to external beam radiotherapy along with short-term androgen deprivation therapy [29]. The risk of lymph node metastasis ranges from 3.7% to 20.1%, and an extended pelvic lymph node dissection should be performed in patients with >5% risk of lymph node metastasis [30]. Nerve sparing can be offered to those with low risk of extracapsular extension, or an individualized decision can be made based on the magnetic resonance imaging findings. The 20-year biochemical recurrence-free survival and cancer-specific survival in men with favorable and unfavorable intermediate-risk prostate cancer were 65% and 44% and 95% and 89%, respectively [31]. 4.7% and 8.2% in the favorable and unfavorable group required adjuvant radiotherapy, whereas 3.6% and 7.7% required adjuvant hormone therapy [31].

16.2.2.3 Radiotherapy

External beam radiotherapy as IMRT with image guidance is a feasible option in patients with intermediate-risk prostate cancer with long expected survival, as an equally effective alternative. A dose of 76–78 Gy is recommended along with 4–6 months of neoadjuvant or adjuvant androgen deprivation therapy. The 10-year biochemical disease-free survival, distant metastasis-free survival, and cancer-specific survival for intermediate-risk disease after IMRT were 78%, 94%, and 97%, respectively [25].

Brachytherapy either LDR or HDR alone or in combination with external beam radiotherapy is also a feasible option for men without a history of transurethral resection of prostate or severe lower urinary tract symptoms. A recent retrospective comparative study found that LDR brachytherapy monotherapy had superior biochemical relapse-free survival rates and similar metastatic-free and cancer-specific survival rates as compared to radical prostatectomy and external beam radiotherapy [32]. HDR brachytherapy monotherapy has also shown convincing results in men with intermediate-risk prostate cancer, although the available data is limited to specialized centers [27].

16.2.3 High-Risk Localized Prostate Cancer

Men with localized prostate cancer and a Gleason score of 8–10 without comorbidities have a 23.9% chance of death from the cancer within 10 years [5]. Even in men with ≥2 comorbidities, the 10-year cancer-specific mortality is 18.4% [5]. Also, there is a high chance of biochemical relapse, need of additional treatment, progression and death despite treatment. Thus, men with high-risk prostate cancer should be offered upfront treatment with a curative intent in the form of either radical prostatectomy or radiotherapy, provided they understand the possible need for additional treatment.

16.2.3.1 Radical Prostatectomy

Men with high-risk localized prostate cancer can opt for radical prostatectomy along with extended pelvic lymph node dissection, as a part of multimodality approach. A decision to spare the nerves can be made on an individualized basis. There is high chance of downgrading of the Gleason score on the final histopathology report. Forty-five percent of the patients with Gleason scores 8–10 were found to have Gleason score 7 or less on the radical prostatectomy specimen [33]. Patients with clinical stage T1c and Gleason score 8 were more likely to be downgraded as compared to T3 and Gleason score 9, and those who were down graded had superior oncologic outcomes as compared to those who were not [33]. The 10-year overall, cancer-specific, and progression-free survival in men with Gleason scores 8–10 undergoing radical prostatectomy is 67%, 85%, and 36%, respectively [33]. Adjuvant therapy may be required in around 45% of the patients, which may improve the progression-free survival [34].

Few retrospective studies have compared radical prostatectomy and radiotherapy in men with high-risk prostate cancer and found a lower risk of metastatic progression and prostate cancer-specific mortality with radical prostatectomy [35, 36]. However, more contemporary reports suggest a similar 10-year prostate cancer-specific survival (97% in radical prostatectomy vs. 95.9% in radiotherapy), distant metastasis-free survival, and overall survival rates [37]. While choosing between radical prostatectomy and radiotherapy as a part of multimodality treatment plan, there are certain advantages of the surgery-first approach. Radical prostatectomy allows for the complete removal of the prostate and final histopathological analysis, which may lead to downgrading of the stage or the Gleason score. Also, after removal of the prostate, the follow-up with PSA levels becomes relatively simple, and any adjuvant therapy, if required, either in form of radiotherapy or hormone therapy can be delivered safely and timely. On the other hand, salvage treatment, either in the form of radical prostatectomy or focal ablation, after radiotherapy is associated with poor functional outcomes and have high complication rates.

16.2.3.2 Radiotherapy

External beam radiotherapy with a dose of 76–78 Gy in the form of IMRT along with 2–3 years of androgen deprivation therapy can be offered to patients with high-risk prostate cancer. The 10-year biochemical disease-free survival, distant metastasis-free survival, and cancer-specific survival for high-risk disease after IMRT were 62%, 90%, and 86%, respectively [25]. Brachytherapy alone is usually not used in men with high-risk prostate cancer; however, a brachytherapy boost combined with external beam radiotherapy and androgen deprivation therapy can be used in select cases.

16.3 Locally Advanced Prostate Cancer

Patients with T3 and T4 disease, irrespective of the PSA level and Gleason score, are classified as locally advanced prostate cancer. Similar to the patients with high-risk disease, men with locally advanced prostate cancer are also at a high risk of biochemical relapse, need of additional treatment, and progression and death despite treatment. These men should be counselled for the need of multimodal treatment, starting either with radical prostatectomy or radiotherapy.

16.3.1 Radical Prostatectomy

Men with clinically T3 prostate cancer can be offered with radical prostatectomy; however, those with invasion of the pelvic wall or the rectum are deemed unresectable. As in patients with high-risk prostate cancer, there are high chances of downstaging of the disease at the final histopathological report. 27–43% of men undergoing radical prostatectomy for a T3 disease were subsequently downstaged into T2 [38, 39]. The reported 10-year overall survival and cancer-specific survival after radical prostatectomy were 60% and 72%, respectively, whereas the clinical progression, local recurrence, and distant metastasis rates were 69%, 44%, and 50%, respectively [40]. Although a high level of evidence comparing radical prostatectomy and radiotherapy is unavailable, a few retrospective studies have compared radical prostatectomy with radiotherapy in men with locally advanced prostate cancer and have reported superior oncological outcomes with radical prostatectomy [41]. Upfront radical prostatectomy can be offered as a part of multimodality approach to men with locally advanced cancer prostate, provided that they understand that around 50–70% will require some adjuvant treatment in the form of radiotherapy or hormone therapy. Post radical prostatectomy, radiotherapy can be delivered either as adjuvant or as salvage therapy, both of which are found to have similar efficacy [42]. An individualized approach, based on the patient and pathological factors, can be pursued while deciding between adjuvant and salvage radiotherapies, and whenever a salvage treatment is planned, it should be initiated as soon as possible [42].

16.3.2 Radiotherapy

External beam radiotherapy with a dose of 76–78 Gy in the form of IMRT along with 2–3 years of androgen deprivation therapy can be offered to patients with locally advanced prostate cancer. Prophylactic pelvic node irradiation has failed to show a survival benefit and thus is not recommended in men with N0 disease [43]. Those who relapse after radiotherapy can be offered with salvage radical prostatectomy, hormone therapy, or focal ablative procedures, as an individualized approach.

16.4 Alternative Treatment Options

16.4.1 Cryoablation

Cryoablation can be performed as whole gland or focal treatment, either in the primary or salvage settings after both radiotherapy and radical prostatectomy. The procedure involves insertion of cryo-needles into the prostate, under transrectal ultrasound guidance, through which pressurized argon gas is passed and allowed to expand resulting in cooling of the prostate tissues to −40 °C. A double freeze-thaw cycle is advocated with either active thawing, with helium, or with passive thawing.

Long-term studies of cryoablation have reported the 10-year biochemical disease-free survival of 80.56%, 74.16%, and 45.54% for low-, moderate-, and high-risk groups, respectively, and a 10-year negative biopsy rate of 76.96% [44]. High-quality evidence comparing cryoablation to the standard treatment is not yet available; however, a recent retrospective matched pair analysis comparing cryoablation (1942 patients) with radical prostatectomy (5826 patients) concluded that cryoablation had lower cancer-specific survival and overall survival as compared to the radical prostatectomy [45]. On the other hand, the reported adverse event profile is favorable as compared to the radical prostatectomy, with 18% chances of erectile dysfunction and 2–20% chances of urinary incontinence [46]. In view of absence of high-quality evidence supporting cryoablation, it is still considered investigational for the treatment of prostate cancer.

16.4.2 High-Intensity Focused Ultrasonography

High-intensity focused ultrasonography (HIFU) uses focused ultrasonic waves to damage the tumor tissues by mechanical, thermal, and cavitation effects. The temperature in the tissues of interest rises to 65 °C resulting in coagulative necrosis.

Long-term single-arm studies have reported the >5-year biochemical disease-free survival, metastasis-free survival, cancer-specific survival, and overall survival from 48–75%, 78–96%, and 98% to 80–88% [47]. The rates of urinary incontinence, impotence, urinary obstruction, retention, and infection were 10%, 44%, 15%, 11%, and 7%, respectively [46]. A retrospective comparison between HIFU and radical prostatectomy showed higher rates of salvage radiotherapy in the HIFU arm, but the cancer-specific survival and metastasis-free survival were similar [48]. In view of the lack of high-quality evidence, HIFU is considered investigational for the treatment of men with prostate cancer.

16.5 Summary

Majority of the patients diagnosed with prostate cancer belong to localized or locally advanced groups. Life expectancy, presence of comorbidities, and the aggressiveness of the disease play a crucial role in treatment planning. Men with shorter life expectancy are best observed, whereas those with >10 years of life expectancy are suitable candidates for cancer-specific treatment.

Men with low-risk disease have low chances of dying from the cancer and thus are best kept under active surveillance, although radical prostatectomy and radiotherapy are also feasible alternatives provided the patient accepts treatment-related adverse events for a reduction in the progression of the disease, as the long-term survival is similar. Selected patients without or with low-volume Gleason 4 disease can also be kept under active surveillance; however, others should be offered with curative treatment with either radiotherapy or radical prostatectomy. Men with high-risk or locally advanced disease have high chances of biochemical relapse, need of additional treatment and progression, and death despite treatment. These men should be counselled for the need of multimodality treatment, starting either with radical prostatectomy or radiotherapy. Focal ablation therapy, in the form of cryoablation or HIFU, is still considered investigational in view of lack of high-quality evidence and should not be offered as the first-line therapy.

References

1. Jemal A, Siegel R, Xu J, Ward E. Cancer statistics, 2010. CA Cancer J Clin. 2010;60:277–300.
2. Siegel DA, O'Neil ME, Richards TB, Dowling NF, Weir HK. Prostate cancer incidence and survival by stage and race/ethnicity—United States, 2001–2017. MMWR Morb Mortal Wkly Rep. 2020;69:1473–80.
3. Adolfsson J, Tribukait B, Levitt S. The 20-year outcome in patients with well- or moderately differentiated clinically localized prostate cancer diagnosed in the pre-PSA era: the prognostic value of tumour ploidy and comorbidity. Eur Urol. 2007;52:1028–35.
4. Lu-Yao GL, Albertsen PC, Moore DF, Shih W, Lin Y, DiPaola RS, et al. Outcomes of localized prostate cancer following conservative management. JAMA. 2009;302:1202–9.
5. Albertsen PC, Moore DF, Shih Wm Lin Y, Hui L, Lu-Yao GL. Impact of comorbidity on survival among men with localized prostate cancer. J Clin Oncol. 2011;29:1335–41.
6. Wilt TJ, No TN, Langsetmo L, Dham P, Wheeler T, Aronson WL, et al. Radical prostatectomy or observation for clinically localized prostate cancer: extended follow-up of the prostate cancer intervention versus observation trial (PIVOT). Eur Urol. 2020;77:713–24.
7. Hamdy FC, Donovan JL, Lane JA, Mason M, Metcalfe C, Holding P, et al. 10-year outcomes after monitoring, surgery, or radiotherapy for localized prostate cancer. N Engl J Med. 2016;375:1415–24.
8. Tosoian JJ, Mamawala M, Epstien JI, Landis P, Macura KJ, Simopoulos DN, et al. Active surveillance of grade group 1 prostate cancer: long-term outcomes from a large prospective cohort. Eur Urol. 2020;77:675–82.
9. Tosoian JJ, Mamawala M, Epstien JI, Landis P, Wolf S, Trock BJ, et al. Intermediate and longer-term outcomes from a prospective active-surveillance program for favorable-risk prostate cancer. J Clin Oncol. 2015;33:3379–85.
10. Schoots IG, Nieboer D, Giganti F, Moore MC, Bangma CH, Roobol M. Is magnetic resonance imaging-targeted biopsy a useful addition to systematic confirmatory biopsy in men on active surveillance for low-risk prostate cancer? A systematic review and meta-analysis. BJU Int. 2018;122:946–58.
11. Klotz L, Pond G, Loblaw A, Sugar L, Moussa M, Berman D, et al. Randomized study of systematic biopsy versus magnetic resonance imaging and targeted and systematic biopsy in men on active surveillance (ASIST): 2-year postbiopsy follow-up. Eur Urol. 2020;77:311–7.
12. Schoots IG, Moore MC, Rouviere O. Role of MRI in low-risk prostate cancer: finding the wolf in sheep's clothing or the sheep in wolf's clothing? Curr Opin Urol. 2017;27:238–45.
13. Osses DF, Drost FJH, Verbeek JFM, Luiting HB, Leenders GJLH, Bangma CH, et al. Prostate cancer upgrading with serial prostate magnetic resonance imaging and repeat biopsy in men on active surveillance: are confirmatory biopsies still necessary? BJU Int. 2020;126:124–32.
14. Chesnut GT, Vertosick EA, Benfante N, Sjoberg DD, Fainberg J, Lee T, et al. Role of changes in magnetic resonance imaging or clinical stage in evaluation of disease progression for men with prostate cancer on active surveillance. Eur Urol. 2020;77:501–7.
15. Lam TBL, MacLennan S, Willemse PPM, Mason MD, Plass K, Sheperd R, Baanders R, et al. EAU-EANM-ESTRO-ESUR-SIOG prostate cancer guideline panel consensus statements for deferred treatment with curative intent for localised prostate cancer from an international collaborative study (DETECTIVE study). Eur Urol. 2019;76:790–813.
16. Ilic D, Evans SM, Allan CA, Jung JH, Murphy D, Frydenberg M. Laparoscopic and robotic-assisted versus open radical prostatectomy for the treatment of localised prostate cancer. Cochrane Database Syst Rev. 2017;9:CD009625.
17. Rosenberg JE, Jung JH, Edgerton Z, Lee H, Lee S, Bakker CJ, et al. Retzius-sparing versus standard robotic-assisted laparoscopic prostatectomy for the treatment of clinically localized prostate cancer. Cochrane Database Syst Rev. 2020;8:CD013641.
18. Cimino S, Reale G, Castelli T, Favilla V, Giardina R, Russo GI, et al. Comparison between Briganti, Partin and MSKCC tools in predicting positive lymph nodes

in prostate cancer: a systematic review and meta-analysis. Scand J Urol. 2017;51:345–50.
19. Fossati N, Willemse PPM, Van den Broeck T, van den Bergh RCN, Yuan CY, Briers E, et al. The benefits and harms of different extents of lymph node dissection during radical prostatectomy for prostate cancer: a systematic review. Eur Urol. 2017;72:84–109.
20. Carlsson S, Jaderling F, Wallerstedt A, Nyberg T, Stranne J, Thorsteinsdottir T, et al. Oncological and functional outcomes 1 year after radical prostatectomy for very-low-risk prostate cancer: results from the prospective LAPPRO trial. BJU Int. 2016;118:205–12.
21. Affenberg GB, Linsell S, Dhir A, Myers SN, Rosenberg B, Miller DC, et al. Comparison of pathological outcomes for men with low risk prostate cancer from diverse practice settings: similar results from immediate prostatectomy or initial surveillance with delayed prostatectomy. J Urol. 2016;196:1415–21.
22. Yu T, Zhang Q, Zheng T, Shi H, Liu Y, Feng S, et al. The effectiveness of intensity modulated radiation therapy versus three-dimensional radiation therapy in prostate cancer: a meta-analysis of the literatures. PLoS One. 2016;11:e0154499.
23. Hickey BE, Lames ML, Daly T, Soh FY, Jeffery M. Hypofractionation for clinically localized prostate cancer. Cochrane Database Syst Rev. 2019;9:CD011462.
24. Widmark A, Gunnlaugsson A, Beckman L, Thellenberg-karlsson C, Hoyer M, Lagerlund M, et al. Ultra-hypofractionated versus conventionally fractionated radiotherapy for prostate cancer: 5-year outcomes of the HYPO-RT-PC randomised, non-inferiority, phase 3 trial. Lancet. 2019;394:385–95.
25. Alicikus ZA, Yamada Y, Zhang Z, Pei X, Hunt M, Kollmeier M, et al. Ten-year outcomes of high dose, intensity modulated radiotherapy for localised prostate cancer. Cancer. 2011;117:1429–37.
26. Potters L, Morgenstern C, Calugaru E, Fearn P, Jassal A, Presser J, et al. 12-year outcomes following permanent prostate brachytherapy in patients with clinically localized prostate cancer. J Urol. 2005;173:1562–6.
27. Zamboglou N, Tselis N, Baltas D, Buhleier T, Martin T, Milickovic N, et al. High-dose-rate interstitial brachytherapy as monotherapy for clinically localized prostate cancer: treatment evolution and mature results. Int J Radiat Oncol Biol Phys. 2013;85:672–8.
28. Musunuru HB, Yamamoto T, Koltz L, Ghanem G, Mamedov A, Sethukavalan P, et al. Active surveillance for intermediate risk prostate cancer: survival outcomes in the Sunnybrook experience. J Urol. 2016;196:1651–8.
29. Sebastian NT, McElroy JP, Martin DD, Sundi D, Diaz DA. Survival after radiotherapy vs. radical prostatectomy for unfavorable intermediate-risk prostate cancer. Urol Oncol. 2019;37:813e11–9.
30. Studer UE, Collette L, Whelan P, Albrecht W, Casselman J, de Reijke T, et al. Using PSA to guide timing of androgen deprivation in patients with T0-4 N0-2 M0 prostate cancer not suitable for local curative treatment (EORTC 30891). Eur Urol. 2008;53:941–9.
31. Meissner VH, Woll M, Ankerst DP, Schiele S, Gschwend JE, Herkommer K. Long term and pathological outcomes of low and intermediate risk prostate cancer after radical prostatectomy: implications for active surveillance. World J Urol. 2021;39:3763–70.
32. Goy BW, Burchette R, Soper MS, Chang T, Cosmatos HA. Ten-year treatment outcomes of radical prostatectomy vs. external beam radiation therapy vs. brachytherapy for 1503 patients with intermediate-risk prostate cancer. Urology. 2020;136:180–9.
33. Donohue JF, Bicano FJ Jr, Kuroiwa K, Vickers AJ, Wheeler TM, Scardino PT, et al. Poorly differentiated prostate cancer treated with radical prostatectomy: long-term outcome and incidence of pathological downgrading. J Urol. 2006;176:991–5.
34. Wk L, Bergstralh EJ, Blute ML, Slezak JM, Zincke H. Radical prostatectomy for pathological Gleason 8 or greater prostate cancer: influence of concomitant pathological variables. J Urol. 2002;167:117–22.
35. Zelefsky MJ, Eastham JA, Cronin AM, Fuks Z, Zhang Z, Yamada Y, et al. Metastasis after radical prostatectomy or external beam radiotherapy for patients with clinically localized prostate cancer: a comparison of clinical cohorts adjusted for case mix. J Clin Oncol. 2010;28:1508–13.
36. Abdollah F, Sun M, Thuret R, Jeldres C, Tian Z, Briganti A, et al. A competing-risks analysis of survival after alternative treatment modalities for prostate cancer patients: 1988–2006. Eur Urol. 2011;59:88–95.
37. Chun SK, Kim JH, Ku JH, Kwak C, Lee ES, Kim S. Comparison of radical prostatectomy and external beam radiotherapy in high-risk prostate cancer. Radiat Oncol J. 2021;39:231–8.
38. Van Poppel H. Surgery for clinical T3 prostate cancer. Eur Urol Suppl. 2005;4:12–4.
39. Van Poppel H, Goethuys H, Callewaert P, Vanuytsel L, Van de Voorde W, Baert L. Radical prostatectomy can provide a cure for well-selected clinical stage T3 prostate cancer. Eur Urol. 2000;38:372–9.
40. van den Ouden D, Hop WC, Schroder FH. Progression in and survival of patients with locally advanced prostate cancer (T3) treated with radical prostatectomy as monotherapy. J Urol. 1998;160:1392–7.
41. Zhou X, Jin K, Qui S, Jin D, Liao X, Zheng X, et al. Comparing effectiveness of radical prostatectomy versus external beam radiotherapy in patients with locally advanced prostate cancer: a population based analysis. Medicine. 2020;99:e21642.
42. Parker CC, Clarke NW, Cook AD, Kynaston HG, Petersen PM, Catton C, et al. Timing of radiotherapy after radical prostatectomy (RADICALS-RT): a randomised, controlled phase 3 trial. Lancet. 2020;396:1413–21.
43. Pommier P, Chabaud S, Lagrange JL, Richaud P, Lesaunier F, Prise EL, et al. Is there a role for pelvic irradiation in localized prostate adenocarcinoma? Preliminary results of GETUG-01. J Clin Oncol. 2007;25:5366–73.

44. Cohen JK, Miller RJ Jr, Ahmed S, Lotz MJ, Baust J. Ten-year biochemical disease control for patients with prostate cancer treated with cryosurgery as primary therapy. Urology. 2008;71:515–8.
45. Guo X, Liu S, Wang M, Hou H, Wang X, Zhang Z, et al. Comparing the oncological outcomes of Cryoablation vs. radical prostatectomy in low-intermediate risk localized prostate cancer. Front Oncol. 2020;10:1489.
46. Ramsay CR, Adewuyi TE, Gray J, Hislop J, Shirley MDF, Jayakody S, et al. Ablative therapy for people with localised prostate cancer: a systematic review and economic evaluation. Health Technol Assess. 2015;19:1–490.
47. He Y, Tan P, He M, Hu L, Ai J, et al. The primary treatment of prostate cancer with high frequency focussed ultrasound: a systematic review and meta-analysis. Medicine. 2020;99:e22601.
48. Gelet A, Crouzet S, Rouviere O, Chapelon JY, Rabilloud M. Radical prostatectomy versus high intensity focused ultrasound for localized prostate cancer: a matched pair comparison. J Ther Ultrasound. 2015;3:O56.

Metastatic Prostate Cancer

17

Sindhu Chitikela, Shuvadeep Ganguly, and Atul Batra

17.1 Introduction

Prostate cancer is the second most common cancer in men worldwide [1]. Risk of prostate cancer increases with age and about 85% of patients are aged >60 years. Its occurrence is more common in the developed countries. It is known to be strongly associated with family history, with up to 9% of patients with a significant family history [2]. Germline mutations involving DNA repair pathway genes have been studied in the pathogenesis of prostate cancer. These include BRCA1, ATM, PALB2, RAD51D, CHEK2, and mismatch repair genes.

Approximately 72% of men are diagnosed at an early stage with disease confined to prostate, 11% with locoregional disease, and 7% with distant metastases [3]. Metastasis of prostate is by either lymphatic spread to locoregional lymph nodes or by hematogenous spread to the bone, bone marrow, and rarely visceral organs. The most common site of metastases in prostate cancer is the bone, predominantly in the axial skeleton, and bone metastases are observed in >80% patients of metastatic prostate cancer. Metastatic prostate cancer is associated with poor outcomes with a 5-year overall survival of 30%. Current treatment options for metastatic prostate cancer include androgen deprivation therapy, chemotherapy, androgen signaling inhibitors, radioligands, PARP inhibitors, and immunotherapy (Fig. 17.1).

Metastatic prostate cancer encompasses a range of advanced diseases that includes the following:

- De novo metastatic castration-sensitive prostate cancer (mCSPC)
- Metastatic castration-resistant prostate cancer (mCRPC) that progressed during or after ADT, with serum testosterone <50 ng/dL (castrate level)

17.2 Androgen Deprivation Therapy (ADT)

The critical role of androgens in the pathogenesis of prostate cancer was identified by Charles Huggins in 1941 [4]. This discovery led to the development of androgen deprivation therapy (ADT) as the prime modality for the treatment of advanced prostate cancer. ADT with surgical orchidectomy or systemic LHRH agonists or antagonists has been the standard of care. ADT was shown to normalize serum PSA (prostate-specific antigen) levels in up to 90% of patients,

S. Chitikela · S. Ganguly · A. Batra (✉)
Department of Medical Oncology, DR.B.R.A. Institute Rotary Cancer Hospital, All India Institute of Medical Sciences (AIIMS), New Delhi, India
e-mail: batraatul85@aiims.edu

P. Singh et al. (eds.), *A Guide to Management of Urological Cancers*,
https://doi.org/10.1007/978-981-99-2341-0_17

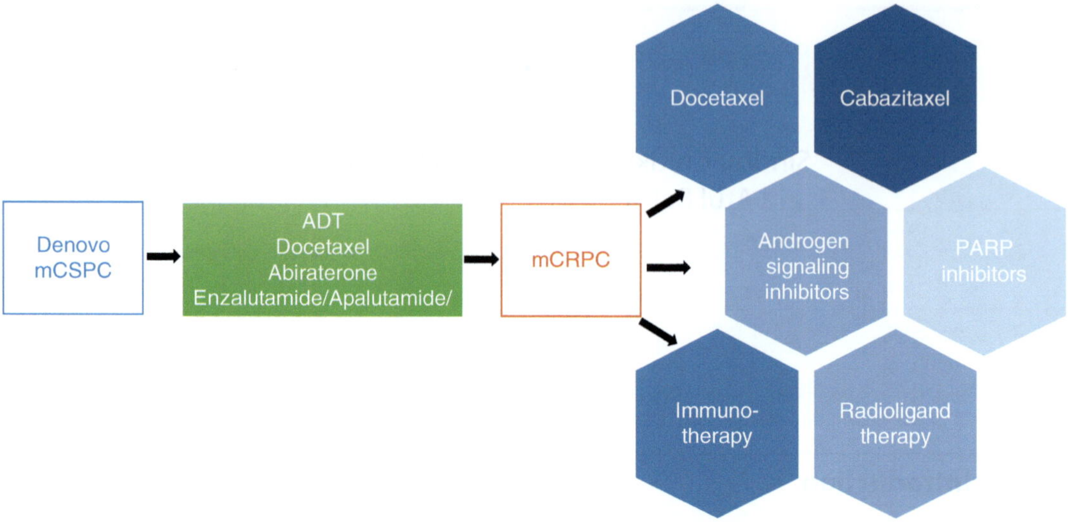

Fig. 17.1 Therapeutic landscape for the management of metastatic prostate cancer

with an objective response rates of 80–90%, and improve symptoms and quality of life.

ADT is the mainstay modality for the management of metastatic prostate cancer. It can be accomplished by surgical castration (bilateral orchiectomy) or by medical castration using either gonadotropin-releasing hormone (GnRH) agonists or antagonists with an aim to lower the serum testosterone level to <50 ng/dL. In a meta-analysis of ten trials that compared bilateral orchiectomy with GnRH agonists, both the modalities have shown to result in comparable outcomes [5].

17.2.1 Surgical Castration

Bilateral orchiectomy is a simpler and a cost-effective mode of ADT. It results in a rapid decline of serum testosterone levels to castrate levels and the resultant faster symptomatic improvement. It carries lower costs and less number of hospital visits and omits from constant adherence to injections for medical castration. However, it has been associated with negative psychosocial impact and effects from irreversible castration.

17.2.2 Medical Castration

This includes administration of either GnRH agonists or antagonists.

17.2.2.1 GnRH Agonists

They bind to GnRH receptors on gonadotropin cells of anterior pituitary, causing an initial release of LH and FSH thereby increasing testosterone production from testicular Leydig cells. After a duration of 1–2 weeks, GnRH receptors on pituitary are downregulated because of negative feedback mechanism resulting in decline in LH and FSH secretion and thereby reducing the levels of testosterone to castrate levels by 3–4 weeks. It requires continued administration for continued suppression of testosterone and to maintain castrate levels. The initial transient rise in LH and testosterone is responsible for the flare phenomenon that occurs as a result of the use of GnRH agonists. This may result in an initial increase in pain, spinal cord compression, and worsening of bladder obstructive symptoms. Hence antiandrogens that block the effect of testosterone are administered along with GnRH agonists for the initial 2–3 weeks of therapy to achieve combined androgen blockade and prevent disease flare.

Doses of GnRH agonists are as follows:

- Leuprolide 7.5 mg monthly or 22.5 mg 3 monthly intramuscular
- Goserelin 3.6 mg every 4 weeks or 10.8 mg every 12 weeks subcutaneous implant
- Triptorelin 3.75 mg every 4 weeks or 11.25 mg every 12 weeks or 22.5 mg every 24 weeks

17.2.2.2 GnRH Antagonists

They bind to GnRH receptors on pituitary gonadotropin-secreting cells and directly inhibit the production of LH and FSH, thereby leading to a relatively rapid decline in serum testosterone level and thereby avoiding the flare phenomenon. When compared to GnRH agonists, GnRH antagonists like degarelix result in a rapid decline in testosterone levels and have shown to result in better progression-free and overall survival.

The downside of using GnRH antagonists is that it requires frequent administration of subcutaneous injections and a higher risk of injection site reactions compared to GnRH agonists. Relugolix is an oral, highly selective GnRH antagonist that is recently approved for use in patients with advanced prostate cancer.

Doses and schedule of GnRH antagonists that can be used are the following:

- Degarelix 240 mg s.c loading dose administered as two 120 mg injections, followed by a maintenance dose of 80 mg s.c every 28 days beginning 28 days after the loading dose
- Relugolix 360 mg on day 1 followed by 120 mg once daily

In a phase III trial of prostate cancer that compared efficacy of degarelix to leuprolide, it was shown that degarelix suppressed testosterone within 3 days and lower incidence of PSA failure (7.7% vs. 12.9%); however, it carried higher risk of injection site reactions (40% vs. 1%) [6]. Two meta-analyses of randomized trials that compared GnRH agonists with antagonists showed that survival outcomes and cardiovascular events were better with degarelix compared to GnRH agonists [7, 8].

Relugolix was evaluated in a phase II HERO study, with comparator arm being leuprolide. It was shown that relugolix resulted in a rapid suppression of testosterone levels with castrate levels attained by day 4 in 56% of patients in relugolix arm versus none in the leuprolide arm. Relugolix also resulted in more consistent medical castration compared to leuprolide (96.7% vs. 88.8%). Major cardiovascular events occurred in 2.9% patients in relugolix arm versus 6.2% of patients in leuprolide arm [9].

GnRH antagonists are preferred in patients with high disease burden, with impending spinal cord compression/pathological fracture.

For patients with symptomatic metastatic prostate cancer, prompt initiation of ADT is recommended to palliate symptoms and prevent bone-related complications. Early ADT versus delayed ADT have been studied in patients with asymptomatic metastatic disease with better treatment-related outcomes in patients started on early ADT. Side effects of ADT include decreased bone mineral density, cardiovascular disease, cognitive dysfunction, and sexual dysfunction.

In addition to androgen production by testes and adrenal gland, it has been studied that several enzymes involved in the androgen synthesis are overexpressed in tumor tissue. With this understanding, various drugs targeting the androgen pathway have been identified and added to the therapeutic armamentarium of prostate cancer.

17.3 Metastatic Castration-Sensitive Prostate Cancer

This category includes patients with newly diagnosed prostate cancer with upfront metastasis or those who develop metastasis after treatment of local prostate primary with or without ADT, when serum testosterone level is more than 50 ng/dL.

Initially ADT was used as monotherapy in treatment of advanced castration-sensitive prostate cancer. However, with the development of effective therapies targeting androgen signaling pathways for treatment of advanced prostate cancer such as abiraterone, docetaxel, enzalutamide, and darolutamide, these agents are now recommended for the front line in combination with ADT for the treatment of CSPC. Randomized trials have shown the benefit of adding docetaxel and androgen signaling inhibitors to ADT. These trials defined different risk categories depending on the burden of the disease as the following:

- *High-volume disease, based upon CHAARTED study*: The presence of visceral metastases or four/more bone metastases with at least one outside the vertebral column and the pelvis [10]
- *High-risk disease, based upon LATITUDE study*: The presence of two out of three factors from a Gleason score of ≥8, the presence of three/more bone metastases, or the presence of visceral metastases

Patients are followed up clinically for any new symptoms or signs of disease progression. Serum PSA is monitored every 3 months. Radiological investigations that include PSMA PET CT or MRI are advised in case of elevated PSA or development of new symptoms.

Various therapeutic options for the treatment of metastatic CSPC include the following (summarized in Table 17.1):

17.3.1 Docetaxel with ADT

Docetaxel with ADT was evaluated in three open-label randomized controlled trials, CHAARTED, STAMPEDE, and GETUG AFU [10–12].

In the CHAARTED trial, it was shown that docetaxel (75 mg per m^2 3 weekly for 6 cycles) had resulted in a significantly longer OS 57.6 versus 47.2 months (HR 0.72), specifically in patients with high-volume disease 51.2 versus 34.4 months, HR 0.63, not in the subgroup with low-volume disease (HR 1.04). Docetaxel plus ADT arm resulted in a longer median time to biochemical, radiographic, or symptomatic progression of 20.2 versus 11.7 months in ADT-alone arm (HR 0.61). In docetaxel arm, 6.2% patients had febrile neutropenia [10].

In the STAMPEDE trial, which is a multi-arm, multi-stage randomized trial that evaluated various therapies including docetaxel (75 mg per m^2 3 weekly for 6 cycles with prednisolone 10 mg daily), the use of docetaxel resulted in better OS compared to ADT, 81 versus 71 months (HR 0.78), and was associated with a higher risk of adverse events with grade 3/grade 4 toxicities in up to 52% patients [11].

GETUG-AFU15 in which nine cycles of docetaxel were allowed had resulted in better biochemical PFS and radiological PFS; however, it has not shown any improvement in overall survival with the use of docetaxel [12]. There was no additional benefit as a result of addition of zoledronic acid.

Cochrane meta-analysis of all the three trials of docetaxel with ADT with 2261 patients had shown to reduce the risk of prostate cancer-specific death by 33%, reduce risk of disease progression, and improve OS regardless of disease burden. Docetaxel carries a higher risk of toxicities and treatment discontinuation (20% vs. 0%) [13].

17.3.2 Abiraterone with ADT

Addition of abiraterone to ADT has demonstrated an increase in OS in two phase III randomized trials LATITUDE and STAMPEDE.

Abiraterone is a cytochrome p450 17A1 (CYP17A1) inhibitor and blocks the activity of enzymes 17-alpha-hydroxylase and 17, 20-lyase, thereby inhibiting androgen synthesis. It decreases the adrenal and intra-tumoral steroid synthesis and increases upstream steroid precursors that can result in symptoms of mineralocorticoid excess such as edema, hypertension, and hypokalemia. Hence, abiraterone has to be administered along with glucocorticoids. Dose of abiraterone is 1000 mg orally on an empty stomach with prednisolone 5 mg daily. In LATITUDE trial, 1199 males with high-risk metastatic castration-sensitive prostate cancer were randomized to abiraterone-prednisolone plus ADT versus ADT alone. Abiraterone arm had resulted in a significantly increased OS of 53.3 versus

Table 17.1 Treatment options for mCSPC

	n	Intervention arm	Control arm	rPFS	mOS
LATITUDE	1199	Abiraterone prednisolone + ADT	ADT	33 vs. 14.8 months (0.47)	53.3 vs. 36.5 months (0.66)
STAMPEDE	1917	Abiraterone prednisolone + ADT	ADT	3 years FFS 75% vs. 45% (0.29)	3 years OS 83% vs. 76% (0.63)
ENZAMET	1125	Enzalutamide + ADT	Nonsteroidal antiandrogens + ADT	3 years 68% vs. 41% (HR 0.4)	5 years OS 67% vs. 57% (0.70)
ARCHES	1150	Enzalutamide plus ADT	ADT	49.8 vs. 38.9 months (0.63)	NR: 4 years OS 71% vs. 57% (0.66)
TITAN	1052	Apalutamide + ADT	Placebo + ADT	2 years 68.2% vs. 47.5% (0.48)	4 years 65% vs. 52% (0.65)
STAMPEDE	1086	Docetaxel plus ADT	ADT	FFS 44.2 vs. 34.8 months	81 vs. 71 months (0.78)
CHAARTED	790	Docetaxel + ADT	ADT	20.2 vs. 11.7 months (0.61)	57.6 vs. 47.2 months (0.72)
ARASENS	1306	Darolutamide + docetaxel + ADT	Docetaxel + ADT + placebo	NA	4 years 62.7% vs. 50.4% (0.68)
PEACE1	1172	Abiraterone + docetaxel + ADT	Docetaxel + ADT	4.46 vs. 2.22 years (0.54)	5.72 vs. 4.72 years (0.82)

36.5 months (HR 0.66). It also resulted in a better time to pain progression, PSA progression, time to skeletal event, and time to subsequent therapy and chemotherapy initiation. The most common serious adverse events (grade 3/grade 4) are hypertension in 21% and hypokalemia in 12% [14, 15].

In STAMPEDE trial, 1917 males were randomized to abiraterone-prednisolone plus ADT versus ADT alone. This trial included newly diagnosed advanced prostate cancer and recurrent cases. Abiraterone arm has resulted in increased OS (3 years OS 83% vs. 76%, HR 0.63) and failure-free survival (3 years FFS 75% vs. 45% with ADT alone, HR 0.29). The benefit was seen irrespective of the risk stratification unlike in LATITUDE trial which recruited only patients with high-risk disease [16]. Abiraterone 250 mg per day given with a low fat meal showed similar pharmacodynamics and resulted in a similar PSA response and PFS and was found to be non-inferior compared to the usual dose in a phase II study of castration-resistant prostate cancer [17].

17.3.3 Second-Generation Antiandrogens with ADT

Enzalutamide, apalutamide, and darolutamide are androgen receptor inhibitors that act by binding to the androgen binding site. Enzalutamide plus ADT was evaluated in two phase III randomized trials: ENZAMET and ARCHES.

In ENZAMET trial, patients of mCSPC were assigned to ADT plus enzalutamide or first-generation antiandrogens like bicalutamide, nilutamide, or flutamide. Around 45% of patients received docetaxel in either arm. Enzalutamide plus ADT had resulted in a better OS (5 years OS 67% vs. 57%, HR 0.70), and this benefit was not seen in patients who received docetaxel. The specific side effects include seizures seen in up to 1% of patients receiving enzalutamide and falls [18].

Enzalutamide plus ADT was also evaluated in a placebo-controlled phase III ARCHES trial. Combined therapy was associated with a better radiologic PFS 49.8 versus 38.9 months with ADT alone (HR 0.63). It also resulted in increased median time to subsequent therapy which was not reached in combined therapy arm versus 40.5 months with ADT alone (0.38). Median OS was not reached in either arms; however, it reached 4 years. OS was significantly better with enzalutamide plus ADT 71% versus 57% (HR 0.66) [19–21].

Apalutamide plus ADT was evaluated in a phase III randomized TITAN trial. Apalutamide plus ADT resulted in an increased 4-year OS 65% versus 52% and median OS not reached versus 52.5 months, HR 0.65. Risk of central nervous system toxicity is lower with apalutamide. Combination therapy was also favored in terms of radiologic PFS, time to first skeletal event, and time to PSA progression compared to ADT alone [22].

For patients with metastatic castration-sensitive prostate cancer, doublet therapy with ADT and docetaxel/abiraterone/second-generation antiandrogens is the preferred regimen. There are limited data directly comparing different combinations. Network meta-analyses were done to compare various combined modalities with varied results. One-network meta-analyses have shown superiority of enzalutamide over docetaxel in low-volume disease with no difference with other drugs. It was consistently proved in the network meta-analyses that docetaxel carried higher risk of adverse events compared to enzalutamide/apalutamide/abiraterone, without any additional survival benefit [23–25]. Given the lack of head-to-head comparison, the appropriate regimen is chosen taking into consideration various factors like patient profile, potential toxicities, availability of drugs, and cost issues.

Recent most updates stem from the use of triplet therapy in the treatment of mCSPC. Two trials have demonstrated OS benefit with the use of ADT with docetaxel plus androgen signaling inhibitor in mCSPC. In ARASENS trial, addition of darolutamide to ADT plus docetaxel has shown an increase in OS with 4-year OS of 62.7% versus 50.4% in ADT plus docetaxel arm (HR 0.68). Triplet therapy also resulted in increased time to castration resistance, time to subsequent anti-neoplastic therapy, time to pain progression, and time to symptomatic skeletal event.

PEACE-1 trial, a phase III trial, evaluated role of addition of abiraterone-prednisolone and/or local RT along with standard of care that is ADT plus docetaxel. Addition of abiraterone to docetaxel plus ADT has resulted in a significantly increased radiologic PFS and OS and median OS not reached versus 4.4 years (HR 0.75) compared to ADT plus docetaxel. Toxicity profile was similar in both the arms except for hepatotoxicity (6% vs. 1%) and hypertension (21% vs. 13%) which were higher in the abiraterone arm [26].

17.4 Metastatic Castration-Resistant Prostate Cancer

Patients with disease progression, clinical or biochemical in the form of rising serum PSA while on ADT and serum testosterone levels in the castrate range (<50 ng/dL), are considered to have castration-resistant prostate cancer. CRPC includes patients with disease progression locoregionally or at metastatic sites or may just be limited to a PSA rise without any obvious radiological progression. Patients in whom the only manifestation of disease progression is a rise in serum PSA without any demonstrable radiologic disease are considered to have nonmetastatic or M0 CRPC. This chapter is limited to metastatic CRPC. Despite high initial response rates to ADT, eventually all patients develop progressive CRPC following ADT. In case of suspected disease progression, imaging with CECT chest abdomen pelvis with bone scan or PSMA PET has to be performed.

Treatment options for metastatic CRPC include (summarized in Tables 17.2 and 17.3) the following:

- Androgen synthesis inhibitor—abiraterone
- Androgen receptor inhibitors—enzalutamide, apalutamide, and darolutamide
- Taxane chemotherapy—docetaxel and cabazitaxel
- Radioisotope therapy—radium 223 for bone-only disease and Lu 177 PSMA-617 PRRT
- PARP inhibitors in patients with patients with germline or somatic DNA mismatch repair genes or homologous recombination repair deficiency
- Immune checkpoint inhibitors in patients with tumors with dMMR/MSI-high or PDL1 overexpression
- Sipuleucel-T and dendritic cell vaccine

Choice of therapy depends on prior systemic therapy, disease burden, tempo of disease progression, patient factors like symptom burden, performance status, and preference for oral or intravenous therapy.

ADT has to be continued in patients with CRPC even after disease progression to maintain castrate levels of testosterone. Discontinuation of GnRH agonists can lead to an increase in testosterone levels over a period of time and can result in disease progression. Hence continuation of ADT is recommended. Temporary stoppage of ADT can be considered if necessary, with stringent monitoring for serum testosterone levels with prompt reinitiation of ADT with rise in serum testosterone levels.

Mitoxantrone with prednisolone was the first therapeutic agent approved for the treatment of metastatic CRPC; however, it has now become obsolete due to approval of various other effective therapies. Currently, approved chemotherapeutic agents for the treatment of mCRPC include docetaxel and cabazitaxel.

17.4.1 Docetaxel

Docetaxel was the first agent that has shown to provide survival benefit in metastatic CRPC. TAX-372 trial compared docetaxel (75 mg/m^2 3 weekly/30 mg/m^2 weekly) to mitoxantrone (12 mg/m^2 3 weekly), with predniso-

Table 17.2 Treatment options for mCRPC

	n	Intervention arm	Control arm	rPFS	mOS
TAX-372	1006	Docetaxel 3 weekly	Mitoxantrone	NA	18.9 vs. 17.4 vs. 16.5 months (0.62)
		Docetaxel weekly			
TROPIC (post-docetaxel)	755	Cabazitaxel + prednisolone	Mitoxantrone + prednisolone	2.8 vs. 1.4	15.1 vs. 12.7 months (0.70)
CARD (post-docetaxel)	255	Cabazitaxel + prednisolone	Abiraterone/enzalutamide	4.4 vs. 2.7 months (0.52)	13.6 vs. 11 months (0.64)
PROSELICA (post docetaxel)	1200	Cabazitaxel 20 mg/m^2	Cabazitaxel 25 mg/m^2	2.9 vs. 3.5 months (1.099)	13.4 vs. 14.5 months (1.024)
COU AA 301 (post docetaxel)	1195	Abiraterone + prednisolone	Placebo + prednisolone	5.6 vs. 3.6 months (0.66)	15.8 vs. 11.2 months (0.74)
COU AA 302	1088	Abiraterone + prednisolone	Placebo + prednisolone	16.5 vs. 8.3 months (0.53)	34.7 vs. 30.3 months (0.81)
AFFIRM (post docetaxel)	1199	Enzalutamide	Placebo	8.3 vs. 2.9 months (0.40)	18.4 vs. 13.6 months (0.63)
PREVAIL	1717	Enzalutamide	Placebo	20 vs. 5.4 months (0.32)	35.5 vs. 31.4 months (0.83)

Table 17.3 PARP inhibitors and ligand therapies approved for treatment of mCRPC

	n	Intervention arm	Control arm	m rPFS (HR)	mOS (HR)
PROFOUND	387	Olaparib	Abiraterone/enzalutamide	Cohort A: 7.6 vs. 3.6 months (0.36)	Cohort A: 19.1 vs. 14.7 months (0.69)
		Cohort A BRCA/ATM		Cohort B:4.8 vs. 3.3 months (0.88)	Cohort B: 14.7 vs. 11.5 months (0.96)
		Cohort B other HRR		Overall: 6.2 vs. 3.5 months (0.51)	Overall: 17.5 vs. 14.3 months (0.67)
TRITON	115	Rucaparib (BRCA 1/2)	NA (single arm phase 2)	9 months	1 year 73%
VISION	831	177 Lu-PSMA 617 + standard of care	Standard of care (excluded chemotherapy, immunotherapy, and radium 223)	8.7 vs. 3.4 months (0.40)	15.3 vs. 11.3 months (0.62)
ALSYMPCA	921	Radium 223 + best supportive care	Placebo + best supportive care	NA	14.9 vs. 11.3 months (0.70)

lone 5 mg in all arms. Median OS was longer in patients treated with docetaxel regimens compared to mitoxantrone (19.2 vs. 17.8 and 16.3 months). Docetaxel resulted in higher PSA response rates in men with mCRPC. Grade 3 or 4 neutropenia was reported to be highest in the docetaxel 3 weekly arm 32% versus 2% in weekly docetaxel arm versus 22% in mitoxantrone arm (PMID 18182665).

In order to minimize the toxicity of 3 weekly docetaxel, an alternative regimen on docetaxel 50 mg/m^2 2 weekly was compared to the original regimen in a phase III trial. This trial reported an increased overall survival (19.5 vs. 17 months) and lesser neutropenia (53% vs. 36%) with 2 weekly regimen making this an alternative regimen for patients in whom toxicity is a concern [27].

17.4.2 Cabazitaxel

Docetaxel was compared to cabazitaxel in first-line treatment setting of mCRPC. A phase III FIRSTANA trial was conducted with patients randomly assigned to one of the three arms, cabazitaxel 20 mg/m^2, cabazitaxel 25 mg/m^2, or docetaxel 75 mg/m^2 3 weekly with prednisolone. Median OS was similar between all the three arms (24.5 vs. 25.2 and 24.3 months). Incidence of grade 3 or 4 toxicity was higher with cabazitaxel 25 mg/m^2 followed by docetaxel arm, and febrile neutropenia was least common in cabazitaxel 20 mg/m^2 dose. Hence, cabazitaxel 20 mg/m^2 can be considered as an option for treatment of patients at higher risk of neutropenia [28].

Cabazitaxel (25 mg/m^2) was compared to mitoxantrone (12 mg/m^2) 3 weekly in patients progressing on docetaxel, with prednisolone 10 mg in both arms in phase III TROPIC trial. Cabazitaxel resulted in an increased OS compared to mitoxantrone (15.1 vs. 12.7 months, HR 0.70) and increased PFS (2.8 vs. 1.4 months, HR 0.74) but with a higher toxicity, with grade 3 or 4 neutropenia in 82% patients [29].

Cabazitaxel was compared to androgen signaling inhibitors (abiraterone or enzalutamide) in third-line setting treatment on mCRPC previously treated with docetaxel or progressed on abiraterone or enzalutamide within 12 months in phase III CARD trial. Cabazitaxel improved response rates (37% vs. 12%), OS (13.6 vs. 11 months), and PSA response and led to better pain response rates and fewer symptomatic skeletal events [30].

Phase III PROSELICA trial also confirmed the non-inferiority of cabazitaxel 20–25 mg/m^2 in later-line setting with lesser toxicity [31].

17.4.3 Abiraterone

Abiraterone/prednisolone was evaluated in phase III trials with activity demonstrated in both chemotherapy naive patients and in those exposed to docetaxel. In COU-AA-301 trial, 1195 patients who received docetaxel chemotherapy and abiraterone/prednisolone was compared to placebo plus prednisolone. Abiraterone has led to a significantly increased OS compared to placebo, 15.8 vs. 11.2 months, HR 0.74. Abiraterone also resulted in increased time to PSA progression, radiologic PFS, and time to first skeletal-related event [32, 33]. In chemotherapy naive setting, abiraterone resulted in better OS and other disease-related outcomes compared to placebo in COU-AA-302 trial [34–36]. In both the trials of mCRPC, dose of prednisolone administered was 5 mg BD. However, it has been shown that abiraterone has a minimal activity in patients progressing on enzalutamide [30, 37].

Enzalutamide was evaluated in phase III trials with proven efficacy in both chemotherapy naive and post-docetaxel setting. In phase III AFFIRM trial, post docetaxel which also included heavily pretreated population and enzalutamide resulted in an increased OS (18.4 vs. 13.6 months) with benefit in response rates, PSA response, radiographic PFS, and time to first symptomatic skeletal events. Enzalutamide resulted in a higher incidence of diarrhea, fatigue, musculoskeletal pain, and seizures compared to placebo [38, 39]. In the phase III PREVAIL trial, in patients not exposed to docetaxel, enzalutamide had shown an increased OS (35.3 vs. 31.3 months, HR 0.77) [40, 41]. On comparison with bicalutamide, enzalutamide improved outcomes in CRPC.

17.4.4 Germline or Somatic Homologous Recombination Repair Deficiency

All patients with metastatic prostate cancer should undergo somatic/tumor and germline molecular testing to identify mutations involving various DNA repair pathways to identify potential molecular targets. PARP inhibitors are a treatment option for mCRPC refractory to androgen signaling inhibitors and taxanes. Testing can be done by next-generation sequencing using different samples as the following:

- Archival or primary tumor tissue
- Biopsy from metastatic site
- Blood and saliva for germline testing
- Circulating tumor DNA

Homologous recombination repair (HRR)-deficient tumors are known to be sensitive to platinum-based chemotherapy and PARP inhibitors. PARP inhibitors act by synthetic lethality. The various genes implicated in homologous recombination repair-deficient prostate cancer include BRCA1, BRCA2, PALB2, ATM, RAD 51D, CHEK2, BRIP1, FANCA, etc. In a study of 692 men with metastatic prostate cancer, unselected for family history or age, germline DNA repair gene mutations were found in 11.8%, with BRCA2 accounting for 5.3%, followed by CHEK2 1.9%, ATM 1.6%, BRCA1 0.9%, RAD51D 0.4%, and PALB2 0.4% [42]. The presence of mutations involving BRCA and ATM is associated with worse prognosis [43].

Two PARP inhibitors, olaparib and rucaparib, are approved for the treatment of mCRPC with HRR deficiency. In phase III PROFOUND trial, olaparib 300 mg BD was compared to physician's choice hormonal therapy abiraterone or enzalutamide in patients with mCRPC with HRR who progressed on at least one line of hormonal therapy irrespective of exposure to docetaxel [44, 45]. Patient population was divided into two cohorts. Cohort A included patients with BRCA1/BRCA2 and ATM. Cohort 2B included patients with non-BRCA/ATM HRR gene alterations. Olaparib had resulted in increased response rates (33% vs. 2%) and significantly prolonged radiologic PFS 7.4 versus 3.6 months (HR 0.34) and overall survival 19.1 versus 14.7 months in cohort of patients with BRCA1/BRCA2 and ATM mutations. Benefit with olaparib was higher in patients with BRCA2 mutation compared to BRCA1 mutation. Olaparib also increased the radiologic PFS (4.8 vs. 3.3 months, HR 0.88) and also overall survival compared to control arm (14.7 vs. 11.5 months, 0.96) in cohort B. The most common adverse events were anemia (46%), nausea, anorexia, and fatigue.

Rucaparib 600 mg BD was evaluated in patients with mCRPC with HRR deficiency in a phase III single-arm TRITON 2 study. In patients with BRCA1/BRCA2 mutations, rucaparib resulted in a response rate of 44% with a PSA response rate of 63% and median radiologic PFS 9 months [46]. In patients with non-BRCA alterations, responses were modest; hence, it was approved only for patients with germline or somatic BRCA mutations.

Niraparib has been evaluated in a phase II GALLAHAD trail in patients with germline or somatic BRCA1/BRCA2 mutation and was found to result in response rates of 34.2% and a 24-month EFS rate of 15% [47].

Combination of PARP inhibitor and abiraterone is now being evaluated in first-line and later-line treatment of mCRPC. Combination of olaparib and abiraterone was evaluated in a phase II trial in comparison to abiraterone in patients who received docetaxel for mCRPC. Patients were biomarker unselected. Olaparib plus abiraterone improved radiologic PFS, median 13.8 versus 8.2 months. Toxicity was higher in the combination arm with higher incidence of grade 3 or 4 adverse events in 54% versus 28%, commonly anemia and pneumonia [48]. Two trials have shown an increase in PFS with the use of PARP inhibitors along with abiraterone in the first-line setting; however, their OS data is not yet mature. These combinations are not yet incorporated into routine clinical practice. In phase III MAGNITUDE trial, of niraparib plus abiraterone versus abiraterone plus placebo, benefit in radiologic PFS was observed in patients with HRR alterations, median 16.5 versus 13.7 months. However, combination was found to be futile in patients without HRR alterations [49]. In phase III PROPEL trail that evaluated role of olaparib plus abiraterone versus abiraterone plus placebo, addition of olaparib resulted in prolongation of median radiologic PFS median 214.8 versus 16.6 months. In this trial, benefit was observed irrespective of the presence of HRR alterations [50].

17.4.5 Aggressive Prostate Cancer Variants

Neuroendocrine or small cell carcinomas of prostate are rare, and account for <2% of all prostate cancers. They are aggressive, carry poor prognosis and are treated similar to other small cell cancers with platinum etoposide combination therapy [51].

However, around 10–20% of prostatic adenocarcinomas develop a neuroendocrine differentiation after treatment with ADT and androgen signaling inhibitors. These cancers are named treatment-related neuroendocrine prostate cancers or aggressive variant prostate cancers [52]. These tumors are aggressive, with bulky primary tumor and lymph nodes, less of bone metastasis, lytic bone metastases, higher visceral metastasis, relatively low PSA in relation to the burden of disease, elevated serum LDH and serum CEA, small cell morphology on histopathology, and presence of neuroendocrine markers on IHC like synaptophysin and chromogranin [53]. Molecular characterization of these tumors has revealed alterations in tumor suppressor genes, TP53, RB1, and PTEN [54]. These tumors can be treated with a combination of platinum etoposide or taxane plus carboplatin with varying response rates of 20–50%.

17.4.6 Immunotherapy

Somatic and germline testing has to be done in all mCRPC cases to look for dMMR/high levels of microsatellite instability (MSI-H) and for overexpression of PDL1 ligand. Prostate cancers are characterized by a low tumor mutational burden, with dMMR/MSI-H in 1–4% of cases.

Pembrolizumab monotherapy was tested in phase III KEYNOTE 199 study. Response with pembrolizumab were modest with response rates of around 5% [55]. Combination of nivolumab and ipilimumab was evaluated in Checkmate 650 trial, which showed a response rate of 17% and a disease control rate of 56% with higher responses in PDL1 > 1%.

17.4.7 Radioligand Therapy

PSMA is a cell membrane protein that is highly expressed in prostate cancer cells. Various ligands of PSMA have been linked to radioisotopes like lutetium-177. Role of 177-Lu-PSMA 617 was evaluated in a phase III VISION trial in patients of mCRPC post one to two lines of taxane-containing regimens and androgen signaling inhibitor [56]. Study arm was 177-Lu-PSMA 617 with standard of care and comparator arm being standard of care alone. Standard of care included steroids, androgen signaling therapies, excluded taxanes, and radium-223 therapy. 177-Lu-PSMA 617 resulted in higher response rates (30% vs. 2%), improved radiologic PFS (8.7 vs. 3.4 months, HR 0.40), and increased OS (15.3 vs. 11.3 months, HR 0.62). However, the toxicity was higher with Lu therapy with bone marrow suppression and cytopenias seen in up to 25% patients.

17.4.8 Radium 223

Radium 223 is an alpha emitter, undergoes decay, and leads to deposition of high energy radiation. It is indicated for patients with mCRPC with bone-only metastases. It has shown to decrease the symptomatic skeletal-related events and increase overall survival.

17.5 Summary

In conclusion, there has been a magnificent pace of drug approvals in treatment of prostate cancer, thereby posing new challenges in treatment selection and sequencing various available options.

References

1. Sung H, Ferlay J, Siegel RL, Laversanne M, Soerjomataram I, Jemal A, et al. Global cancer statistics 2020: GLOBOCAN estimates of incidence and mortality worldwide for 36 cancers in 185 countries. CA Cancer J Clin. 2021;71(3):209–49.
2. Hemminki K, Li X. Familial risk for lung cancer by histology and age of onset: evidence for recessive inheritance. Exp Lung Res. 2005;31(2):205–15.
3. Siegel RL, Miller KD, Fuchs HE, Jemal A. Cancer statistics, 2022. CA Cancer J Clin. 2022;72(1):7–33.
4. Huggins C. Effect of orchiectomy and irradiation on cancer of the prostate. Ann Surg. 1942;115(6):1192–200.
5. Seidenfeld J, Samson DJ, Hasselblad V, Aronson N, Albertsen PC, Bennett CL, et al. Single-therapy androgen suppression in men with advanced prostate cancer. Ann Intern Med. 2000;132(7):566–77.
6. Klotz L, Boccon-Gibod L, Shore ND, Andreou C, Persson BE, Cantor P, Jensen JK, Olesen TK, Schröder FH. The efficacy and safety of degarelix: a 12-month, comparative, randomized, open-label, parallel-group phase III study in patients with prostate cancer. BJU Int. 2008;102(11):1531–8. https://doi.org/10.1111/j.1464-410X.2008.08183.x.
7. Klotz L, Miller K, Crawford ED, Shore N, Tombal B, Karup C, et al. Disease control outcomes from analysis of pooled individual patient data from five comparative randomised clinical trials of degarelix versus luteinising hormone-releasing hormone agonists. Eur Urol. 2014;66(6):1101–8.
8. Abufaraj M, Iwata T, Kimura S, Haddad A, Al-Ani H, Abusubaih L, et al. Differential impact of gonadotropin-releasing hormone antagonist versus agonist on clinical safety and oncologic outcomes on patients with metastatic prostate cancer: a meta-analysis of randomized controlled trials. Eur Urol. 2021;79(1):44–53.
9. Shore ND, Saad F, Cookson MS, George DJ, Saltzstein DR, Tutrone R, et al. Oral Relugolix for androgen-deprivation therapy in advanced prostate cancer. N Engl J Med. 2020;382(23):2187–96.
10. Sweeney CJ, Chen YH, Carducci M, Liu G, Jarrard DF, Eisenberger M, et al. Chemohormonal therapy in metastatic hormone-sensitive prostate cancer. N Engl J Med. 2015;373(8):737–46.
11. James ND, Sydes MR, Clarke NW, Mason MD, Dearnaley DP, Spears MR, et al. Addition of docetaxel, zoledronic acid, or both to first-line long-term hormone therapy in prostate cancer (STAMPEDE): survival results from an adaptive, multiarm, multistage, platform randomised controlled trial. Lancet. 2016;387(10024):1163–77.
12. Gravis G, Fizazi K, Joly F, Oudard S, Priou F, Esterni B, et al. Androgen-deprivation therapy alone or with docetaxel in non-castrate metastatic prostate cancer (GETUG-AFU 15): a randomised, open-label, phase 3 trial. Lancet Oncol. 2013;14(2):149–58.
13. Sathianathen NJ, Philippou YA, Kuntz GM, Konety BR, Gupta S, Lamb AD, et al. Taxane-based chemohormonal therapy for metastatic hormone-sensitive prostate cancer. Cochrane Database Syst Rev. 2018;10(10):CD012816. https://doi.org/10.1002/14651858.CD012816.pub2/full.
14. Fizazi K, Tran N, Fein L, Matsubara N, Rodriguez-Antolin A, Alekseev BY, et al. Abiraterone acetate plus prednisone in patients with newly diagnosed high-risk metastatic castration-sensitive prostate cancer (LATITUDE): final overall survival analysis of a randomised, double-blind, phase 3 trial. Lancet Oncol. 2019;20(5):686–700.
15. Fizazi K, Tran N, Fein L, Matsubara N, Rodriguez-Antolin A, Alekseev BY, et al. Abiraterone plus prednisone in metastatic, castration-sensitive prostate cancer. N Engl J Med. 2017;377(4):352–60.
16. James ND, de Bono JS, Spears MR, Clarke NW, Mason MD, Dearnaley DP, et al. Abiraterone for prostate cancer not previously treated with hormone therapy. N Engl J Med. 2017;377(4):338–51.
17. Szmulewitz RZ, Peer CJ, Ibraheem A, Martinez E, Kozloff MF, Carthon B, et al. Prospective international randomized phase II study of low-dose abiraterone with food versus standard dose abiraterone in castration-resistant prostate cancer. J Clin Oncol. 2018;36(14):1389–95.
18. Davis ID, Martin AJ, Stockler MR, Begbie S, Chi KN, Chowdhury S, et al. Enzalutamide with standard first-line therapy in metastatic prostate cancer. N Engl J Med. 2019;381(2):121–31.
19. Armstrong AJ, Szmulewitz RZ, Petrylak DP, Holzbeierlein J, Villers A, Azad A, et al. ARCHES: a randomized, phase III study of androgen deprivation therapy with enzalutamide or placebo in men with metastatic hormone-sensitive prostate cancer. J Clin Oncol. 2019;37(32):2974–86.
20. Armstrong AJ, Azad AA, Iguchi T, Szmulewitz RZ, Petrylak DP, Holzbeierlein J, et al. Improved survival with enzalutamide in patients with metastatic hormone-sensitive prostate cancer. J Clin Oncol. 2022;40(15):1616–22.
21. Armstrong AJ, Iguchi T, Azad A, Szmulewitz RZ, Holzbeierlein J, Villers A, et al. Overall survival (OS) in patients (pts) with metastatic hormone-sensitive prostate cancer (mHSPC) treated with enzalutamide (ENZA) + androgen deprivation therapy (ADT) by high or low disease volume and progression to mHSPC (M0 at diagnosis) or de novo mHSPC (M1 at diagnosis): post hoc analysis of the phase 3 ARCHES trial. J Clin Oncol. 2022;40(6_Suppl):115.
22. Chi KN, Chowdhury S, Bjartell A, Chung BH, Pereira de Santana Gomes AJ, Given R, et al. Apalutamide in patients with metastatic castration-sensitive prostate cancer: final survival analysis of the randomized, double-blind, phase III TITAN study. J Clin Oncol. 2021;39(20):2294–303.
23. Sathianathen NJ, Koschel S, Thangasamy IA, Teh J, Alghazo O, Butcher G, et al. Indirect comparisons of efficacy between combination approaches in

metastatic hormone-sensitive prostate cancer: a systematic review and network meta-analysis. Eur Urol. 2020;77(3):365–72.
24. Wang L, Paller CJ, Hong H, De Felice A, Alexander GC, Brawley O. Comparison of systemic treatments for metastatic castration-sensitive prostate cancer: a systematic review and network meta-analysis. JAMA Oncol. 2021;7(3):412–20.
25. Marchioni M, Di NM, Primiceri G, Novara G, Castellan P, Paul AK, et al. New antiandrogen compounds compared to docetaxel for metastatic hormone sensitive prostate cancer: results from a network meta-analysis. J Urol. 2020;203(4):751–9.
26. Fizazi K, Foulon S, Carles J, Roubaud G, McDermott R, Fléchon A, et al. Abiraterone plus prednisone added to androgen deprivation therapy and docetaxel in de novo metastatic castration-sensitive prostate cancer (PEACE-1): a multicentre, open-label, randomised, phase 3 study with a 2×2 factorial design. Lancet. 2022;399(10336):1695–707.
27. Kellokumpu-Lehtinen PL, Harmenberg U, Joensuu T, McDermott R, Hervonen P, Ginman C, et al. 2-weekly versus 3-weekly docetaxel to treat castration-resistant advanced prostate cancer: a randomised, phase 3 trial. Lancet Oncol. 2013;14(2):117–24.
28. Oudard S, Fizazi K, Sengeløv L, Daugaard G, Saad F, Hansen S, Hjälm-Eriksson M, Jassem J, Thiery-Vuillemin A, Caffo O, Castellano D, Mainwaring PN, Bernard J, Shen L, Chadjaa M, Sartor O. Cabazitaxel versus docetaxel as first-line therapy for patients with metastatic castration-resistant prostate cancer: a randomized phase III trial—FIRSTANA. J Clin Oncol. 2017;35(28):3189–97.
29. de Bono JS, Oudard S, Ozguroglu M, Hansen S, Machiels JP, Kocak I, et al. Prednisone plus cabazitaxel or mitoxantrone for metastatic castration-resistant prostate cancer progressing after docetaxel treatment: a randomised open-label trial. Lancet. 2010;376(9747):1147–54.
30. de Wit R, de Bono J, Sternberg CN, Fizazi K, Tombal B, Wülfing C, et al. Cabazitaxel versus abiraterone or enzalutamide in metastatic prostate cancer. N Engl J Med. 2019;381(26):2506–18.
31. Eisenberger M, Hardy-Bessard AC, Kim CS, Géczi L, Ford D, Mourey L, Carles J, Parente P, Font A, Kacso G, Chadjaa M, Zhang W, Bernard J, de Bono J. Phase III study comparing a reduced dose of cabazitaxel (20 mg/m2) and the currently approved dose (25 mg/m2) in postdocetaxel patients with metastatic castration-resistant prostate cancer—PROSELICA. J Clin Oncol. 2017;35(28):3198–206.
32. de Bono JS, Logothetis CJ, Molina A, Fizazi K, North S, Chu L, et al. Abiraterone and increased survival in metastatic prostate cancer. N Engl J Med. 2011;364(21):1995–2005.
33. Fizazi K, Scher HI, Molina A, Logothetis CJ, Chi KN, Jones RJ, et al. Abiraterone acetate for treatment of metastatic castration-resistant prostate cancer: final overall survival analysis of the COU-AA-301 randomised, double-blind, placebo-controlled phase 3 study. Lancet Oncol. 2012;13(10):983–92.
34. Rathkopf DE, Smith MR, de Bono JS, Logothetis CJ, Shore ND, de Souza P, et al. Updated interim efficacy analysis and long-term safety of abiraterone acetate in metastatic castration-resistant prostate cancer patients without prior chemotherapy (COU-AA-302). Eur Urol. 2014;66(5):815–25.
35. Ryan CJ, Smith MR, de Bono JS, Molina A, Logothetis CJ, de Souza P, et al. Abiraterone in metastatic prostate cancer without previous chemotherapy. N Engl J Med. 2013;368(2):138–48.
36. Ryan CJ, et al. Abiraterone acetate plus prednisone versus placebo plus prednisone in chemotherapy-naive men with metastatic castration-resistant prostate cancer (COU-AA-302): final overall survival analysis of a randomised, double-blind, placebo-controlled phase 3 study. Lancet Oncol. 2015;16(2):152–60.
37. Attard G, Borre M, Gurney H, Loriot Y, Andresen-Daniil C, Kalleda R, Pham T, Taplin ME, PLATO Collaborators. Abiraterone alone or in combination with enzalutamide in metastatic castration-resistant prostate cancer with rising prostate-specific antigen during enzalutamide treatment. J Clin Oncol. 2018;36(25):2639–46.
38. Fizazi K, Scher HI, Miller K, Basch E, Sternberg CN, Cella D, et al. Effect of enzalutamide on time to first skeletal-related event, pain, and quality of life in men with castration-resistant prostate cancer: results from the randomised, phase 3 AFFIRM trial. Lancet Oncol. 2014;15(10):1147–56.
39. Scher HI, Fizazi K, Saad F, Taplin ME, Sternberg CN, Miller K, et al. Increased survival with enzalutamide in prostate cancer after chemotherapy. N Engl J Med. 2012;367(13):1187–97.
40. Beer TM, Armstrong AJ, Rathkopf DE, Loriot Y, Sternberg CN, Higano CS, et al. Enzalutamide in metastatic prostate cancer before chemotherapy. N Engl J Med. 2014;371(5):424–33.
41. Beer TM, Armstrong AJ, Rathkopf D, Loriot Y, Sternberg CN, Higano CS, et al. Enzalutamide in men with chemotherapy-naïve metastatic castration-resistant prostate cancer: extended analysis of the phase 3 PREVAIL study. Eur Urol. 2017;71(2):151–4.
42. Pritchard CC, et al. Inherited DNA-repair gene mutations in men with metastatic prostate cancer. N Engl J Med. 2016;375(5):443–53.
43. Castro E, Romero-Laorden N, del Pozo A, Lozano R, Medina A, Puente J, et al. PROREPAIR-B: a prospective cohort study of the impact of germline DNA repair mutations on the outcomes of patients with metastatic castration-resistant prostate cancer. J Clin Oncol. 2019;37(6):490–503.
44. de Bono J, Mateo J, Fizazi K, Saad F, Shore N, Sandhu S, et al. Olaparib for metastatic castration-resistant prostate cancer. N Engl J Med. 2020;382(22):2091–102.
45. Hussain M, Mateo J, Fizazi K, Saad F, Shore N, Sandhu S, et al. Survival with olaparib in metastatic

castration-resistant prostate cancer. N Engl J Med. 2020;383(24):2345–57.
46. Abida W, Patnaik A, Campbell D, Shapiro J, Bryce AH, McDermott R, et al. Rucaparib in men with metastatic castration-resistant prostate cancer harboring a BRCA1 or BRCA2 gene alteration. J Clin Oncol. 2020;38(32):3763–72.
47. Smith MR, Scher HI, Sandhu S, Efstathiou E, Lara PN, Yu EY, et al. Niraparib in patients with metastatic castration-resistant prostate cancer and DNA repair gene defects (GALAHAD): a multicentre, open-label, phase 2 trial. Lancet Oncol. 2022;23(3):362–73.
48. Clarke N, Wiechno P, Alekseev B, Sala N, Jones R, Kocak I, et al. Olaparib combined with abiraterone in patients with metastatic castration-resistant prostate cancer: a randomised, double-blind, placebo-controlled, phase 2 trial. Lancet Oncol. 2018;19(7):975–86.
49. Chi KN, Rathkopf DE, Smith MR, Efstathiou E, Attard G, Olmos D, et al. Phase 3 MAGNITUDE study: First results of niraparib (NIRA) with abiraterone acetate and prednisone (AAP) as first-line therapy in patients (pts) with metastatic castration-resistant prostate cancer (mCRPC) with and without homologous recombination repair (HRR) gene alterations. J Clin Oncol. 2022;40(6_Suppl):12.
50. Saad F, Armstrong AJ, Thiery-Vuillemin A, Oya M, Loredo E, Procopio G, et al. PROpel: phase III trial of olaparib (ola) and abiraterone (abi) versus placebo (pbo) and abi as first-line (1L) therapy for patients (pts) with metastatic castration-resistant prostate cancer (mCRPC). J Clin Oncol. 2022;40(6_Suppl):11.
51. Beltran H, Rickman DS, Park K, Chae SS, Sboner A, MacDonald TY, et al. Molecular characterization of neuroendocrine prostate cancer and identification of new drug targets. Cancer Discov. 2011;1(6):487–95.
52. Turbat-Herrera EA, Herrera GA, Gore I, Lott RL, Grizzle WE, Bonnin JM. Neuroendocrine differentiation in prostatic carcinomas. A retrospective autopsy study. Arch Pathol Lab Med. 1988;112(11):1100–5.
53. Aparicio AM, Harzstark AL, Corn PG, Wen S, Araujo JC, Tu SM, et al. Platinum-based chemotherapy for variant castrate-resistant prostate cancer. Clin Cancer Res. 2013;19(13):3621–30.
54. Aparicio AM, Shen L, Tapia ELN, Lu JF, Chen HC, Zhang J, et al. Combined tumor suppressor defects characterize clinically defined aggressive variant prostate cancers. Clin Cancer Res. 2016;22(6):1520–30.
55. Antonarakis ES, Piulats JM, Gross-Goupil M, Goh J, Ojamaa K, Hoimes CJ, et al. Pembrolizumab for treatment-refractory metastatic castration-resistant prostate cancer: multicohort, open-label phase II KEYNOTE-199 study. J Clin Oncol. 2020;38(5):395–405.
56. Sartor O, et al. Lutetium-177–PSMA-617 for metastatic castration-resistant prostate cancer. N Engl J Med. 2021;385(12):1091–103.

18 Adjuvant Treatment and Follow Up after Radical Prostatectomy in Prostate Cancer

K. P. Haresh and V. R. Anjali

18.1 Introduction

Prostate cancer (PCa) is the second most common cancer among men, with an estimated new case of 1.4 million patients worldwide. It is the fifth leading cause of cancer death among men with 375,000 deaths worldwide [1]. The risk factors include age, race, family history and certain germline mutations. The incidence of PCa increases sharply as age advances, with the median age of presentation at 68 years. For prostate carcinogenesis and disease progression, androgen and androgen receptors play a pivotal role. Various treatment options for localised prostate cancer are available depending on the risk of the disease (Table 18.1).

The treatment options for low-risk PCa include active surveillance, radical prostatectomy (RP) or radical radiotherapy. In patients with high-risk disease, the multimodality treatment options include radical radiotherapy with long-term androgen deprivation therapy (ADT) or RP with pelvic lymph node dissection (PLND) and adjuvant radiotherapy (aRT). The treatment options are individualised for each patient and depends on various factors like medical co-morbidity, life expectancy, tumour burden, performance status and general condition of the patient and the expected side effects the patient i ready to accept. The treatment options are summarised in Table 18.1.

For localised PCa, the main surgical treatment is RP, which has shown cause-specific cancer survival. But about 25–35% of patients can have biochemical recurrence (BCR) [2], over a period of 10 years. The rates of BCR increase in patients with intermediate- and high-risk disease. BCR is an early marker of distant relapse, poor prognosis and cancer death [3, 4]. Identifying the prognostic factors of BCR can help in defining the patients who require adjuvant treatment. The risk factors for BCR in PCa include adverse features like positive surgical margins (PSM), seminal vesicle invasion (SVI), lymph node involvement, extra-prostatic extension (EPE), high Gleason score and PSA value.

As already mentioned, not all patients after RP recur; about one-third of them will have BCR. BCR may not translate into clinical progression in all patients.

K. P. Haresh (✉) · V. R. Anjali
Radiation Oncology, Dr B R Ambedkar Institute Rotary Cancer Hospital, All India Institute of Medical Sciences (AIIMS), New Delhi, India

P. Singh et al. (eds.), *A Guide to Management of Urological Cancers*,
https://doi.org/10.1007/978-981-99-2341-0_18

Table 18.1 Treatment options for localised prostate cancer

NCCN risk group (localised disease)		Treatment options
Low risk	T1–T2a	Active surveillance
	GS ≤ 6	Radical prostatectomy
	PSA < 10	Radical brachytherapy
		Radical EBRT
Intermediate risk	T2b–T2c	Radical EBRT+ short-term ADT
	GS = 7	EBRT+ brachytherapy boost+ short-term ADT
	PSA 10–20	Radical prostatectomy +/− PLND
		Radical brachytherapy
High risk	T3a	EBRT+ brachytherapy boost+ long-term ADT
	GS 8–10	Radical EBRT+ long-term ADT
	PSA > 20	Radical prostatectomy +PLND+/− PORT

EBRT external beam radiotherapy, *PLND* pelvic lymph node dissection, *ADT* androgen deprivation therapy, *PORT* postoperative radiotherapy

18.2 Prognostic Factors After Radical Prostatectomy

The pathological risk factors are positive surgical margin, seminal vesicle invasion, extra prostatic extension, lymph nodal involvement, high Gleason score and the PSA kinetics. Positive surgical margin PSM is the histological presence of prostate cancer cells at the inked margins. After RP, the occurrence of PSM is 11–48% [5, 6] and the chances are higher in advanced pathological stage. Systematic review by Yossepowitch reported that positive margins were associated with a twofold increased hazard of BCR [7]. Meta-analysis from retrospective studies by Zhang et al. showed PSM as an independent prognostic factor associated with higher BCR risk. A study by Pressie et al. with more than 8000 patients showed that Gleason pattern ≥4 at the margin and length of positive margin ≥3 mm were associated with the highest risk of BCR. Tumour grade and cumulative length at margins were important independent predictors for BCR-free survival. Although positive margin in prostate cancer is a high risk factor and increases the risk for BCR, the long-term impact on survival as end point is controversial. Seminal vesical involvement and extracapsular extension are independent poor prognostic factors for BCR and metastasis. In patients with SVI, there is 2.3-fold risk of BCR and 22% increased PCa-specific mortality [8]. PSA is the most sensitive and specific biomarker for disease persistence and recurrence. Postoperative PSA value is critical, with high association between PSA value and BCR. But PSA cannot detect recurrence smaller than 10^7–10^8 cells. Shorter PSA doubling time, persistence of PSA and less time interval to PSA failure are poor prognostic factors for BCR and risk of metastasis. PSA persistence after surgery is the worst prognostic predictor of BCR. PSA persistence is defined when PSA is ≥0.1 ng/mL at 1 month after RP.

18.3 Biochemical Recurrence After Radical Prostatectomy

During radical prostatectomy when the entire prostate gland is removed, the PSA should fall below undetectable levels. A detectable or rising PSA after radical treatment is called BCR which is a forerunner of disease recurrence. With newer techniques, ultrasensitive PSA test can be done which can detect PSA values below 0.1 ng/mL. Monitoring of PSA helps to detect BCR, which is a precursor of disease metastasis and cancer-specific mortality by almost 7 and 15 years, respectively. But it must be noted that the BCR need not to correlate to these endpoints in all patients. Uniform consensus for defining BCR after radical prostatectomy is not available. On analysis with 2782 patients with PSA 0.2, 0.3 and 0.4 ng/mL cut-offs, the biochemical progression-free percentages were 62%, 72% and 76% at 5 years, and subsequent PSA rise was seen in 49%, 62% and 72%, respectively [9]. Postoperative PSA assessment is usually done after 6 weeks of surgery. Commonly used BCR definition criteria following radical prostatectomy are the following:

- An initial PSA of ≥0.2 ng/mL, with a second confirmatory level of PSA >0.2 ng/mL, is defined as BCR by the European Association of Urology [10] and American Urological Association [11].
- A PSA of at least 0.4 ng/mL, followed by another rise, is defined as BCR according to the American Society of Clinical Oncology (ASCO) [12] as it correlated well with the development of distant metastasis.

18.3.1 Post Radical Prostatectomy Risk Stratification for BCR

Various risk stratification tools and nomograms are developed to identify the patients who are high risk of BCR. One of the commonly used scoring systems is Cancer of Prostate Risk Assessment (CAPRA) score, which used pre-treatment clinical parameters including PSA, Gleason score, T-stage, percentage of biopsy-positive core and age. The CAPRA-S score is used in post-RP setting, with six variables, which include preoperative PSA and pathologic parameters like pGS, pSM, pSVI, pECE and pLNI. The CAPRA-S score was developed to predict BCR and systemic progression (Table 18.2).

18.3.2 Adjuvant Treatment

Adjuvant treatment is defined as the treatment added (adjunct) to the primary therapy, to reduce the risk of relapse. In PCa patients who are undergoing radical prostatectomy as the primary treatment, the adjuvant treatment given is external beam radiotherapy. The decision for adjuvant treatment depends on the chance of disease recurrence.

Table 18.2 CAPRA-s scoring system

Variable		Points	Variable		Points
PSA	0–6	0	pGS	2–6	0
	6.01–10	1		3+4	1
	10.1–20	2		4+3	2
	>20	3		8–10	3
pSM	Negative	0	ECE	No	0
	Positive	2		Yes	2
SVI	No	0	LNI	No	0
	Yes	2		Yes	2

18.3.2.1 Timing of Postoperative Radiotherapy

The optimum timing of postoperative radiotherapy after radical prostatectomy is debatable. The timings at which postoperative radiotherapy given are (1) adjuvant radiotherapy and (2) salvage radiotherapy.

Adjuvant radiotherapy is given to patients with adverse pathological factors after the postoperative side effects have settled or stabilised, without a PSA failure (<0.2) and in the absence of disease persistence or progression. Salvage radiotherapy is given when the postoperative patients have biochemical recurrence or PSA persistence without distant metastasis. Early salvage radiotherapy is defined when radiation is delivered to postoperative patients when an undetectable PSA becomes eventually detectable at a relatively low PSA level, or at the time of increasing PSA, with no evidence of distant metastasis. The cut-off level for early salvage varies but is usually taken as less than 0.5 ng/dL.

18.3.2.2 Evidence Supporting Adjuvant Radiotherapy

The role of adjuvant RT versus observation after radical prostatectomy was addressed in the randomised controlled trials – SWOG S8794 [13], EORTC 22911 and ARO 96-02/AUO AP 09/95 and Finn Prostate Group. However, the three RCTs had different inclusion criteria and assessed different primary outcomes. The primary outcome for the SWOG 8794 trial was metastasis-free survival. EORTC 22911 used biochemical RFS as the primary outcome while biochemical PFS was the outcome in the ARO study. All the three trials met their primary endpoints. The trials are summarised below, table SWOG8794, EORTC22911 and ARO trial (Table 18.3).

Cochrane meta-analysis [14] including the three trials (SWOG S8794, EORTC 22911, ARO 96-02/AUO AP 09/95) showed post prostatectomy adjuvant RT:

Table 18.3 Trials supporting adjuvant treatment

SWOG 8794	Criteria	Adjuvant arm showed
Thompson et al.	• cT1–T2, post RP	– Improved MFE ($p = 0.016$)
August 1988–January 1997	• pT3 (any one feature extracapsular extension, positive margins or seminal vesicle invasion)	– Improved OS ($p = 0.023$)
$N = 425$	• Randomisation at 16 weeks, into RT and observation	– Reduced risk of PSA recurrence
Median follow-up 12.7 years in 2009	• RT started within 10 days of randomisation	– Reduced need for hormonal treatment
	• RT dose 60–64 Gy to tumour bed	– Higher GI and GU toxicity
	• Postoperative undetectable PSA level was not required	– No difference in rate of erectile dysfunction
		– Global QOL is similar at 2 years and became superior in following 3 years

EORTC 22911	Criteria	Adjuvant RT arm
Bolla et al.	• cT0–T3, N0M0, post RP	– Improved biochemical PFS (60% vs. 41%; $p < 0.0001$)
November 1992–December 2001	• pT2–3 N0 (with at least one risk factor: capsule perforation, positive surgical margins or seminal vesicle invasion)	– Improved LC (16.6% vs. 7.3%; $p < 0.0001$)
$N = 1005$	• Radiotherapy began within 16 weeks after surgery	– Clinical PFS benefitted only in patients<70 years and with positive margins (70.3% vs. 64.8%; $p = 0.0539$)
Median follow-up 10.6 years in 2012	• RT dose 60 Gy/30 fractions	– No difference in OS
		– Better prostate cancer mortality rate (3.9% vs. 5.4%)
		– Late adverse effects more in RT arm (70.8% vs. 59.7%; $p = 0.001$)

ARO 96-02/AUO AP 09/95	Criteria	Adjuvant RT arm
Wiegel et al.	• cT1–cT3 N0	– Improved biochemical PFS (56% vs. 35%; $p < 0.0001$)
April 1997–September 2004	• Post RP and PLND	– One grade 3 and five grade 2 late toxicity
$N = 388$	• pT3–4 pN0 with undetectable PSA after RP (<0.5 ng/mL was mandatory)	
Median follow-up 10 years in 2014	• RT (3DCRT) began between 6 and 12 weeks after surgery	
	• RT dose – 60 Gy in 30 fractions	

- Improved survival at 10 years ($p = 0.02$).
- Improved MFS at 10 years ($p = 0.03$).
- Decreased local recurrence at 10 years ($p = 0.00001$).
- Biochemical PFS improved at 5 years ($p < 0.00001$) and 10 years ($p < 0.00001$).
- Prostate cancer-specific mortality at 5 years was not improved by aRT.
- A significant increase in mild acute and late GU and GI toxicity with aRT.

18.4 Adjuvant RT Versus Early Salvage Radiotherapy

After radical prostatectomy rather than adjuvant RT, patients with low rising levels of PSA are considered for early salvage RT, aimed to reduce GI and GU toxicities with similar outcomes. The use of early salvage RT was initially supported by multi-institutional retrospective studies. The three randomised controlled trials that evaluated the benefit of adjuvant RT over early salvage RT are RADICALS-RT [15], GETUG-AFU17 [16] and RAVES [17]. The primary endpoints were different for three trials. The primary endpoints are time free of metastases (RADICALS-RT), event-free survival (GETUG-AFU) and biochemical progression (RAVES). The trials are summarised in Table 18.4.

Outcomes are better when the salvage RT is started when PSA is <0.5 ng/mL [18], than with >0.5 ng/mL [19]. Patients with at least two pathological risk factors (pT3b/pT4, pathological GS ≥ 8 or negative surgical margin) showed an increased risk of 5-year BCR as high as 10% per 0.1 ng/mL of PSA level, as compared with 1.5% in patients with one or no risk features [20]. The effect on metastasis-free survival decreased when PSA increased >1 ng/mL, and the window of opportunity for disease control is reduced. For every 0.1 μg/L increase in PSA, it is estimated to correspond to an expected loss of 4% in a 5-year biochemical progression-free survival [21].

The artistic meta-analysis to evaluate the effect of adjuvant RT versus salvage RT included the three trials (RADICALS-RT, GETUG-AFU, RAVES), with a median follow-up of 60–78 months. The results showed no improvement in event-free survival with adjuvant RT as compared to early salvage RT. It was commented until the long-term outcomes are available; early salvage treatment seems preferable, to spare many patients from RT and its side effects.

Table 18.4 Trials comparing adjuvant versus salvage treatment

Radicals	Criteria	Results
Parker et al.	At least one risk factor post RP	– Primary outcome – freedom from distant metastases – not sufficiently mature
$N = 1396$	• pT3 or pT4	– Similar biochemical PFS (88% vs. 85%; $p = 0.56$)
Superiority trial design	• GS 7–10	– Grade 3–4 urethral stricture 6%(aRT) versus 4% (early sRT) ($p = 0.020$)
November 2007–December 2016	• Margin positive	
Median follow up 4.9 years in 2020	• Preoperative PSA ≥10 ng/mL	
	• Postoperative PSA ≤ 0.2 ng/mL	
	• Biochemical progression (PSA ≥0.1 ng/mL or three consecutive rises)	

TROG 08.03/ANZUP RAVES	Criteria	Results
Kneebone et al.	• Post RP with high-risk feature	– Primary endpoint: freedom from biochemical progression 86% (aRT) vs. 87%(sRT)
$N = 333$	• Positive surgical margins, extra prostatic extension or seminal vesicle invasion	– Lower GU toxicity in sRT [54%] than aRT [70%]
Non-inferiority trial	• Postoperative PSA ≤ 0.10 ng/mL	– Similar GI toxicity 10% (sRT) and 14% (aRT)
March 2009–December 2015	• Early salvage radiotherapy if PSA is ≥0.20 ng/mL	
Median follow-up 6.1 years in 2020		

GETUG-AFU 17	Criteria	Results
Sargos et al.	• Post RP	– Primary endpoint – event-free survival 92% (aRT) and 90% (sRT) (HR 0.81)
$N = 424$	• pT3 or pT4a (with bladder neck invasion), pNx or pN0 disease, positive surgical margins	– Acute toxicity 3% (aRT) and 2% (sRT)
Superiority	• All patients received 6 months of triptorelin	– Late GU toxicity and erectile dysfunction was increased in aRT group
March 2008–June 2016		
Median follow-up 75 months in 2020		

It is important to consider that the benefits of adjuvant RT were not significant in the early follow-up results. Only with long-term follow-up the benefit was statistically significant for MFS, OS, PFS and LC. The results of early salvage RT trials have median follow-up of only 4.9, 6.1 and 6.3 years while adjuvant RT trials had median follow-up of 12.7, 10.6 and 9.4 years.

18.5 Role of Adding Hormonal Therapy to Adjuvant or Salvage Radiotherapy

The role of the addition of hormonal therapy to adjuvant or salvage radiotherapy in prostate cancer is coming up in a big way.

GETUG AFU 16 study [22] enrolled stage pT2, pT3 or pT4a (bladder neck involvement only) in patients who had rising PSA of 0.2 to less than 2.0 μg/L following radical prostatectomy. Patients were randomised (1:1) to standard salvage radiotherapy of 66 Gy in 33 fractions or radiotherapy plus short-term androgen suppression using 10.8 mg goserelin by subcutaneous injection on the first day of irradiation and 3 months later. Seven hundred forty-three patients were randomly assigned, 374 to radiotherapy alone and 369 to radiotherapy plus goserelin. Patients assigned to radiotherapy plus goserelin were significantly more likely than patients in the radiotherapy-alone group to be free of biochemical progression or clinical progression at 5 years (80% [95% CI 75–84] vs. 62% [57–67]; hazard ratio [HR] 0·50, 95% CI 0.38–0.66; $p < 0.0001$). Further GETUG AFU 17 [23] which randomised between adjuvant and salvage RT used short course of ADT with inj triptorelin for 6 months in both arms of the trial.

In RTOG 9601 trial [24], 760 patients receiving salvage radiotherapy were randomised to 24 months of bicalutamide 150 mg daily versus placebo. The actuarial rate of overall survival at 12 years was 76.3% in the bicalutamide group, as compared with 71.3% in the placebo group (hazard ratio for death, 0.77; 95% confidence interval, 0.5–0.99; $p = 0.04$). The 12-year incidence of death from prostate cancer was 5.8% in the bicalutamide group, as compared with 13.4% in the placebo group ($p < 0.001$). The cumulative incidence of metastatic prostate cancer at 12 years was 14.5% in the bicalutamide group, as compared with 23.0% in the placebo group ($p = 0.005$). Gynecomastia was recorded in 69.7% of the patients in the bicalutamide group, as compared with 10.9% of those in the placebo group ($p < 0.001$). In a post-hoc analysis, men with a PSA <0.7 ng/mL did not benefit by addition of bicalutamide.

RTOG 0534- SPPORT trial [25] was done in patients who had a persistently detectable or an initially undetectable and rising PSA of between 0.1 and 2.0 ng/mL. 1792 eligible patients were enrolled and randomly assigned to the 3 treatment groups (592 to group 1 [PBRT alone], 602 to group 2 [PBRT plus short-term ADT] and 598 to group 3 [PLNRT plus PBRT plus short-term ADT]). At a median follow-up of 8.2 years, the 5-year freedom from progression rates in all 1716 eligible patients were 70.9% (95% CI 67.0–74.9) in group 1, 81.3% (78.0–84.6) in group 2 and 87.4% (84.7–90.2) in group 3. The presence of extensive extraprostatic disease, seminal vesicle insolvent, high presalvage RT PSA level and grade group 4/group 5 support the addition of short-term concurrent ADT to radiotherapy.

For those patients with pathological lymph node-positive disease, we prefer adjuvant radiotherapy with long-term ADT for 2–3 years.

The RADICALS-HD trial (NCT00541047) is currently randomising patients between 6 months and 24 months and no GnRH agonist. It will help clarify the optimal ADT duration in the postoperative setting. The LOBSTER trial (NCT04242017) is also comparing 6 versus 24 months of ADT in case of salvage RT for BCR after pN0 PCa.

18.6 Radiotherapy Treatment Planning

Radiation treatment in the era of intensity-modulated radiotherapy (IMRT), volumetric modulated arc therapy (VMAT) and image-guided radiotherapy (IGRT) necessitates the need to delineate the target volumes accurately to obtain maximum local control, simultaneously sparing the organs at risk to reduce the toxicity.

18.6.1 Patient Positioning and Immobilisation

Patient supine, arms over chest and immobilised with pelvic orfit or patient may be positioned with knee rest and ankle rest which obliviates the need for pelvic immobilisation. Planning CT scan is taken in the treatment position and must be reproducible without discomfort to the patient. Institutional bladder filling protocol is maintained. Usually comfortably full bladder is obtained. Bladder protocol is maintained during the entire treatment. Variation in the daily rectal filling can lead to changes in prostate position. Patient is advised with low residue diet, and measures are taken to prevent overdistension (≥4 cm in AP diameter) of the rectum along the region of interest. If over-distended, repeat planning CT scan is mandated with proper rectal protocol. CT scan slices of 3–5 mm are taken from the level of L3 vertebrae to 5 cm below ischium. Routinely for postoperative tumour bed irradiation, intravenous or rectal contrast is not used. Intravenous contrast helps only when nodal volume delineation is required.

18.6.2 Target Volume Delineation

After radical surgery, the macroscopic disease has been removed completely, so there is no gross tumour volume. The postoperative tumour bed with risk of microscopic disease forms the clinical tumour volume (CTV). The CTV volumes to be encompassed and the contouring guidelines have been given by RTOG, EORTC and FROGG-ANZ. It is equally important to know the most common sites of local relapse after surgery and to include them in the CTV. The common sites of local relapse are vesicourethral anastomosis (VUA), retro vesical space, residual seminal vesicle, perianastomotic, bladder neck and surgical margins [26, 27].

The organs at risk are the rectum, bladder, penile bulb and femoral head. Small bowel becomes OAR when pelvic lymph nodal volumes are irradiated. After contouring, treatment planning is performed. Usually, VMAT or IMRT plans are made. RT dose of 60–66 Gy in 30–33 fractions (conventional fractionation) or 54 Gy in 18 fractions (moderate hypo fractionated) is planned. The treatment plans are verified, and the accepted plan is sent to the treatment system. On all the days of treatment, patient is simulated like planning CT protocol. Cone beam CT (CBCT) or electronic portal imaging devices (EPIDs) are used for treatment position verification. Treatment can also be delivered under image guidance by real-time transperineal ultrasound monitoring (if available).

18.7 Gene Signature Risk Prediction Model

Decipher prostate cancer test post prostatectomy is the commercially available gene signature risk prediction model to predict systemic progression after definitive surgery. It is based on the 22 gene expression markers in biopsy or prostatectomy specimen. Validation studies have confirmed the use of Decipher test in post prostatectomy patients in decision-making for adjuvant treatment. In post RP patients, Decipher test can predict a 5-year metastasis-free survival and 10-year prostate cancer-specific survival and stratify the patient into low risk (<0.45), intermediate risk (0.45–0.60) or high risk (>0.60). Low-risk patients may be kept on observation with serial PSA monitoring and intervene on PSA rise, with salvage RT. High-risk patients may be considered for adjuvant RT.

18.8 Follow-Up

We usually call the patients for follow-up every 6 months for first 5 years and then annually. During the follow-up history, physical findings and the bowel, bladder and sexual side effects of treatment are enquired and recorded. PSA evaluation is done every 6 months for first 5 years and then annually. We do not advice any other imaging like ultrasound, bone scan, CT scan, MRI or PSMA PET unless there is a rising PSA or specific symptoms suggesting recurrence of disease.

References

1. Sung H, Ferlay J, Siegel RL, Laversanne M, Soerjomataram I, Jemal A, Bray F. Global cancer statistics 2020: GLOBOCAN estimates of incidence and mortality worldwide for 36 cancers in 185 countries. CA Cancer J Clin. 2021;71(3):209–49. https://doi.org/10.3322/caac.21660.
2. Kumar A, Samavedi S, Mouraviev V, Bates AS, Coelho RF, Rocco B, Patel VR. Predictive factors and oncological outcomes of persistently elevated prostate-specific antigen in patients following robot-assisted radical prostatectomy. J Robot Surg. 2017;11:37–45.
3. Van den Broeck T, et al. Prognostic value of biochemical recurrence following treatment with curative intent for prostate cancer: a systematic review. Eur Urol. 2019;75(6):967–87. https://doi.org/10.1016/j.eururo.2018.10.011.
4. Pagano MJ, Whalen MJ, Paulucci DJ, Reddy BN, Matulay JT, Rothberg M, Scarberry K, Patel T, Shapiro EY, RoyChoudhury A, et al. Predictors of biochemical recurrence in pT3b prostate cancer after radical prostatectomy without adjuvant radiotherapy. Prostate. 2016;76:226–34.
5. Hsu M, Chang SL, Ferrari M, Nolley R, Presti JC Jr, Brooks JD. Length of site-specific positive surgical margins as a risk factor for biochemical recurrence following radical prostatectomy. Int J Urol. 2011;18:272–9.
6. Alkhateeb S, Alibhai S, Fleshner N, Finelli A, Jewett M, Zlotta A, Nesbitt M, Lockwood G, Trachtenberg J. Impact of positive surgical margins after radical prostatectomy differs by disease risk group. J Urol. 2010;183:145–50.
7. Yossepowitch O, Briganti A, Eastham JA, Epstein J, Graefen M, Montironi R, Touijer K. Positive surgical margins after radical prostatectomy: a systematic review and contemporary update. Eur Urol. 2014;65:303–13.
8. Tourinho-Barbosa R, Srougi V, Nunes-Silva I, Baghdadi M, Rembeyo G, Eiffel SS, Barret E, Rozet F, Galiano M, Cathelineau X, Sanchez-Salas R. Biochemical recurrence after radical prostatectomy: what does it mean? Int Braz J Urol. 2018;44(1):14–21.
9. Amling CL, Bergstralh EJ, Blute ML, Slezak JM, Zincke H. Defining prostate specific antigen progression after radical prostatectomy: what is the most appropriate cut point? J Urol. 2001;165:1146–51.
10. Heidenreich A, Bastian PJ, Bellmunt J, Bolla M, Joniau S, van der Kwast T, et al. European Association of Urology guidelines on prostate cancer. Part II: treatment of advanced, relapsing, and castration-resistant prostate cancer. Eur Urol. 2014;65:467–79.
11. Cookson MS, Aus G, Burnett AL, Canby-Hagino ED, D'Amico AV, Dmochowski RR, et al. Variation in the definition of biochemical recurrence in patients treated for localized prostate cancer: the American urological association prostate guidelines for localized prostate cancer update panel report and recommendations for a standard in the reporting of surgical outcomes. J Urol. 2007;177:540–5.
12. Stephenson AJ, Kattan MW, Eastham JA, Dotan ZA, Bianco FJ Jr, Lilja H, Scardino PT. Defining biochemical recurrence of prostate cancer after radical prostatectomy: a proposal for a standardized definition. J Clin Oncol. 2006;24(24):3973–8.
13. Thompson IM, Tangen CM, Paradelo J, Lucia MS, Miller G, Troyer D, Messing E, Forman J, Chin J, Swanson G, et al. Adjuvant radiotherapy for pathological T3N0M0 prostate cancer significantly reduces risk of metastases and improves survival: long-term followup of a randomized clinical trial. J Urol. 2009;181:956–62.
14. Daly T, Hickey BE, Lehman M, Francis DP, See AM. Adjuvant radiotherapy following radical prostatectomy for prostate cancer. Cochrane Database Syst Rev. 2011;12:CD007234.
15. Parker CC, Clarke NW, Cook AD, Kynaston HG, Petersen PM, Catton C, Cross W, Logue J, Parulekar W, Payne H, et al. Timing of radiotherapy after radical prostatectomy (RADICALS-RT): a randomised, controlled phase 3 trial. Lancet. 2020;396:1413–21.
16. Sargos P, Chabaud S, Latorzeff I, Magne N, Benyoucef A, Supiot S, Pasquier D, Abdiche MS, Gilliot O, GraffCailleaud P, et al. Adjuvant radiotherapy versus early salvage radiotherapy plus short-term androgen deprivation therapy in men with localised prostate cancer after radical prostatectomy (GETUG-AFU 17): a randomised, phase 3 trial. Lancet Oncol. 2020;21:1341–52.
17. Kneebone A, Fraser-Browne C, Duchesne GM, Fisher R, Frydenberg M, Herschtal A, Williams SG, Brown C, Delprado W, Haworth A, et al. Adjuvant radiotherapy versus early salvage radiotherapy following radical prostatectomy (TROG 08.03/ANZUP RAVES): a randomised, controlled, phase 3, non-inferiority trial. Lancet Oncol. 2020;21:1331–40.
18. Van den Broeck T, van den Bergh RCN, Arfi N, et al. Prognostic value of biochemical recurrence following treatment with curative intent for prostate cancer: a systematic review. Eur Urol. 2019;75:967e987.
19. Pfister D, Bolla M, Briganti A, Carroll P, Cozzarini C, Joniau S, et al. Early salvage radiotherapy following radical prostatectomy. Eur Urol. 2014;65:103443.
20. Fossati N, Karnes RJ, Cozzarini C, Fiorino C, Gandaglia G, Joniau S, et al. Assessing the optimal timing for early salvage radiation therapy in patients with prostate-specific antigen rise after radical pros-

tatectomy. Eur Urol. 2016;69:728–33. https://doi.org/10.1016/j.eururo.2015.10.009.
21. King CR. Adjuvant radiotherapy after prostatectomy: does waiting for a prostate specific antigen level make sense? Int J Radiat Oncol Biol Phys. 2011;80:1–3.
22. Carrie C, Hasbini A, de Laroche G, Richaud P, Guerif S, Latorzeff I, Supiot S, Bosset M, Lagrange JL, Beckendorf V, Lesaunier F, Dubray B, Wagner JP, N'Guyen TD, Suchaud JP, Créhange G, Barbier N, Habibian M, Ferlay C, Fourneret P, Ruffion A, Dussart S. Salvage radiotherapy with or without short-term hormone therapy for rising prostate-specific antigen concentration after radical prostatectomy (GETUG-AFU 16): a randomised, multicentre, open-label phase 3 trial. Lancet Oncol. 2016;17(6):747–56.
23. Sargos P, Chabaud S, Latorzeff I, Magné N, Benyoucef A, Supiot S, Pasquier D, Abdiche MS, Gilliot O, Graff-Cailleaud P, Silva M, Bergerot P, Baumann P, Belkacemi Y, Azria D, Brihoum M, Soulié M, Richaud P. Adjuvant radiotherapy versus early salvage radiotherapy plus short-term androgen deprivation therapy in men with localised prostate cancer after radical prostatectomy (GETUG-AFU 17): a randomised, phase 3 trial. Lancet Oncol. 2020;21(10):1341–52.
24. Shipley WU, Seiferheld W, Lukka HR, Major PP, Heney NM, Grignon DJ, Sartor O, Patel MP, Bahary JP, Zietman AL, Pisansky TM, Zeitzer KL, Lawton CA, Feng FY, Lovett RD, Balogh AG, Souhami L, Rosenthal SA, Kerlin KJ, Dignam JJ, Pugh SL, Sandler HM, NRG Oncology RTOG. Radiation with or without antiandrogen therapy in recurrent prostate cancer. N Engl J Med. 2017;376(5):417–28.
25. Pollack A, Karrison TG, Balogh AG, Gomella LG, Low DA, Bruner DW, Wefel JS, Martin AG, Michalski JM, Angyalfi SJ, Lukka H, Faria SL, Rodrigues GB, Beauchemin MC, Lee RJ, Seaward SA, Allen AM, Monitto DC, Seiferheld W, Sartor O, Feng F, Sandler HM. The addition of androgen deprivation therapy and pelvic lymph node treatment to prostate bed salvage radiotherapy (NRG oncology/RTOG 0534 SPPORT): an international, multicentre, randomised phase 3 trial. Lancet. 2022;399(10338):1886–901.
26. Sella T, Schwartz LH, Swindle PW, Onyebuchi CN, Scardino PT, Scher HI, et al. Suspected local recurrence after radical prostatectomy: endorectal coil MR imaging. Radiology. 2004;231(2):379–85. https://doi.org/10.1148/radiol.2312030011.
27. Park JS, Park W, Pyo HR, Park BK, Park SY, Choi HY, et al. Suggestion for the prostatic fossa clinical target volume in adjuvant or salvage radiotherapy after a radical prostatectomy. Radiother Oncol. 2014;110(2):240–4. https://doi.org/10.1016/j.radonc.2014.01.001.

Part V

Penile Cancer

19 Diagnosis and Clinical Staging

Jyoti Mohan Tosh, Vikas Kumar Panwar, and Ankur Mittal

19.1 Introduction

Squamous cell carcinoma (SCC) of the penis is a common malignancy in Southeast Asian countries. Proper history with relevant diagnostic and management strategies improves survival outcomes in patients. Appropriate management and treatment outcomes in men with SCC of the penis depend on the correct diagnosis, grading and staging of the malignancy.

19.2 Diagnosis

Carcinoma penis clinical presentation ranges from skin ulceration to palpable abnormalities, which may be associated with erythema, penile pain, discharge and foul odour. Most common presentation is mass (45%), ulcer (35%) and inflammatory lesion (17%). In men with penile mass or an ulcer, a high degree of clinical suspicion should always be kept [1]. A thorough clinical history should include the initial time of presentation, progression of lesion, any traumatic history, multiple sexual contacts in the recent past, smoking or tobacco use and any previous local treatment. Metastatic symptoms like weight loss, cachexia, loss of appetite, fatigue and systemic malaise should also be accounted. Primary penile tumours should be evaluated clinically for number, size, location (foreskin, glans, shaft), colour, form (flat, papillary, nodular, ulcerative), involvement of nearby structures (corpus spongiosum, corpora cavernosa, urethra, pubic bone) and borders (edges). The base of the penis and scrotum should also be thoroughly inspected for any induration. Digital rectal examination and bimanual examination help to detect perineal body involvement and pelvic mass.

About 26% of individuals will have an erroneous clinical staging of their initial tumour (T stage). Over-staging from oedema and infection, as well as histologic infiltration that is not clinically visible, might lead to under staging [2].

Additionally, the clinical assessment includes an examination of the enlarged inguinal lymph nodes present in more than 28–64% of the patients [3], with the majority having reactive lymphadenopathy. However, metastases are seen in around 47–85% of palpable inguinal lymph nodes and 20% non-palpable inguinal lymph nodes [4].

Most men have a delayed presentation due to the fear of social stigma and loss of self-esteem. About 15–50% patients present 1 year after the start of first symptom. Penile cancer is a fatal disease, and delay in presentation and diagnosis subsequently makes it lethal [5–9].

Basic lab investigations to detect anaemia, leucocytosis, hypoalbuminemia, hypercalcemia,

J. M. Tosh · V. K. Panwar · A. Mittal (✉)
Department of Urology, AIIMS Rishikesh, Rishikesh, India

P. Singh et al. (eds.), *A Guide to Management of Urological Cancers*,
https://doi.org/10.1007/978-981-99-2341-0_19

azotaemia and raised parathyroid hormone-related substances should be carried out.

19.3 Histopathological Examination

According to the International Guidelines, histopathological evaluation is the gold standard investigation for the confirmation of any suspicious malignant lesions in the penis. Techniques of biopsy include incision, excision, core biopsy or fine needle aspiration cytology (FNAC). An incision or wedge biopsy is the most common, in which a wedge of tissue is incised, including normal and tumour tissue [10–12].

Histopathology report should include information on all factors that are relevant to treatment and prognosis like the anatomic site, tumour size, histologic type or subtype, grade, growth pattern, front of invasion, depth of invasion, tumour thickness and resection margins. It should also include information on lymphovascular invasion and perineural invasion [13–17]. For correct staging, a deep biopsy specimen must be obtained; hence, superficial or shave biopsies are not suitable, and the physician must be cautious as the grade and stage of the initial specimen may vary from those of the final [18]. Cubilla et al., in a retrospective review, classified the histological types into usual type (59%), papillary (15%), basaloid (10%), condylomatous (10%), verrucous (3%) and sarcomatoid (3%). Basaloid and sarcomatoid variants were associated with poor prognosis.

19.3.1 Grade

In SCC of the penis, the grade of the lesion is an important predictive factor for lymph node metastases and outcomes [19]. The degree of anaplasia determines the grading. Velazquez et al. classified the grading into low grade, intermediate and high grade according to the degree of differentiation [20].

According to the recent WHO (World Health Organisation) histopathological classification, penile cancer is graded into three groups [21]:

Grade 1 – Well differentiated
Grade 2 – Moderately differentiated
Grade 3 – Poorly differentiated

Grading is also important for improving the tumour-free margin and decreasing local recurrence after excision of the penile mass. Aggarwal et al. revealed that for grade 1 and 2 tumours, 1 cm clearance is ample and for grade 3 lesion 1.5 cm clearance [22]. The achievement of minimal negative surgical margins has made the organ-sparing approach effectively.

The WHO has recently adopted the International Society of Urologic Pathology (ISUP) grading system after revising the WHO classification. The patient is classified into grade 3 if there is any suspicion of anaplasia [23].

19.4 Staging

19.4.1 Clinical Examination

A complete physical examination, including the location, size, number, involvement of corporal bodies, urethra, prostate, scrotum and pubic bone, helps to assess the local extent of disease. The physical examination also gives a better idea for the corporal invasion, but to perform an organ-preserving approach and to assess the invasiveness accurately, the radiological investigation may be required. Radiological investigations like ultrasonography (USG), computed tomography (CT) and magnetic resonance imaging (MRI) also help in diagnosis, especially in obese patients.

19.4.2 Radiological Investigations

19.4.2.1 Ultrasonography (USG)

Primary Tumour Staging

High-resolution USG has facilitated the depiction of the local extent of tumour, corporal and urethral involvement, which further helps in better planning of surgical management. Aggarwal et al. revealed that the USG was better than physical examination in diagnosing lesions restricted to glans [24]. But Lont et al. showed USG to be useful in diagnosing corporal involvement, which were difficult to determine on clinical examination [25].

Restaging and Post Surveillance

National Comprehensive Cancer Network (NCCN) guidelines recommend serial clinical examination post-surgery for assessment of recurrence. USG is not recommended for surveillance post-surgery; however, in cases of suspicion of recurrence in the nodal basin or penectomy bed, an USG-guided percutaneous biopsy is required to confirm the diagnosis [26].

19.4.2.2 Computed Tomography (CT)

Primary Tumour Staging

CT of the abdomen, pelvis and chest is a good imaging modality for staging tumours and detecting lymph node status. According to NCCN guidelines, patients with low-risk tumours (T1a, Tis, Ta) and non-palpable lymph nodes do not require imaging. NCCN recommends imaging with CT for intermediate-risk tumours (T1b or >T2) or palpable lymph nodes [26, 27].

Restaging and Post Surveillance

NCCN guidelines recommend surveillance with CT abdomen and pelvis in patients with N0 and N1 disease every 6 months for the first 2 years and then yearly for the next 2 years. In N2 and N3 disease, surveillance for recurrence post-surgery is recommended every 3 months for the first 2 years and then every 6 months for the next 2 years [26]. In patients with metastatic disease, CT abdomen, pelvis and chest are essential to assess the response of disease post systemic chemotherapy [26].

19.4.2.3 Magnetic Resonance Imaging (MRI)

Primary Tumour Staging

MRI is now considered as a one-stop imaging modality of choice and is superior to clinical palpation for local staging of penile cancer. It helps to delineate local extension to corpora, tunica albuginea, urethra and distant spread [28]. MRI combined with pharmacologically induced penile erection (PIPE) by injecting 10 µg of prostaglandin E1 has been used for assessing the local staging of penile cancer [29, 30]. On MRI, the penile mass appears hypointense (relative to corpora) on T1W and T2W images and hyperintense (relative to the fascia and tunica) on T2W images [28]. Petralia et al. compared physical examination, USG and MRI in 13 patients and found MRI-PIPE to be better than clinical examination, accurately diagnosing 12 patients, further leading to appropriate management [31].

Restaging and Post Surveillance

MRI is an excellent tool for detecting local recurrences, especially in obese and organ-sparing therapy. It can also detect recurrence post inguinal lymphadenectomy or radiation therapy [32].

19.4.2.4 Positron Emission Tomography-Computed Tomography (PET-CT)

Primary Tumour Staging

18F-Fluorodeoxyglucose (FDG) PET imaging has also shown promises for accurate detection of nodal metastases by providing both anatomical information and functional imaging [33, 34]. It can be used in patients with allergy to contrast or those with low glomerular filtration rate, which hinders the use of contrast. PET-CT is not advised for the staging of primary penile cancers, despite the fact that they are almost all FDG-avid. This is because of the low spatial resolution of the scan and is hampered by urine FDG excretion [33].

Sadeghi et al., in a meta-analysis, demonstrated a pooled sensitivity per groin with PET-CT to be just 57% in the N0 group of patients. PET-CT is not recommended for staging in non-palpable lymph nodes [35]. PET-CT is preferable in patients with inguinal metastases. It can be used in detecting pelvic node metastases and occult distant metastases before administering systemic chemotherapy [33].

Restaging and Post Surveillance

According to NCCN guidelines, PET-CT can be used for systemic staging in patients with recurrent and metastatic disease [26].

19.5 Nodal Staging

The most important prognostic factor for survival in penile cancer patients is the existence and spread of metastases. They have a constant pattern of spread initially to inguinal and then to pelvic and further to distant organs. Appropriate staging is of prime importance for proper clinical staging in these patients. Patients with non-palpable nodes have a good prognosis, whereas those with higher stage of lymph node involvement have a worse prognosis [35, 36].

19.5.1 Clinical Examination

Around 28–64% of penile carcinoma patients have clinically enlarged lymph nodes. Less than 50% of patients have inflammatory lymph nodes, and 47–85% of patients with lymph nodes have a metastatic invasion. Metastatic nodes are unilateral in 75% of cases, and the rest are bilateral [10, 37, 38]. Clinical examination of inguinal lymph nodes, including size, number and fixity, is paramount in the initial evaluation for a patient with penile mass, which helps in further management, but has a high false-negative rate. In obese patients and in whom the clinical examination is doubtful, radiological imaging is often helpful.

19.5.2 Radiological Investigations

19.5.2.1 Ultrasound (USG)

USG can be the initial evaluation of non-palpable lymph nodes. In non-palpable lymph nodes, the chance of micro-metastasis is approximately 25%. It can reveal abnormal nodes with some enlargement. The short to long axis ratio <2, abnormal shape, eccentric cortical hypertrophy and loss of fatty hilum in a node have high specificity to characterize metastatic nodes [39]. A negative inguinal ultrasound does not rule out the need for nodal dissection [27, 40].

In palpable lymphadenopathy, USG helps in diagnosis, and percutaneous biopsy helps in confirming the metastases with a sensitivity of 93%, which expedites surgical dissection [41, 42].

19.5.2.2 CT and MRI Imaging

In non-palpable lymph nodes, CT/MRI imaging has not shown any advantage to delineate the extent of lymphadenopathy. But its role may be evident in obese patients, in prior inguinal surgery or in whom the clinical examination is doubtful [43].

19.5.2.3 Positron Emission Tomography (PET)

Metastatic lymph nodes have a tendency for increased uptake of FDG, which facilitates detection, but smaller-size <2 mm micro-metastases are underreported [44]. Sadeghi et al., in a meta-analysis, demonstrated a pooled sensitivity per groin with PET-CT to be just 57% in the N0 group of patients. PET-CT is not recommended for staging in non-palpable lymph nodes [35]. PET-CT is preferable in patients with inguinal metastases. It can be used in detecting pelvic node metastases and distant metastases before administering systemic chemotherapy [33].

19.5.2.4 Lymphotropic Nano-particle-Enhanced Magnetic Resonance Imaging (LNMRI)

LNMRI is a novel technique that uses ultrasmall super magnetic iron oxide particles like ferumoxtran-10 or ferumoxytol. These nano-particles get deposited in the lymph nodes and are phagocytosed by macrophages resulting in accumulation of contrast, but malignant nodes reveal low contrast accumulation due to fewer macrophages. So the benign nodes have low T2 intensity, but malignant nodes show a high T2 intense image. It is an important diagnostic tool in detecting microscopic metastases [45]. Tabatabaei et al. compared standard MRI and LNMRI and revealed a significant advantage of LNMRI over MRI with a sensitivity (100%), specificity (97%), PPV (81%) and NPV (100%), respectively [34].

19.5.2.5 Minimally Invasive Staging

Sentinel Lymph Node Biopsy (SLNB)

The role of invasive imaging to detect micrometastases becomes vital due to the unpredictability and low sensitivity of noninvasive modality. In the year 1977, Cabana demonstrated the first echelon node, located superomedial to junction of saphenous and femoral veins in the area of superficial epigastric region [46]. Conventional histopathological approaches may miss metastases in the sentinel lymph node (SLN) that may be diagnosed with a more targeted approach. But the reliability of SLN was questioned because of high false-negative rate of 25% for the anatomical variation in the SLN position [47].

Dynamic Sentinel Node Biopsy (DSNB)

It uses a combination of injection of dye (technetium-99 m nano-colloid or vital blue) and visualization of SLN using handheld gamma camera. It has a minimal role in clinically palpable nodes but has a sensitivity of 80% in occult lymph node metastases [48]. The histopathological examination includes serial sectioning of involved nodes along with cytokeratin immunohistochemical staining [48]. It accurately reveals the SLN with minimal complication and acceptable sensitivity.

19.5.2.6 Modified Inguinal Lymphadenectomy

Modified inguinal lymphadenectomy includes a small skin incision, limited field of inguinal dissection, preservation of saphenous vein and avoiding transposition of sartorius muscle over the exposed femoral vessels [49]. It is associated with a high complication rate over DSNB, and its oncological safety has also been questioned, although its false-negative rate seems comparable with that of SNB [50]. Nowadays, the modified inguinal lymphadenectomy is largely replaced by the SNB procedure, but it can be used as an alternative if the identification of a sentinel node fails [51].

19.6 Metastatic Staging

19.6.1 Assessment for Distant Metastatic Disease

Distant metastases are uncommon in the carcinoma penis, and patients who present with the node-positive disease need further evaluation. In patients with metastatic symptoms and clinically enlarged nodes, CT of the abdomen and pelvis with chest X-ray or CT chest should be done. PET/CT is also a sensitive and alternate imaging option that should be considered for pelvic nodal and distant metastases in penile cancer patients with positive inguinal nodes [36] (Fig. 19.1).

19.7 TNM Staging

In 1966, the Jackson staging system was initially used, but subsequently, the first TNM classification was developed in 1968, and since then, many modifications have been done [52]. The TNM staging is used to prognosticate and plan the best management options. Now the eighth edition of the American Joint Committee

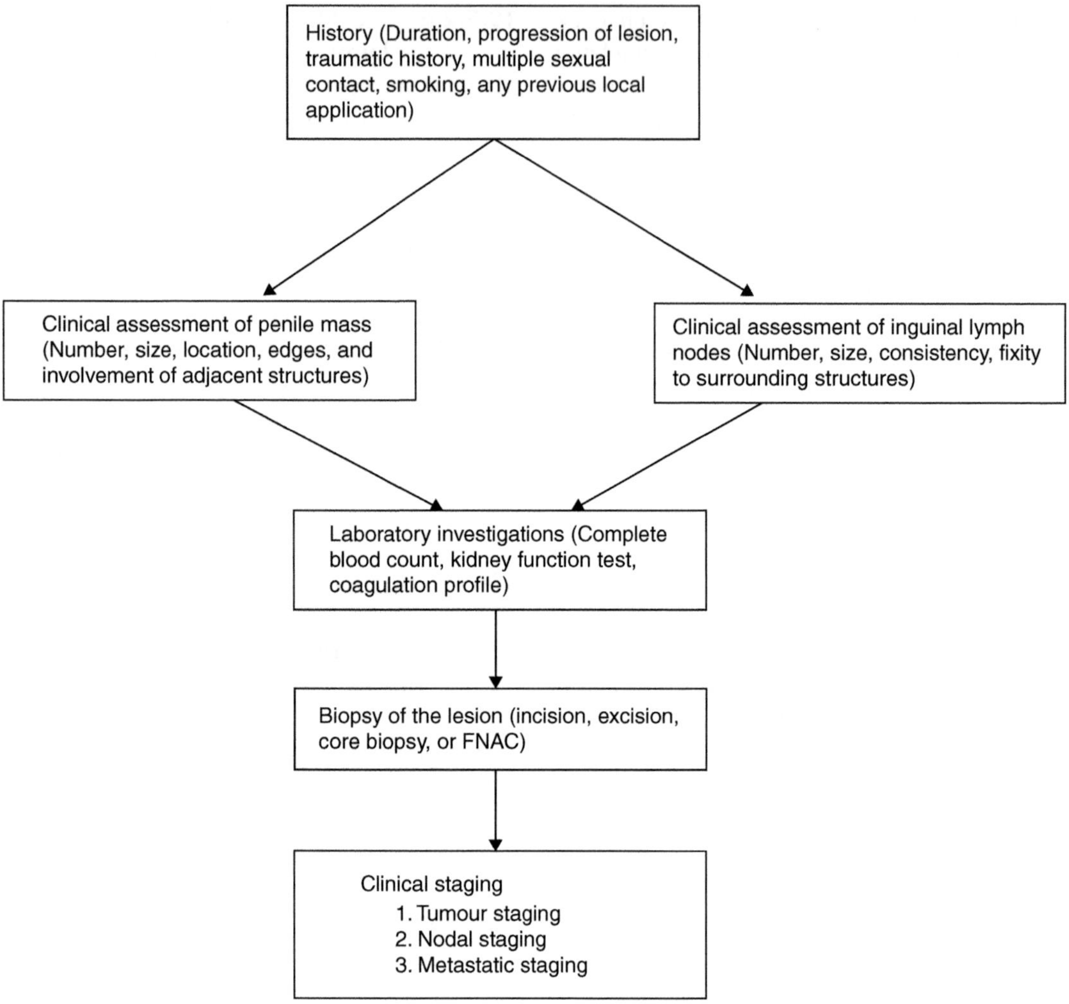

Fig. 19.1 Flow chart: diagnosis and staging

on Cancer (AJCC) and Union for International Cancer Control (UICC) tumour, node and metastasis (TNM) staging system is used for staging carcinoma of the penis (Table 19.1). In the seventh edition of AJCC, involvement of corpora cavernosa or spongiosa was classified as T2 whereas involvement of urethra was classified as T3 stage. However, in the recent eighth edition of AJCC TNM staging, involvement of corpora spongiosa with or without urethral involvement was revised as T2 stage whereas involvement of corpora cavernosa with or without urethral involvement was classified as T3 stage. In seventh edition of nodal staging, single lymph node metastasis was classified as pN1, and multiple or bilateral inguinal lymph node (ILN) metastases was classified as pN2 whereas in the eighth edition, ≤ 2 unilateral ILN metastasis without extranodal extension was classified as pN1 and ≥ 3 unilateral or bilateral ILN metastasis was classified as pN2 [53].

Key Points

1. SCC of the penis is a common malignancy in Southeast Asian countries.

Table 19.1 Staging of primary tumour

pT category	T criteria
Tx	Primary tumour cannot be assessed
T0	No evidence of primary tumour
Tis	Carcinoma in situ (penile intraepithelial neoplasia – PeIN)
Ta	Noninvasive localized squamous cell carcinoma
T1	Glans: Tumour invades the lamina propria
	Foreskin: Tumour invades the dermis, lamina propria or dartos fascia
	Shaft: Tumour invades connective tissue between the epidermis and corpora regardless of location
	All sites with or without lymphovascular invasion or perineural invasion are and/or are not high grade
T1a	Tumour is without lymphovascular invasion or perineural invasion and is not high grade (i.e. grade 3 or sarcomatoid)
T1b	Tumour exhibits lymphovascular invasion and/or perineural invasion or is high grade (i.e. grade 3 or sarcomatoid)
T2	Tumour invades into the corpus spongiosum (either glans or ventral shaft) with or without urethral invasion
T3	Tumour invades into the corpora cavernosum (including tunica albuginea) with or without urethral invasion
T4	Tumour invades into adjacent structures (i.e. scrotum, prostate, pubic bone)

pN category	N criteria
Nx	Lymph node metastasis cannot be established
N0	No lymph node metastasis
N1	≤2 unilateral inguinal metastases, no extranodal extension
N2	≥3 unilateral inguinal metastases or bilateral metastases, no extranodal extension
N3	Extranodal extension of lymph node metastases or pelvic lymph node metastases

M category	M criteria
M0	No distant metastases present
M1	Distant metastases present

GROUP	T	N	M
Stage 0is	Tis	N0	M0
Stage 0a	Ta	N0	M0
Stage I	T1a	N0	M0
Stage IIA	T1b	N0	M0
Stage IIA	T2	N0	M0
Stage IIB	T3	N0	M0
Stage IIIA	T1–T3	N1	M0
Stage IIIB	T1–T3	N2	M0
Stage IV	T4	Any N	M0
Stage IV	Any T	N3	M0
Stage IV	Any T	Any N	M1

2. Appropriate history and meticulous clinical examination are key to early diagnosis and management.
3. Histopathological biopsy is the gold standard for the diagnosis of penile cancer.
4. Radiological investigations like USG, CT, MRI, PET-CT and LNMRI act as adjuncts for clinical staging of tumour mass, nodes and metastases.
5. Sentinel lymph node biopsy has shown role in detecting micro-metastases.

References

1. Barocas D, Chang S. Penile cancer: clinical presentation, diagnosis, and staging. Urol Clin N Am. 2010;37(3):343–52.
2. Horenblas S, Van Tinteren H, Delemarre JF, et al. Squamous cell carcinoma of the penis: accuracy of tumor, nodes and metastasis classification system, and role of lymphangiography, computerized tomography scan and fine needle aspiration cytology. J Urol. 1991;146(5):1279–83.
3. Sufrin G, Huben R. Benign and malignant lesions of the penis. In: Gillenwater JY, Grayhack JT, Howards SS, Duckett JW, editors. Adult and pediatric urology. 2nd ed. Chicago: Mosby Year Book Medical Publishers; 1991. p. 1997–2042.
4. Penile cancer lymph nodes, illustration. The British Association of Urological Surgeons. https://www.baus.org.uk/professionals/sections/penile_cancer.aspx.
5. Carver BS, Mata JA, Venable DD, Eastham JA. Squamous cell carcinoma of the penis: a retrospective review of forty-five patients in Northwest Louisiana. South Med J. 2002;95(8):822–5.
6. Burgers JK, Badalament RA, Drago JR. Penile cancer. Clinical presentation, diagnosis, and staging. Urol Clin North Am. 1992;19(2):247–56.
7. Gursel E, Georgountzos C, Uson A, Melicow M, Veenema R. Penile cancer Clinicopathologic study of 64 cases. Urology. 1973;1(6):569–78.
8. Hardner G, Bhanalaph T, Murphy G, Albert D, Moore R. Carcinoma of the penis: analysis of therapy in 100 consecutive cases. J Urol. 1972;108(3):428–30.
9. Lynch HT, Krush AJ. Delay factors in detection of cancer of the penis. Nebr State Med J. 1969;54(6):360–7.
10. Solsona E, Algaba F, Horenblas S, Pizzocaro G, Windahl T. EAU guidelines on penile cancer. Eur Urol. 2004;46(1):1–8.
11. Edge S, Compton C. The American joint committee on cancer: the 7th edition of the AJCC cancer staging manual and the future of TNM. Ann Surg Oncol. 2010;17(6):1471–4.
12. Sobin L, Gospodarowicz M, Wittekind C. TNM classification of malignant tumours. Chichester: Wiley-Blackwell; 2009.
13. Cubilla A. The role of pathologic prognostic factors in squamous cell carcinoma of the penis. World J Urol. 2008;27(2):169–77.
14. Lopes A, Hidalgo G, Kowalski L, Torloni H, Rossi B, Fonseca F. Prognostic factors in carcinoma of the penis: multivariate analysis of 145 patients treated with amputation and lymphadenectomy. J Urol. 1996;156(5):1637–42.
15. Villavicencio H, Rubio-Briones J, Regalado R, et al. Grade, local stage and growth pattern as prognostic factors in carcinoma of the penis. Eur Urol. 1997;32(4):442–7.
16. Emerson R, Ulbright T, Eble J, Geary W, Eckert G, Cheng L. Predicting cancer progression in patients with penile squamous cell carcinoma: the importance of depth of invasion and vascular invasion. Mod Pathol. 2001;14(10):963–8.
17. Slaton JW, Morgenstern N, Levy DA, et al. Tumor stage, vascular invasion and the percentage of poorly differentiated cancer: independent prognosticators for inguinal lymph node metastasis in penile squamous cancer. J Urol. 2001;165(4):1138–42.
18. Velazquez E, Barreto J, Rodriguez I, Piris A, Cubilla A. Limitations in the interpretation of biopsies in patients with penile squamous cell carcinoma. Int J Surg Pathol. 2004;12(2):139–46.
19. Aita G, Zequi S, Costa W, Guimarães G, Soares F, Giuliangelis T. Tumor histologic grade is the most important prognostic factor in patients with penile cancer and clinically negative lymph nodes not submitted to regional lymphadenectomy. Int Braz J Urol. 2016;42(6):1136–43.
20. Velazquez E, Ayala G, Liu H, Chaux A, Zanotti M, Torres J, et al. Histologic grade and Perineural invasion are more important than tumor thickness as predictor of nodal metastasis in penile squamous cell carcinoma invading 5 to 10 mm. Am J Surg Pathol. 2008;32(7):974–9.
21. Cubilla A, Velazquez E, Amin M, Epstein J, Berney D, Corbishley C. The World Health Organisation 2016 classification of penile carcinomas: a review and update from the International Society of Urological Pathology expert-driven recommendations. Histopathology. 2018;72(6):893–904.
22. Agrawal A, Pai D, Ananthakrishnan N, Smile S, Ratnakar C. The histological extent of the local spread of carcinoma of the penis and its therapeutic implications. BJU Int. 2000;85(3):299–301.
23. Sanchez D, Fernandez-Nestosa M, Canete-Portillo S, Rodriguez I, Cubilla A. What is new in the pathologic staging of penile carcinoma in the 8th edition of AJCC TNM model: rationale for changes with practical stage-by-stage Category diagnostic considerations. Adv Anat Pathol. 2021;28(4):209–27.
24. Agrawal A, Pai D, Ananthakrishnan N, et al. Clinical and sonographic findings in carcinoma of the penis. J Clin Ultrasound. 2000;28(8):399–406.
25. Lont A, Besnard A, Gallee M, Van Tinteren H, Horenblas S. A comparison of physical examination and imaging in determining the extent of primary penile carcinoma. BJU Int. 2003;91(6):493–5.
26. Treatment by cancer type [Internet]. NCCN. 2022. https://www.nccn.org/guidelines/category_1.
27. Heyns C, Mendoza-Valdes A, Pompeo A. Diagnosis and staging of penile cancer. Urology. 2010;76(2):S15–23.
28. Krishna S, Shanbhogue K, Schieda N, Morbeck F, Hadas B, Kulkarni G, et al. Role of MRI in staging of penile cancer. J Magn Reson Imaging. 2020;51(6):1612–29.

29. Scardino E, Villa G, Bonomo G, Matei D, Verweij F, Rocco B, et al. Magnetic resonance imaging combined with artificial erection for local staging of penile cancer. Urology. 2004;63(6):1158–62.
30. Kayes O, Minhas S, Allen C, Hare C, Freeman A, Ralph D. The role of magnetic resonance imaging in the local staging of penile cancer. Eur Urol. 2007;51(5):1313–9.
31. Petralia G, Villa G, Scardino E, Zoffoli E, Renne G, de Cobelli O, et al. Local staging of penile cancer using magnetic resonance imaging with pharmacologically induced penile erection. Radiol Med. 2008;113(4):517–28.
32. Graafland N, Moonen L, van Boven H, van Werkhoven E, Kerst J, Horenblas S. Inguinal recurrence following therapeutic lymphadenectomy for node positive penile carcinoma: outcome and implications for management. J Urol. 2011;185(3):888–94.
33. Ottenhof S, Vegt E. The role of PET/CT imaging in penile cancer. Transl Androl Urol. 2017;6(5):833–8.
34. Tabatabaei S, Harisinghani M, McDougal WS. Regional lymph node staging using lymphotropic nanoparticle enhanced magnetic resonance imaging with ferumoxtran-10 in patients with penile cancer. J Urol. 2005;174(3):923–7.
35. Sadeghi R, Gholami H, Zakavi S, Kakhki V, Horenblas S. Accuracy of 18F-FDG PET/CT for diagnosing inguinal lymph node involvement in penile squamous cell carcinoma. Clin Nucl Med. 2012;37(5):436–41.
36. Hakenberg O, Compérat E, Minhas S, Necchi A, Protzel C, Watkin N. EAU guidelines on penile cancer: 2014 update. Eur Urol. 2015;67(1):142–50.
37. Horenblas S, Van Tinteren H. Squamous cell carcinoma of the penis. IV. Prognostic factors of survival: analysis of tumor, nodes and metastasis classification system. J Urol. 1994;151(5):1239–43.
38. Ficarra V, Galfano A. Should the dynamic sentinel node biopsy (DSNB) be considered the gold standard in the evaluation of lymph node status in patients with penile carcinoma? Eur Urol. 2007;52(1):17–9.
39. Krishna R, Sistla S, Smile R, Krishnan R. Sonography: an underutilized diagnostic tool in the assessment of metastatic groin nodes. J Clin Ultrasound. 2008;36(4):212–7.
40. Kochhar R, Taylor B, Sangar V. Imaging in primary penile cancer: current status and future directions. Eur Radiol. 2009;20(1):36–47.
41. Kroon B, Horenblas S, Deurloo E, Nieweg O, Teertstra H. Ultrasonography-guided fine-needle aspiration cytology before sentinel node biopsy in patients with penile carcinoma. BJU Int. 2005;95(4):517–21.
42. Saisorn I, Lawrentschuk N, Leewansangtong S, Bolton DM. Fine-needle aspiration cytology predicts inguinal lymph node metastasis without antibiotic pretreatment in penile carcinoma. BJU Int. 2006;97(6):1225–8.
43. Hughes B, Leijte J, Shabbir M, Watkin N, Horenblas S. Non-invasive and minimally invasive staging of regional lymph nodes in penile cancer. World J Urol. 2008;27(2):197–203.
44. Scher B, Seitz M, Reiser M, et al. 18F-FDG PET/CT for staging of penile cancer. J Nucl Med. 2005;46(9):1460–5.
45. Eisner BH, Feldman AS. Nanoparticle imaging for genitourinary cancers. Cancer Biomark. 2009;5(2):75–9.
46. Cabanas R. An approach for the treatment of penile carcinoma. Cancer. 1977;39(2):456–66.
47. Pettaway C, Pisters L, Dinney C, Jularbal F, Swanson D, von Eschenbach A, et al. Sentinel lymph node dissection for penile carcinoma: the M. D. Anderson cancer center experience. J Urol. 1995;154(6):1999–2003.
48. Tanis P, Lont A, Meinhardt W, Olmos R, Nieweg O, Horenblas S. Dynamic sentinel node biopsy for penile cancer: reliability of a staging technique. J Urol. 2002;168(1):76–80.
49. Catalona W. Modified inguinal lymphadenectomy for carcinoma of the penis with preservation of saphenous veins: technique and preliminary results. J Urol. 1988;140(2):306–10.
50. d'Ancona CAL, de Lucena RG, Querne FA, et al. Long-term followup of penile carcinoma treated with penectomy and bilateral modified inguinal lymphadenectomy. J Urol. 2004;172:498–501.
51. Ferreira U, Ribeiro M, Reis L, Prudente A, Matheus W. Sentinel lymph node biopsy in penile cancer: a comparative study using modified inguinal dissection. Int Braz J Urol. 2008;34(6):725–33.
52. Jackson S. The treatment of carcinoma of the penis. Br J Surg. 1966;53(1):33–5.
53. Kandori S, Kojima T, Nishiyama H. The updated points of TNM classification of urological cancers in the 8th edition of AJCC and UICC. Jpn J Clin Oncol. 2019;49(5):421–5.

Pathology and Staging

20

Subhash Yadav, Santosh Menon,
and Sangeeta Desai

20.1 Introduction and Epidemiology

Penile cancers have a heterogeneous distribution worldwide, ranging from age-standardised incidence of >2 per 100,000 in Africa, South America and South Asia to incidence of <0.5 per 100,000 in the Middle East and East Asia [1]. Penile cancer (PC) is an extremely uncommon disease with an incidence as low as 0.29/100,000 in the United States [2].The World Health Organization (WHO) estimated a total of 36,068 new cases in 2020 with an incidence of 0.8 per 100,000 men worldwide [3]. Penile squamous cell carcinoma (PSCC) is the fourth least common cancer by incidence and is classified under "rare tumour" as per the definition by the National Cancer Institute [4]. The incidence is higher in certain African and South American countries such as Uganda with an incidence of 4.4 per 100,000 and Paraguay with an incidence of 4.2 per 100,000 [2]. This heterogeneity is attributed to various risk factors such as socioeconomic status, history of penile injuries and inflammation, tobacco smoking, hygiene, genetic predisposition, the prevalence of practice of circumcision and human papillomavirus (HPV) infection [5, 6].

S. Yadav · S. Menon (✉) · S. Desai
Department of Pathology, Tata Memorial Centre, Mumbai, India

Penile cancers occur predominantly in the elderly age group, with a peak incidence in the sixth decade of life [6]. Cancer registry data from urban India from 2006 to 2008 revealed an age-specific incidence of 0.7–3 per 100,000 person in India and with increasing incidence with age [7]. The incidence rates were 1.8, 3.8 and 6.6 for age group 45–54, 55–64 and >65 years, respectively [7]. The International Agency for Research on Cancer (IARC) has published the relative frequency of penile cancer among males and the incidence rates in different parts of the world by gleaning data from different cancer registries [8, 9]. Indian cancer registry data in volumes VIII (1993–1997) and X (2003–2007) showed a decline in relative frequency and age-standardised ratio in the urban population. Incidence is higher in the rural parts of India [7].

Similar to head and neck carcinoma and cervical/vulvar carcinoma, PSCC also shows two major pathogenic mechanisms: one related to HPV and the other independent of HPV. However, unlike the uterine cervix where the majority are HPV-associated cancers, only 30–50% of penile cancers are HPV-related cancers [6]. Male circumcision is known to be protective against PC, although it has never been systematically evaluated. In African countries, circumcision drives have been carried out for HIV prevention, which in turn has shown benefit in the prevention of PC also [10].

P. Singh et al. (eds.), *A Guide to Management of Urological Cancers*,
https://doi.org/10.1007/978-981-99-2341-0_20

20.2 Risk Factors for Penile Cancer

The most important risk factor for penile cancer is **phimosis** or the presence of an intact tight foreskin. Penile cancer is almost unknown in Jews who are circumscribed at birth. Around 25–60% of the patients with PC have a history of phimosis signifying its causal effect [11]. The odds ratio (OR) varies from 2.3 to 16 in various studies for the association of phimosis with invasive PC [12–14]. Phimosis was significantly associated with invasive PC in the study by Maden et al. [14] with an OR of 3.39 [14]. Similar associations have been observed by Tseng et al. [13] with an adjusted OR of 16. However, there was no increased risk for carcinoma in situ with phimosis (OR 1.7). Circumcision in infancy was inversely associated with invasive cancer (OR 0.41) [13]. The lowest incidence of penile cancer is seen in Israeli Jews who practise neonatal circumcision. Pathogenesis for the development of malignancy in cases with phimosis relates to the associated chronic infection and inflammation secondary to poor penile hygiene. Smegma, a putative factor suspected of contributing to PC, is not a proven carcinogen as such [15].

The relative risk of PC in uncircumcised men is 22:1 as compared to circumcised men [16]. Also, the incidence of PC in uncircumcised men was 3.2 times greater than those who are circumcised at birth and was 3 times more than those circumcised in the neonatal period [14]. Hence, the benefit of circumcision in the prevention of PC appears to be in the immediate neonatal period of birth [14].

Lichen sclerosus, a common inflammatory dermatological condition, is a known risk factor for PSCC; penile lichen sclerosus has an estimated risk of malignant transformation of 4–8% [17]. Another dermatological disease, **psoriasis**, in which patients are treated with psoralens and ultraviolet A radiation therapy (PUVA), is known to carry a high risk of development of invasive PC. The risk was as high as 286 times with high-dose exposure to PUVA and 16.3 times for low-dose exposure [18]. **Smoking** also increases the risk of invasive PC by fivefold and an OR of 1.44 [12, 14, 19]. Also, the risk of invasive PC has been demonstrated to be more in those who smoked >10 cigarettes/day (OR 1.44), those more than 5 years (OR 1.43) and a lifetime exposure risk of >30 packs/year (OR 1.86). Tobacco chewing is also an important etiological factor with an OR 3.11. The combination of smoking and tobacco chewing carried a higher risk with an OR 3.39 [19]. In India, tobacco chewing is rampant, and this might be an associated factor for the higher incidence as compared to the West [19].

The unmarried population has a higher likelihood of occurrence and advanced disease in an analysis of 1884 patients from the SEER (Surveillance, Epidemiology, and End Results) database [20]. The incidence of locally advanced disease was significantly higher in unmarried men as compared to married [20].

Epidemiological studies have found a direct correlation of **poor socio-economic status** as an important risk factor for penile cancer development [21]. Early first intercourse and multiple sexual partners also contribute to a 3–5-time higher incidence of penile cancer [14]. A Danish population-based analysis of 1292 patients with invasive penile cancer showed that patients who were unmarried, divorced and widowed had a higher incidence of invasive PC [22]. Injury to the penis in the form of **tear or abrasion and chronic balanitis/balanoposthitis** are risk factors for malignancy [12–14]. Patients infected with the **human immunodeficiency virus (HIV)** are also at an increased risk of invasive PC [23].

Role of human papilloma virus (HPV)—Penile carcinogenesis involves two major pathogenetic pathways: one HPV-driven and the other HPV-independent [24]. Approximately, one-third to half of the cases of invasive PC is associated with HPV infection, the majority being associated with strain HPV16 and HPV18 [25]. The HPV-mediated oncogenic effect lies in the expression of E6 and E7 oncoproteins impacting cellular proliferation and differentiation [24]. To determine the prevalence of HPV infection, a large international multicentric study involving 25 countries demonstrated an incidence of 33.1% in invasive PC and 87.1% in pre-malignant conditions. The highest prevalence was seen in the warty-basaloid variants [25]. Around 76% of basaloid variants and 82% of warty-basaloid variants of penile squamous carcinoma are known to harbour HPV infection [26]. Another multi-institutional study analysed the presence of HPV DNA in a large cohort of invasive cancer, dysplasia and condyloma. HPV DNA was isolated in 42% of invasive cancers, 90% dysplasia and 100% condyloma specimens. This study also emphasised the relative frequency of occurrence of different strains of HPV in specimens of dysplasia as follows: HPV16—40.7%, HPV6—22.2%, HPV52—14.8% and HPV11—3.7%. HPV18 was typically absent in all specimens of dysplasia [2]. The risk of PC is increased in patients with condyloma acuminata [27]. Although most HPV infections are transient, patients who develop condyloma/warts persistently harbour these infections and increase the risk for PC [27].

20.3 Pathology of Premalignant Conditions and their Recent Terminologies

The premalignant/precursor lesions of PSCC have been termed variably as Erythroplasia of Queyrat, penile Bowen's disease, penile carcinoma in situ and bowenoid papulosis. This nomenclature with multiple terminologies for the same entity creates confusion for pathologists and clinicians, especially as they do not describe the grade of the premalignant changes and their consequent prognosis and progression to malignancy [28]. The standardised term penile intraepithelial neoplasia (PeIN) is now preferred as per WHO classification, over previous terms [29]. Clinically they present as flat or slightly raised pale, white or erythematous lesions on the prepuce or the glans penis.

PeIN is divided into two subtypes: a differentiated subtype, which is typically lichen sclerosus-associated, and an undifferentiated HPV-associated subtype [30–32]. Some even propose a three-tier grading for undifferentiated HPV-associated PeIN [28]. A registry-based study in the Netherlands found that 7% of PeIN 3 (severe dysplasia), 8% of PeIN 2 (moderate dysplasia) and 2% of PeIN 1 progressed to malignancy [28]. PeIN lesions are commonly noted on the prepuce (45%) or glans (38%) [28]. The majority of PeIN lesions are HPV positive, and they predominantly harbour several HPV genotypes (HPV6, HPV11 or HPV16). Undifferentiated PeINs, of which 80% are HPV positive, are mostly associated with HPV16 [32]. Progression of HPV16 infection to PeIN is believed to occur in up to 2% of cases and typically occurs over a longer period (within 2 years) [27].

Morphologically, a differentiated PeIN shows thickened squamous epithelium with elongated, anastomosing rete ridges, abnormal maturation with some squamous cells having striking eosinophilic cytoplasm, basal layer atypia, parakeratosis, prominence of intercellular bridges and presence of basal and suprabasal mitotic figures. The undifferentiated PeIN, on the other hand, are divided morphologically into warty type characterised by prominent pleomorphism and koilocytosis and basaloid type which has full thickness of immature and atypical squamous cells with small, monotonous basophilic appearance. A warty-basaloid PeIN may be seen which has an admixture of warty and basaloid cells [28, 29].

P16 is negative in differentiated PeIN while it is positive in warty and basaloid PeIN. Basaloid PeIN is commonly associated with HPV16 while the warty ones can have a heterogeneous HPV genomic profile [33]. The differentiated PeIN are usually associated with low-grade keratinising squamous carcinoma while the basaloid and warty subtypes develop invasive basaloid and warty carcinomas [28, 29].

20.4 Pathogenetic Mechanisms of Penile Carcinogenesis

PSCC can develop along HPV-dependent and HPV-independent pathogenetic pathways. In the HPV-related pathway, a persistent and/or recurrent exposure of the penile epithelium to HPV leads to the integration of HPV DNA into the host genome and eventual transformation of the host cell. This triggers an overexpression of viral oncoproteins E6 and E7 and subsequent host genomic instability through interaction with p53 and pRb, respectively. The association of E7 with pRb results in overexpression of p16INK4a, which is a useful surrogate biomarker of HPV-related PSCC [34, 35].

Through a complex downstream pathway involving p21 and p27 along with cyclins A and E, this E7 protein promotes cell proliferation and aids cellular immortalisation/carcinogenesis. The inhibitory effects of E6 on p53 and BCL-2 homologous antagonist/killer (BAK) lead to suppression of apoptosis and induction of chromosomal instability and activates telomerase and SRC kinases, leading to cell immortalisation and dysregulated growth [36].

In contrast to genomic events in HPV-induced carcinogenesis, pathways relating to non-HPV-related penile carcinogenesis and progression are not very well understood. However, few studies have implicated chemical mediators of chronic inflammation and somatic gene alterations [34]. Chronic inflammation, in long term, causes malignant transformation via the production of reactive oxygen species and reactive nitrogen intermediates that can induce DNA damage and genomic instability. As alluded earlier, many chronic inflammatory conditions, including balanoposthitis, phimosis and lichen sclerosus, which are important risk factors for the development of penile cancer, converge on acting via a common pathway of inducing cyclooxygenase 2 (COX2) expression, which is implicated in the development of differentiated PeIN and primary PSCC. COX2 overexpression, in turn, drives the overproduction of prostaglandins (most notably prostaglandin E2) and thromboxanes, promoting angiogenesis, proliferation and invasion [37–39].

Somatic gene alterations in tumour suppressor genes of the p16INK4a/cyclin D/Rb apoptotic pathways are the other alternate mechanisms of carcinogenesis in HPV-independent pathway [40, 41]. Tumour microenvironment, including tumour-infiltrating lymphocytes, may also influence and modify the unique biology of each individual penile cancer both in HPV-positive and HPV-negative tumours [42].

In recent years, understanding of expression of programmed cell death 1 ligand 1 (PDL1) expression on tumour cells, CD163-positive macrophages within the tumour, non-classical HLA class 1 upregulation and low stromal CD8-positive T cell infiltration has offered unique insights into tumour microenvironment, and this promises to improve personalised targeted therapy [43, 44].

20.5 Pathology and Staging of Invasive Squamous Carcinoma

A formal biopsy is necessary in all cases of suspected PC. Some penile lesions that appear ulcerative or inflammatory may be a benign disease and hence mandate a biopsy before any radical procedure is planned. The aim on a biopsy is to diagnose cancer and ascertain its grade and depth and extent of invasion. Based on the grade and depth of invasion, the decision on the extent of resection is taken by the urologist as per risk stratification [45].

For a partial or complete penile amputation specimen, a standardised grossing protocol is required to be employed to precisely stage the tumour (Fig. 20.1). Further management, especially addressing the nodal basin in the inguinal region, is based on final staging on a resection specimen [46]. Lymph node metastasis is the single most important predictor of survival analysis in patients with penile squamous carcinoma [46]. Penile carcinoma metastasises to the regional group of lymph nodes via the penile lymphatic vessels. The regional group includes the superficial and the deep inguinal nodes and subsequently the iliac group of the lymph nodes [47].

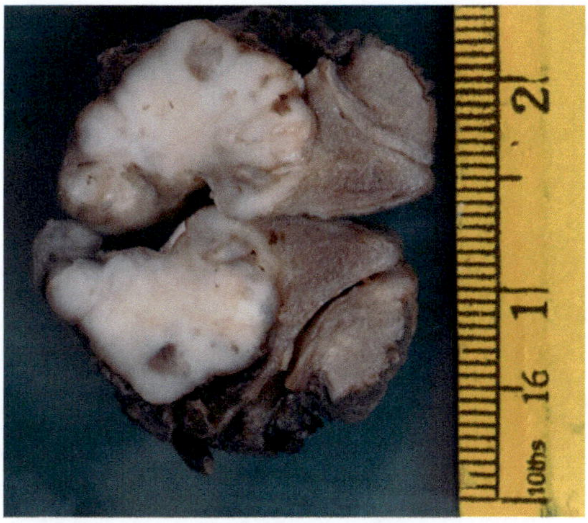

Fig. 20.1 Gross images of a partial penectomy specimen showing a whitish solid tumour involving the glans penis with infiltration of the glans

Ultrasonography combined with fine needle aspiration (FNA) for lymph node status may be deemed necessary in clinically suspicious nodal findings. A positive FNA finding indicate nodal metastasis requiring inguinal lymph node dissection; however, a negative result does not entirely rule out lymph node metastasis [48, 49].

Most classification schemes of PSCC before the year 2016 were morphology-based. The 2016 WHO classification organised a new classification based on clinicopathological distinctiveness and relation to HPV infection. An overview of subtypes and salient histopathological features is as follows [29, 50].

20.5.1 HPV-Independent Squamous Cell Carcinoma

1. Squamous cell carcinoma, usual type (Fig. 20.2a, b): This constitutes nearly 45–75% of all squamous carcinomas. Various degrees of squamous differentiation and keratinisation are noted in these tumours based on their grade which follows a three-tiered WHO/ISUP grading system.
2. Verrucous carcinoma: Papillomatosis, hyperkeratosis, acanthosis, extreme squamous differentiation, no koilocytosis, broad-based and pushing tumour front.
3. Papillary carcinoma, NOS: Variable and complex papillae with or without fibrovascular core, hyperkeratosis, maturing squamous cells with minimal to moderate atypia, no koilocytosis and irregular and jagged tumour-stromal interface.
4. Sarcomatoid carcinoma: Biphasic epithelial-spindle cell neoplasm, composed of atypical spindle cells arranged in fascicles or bundles, with or without foci of carcinoma, sometimes pleomorphic or giant cells or heterologous bone and cartilaginous formation.

Other rare types of non-HPV-/HPV-independent squamous carcinoma variants include pseudohyperplastic carcinoma, pseudoglandular carcinoma, carcinoma cuniculatum and adenosquamous carcinoma.

20.5.2 HPV-Related Squamous Carcinomas

1. Basaloid carcinoma forms approximately 4–10% of squamous carcinomas. Solid or centrally necrotic (comedo necrosis) nests and islands of small uniform basaloid cells, abrupt keratinisation, abundant mitosis and apoptosis (Fig. 20.3a, b).
2. Warty carcinoma composed of a condylomatous pattern of papillae with prominent fibrovascular cores, with hyper- and parakeratosis, with pleomorphic koilocytosis and with irregular and jagged tumour-stromal interface. These form around 5–10% of squamous carcinomas.
3. Warty-basaloid carcinoma—Intermixed varying proportions of warty-type and basaloid-type squamous carcinoma.

Other rare types of HPV-related penile carcinoma include lymphoepithelioma like, clear cell and papillary basaloid types.

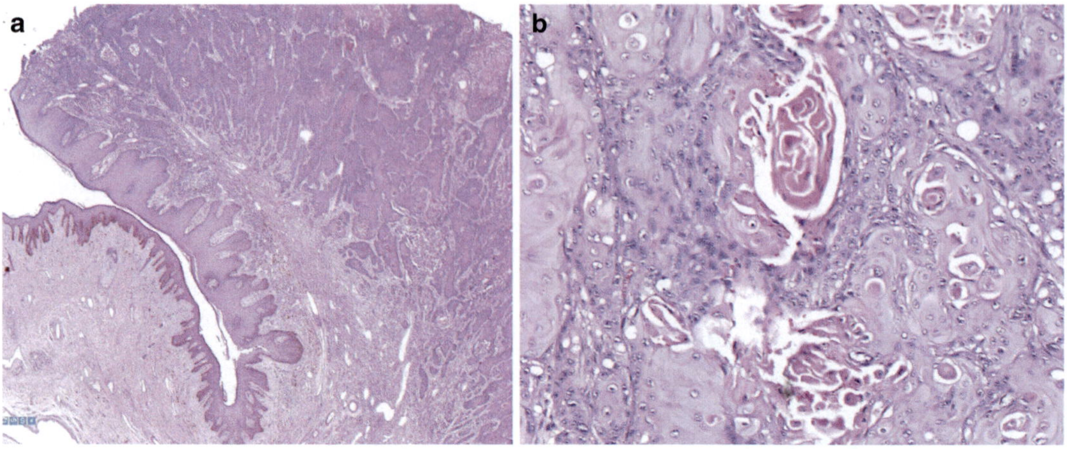

Fig. 20.2 (**a**) HPV-independent: Usual squamous carcinoma islands noted with abundant keratinisation arising in relation to preputial mucosa. (**b**) Higher power view to show a grade 2 squamous carcinoma with keratin pearls

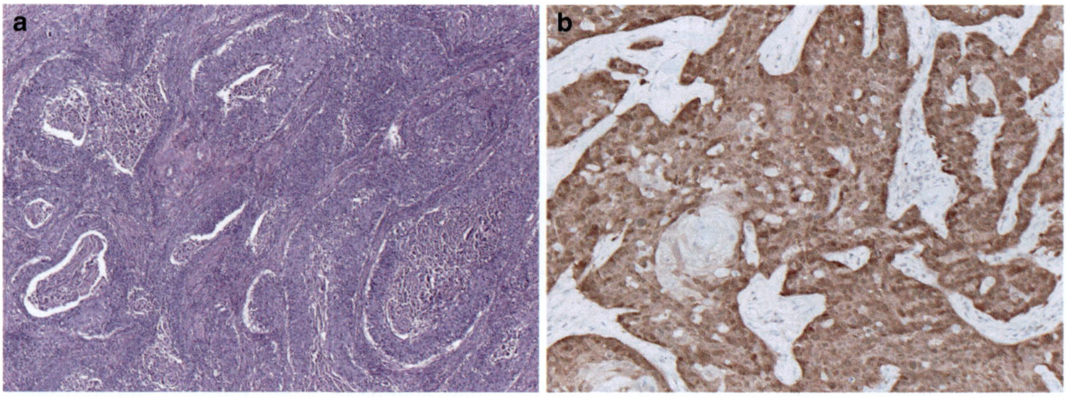

Fig. 20.3 (**a**) Histology showing HPV-associated squamous carcinoma. Basaloid morphology comprised of cells with high N/C ratio with blue basaloid nuclei. (**b**) Immunohistochemistry for p16 showing strong block positivity in HPV-associated squamous carcinoma

20.6 Grossing and Reporting of Penile Resection Specimen

The most common specimen is a partial or a total penectomy depending on the size of the tumour. Circumcision is done for preputial cancers which are also common specimens. The aim of surgical treatment is the complete removal of the penile carcinoma with negative surgical margins. The width of negative surgical margins should follow a risk-adapted strategy based on tumour grade and also based on achieving a functional penile stump. Negative surgical margins may be confirmed intra-operatively by frozen section. The surgical margins taken and studied at the frozen section include the urethral, corporal and skin cut margins. Only 5 mm of tumour-free tissue is sufficient to consider the surgical margins to be negative [51].

After the surgery, the specimen should be either transferred immediately to the pathology department or placed in adequate formalin for fixation. Except for large en bloc resections, it is generally not necessary to section the specimens to achieve optimum fixation. Ink the resected proximal margins before sectioning. Divide the specimen in two halves with the urethra as the landmark. It is imperative that a standardised protocol of examination and grossing of penile resections is followed [52–54]. The staging of a specimen is based on gauging the extent of tumour on gross specimen and taking adequate sections. The four most important landmarks in penile specimen include the following:

1. The epithelium/mucosa
2. The underlying lamina propria
3. The corpus spongiosum—with the urethra
4. The corpora cavernosa

The involvement of each of these anatomical compartments has an important clinical connotation as regards to staging as well as in planning the nodal dissection based on risk stratification [55].

The final histopathology report should also follow a standardised dataset/synoptic format of reporting and should include (Table 20.1) the following:

Table 20.1 The core (essential) and conditional (optional) elements of a histopathology report of a penectomy specimen

Core data elements	Conditional data elements
Type of specimen	Clinical and radiological details
Site of tumour	Gross appearance of tumour
Maximum tumour dimensions	Tumour distribution/ focality
Histology	Edges/borders of the tumour
Grade of the tumour	Depth of invasion/ thickness in millimetres
Tumour extent/ involvement	Closest margin distance from the invasive tumour in millimetres
Lymphovascular space invasion (LVSI)	Size of the largest metastatic nodal deposit
Perineural invasion	Size of the largest involved lymph node
Status of margins	Adjacent epithelium status and hyperplasia/dysplasia/ in situ carcinoma
Lymph node levels and involvement	Any other additional findings
Pathological staging (AJCC TNM eighth edition)	
Ancillary studies, for example, p16 status	

- Histological type
- Histological grade
- Tumour site
- Anatomic levels of invasion
- Depth of invasion (in mm from the basement membrane to the deepest point of invasion)
- Lymphovascular invasion
- Perineural invasion
- Margins of resection (usually sampled in the frozen section)
- Immunohistochemistry with p16 is mandatory, as a surrogate marker, for documenting HPV- or non-HPV-related cancer
- Lymph nodal involvement (if sent with the main specimen for pN status) would need an adequate description on the number, size of nodes, extra-capsular spread

20.7 Staging of Penile Cancers

Staging is an important parameter in cancer management and prognostication. First developed in France by Pierre Denoix in 1940, the cancer staging was based on anatomical extent of any cancer, that is, the TNM (tumour, node and metastasis) staging system, and is well accepted globally till date [56].The American Joint Committee for Cancer (AJCC) was formed in 1959, and the first staging manual was published in 1977. In 1987, the International Union Against Cancer (UICC) and AJCC TNM classification systems were unified resulting in the simultaneous release of AJCC Staging Manual and the TNM Classification of Malignant Tumors by the UICC. Since then, the revisions are made every 6–8 years based upon the research and evidence synthesis [57].The AJCC and TNM staging system is used for guiding treatment, for patient prognosis and for ensuring uniformity and comparability of the data across the world. The AJCC published its eighth edition of the staging manual with effect from January 2018 for clinical use and has been discussed in previous chapter [55, 58, 59].

PC was included in the AJCC staging system much later since inception and no changes were made in the staging since 1988, that is, from the third to the sixth editions of AJCC. Major changes were introduced in the recent seventh and eighth editions of the AJCC classification [57]. In comparison to the previous editions, AJCC seventh edition was proposed to be better in predicting patient outcomes. Over the years, with accumulating evidence, this staging failed to demonstrate survival difference in the patients of stage 2 and stage 3 disease, thus highlighting its fallacies and shortcomings [60].There have been significant changes in the eighth edition as compared to the seventh edition of AJCC cancer staging manual, both in the pT and pN staging, and it has resulted in a change in the management of PC with respect to neoadjuvant or adjuvant therapies and in addressing the inguinal lymph nodes, surgically [55]. It is therefore necessary to stratify the patients as per the latest AJCC for the best possible and universally accepted treatment guidelines and research.

From the third to seventh edition, pTis was referred to as carcinoma in situ [57]. In the eighth edition of AJCC staging, PeIN finds its presence signifying Tis. As discussed before, PeIN is classified as differentiated and undifferentiated as per the HPV status with further morphological subcategorisation [55]. Staging of penile skin-derived non-urethral tumour was revised to incorporate all localised noninvasive squamous cell carcinomas (Ta). In current staging, pTa does not permit to include tumours with destructive invasion in a well-sampled carcinoma. This new definition is also applicable to other noninvasive SCC such as basaloid, warty, papillary and mixed type without destructive invasion [58, 59]. In contrast, stage pTa in the seventh edition of AJCC exclusively referred only to noninvasive verrucous carcinoma [55]. In the eighth edition of AJCC, pT1 is further subdivided into two tiers—pT1a and pT1b as per the grade of tumour, lymphovascular space invasion (LVSI) and/or perineural invasion (PNI) status. Recent studies have indicated that in addition to histologic grade and LVSI, the presence of PNI also predicts the risk of lymph node metastasis and is therefore now included in the eighth edition of AJCC [55, 57–59]. Thus, a subepithelial non-corporal invasive tumour with PNI would have been staged as pT1a in the seventh edition; however, it is now staged as pT1b in the eighth edition of AJCC.

There have been changes in the pT2 and pT3 stages of penile cancers. Formerly, involvement of either or both corpora was staged as pT2 while urethral involvement was defined as pT3 in the seventh edition of AJCC [55]. Leitje et al. [61] reviewed a large cohort of penile cancers over a 50-year period and staged them as per the seventh edition of AJCC staging system. They did not find a statistical difference in the 5-year survival between pT2 and pT3 diseases, indicating the urethral involvement does not affect survival. Depending upon the extent of involvement, they subdivided their tumours as pT2a (corpora spongiosa, CS) and pT2b (corpora cavernosa, CC) and found a significant difference in survival between the two [61]. Sun et al. [62] observed that the risk of inguinal lymph node involvement with CS involvement is lower than tumours involving the CC (33–35.8% vs. 48.6–52.5%) [62]. These studies supported the evidence to segregate the corporal tumours into pT2 (corpora spongiosa) and pT3 (corpora cavernosa) stage irrespective of urethral involvement in the eighth edition of the AJCC staging manual [57]. Recently, Sali et al. have recommended inclusion of histologic grade, LVSI and PNI also in pT2/pT3 stage for better prediction of nodal metastasis when compared to the current eighth edition of AJCC staging [63, 64]. In the seventh edition, prostate involvement was included as stage pT4 while the eighth edition clearly defines that involvement of either the prostate, scrotum and pubic bone should be considered as pT4 [57].

Changes in the AJCC staging is not limited only to the pT stage; the pN stage also has witnessed changes and modification in the recent AJCC staging. Till the sixth edition of AJCC, pN1 referred to the involvement of a single superficial inguinal lymph node, which was changed to a single superficial or deep inguinal lymph node in the seventh edition of AJCC as skip metastasis bypassing the superficial nodes was identified [57]. Currently, in the eighth edition of AJCC, pN1 corresponds to involvement of up to two inguinal lymph nodes irrespective of whether superficial or deep levels while pN2 refers to ≥ 3

unilateral or bilateral inguinal lymph node metastasis without extranodal extension. This was based on the observation that the survival of patients with ≤2 lymph node metastasis without extranodal extension was similar to those with a single metastatic lymph node without extranodal extension [62–65]. Also, patients with three or more unilateral or bilateral inguinal lymph node metastases had poorer prognoses when compared with those with one or two unilateral inguinal lymph node metastasis with a 3-year cancer-specific survival of 60.5% versus 90.7% [62, 65]. Lymph node density and yield are two important factors for predicting patient outcomes, and it is recommended that more than 15 groin lymph nodes should be sampled for the adequate N staging of the patients [57]. Involvement of deep inguinal and pelvic lymph nodes was staged as pN3 in the third–sixth edition of the AJCC staging manual. This concept no longer exists, and the presence of extranodal extension was introduced in the seventh and eighth editions of the AJCC staging manual. The presence of extranodal extension and pelvic lymph node involvement are poor prognostic indicators with a 3-year cancer free survival of 32–33% and is also a strong indicator for adjuvant chemotherapy [65, 66].

References

1. Bandini M, Ahmed M, Basile G, et al. A global approach to improving penile cancer care. Nat Rev Urol. 2022;19(4):231–9.
2. Rubin MA, Kleter B, Zhou M, et al. Detection and typing of human papillomavirus DNA in penile carcinoma: evidence for multiple independent pathways of penile carcinogenesis. Am J Pathol. 2001;159(4):1211–8.
3. International Agency for Research on Cancer, WHO. Cancer today. GCO. 2020. http://gco.iarc.fr/today/home.
4. National Cancer Institute. Definition of rare cancer. NCI Dictionary of Cancer Terms.
5. Douglawi A, Masterson TA. Penile cancer epidemiology and risk factors: a contemporary review. Curr Opin Urol. 2019;29(2):145–9.
6. Chaux A, Netto GJ, Rodríguez IM, et al. Epidemiologic profile, sexual history, pathologic features, and human papillomavirus status of 103 patients with penile carcinoma. World J Urol. 2013;31(4):861–7.
7. Takiar R, Kumar S. Pattern of reproductive cancers in India. Asian Pac J Cancer Prev. 2014;15(2):599–603.
8. Parkin DM, Whelan SL, Ferlay J, Teppo L, Thomas DB. Cancer incidence in five continents volume VIII. IARC Scientific Publications No. 155. Lyon: The International Agency for Research on Cancer; 2002.
9. Forman D, Bray F, Brewster DH, Gombe Mbalawa C, Kohler B, Piñeros M, Steliarova-Foucher E, Swaminathan R, Ferlay J. Cancer incidence in five continents volume X. IARC Scientific Publications No. 164. Lyon: The International Agency for Research on Cancer; 2014.
10. Larke NL, Thomas SL, Dos Santos SI, Weiss HA. Male circumcision and penile cancer: a systematic review and meta-analysis. Cancer Causes Control. 2011;22(8):1097–110.
11. Pow-Sang MR, Ferreira U, Pow-Sang JM, Nardi AC, Destefano V. Epidemiology and natural history of penile cancer. Urology. 2010;761:S2.
12. Daling JR, Madeleine MM, Johnson LG, et al. Penile cancer: importance of circumcision, human papillomavirus and smoking in in situ and invasive disease. Int J Cancer. 2005;116(4):606–16.
13. Tseng HF, Morgenstern H, Mack T, Peters RK. Risk factors for penile cancer: results of a population-based case-control study in Los Angeles County (United States). Cancer Causes Control. 2001;12(3):267–77.
14. Maden C, Sherman KJ, Beckmann AM, et al. History of circumcision, medical conditions, and sexual activity and risk of penile cancer. J Natl Cancer Inst. 1993;85(1):19–24.
15. Van Howe RS, Hodges FM. The carcinogenicity of smegma: debunking a myth. J Eur Acad Dermatol Venereol. 2006;20(9):1046–54.
16. Schoen EJ, Oehrli M, Colby C, Machin G. The highly protective effect of newborn circumcision against invasive penile cancer. Pediatrics. 2000;105(3):E36.
17. Clouston D, Hall A, Lawrentschuk N. Penile lichen sclerosus (balanitis xerotica obliterans). BJU Int. 2011;108(Suppl 2):14–9.
18. Stern RS. Genital tumors among men with psoriasis exposed to psoralens and ultraviolet a radiation (PUVA) and ultraviolet B radiation. The photochemotherapy follow-up study. N Engl J Med. 1990;322(16):1093–7.
19. Harish K, Ravi R. The role of tobacco in penile carcinoma. Br J Urol. 1995;75(3):375–7.
20. Thuret R, Sun M, Budaus L, et al. A population-based analysis of the effect of marital status on overall and cancer-specific mortality in patients with squamous cell carcinoma of the penis. Cancer Causes Control. 2013;24(1):71–9.
21. Koifman L, Vides AJ, Koifman N, Carvalho JP, Ornellas AA. Epidemiological aspects of penile cancer in Rio de Janeiro: evaluation of 230 cases. Int Braz J Urol. 2011;37(2):231–40.
22. Ulff-Møller CJ, Simonsen J, Frisch M. Marriage, cohabitation and incidence trends of invasive penile

squamous cell carcinoma in Denmark 1978–2010. Int J Cancer. 2013;133(5):1173–9.
23. Engels EA, Pfeiffer RM, Goedert JJ, et al. Trends in cancer risk among people with AIDS in the United States 1980–2002. AIDS. 2006;20(12):1645–54.
24. D'Hauwers KWM, Depuydt CE, Bogers JJ, et al. Human papillomavirus, lichen sclerosus and penile cancer: a study in Belgium. Vaccine. 2012;30(46):6573–7.
25. Alemany L, Cubilla A, Halec G, et al. Role of human papillomavirus in penile carcinomas worldwide. Eur Urol. 2016;69(5):953–61.
26. Da Costa Nunes JF, Pires S, Chade DC. Human papillomavirus vaccination and prevention of intraepithelial neoplasia and penile cancer: review article. Curr Opin Urol. 2020;30(2):208–12.
27. Nordenvall C, Chang ET, Adami HO, Ye W. Cancer risk among patients with condylomata acuminata. Int J Cancer. 2006;119(4):888–93.
28. Hoekstra RJ, Trip EJ, ten Kate FJW, Horenblas S, Lock MT. Penile intraepithelial neoplasia: nomenclature, incidence and progression to malignancy in The Netherlands. Int J Urol. 2019;26(3):353–7.
29. Moch H, Cubilla AL, Humphrey PA, Reuter VE, Ulbright TM. The 2016 WHO classification of tumours of the urinary system and male genital organs—part a: renal, penile, and testicular tumours. Eur Urol. 2016;70(1):93–105.
30. Ingles DJ, Pierce Campbell CM, Messina JA, et al. Human papillomavirus virus (HPV) genotype-and age-specific analyses of external genital lesions among men in the HPV infection in men (HIM) study. J Infect Dis. 2015;211(7):1060–7.
31. Sudenga SL, Ingles DJ, Pierce Campbell CM, et al. Genital human papillomavirus infection progression to external genital lesions: the HIM study. Eur Urol. 2016;69(1):166–73.
32. Akogbe GO, Ajidahun A, Sirak B, et al. Race and prevalence of human papillomavirus infection among men residing in Brazil, Mexico and the United States. Int J Cancer. 2012;131(3):1–10.
33. Fernández-Nestosa MJ, Guimerà N, Sanchez DF, et al. Human papillomavirus (HPV) genotypes in condylomas, intraepithelial neoplasia, and invasive carcinoma of the penis using laser capture microdissection (LCM)-PCR: a study of 191 lesions in 43 patients. Am J Surg Pathol. 2017;41(6):820–32.
34. Emmanuel A, Nettleton J, Watkin N, Berney DM. The molecular pathogenesis of penile carcinoma—current developments and understanding. Virchows Arch. 2019;475(4):397–405.
35. Steinestel J, Al Ghazal A, Arndt A, et al. The role of histologic subtype, p16INK4a expression, and presence of human papillomavirus DNA in penile squamous cell carcinoma. BMC Cancer. 2015;15(1): 1–9.
36. Gewin L, Myers H, Kiyono T, Galloway DA. Identification of a novel telomerase repressor that interacts with the human papillomavirus type-16 E6/E6-AP complex. Genes Dev. 2004;18(18):2269–82.
37. Khansari N, Shakiba Y, Mahmoudi M. Chronic inflammation and oxidative stress as a major cause of age- related diseases and cancer. Recent Patents Inflamm Allergy Drug Discov. 2009;3(1):73–80.
38. De Paula AAP, Motta ED, Alencar RDC, et al. The impact of cyclooxygenase-2 and vascular endothelial growth factor C immunoexpression on the prognosis of penile carcinoma. J Urol. 2012;187(1):134–40.
39. Greenhough A, Smartt HJM, Moore AE, et al. The COX-2/PGE2 pathway: key roles in the hallmarks of cancer and adaptation to the tumour microenvironment. Carcinogenesis. 2009;30(3):377–86.
40. Poetsch M, Hemmerich M, Kakies C, et al. Alterations in the tumor suppressor gene p16 INK4A are associated with aggressive behavior of penile carcinomas. Virchows Arch. 2011;458(2):221–9.
41. Ferreux E, Lont AP, Horenblas S, et al. Evidence for at least three alternative mechanisms targeting the p16INK4A/cyclin D/Rb pathway in penile carcinoma, one of which is mediated by high-risk human papillomavirus. J Pathol. 2003;201(1):109–18.
42. Lohneis P, Boral S, Kaufmann AM, et al. Human papilloma virus status of penile squamous cell carcinoma is associated with differences in tumour-infiltrating T lymphocytes. Virchows Arch. 2015;466(3):323–31.
43. Chu C, Yao K, Lu J, et al. Immunophenotypes based on the tumor immune microenvironment allow for unsupervised penile cancer patient stratification. Cancers (Basel). 2020;12(7):1–17.
44. Ottenhof SR, Djajadiningrat RS, Thygesen HH, et al. The prognostic value of immune factors in the tumor microenvironment of penile squamous cell carcinoma. Front Immunol. 2018;9:1253.
45. Hakenberg OW, Compérat E, Minhas S, Necchi A, Protzel C, Watkin N, Robinson R. EAU guidelines. Amsterdam: EAU Annual Congress; 2020.
46. Alkatout I, Naumann CM, Hedderich J, et al. Squamous cell carcinoma of the penis: predicting nodal metastases by histologic grade, pattern of invasion and clinical examination. Urol Oncol. 2011;29(6):774–81.
47. Schlenker B, Scher B, Tiling R, et al. Detection of inguinal lymph node involvement in penile squamous cell carcinoma by 18F-fluorodeoxyglucose PET/CT: a prospective single-center study. Urol Oncol. 2012;30(1):55–9.
48. Letendre J, Saad F, Lattouf JB. Penile cancer: what's new? Curr Opin Support Palliat Care. 2011;5(3):185–91.
49. Petralia G, Villa G, Scardino E, et al. Stadiazione locale del tumore del pene con risonanza magnetica abbinata a test di farmacoinfusione intracavernosa (RM-TFI). Radiol Med. 2008;113(4):517–28.
50. Cubilla AL, Velazquez EF, Amin MB, Epstein J, Berney DM, Corbishley CM, Members of the ISUP Penile Tumor Panel. The World Health Organisation 2016 classification of penile carcinomas: a review and update from the International Society of Urological Pathology expert-driven recommendations. Histopathology. 2018;72:893–904.

51. Danakas AM, Bsirini C, Miyamoto H. The impact of routine frozen section assessment during penectomy on surgical margin status and long-term oncologic outcomes. Pathol Oncol Res. 2018;24(4):947–50.
52. The Royal College of Pathologist. Cancer datasets and tissue pathways. https://www.rcpath.org/profession/guidelines/cancer-datasets-and-tissue-pathways.html.
53. Corbishley C, Chaux A, Colecchia M, Cubilla AL, Shanks J, Velazquez EF, Watkin N, Srigley JR. Carcinoma of the penis and distal urethra histopathology reporting guide 1st edition. International collaboration on cancer reporting; Sydney, Australia. 2017. ISBN: 978-1-925687-05-7.
54. College of American Pathologist. Cancer protocol templates. https://www.cap.org/protocols-and-guidelines/cancer-reporting-tools/cancer-protocol-templates.
55. Khalil MI, Kamel MH, Dhillon J, et al. What you need to know: updates in penile cancer staging. World J Urol. 2021;39(5):1413–9.
56. Brierley J. National Cancer Institute of Canada committee on cancer staging. The evolving TNM cancer staging system: an essential component of cancer care. CMAJ. 2006;174:155–6.
57. Sanchez DF, Fernandez-Nestosa MJ, Canete-Portillo S, Rodriguez I, Cubilla AL. What is new in the pathologic staging of penile carcinoma in the 8th edition of AJCC TNM model: rationale for changes with practical stage-by-stage category diagnostic considerations. Adv Anat Pathol. 2021;28(4):209–27.
58. Paner GP, Stadler WM, Hansel DE, Montironi R, Lin DW, Amin MB. Updates in the eighth edition of the tumor-node-metastasis staging classification for urologic cancers. Eur Urol. 2018;73(4):560–9.
59. Cornejo KM, Rice-Stitt T, Wu CL. Updates in staging and reporting of genitourinary malignancies. Arch Pathol Lab Med. 2020;144(3):305–19.
60. Li ZS, Ornellas AA, Schwentner C, et al. A modified clinicopathological tumor staging system for survival prediction of patients with penile cancer ChiCTR16008041 ChiCTR 11 medical and health sciences 1112 oncology and carcinogenesis. Cancer Commun. 2018;38(1):1–10.
61. Leijte JAP, Gallee M, Antonini N, Horenblas S. Evaluation of current TNM classification of penile carcinoma. J Urol. 2008;180(3):933–8.
62. Sun M, Djajadiningrat RS, Alnajjar HM, et al. Development and external validation of a prognostic tool for prediction of cancer-specific mortality after complete loco-regional pathological staging for squamous cell carcinoma of the penis. BJU Int. 2015;116(5):734–43.
63. Sali AP, Menon S, Murthy V, et al. A modified Histopathologic staging in penile squamous cell carcinoma predicts nodal metastasis and outcome better than the current AJCC staging. Am J Surg Pathol. 2020;44(8):1112–7.
64. Sali AP, Prakash G, de Cássio ZS, et al. A comparative study of AJCC and the modified staging system in pT2/pT3 penile squamous cell carcinoma—a validation on an external data set. Histopathology. 2022;80(3):566–74.
65. Li ZS, Yao K, Chen P, et al. Modification of N staging systems for penile cancer: a more precise prediction of prognosis. Br J Cancer. 2015;112(11):1766–71.
66. Zhu Y, Ye DW, Yao XD, Zhang SL, Dai B, Zhang HL. New N staging system of penile cancer provides a better reflection of prognosis. J Urol. 2011;186(2):518–23.

Management

21

Kevin Arulraj, Brusabhanu Nayak, Prabhjot Singh, and Sridhar Panaiyadiyan

21.1 Introduction

The management of penile carcinoma (PeCa) can be broadly categorized into management of the primary tumor and management of the inguinal nodes. Management of the primary tumor relies on the extent and location of the growth. Organ-preserving modalities are considered whenever feasible. Partial or total penile amputation is offered in large growths where organ preservation is not attainable. Management of inguinal nodes is based upon the laterality, size, and mobility of inguinal nodes. A radical inguinal lymph node dissection with or without a pelvic lymph node dissection is the standard of care for node-positive disease. Adjuvant chemotherapy is offered in pN2 and pN3 disease whereas neoadjuvant chemotherapy is preferred in N3 disease. Intensive follow-up for recurrences is advised in the first 2 years following treatment. Palliative chemotherapy and radiotherapy are mainstay in unresectable and metastatic disease.

21.2 Management of Penile Intraepithelial Neoplasia (PeIN)

Penile intraepithelial neoplasia (PeIN/PIN) or carcinoma in situ (CIS) of the penis includes erythroplasia of Queyrat (EQ), Bowen's disease (BD), and Bowenoid papulosis (BP). The characteristic feature includes epithelial dysplasia like squamous cell CIS. While BP has <1% risk of malignant progression, EQ and BD have a 10–20% risk of progression into invasive malignancy [1]. PIN is also classified into mild (PIN I), moderate (PIN II), and severe dysplasia (PIN III). PIN II includes BP whereas PIN III consists of EQ and BD [2]. All types of PIN have an HPV association of 70–100% [3].

Management goal of PIN is focused on disease elimination balanced with penile preservation. Topical, ablative, and excisional therapies are described. Histologic confirmation is necessary with deep biopsies to exclude invasive disease prior to initiation of treatment. A repeat biopsy at completion of treatment is necessary due to the risk of persistent disease. Inadequate response to therapy indicates invasive disease.

Circumcision is vital in the management of PIN. In addition to being curative for lesions limited to the prepuce, it eliminates the environment for persistent HPV infection and facilitates surveillance and self-examination [4].

K. Arulraj · B. Nayak · P. Singh · S. Panaiyadiyan (✉)
Department of Urology, AIIMS, New Delhi, India

P. Singh et al. (eds.), *A Guide to Management of Urological Cancers*,
https://doi.org/10.1007/978-981-99-2341-0_21

21.2.1 Topical Chemotherapy

Topical chemotherapy includes 5-fluorouracil (5-FU) cream or 5% imiquimod cream. 5-FU is an antimetabolite (thymidylate synthetase inhibitor) whereas imiquimod (IQ) is an immunomodulator [5]. Complete response with minimal toxicity was observed in 50% of patients treated with 5-FU cream and in 44% treated with IQ [4].

21.2.2 Ablative Therapy

Ablative therapy entails laser vaporization with Nd:YAG or CO_2 which allows destruction of PIN while minimizing collateral damage to healthy penile tissue. Recurrence rates after laser vaporization range from 0% to 33% [6]. Both topical and ablative therapies require long-term surveillance after a posttreatment biopsy to document treatment response [6].

21.2.3 Excisional Therapy

Excisional therapy for PIN consists of partial or total glans resurfacing where the glanular epithelium and subepithelial tissue are excised followed by a split skin graft or a buccal mucosal graft to cover the defect. It can either be done as a primary treatment for PIN or as a secondary procedure for cases with recurrence following topical or ablative therapies. The recurrence rate following glans resurfacing is reported to be 4%, and up to 20% of patients had invasive disease on histopathologic examination [7].

21.3 Management of the Primary Tumor

The surgical management of the primary growth rests upon tumor size and grade. Penile preservation has gained momentum of late and is suitable for patients with favorable histologic features and lower risk for metastases [8]. Penile preservation includes laser therapy, Mohs' micrographic surgery (MMS), glans resurfacing, and glansectomy. Penile amputation, either a partial or total penectomy, is ideal for patients with high risk factors such as a tumor size of 4 cm or more, high-grade tumors, and lesions involving the corpora cavernosa [9, 10] (Table 21.1).

Table 21.1 Management options

Stage	Management options
Tis	Topical therapy, laser ablation, and penile preservation
Ta and T1a (G1 and G2)	Laser ablation, penile preservation, and radiotherapy[a] (<4 cm)
T1b (G3) and T2	Wide local excision with reconstruction, glansectomy with reconstruction, and radiotherapy[a] (<4 cm)
T3	Glansectomy with distal corporectomy, partial penectomy, and total penectomy (if urethral involvement)
T4	Total penectomy, neoadjuvant chemotherapy[a] followed by surgery in unresectable, and palliative chemotherapy

[a] Details of radiotherapy and/or chemotherapy have been described in Chap. 22

21.3.1 Penile Preservation

Thirty percent of patients with penile cancer are younger than 55 years [11]. Penile amputation is the oncologic gold standard for the primary tumor. However, it leads to a significant decrease in the sexual quality of life in patients [12]. Thus, penile preservation is recommended for patients with primary tumors with a favorable histopathology (Ta, T1, G1/G2). Goals of treatment include preservation of glans sensation and maximal preservation of penile shaft length. Various approaches to organ preservation include local ablative therapy, circumcision, wide local excision, glansectomy, or radiotherapy (details of radiotherapy have been described in Chap. 22). The selection of procedure depends upon the location, size, grade of tumor, and nearness to the meatus.

21.3.1.1 Circumcision

For lesions which are confined to the prepuce, a radical circumcision is considered effective for local control.

21.3.1.2 Laser Therapy

Laser ablation when performed in select cases can provide outcomes similar to surgery. There is a higher overall sexual satisfaction and higher rates of resumption to sexual activity following laser ablation [13]. Following CO_2 laser for T1 tumors, local recurrence rate is reported to be 23% [14] with a secondary partial penectomy rate of 10% [15]. Nd:YAG laser with a deeper penetration of 6 mm has a lower recurrence rate of 7% [16].

21.3.1.3 Mohs' Micrographic Surgery (MMS)

Introduced by Frederic E. Mohs, this technique involves in sequential layer-by-layer excision of tumor guided by microscopic examination to achieve a negative margin [17]. Mohs initially used a zinc chloride cream to fix the tumor tissue (hence the term chemosurgery). However, due to severe patient discomfort and the need for multiple sessions for complete tumor resection, frozen sections were used to hasten the process of microscopic examination. MMS is most useful for tumors expanding in a contiguous manner. The visible tumor is curetted out and resection starts at the base with 2–3 mm margin. Beveling incisions are given toward to the center of the defect at 45°. The excised tissue is marked, oriented, and covered in freezing media. Thin sections are taken from the margins and are stained with hematoxylin and eosin prior to microscopic examination. Residual tumor, if present, is noted and its location is correlated to the bed of resection. The surgeon returns back to take deeper cuts where margins were positive in the frozen section [18]. With frozen section, Mohs reported no recurrences in 5 years for penile tumors less than 1 cm, 17% for tumors between 1 and 2 cm, and 25% for tumors between 2 and 3 cm. A recurrence rate of greater than 50% was observed when the tumor size exceeds 3 cm [19]. Machan et al. in a recent series of 48 cases reproduced Mohs' technique with a cure rate of 100% in invasive SCC and 94% in PIN [20].

21.3.1.4 Glans Resurfacing

This technique, also known as glans stripping, involves the excision of glanular epithelium and subepithelial tissue off the underlying corpora by subdermal dissection. The resultant defect is managed with a split skin graft or a buccal mucosal graft. Shabbir et al. described this procedure in 25 patients with PIN with an overall recurrence rate of 4% [7]. Ayres et al. applied the concept of glans resurfacing in 33 patients with invasive disease. No recurrences were observed in patients with a negative margin. Nonetheless, in patients with a positive margin (21%), the recurrence rate was reported to be 6% [21].

21.3.1.5 Surgical Margin for Penile Cancer

Traditionally, a surgical margin of 2 cm was considered essential for disease control. However, this has been challenged by recent studies which show acceptable outcomes with lesser margins. Agrawal et al. studied 64 penectomy specimens and showed that the maximum tumor spread was 5 mm for grade I tumors and 10 mm for tumor grades II and III [22]. Philippou et al. followed up 179 patients who underwent limited margin excision, and the local recurrence rate was 8.9% [23]. These findings suggest that a 2 cm margin might not be always necessary, especially in small low-grade tumors. Guidelines currently recommend a 3–5 mm margin which is tailored based on the grade of tumor (grade I, 3 mm; grade II, 5 mm; grade III, 8 mm) [8].

21.3.1.6 Glansectomy

Most penile growths occur at the glans. Naturally, these patients are candidates for penile preservation in the form of glansectomy. This can be either a partial glansectomy where the tumor is excised with negative margins confirmed by frozen section or a total glansectomy where the entire glans is excised. Reconstruction following partial glansectomy can be either primary closure if the defect is small or a lateral preputial skin flap in larger defects [24–26]. A split-thickness skin graft can also be utilized. If the primary closure is within 5 mm from the meatus, excision must include the meatus, and negative margins should be confirmed in frozen section. Following total glansectomy, SSG and cavernosal tip reconstruction are required. If the tunica albuginea of the corpora cavernosum is involved, distal corporectomy should be a part of the procedure [26]. The recurrence rate following glansectomy is close to 7%, and regular follow-up is essential postoperatively [23].

21.3.1.7 Local Recurrence Following Organ-Conserving Surgery

A repeat penile preservation procedure can be done if there is no corpus cavernosum invasion. In case of extensive recurrences, penile amputation is required [8].

21.3.2 Penile Amputation

21.3.2.1 Partial Penectomy

Partial penectomy provides local control, enables patient to void in a standing position, and might allow satisfactory sexual performance. The procedure is performed under a tourniquet control to reduce blood loss. The distal growth is wrapped with a surgical glove and isolated to avoid wound seeding. A periurethral catheter is placed, and the skin is incised circumferentially proximal to the growth after preserving adequate skin for closure. The dorsal neurovascular bundles are ligated, and the corpora is transected. The urethra is transected 1–1.5 cm distal to the corporal bodies. A horizontal mattress closure of the corporal bodies is done with 3-0 sutures. The urethra is spatulated and is sutured to the penile skin with 4-0 absorbable sutures (Fig. 21.1). Spatulation prevents the late complication of neomeatal stenosis which is seen in 6% of patients [27]. The local recurrence following partial penectomy ranges from 4% to 13% [28, 29]. Ruslan et al. followed 32 patients who underwent a partial penectomy, out of which one developed local recurrence (3%) [30].

21.3.2.2 Total Penectomy

A total penile amputation is indicated in penile tumors which are large and are extend proximally (Fig. 21.2). This would not facilitate a negative margin as well as an adequate stump for upright voiding. A perineal urethrostomy is fashioned for urinary diversion. Unlike radical penectomy where the corporal bodies are excised entirely, total penectomy involves amputation of the penis at the level of the suspensory ligament of the penis. A diamond-shaped incision is given at the base of the penis. Following which, the suspensory ligament is divided and proximal crural

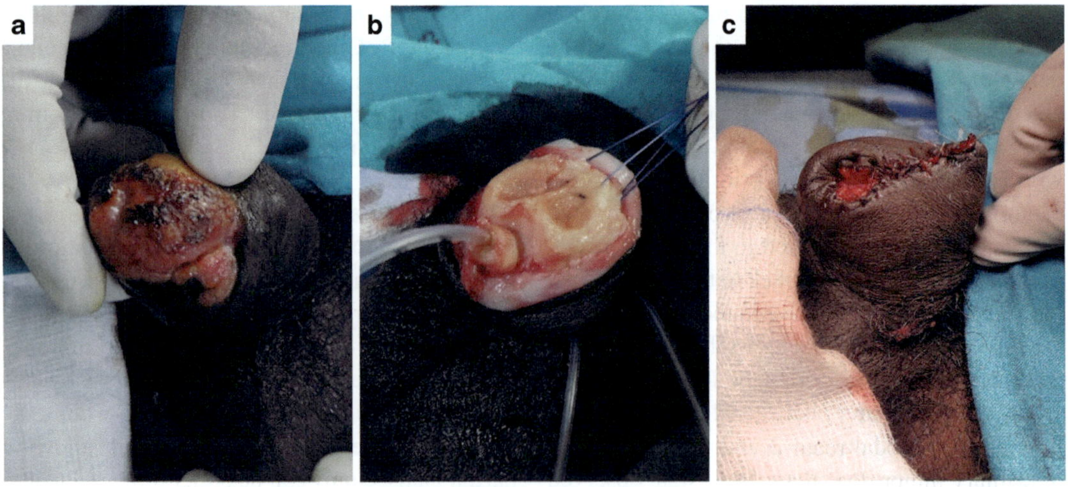

Fig. 21.1 (**a**) Distal penile growth involving corona, (**b**) post excision of growth, and (**c**) spatulated urethra with skin closure

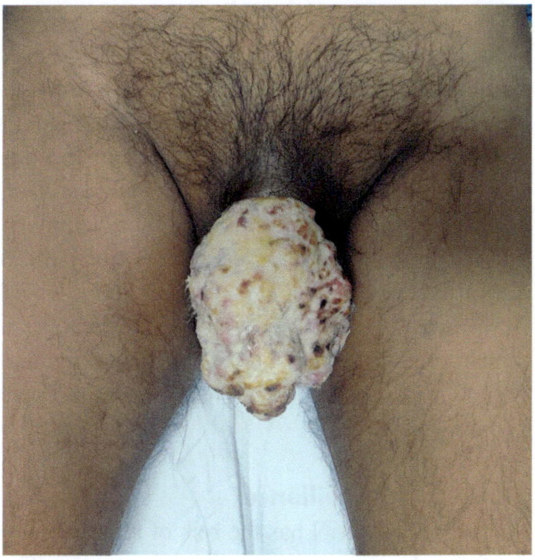

Fig. 21.2 Penile growth involving entire shaft

amputation is achieved. The urethra is mobilized ventrally until adequate length is obtained to reach the perineum. A perineal skin flap is raised and is sutured to the full-thickness spatulated urethra with 3-0 sutures over a periurethral catheter which is removed after a week. The diamond-shaped skin defect is closed transversely. Local recurrences following total penectomy are less than 10% [3, 31].

21.3.2.3 Penile Preservation vs. Amputation

Although organ-sparing techniques improve QOL and sexual satisfaction, the local recurrence is higher than that of penile amputation. Rosa et al. followed up 859 patients who underwent surgery for penile carcinoma from 1956 to 2012 and found a local recurrence of 27% for penile preservation strategies whereas it was 3.8% in patients who underwent penile amputation. However, there was no significant difference in the survival between both groups [32].

21.3.2.4 Local Recurrence of Primary Tumor

In contrast to nodal recurrence, local recurrence of primary tumor does not affect overall survival if promptly managed [33, 34]. Recurrences are commoner with organ-preserving strategies. In the first 2 years posttreatment, up to 27% of patients developed recurrences after organ-preserving modalities. Following penile amputation, the risk of recurrence is 4–5% [32–34].

21.4 Management of Inguinal Lymph Nodes (ILN)

Inguinal lymph nodal metastasis is the most important prognostic factor for survival in penile cancer. At index presentation, palpable inguinal lymphadenopathy is noted in 60% of patients, and up to 85% of them end up having nodal metastasis. On the other hand, up to 30% of patients who have no clinically palpable inguinal lymph nodes are shown to have occult inguinal micrometastasis. Bilateral inguinal nodal involvement is seen in up to 80% of patients [35–38]. It is imperative to understand the natural history of penile cancer to provide optimal management in patients with nodal metastasis. Squamous cell carcinoma of the penis has a prolonged locoregional phase prior to distant spread. This window offers an opportunity and for the clinician to intervene and provide surgical cure with lymphadenectomy. Moreover, the lymphatic spread occur in a predictable manner. It follows a distinct pathway—initially to the superficial inguinal nodes and then to deep inguinal nodes and finally to the pelvic nodes [38]. Unlike other urologic cancers where lymphadenectomy helps in staging and prognosticating the disease, lymphadenectomy in penile cancer, when performed appropriately, in select patients with limited nodal disease has a curative potential. Historically, a course of antibiotics was recommended for patients with suspicious nodes to differentiate from infective adenopathy [39]. However, this causes significant delay of curative treatment and is not recommended at present.

The 5-year survival in node-negative patients is 90–100%. This reduces to 60% in patients with positive inguinal nodal metastasis which are resected [40]. Survival in node-positive patients also depends upon the number, size, and histopathologic features. There is an 80% survival after lymphadenectomy in patients with unilateral, limited (up to two nodes) disease with no extra nodal extension or pelvic nodes. This figure drops to 25% in patients with more than two positive nodes or presence of extra nodal extension. The survival in patients with positive pelvic nodes is less than 10% [36, 41–43].

There are three possible scenarios in the management of regional lymph nodes—clinically node negative patients, clinically palpable lymph nodes, and enlarged fixed or ulcerated lymphadenopathy (Fig. 21.3).

21.4.1 cN0 Stage

Up to 25–30% of patients with clinically negative groins will harbor micrometastatic disease. An invasive lymph node staging is required since no imaging technique can reliably detect or exclude micrometastatic disease. Treating all patients with lymphadenectomy results in unwarranted morbidity of the surgery in the truly node-negative population. Surveillance of regional nodes has the risk of recurrence in the future from pre-existing micrometastasis [44]. Hence, it is essential to identify the patients who have a high risk of harboring occult nodal metastases so that patients with truly negative nodes are spared from the morbidity of inguinal lymph node dissection.

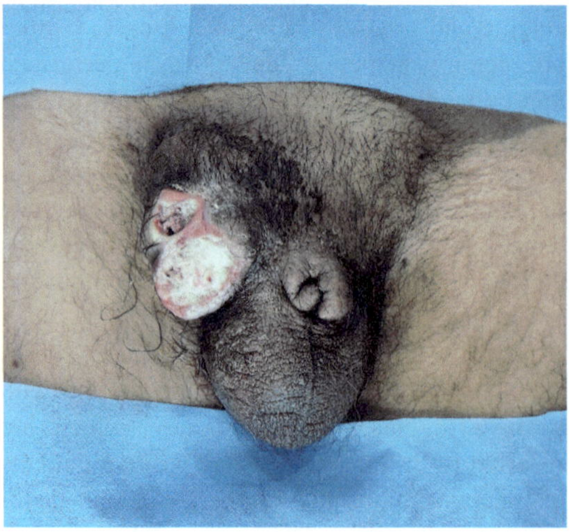

Fig. 21.3 Ulcerated lymphadenopathy

21.4.1.1 Risk Stratification in cN0

Risk stratification for micrometastatic inguinal lymph node disease involves in considering disease stage, tumor grade, and the presence or absence of lymphovascular invasion in the primary tumor. *Low-risk category* includes pTa, pTis, and pT1 well-differentiated (GI) tumors. pT1G2 tumors have an *intermediate risk*. pT1G3 and all stages above are considered *high risk* [35]. Ficarra et al. have developed a nomogram which predicts the risk of metastatic inguinal lymph nodes based on eight clinicopathologic variables [45].

21.4.1.2 Surveillance

Surveillance of ILN has the risk of recurrence in the future from pre-existing micrometastasis. The survival significantly drops from 84% in patients who receive immediate lymphadenectomy to 35% in patients who undergo delayed lymphadenectomy [44]. Hence, surveillance of ILN is recommended only for the low-risk category (pTis/pTa/pT1G1). Patients must be well educated and compliant to follow-up if surveillance is considered.

21.4.1.3 Invasive Nodal Staging

Invasive nodal staging is required for intermediate- and high-risk categories. It can either be a dynamic sentinel node biopsy (DSNB) or a modified inguinal lymphadenectomy. DSNB is based on the principle of sequential spread of malignancy from the primary tumor to the nodal basins. It involves in injecting a technetium-99 nanocolloid around the primary tumor the day prior to surgery along with a blue dye. Intraoperatively, a gamma-ray probe is used to detect the sentinel nodes which are biopsied. Patients with positive lymph nodes undergo ILND while patients with negative sentinel nodes are kept on surveillance [46]. The cumulative false-negative rate in DSNB is 5%. In a meta-analysis by Zou et al., the sensitivity of DSNB was 88% with a negative predictive value of 99% [47–49]. Despite being less invasive, there is a significant learning curve for DSNB. There is also inconsistency in the reproducibility of the results in other centers.

Therefore, DSNB is best performed in high-volume and experienced centers [50–52].

Modified ILND introduced by Catalona has supplanted the classic ILND as a staging procedure in cN0 disease. The four modifications include a smaller skin incision, limitation of dissection medial to the femoral artery, preservation of the saphenous vein, and omitting the transposition of the sartorius muscle. Superficial and deep nodes within this region including the Cloquet node are removed bilaterally and sent for histopathological examination. If metastasis is present, the procedure is converted to standard LND on the corresponding side [53].

21.4.2 cN1/cN2 Stage

Metastatic nodal disease is seen in 85% of patients with palpable lymph nodes which are not fixed [35, 36]. Antibiotic trial prior to LND is not recommended and it delays curative treatment. In clinically doubtful cases, ultrasound-guided fine needle aspiration cytology (FNAC) can be considered. The false-negative rate of FNAC is 5–15%. Hence, a negative FNAC should be approached with caution [35, 54, 55]. Up to 50% of clinically negative contralateral groins in patients with N1 or N2 disease are found to have occult metastasis [56]. Hence, a bilateral inguinal LND is offered in all patients with N1 and N2 disease.

21.4.2.1 Procedure of ILND

The boundaries include the medial edge of sartorius laterally, the lateral edge of the adductor muscle medially, the fossa ovalis inferiorly, the muscular floor of the femoral triangle posteriorly, and the inguinal ligament superiorly [57–59]. The skin incision in radical inguinal LND is 2 cm inferior and parallel to the inguinal ligament. Alternatively, a lazy S incision can also be used in case of concomitant PLND. Skin flaps are raised below the Scarpa fascia. The areolar tissue is dissected from the external oblique aponeurosis and the spermatic cord till the inferior border of the inguinal ligament. This forms the superior nodal pocket. The femoral vessels are identified at the apex of the femoral triangle which is the inferior nodal pocket. The saphenous vein is usually divided. Laterally, the dissection is limited up to the femoral artery to avoid injury to the femoral nerve. Within these boundaries, all lymphatic tissue, superficial and deep, including the Cloquet node are removed. A sartorius transposition is usually performed to cover the femoral vessels [40].

ILND results in impaired lymphatic drainage from the lower limbs. The morbidity following ILND is as high as 50%. BMI is a significant risk factor for wound complications [60]. Contemporary series show a reduced morbidity of 25% [61, 62]. Meticulous tissue handling and ligation of all lymphatic channels are recommended [63, 64]. Postoperatively, compression stockings, bandages, inguinal compression dressings, and suction drains can be used to mitigate morbidity [65]. Common complications include surgical site infection (1.4%), flap necrosis (4.7%) (Fig. 21.4), lymphedema (13.9%), and lymphocele formation (4%) [61, 62].

21.4.2.2 PLND in N1/N2

The probability of PLN involvement in solitary inguinal nodal involvement is up to 5%. This increases to 25% when two or more inguinal lymph nodes are positive and further to 56% with more than three positive nodes or extracapsular extension [66, 67]. Patients with three or more positive inguinal nodes or extracapsular nodal

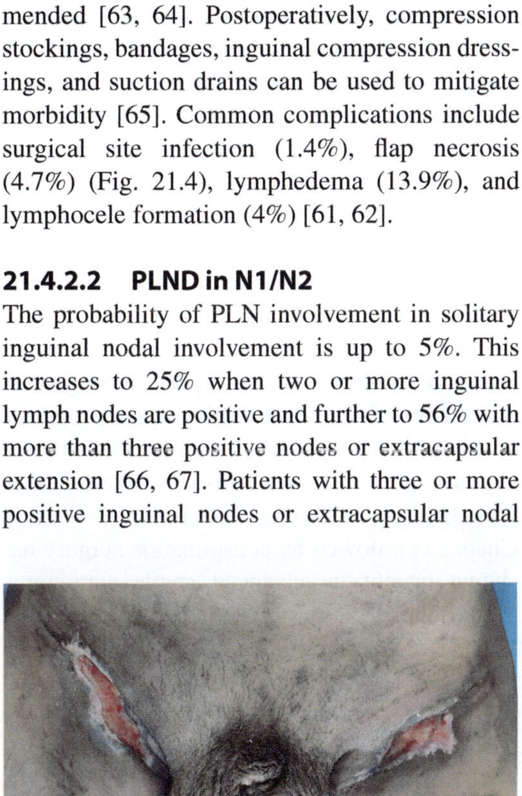

Fig. 21.4 Flap necrosis following inguinal lymph node dissection

extension are recommended to undergo ipsilateral PLND (EAU). Nodal metastases more than 4 cm are associated with extranodal extension. These patients should also undergo a PLND [42]. PLND can be either done along with ILND or as a secondary procedure. In case of bilateral PLND, a midline suprapubic extraperitoneal incision is used [68].

21.4.2.3 Laparoscopic or Robot-Assisted ILND

The advantages of minimally invasive ILND include reduced local complication rate, hastened recovery, and decreased length of hospitalization. Video-endoscopic inguinal lymph node dissection (VEILND), when compared to open ILND, has a comparable nodal yield, number of positive nodes, and density. Wound complications were significantly lower in VEILND group (6%) compared to open ILND (68%) [69, 70].

21.4.3 cN3 Stage

Survival in patients with bulky fixed nodal metastasis is dependent upon complete eradication of the disease. This is seldom achieved by surgery or chemotherapy as standalone management options [66]. N3 disease carries a poor prognosis and multimodal therapy is recommended in these patients [71–73]. Neoadjuvant chemotherapy (details of chemotherapy have been described in Chap. 22) followed by consolidation surgery has shown benefit in advanced penile carcinoma. Studies have shown up to 60% response rates with chemotherapy and up to 20% showing complete response in patients undergoing consolidative ilioinguinal LND [72–74]. Neoadjuvant paclitaxel, ifosfamide, and cisplatin (TIP) chemotherapy (four cycles) resulted in an overall response rate of 50% with 30% pathologic complete response. TIP regimen was better tolerated and had a higher response rate compared to single agent cisplatin chemotherapy [75]. Thus, a four-cycle course of platinum- and taxane-based triple combination regimen is recommended [75, 76]. The management of lymph nodal metastasis is tabulated in Table 21.2.

Table 21.2 Management of lymph node metastasis

Nodal status	Management
cN0 (no palpable inguinal nodes)	Tis, ta, and T1G1: Surveillance
	T1G2 and above: Invasive lymph node staging (dynamic sentinel node biopsy or bilateral modified inguinal lymphadenectomy)
cN1/cN2 (palpable inguinal nodes)	Radical inguinal lymphadenectomy
cN3 (fixed inguinal nodes)	Neoadjuvant chemotherapy followed by radical inguinal lymphadenectomy if responsive
Pelvic nodes	Ipsilateral pelvic lymphadenopathy if two or more inguinal nodes are positive (pN2) or in extracapsular extension (pN3)

21.4.4 Adjuvant Therapy in Node-Positive Disease

Patients with pN2/pN3 disease require adjuvant chemotherapy following LND. Pizzocaro et al. showed that the disease-free survival in patients undergoing adjuvant chemotherapy was 84% as compared to 39% in historical controls without any adjuvant therapy. In this study, 25 patients received vincristine, bleomycin, and methotrexate for 12 courses [71]. Better toxicity profile and outcomes were found with 3–4 cycles of a cisplatin, 5-FU, and taxane (paclitaxel or docetaxel) regimen (TPF). At a median follow-up of 42 months, 52% of patients were disease free with TPF chemotherapy [76]. For patients with pN1 disease, no data exists concerning adjuvant therapy as is therefore not routinely provided. Further details on chemotherapy and radiotherapy are discussed in Chap. 22.

21.4.5 Nodal Recurrence

Patients who have a nodal recurrence should be managed the same way as cN1/cN2 disease. Among patients with prior DSNB or a modified ILND, the natural lymphatic drainage is absent, and the disease spread is erratic. The survival of patients who have a recurrence after radical ILND is 16%, and multimodal therapy is recommended in these patients (EAU). In patients who are under observation, new-onset unilateral lymphadenopathy signifies metastatic spread. Contralateral nodal disease is reported in up to 30% of patients with an ipsilateral bulky recurrence. Therefore, in addition to radical ILND on the ipsilateral side, a contralateral modified ILND is recommended in these patients [59].

21.5 Advanced Penile Cancer and Relapsed Disease

The presence of visceral metastases and an ECOG score of greater than one are considered as independent prognostic factors for advanced penile cancer. Cisplatin-based regimen is preferable and has better outcomes.

Hass et al. from SWOG (Southwest Oncology Group) used BEP (bleomycin, etoposide, cisplatin) chemotherapy for locally advanced and metastatic penile carcinoma. The response rate was 32.5%. This was not superior to single-agent cisplatin therapy [77]. Theodore et al. reported an EORTC (European Organization for Research and Treatment of Cancer) study where 28 patients were treated with cisplatin and irinotecan chemotherapy. Objective response rate was 30.8% [78]. Pagliaro et al. used TIF (paclitaxel, ifosfamide, and cisplatin) chemotherapy in patients with N2 N3 disease. Overall response rate was 50% and pathologic complete response rate was 10% with acceptable toxicity [75]. Nicholson et al. evaluated the combination of docetaxel, cisplatin, and 5-FU in locally advanced and metastatic penile carcinoma. Response rate was 38% but 65% of patients had grade III or grade IV toxicity. Addition of docetaxel was shown to increase the toxicity [79]. These data suggest that in advanced and metastatic penile cancer, a cisplatin-based chemotherapy is recommended.

21.6 Follow-Up in Penile Cancer

Recurrent penile cancer can be local or regional which usually occurs within the first 2 years of primary treatment. Early detection of local recurrences and prompt treatment before metastasis to inguinal nodes have survival advantage [33, 34]. This calls for an intensive follow-up in the first 2 years followed by 3 years of less intensive follow-up amounting to a total of 5 years. In patients with cN0 disease, physical examination of the penis and groins is recommended. Imaging does not provide an added advantage. In patients who underwent laser ablation or topical therapy, confirmatory biopsies are taken following completion of treatment course. Following management of node-positive disease, cross-sectional imagining is recommended every 3 months for the first 2 years. After 5 years, surveillance can be omitted provided the patient is educated about self-examination [34].

References

1. Porter WM, Francis N, Hawkins D, Dinneen M, Bunker CB. Penile intraepithelial neoplasia: clinical spectrum and treatment of 35 cases. Br J Dermatol. 2002;147(6):1159–65.
2. Malek RS, Goellner JR, Smith TE, Espy MJ, Cupp MR. Human papillomavirus infection and intraepithelial, in situ, and invasive carcinoma of penis. Urology. 1993;42(2):159–70.
3. Horenblas S, von Krogh G, Cubilla AL, Dillner J, Meijer CJLM, Hedlund PO. Squamous cell carcinoma of the penis: premalignant lesions. Scand J Urol Nephrol. 2000;34(203):187–8.
4. Alnajjar HM, Lam W, Bolgeri M, Rees RW, Perry MJA, Watkin NA. Treatment of carcinoma in situ of the glans penis with topical chemotherapy agents. Eur Urol. 2012;62(5):923–8.
5. Manjunath A, Brenton T, Wylie S, Corbishley CM, Watkin NA. Topical therapy for non-invasive penile cancer (tis)-updated results and toxicity. Transl Androl Urol. 2017;6(5):803–8.
6. Crispen PL, Mydlo JH. Penile intraepithelial neoplasia and other premalignant lesions of the penis. Urol Clin North Am. 2010;37(3):335–42.
7. Shabbir M, Muneer A, Kalsi J, Shukla CJ, Zacharakis E, Garaffa G, et al. Glans resurfacing for the treatment of carcinoma in situ of the penis: surgical technique and outcomes. Eur Urol. 2011;59(1):142–7.
8. Solsona E, Algaba F, Horenblas S, Pizzocaro G, Windahl T. EAU guidelines on penile Cancer. Eur Urol. 2004;46(1):1–8.
9. Gotsadze D, Matveev B, Zak B, Mamaladze V. Is conservative organ-sparing treatment of penile carcinoma justified? Eur Urol. 2000;38(3):306–12.
10. Kiltie AE, Elwell C, Close HJ, Ash DV. Iridium-192 implantation for node-negative carcinoma of the

penis: the Cookridge hospital experience. Clin Oncol (R Coll Radiol). 2000;12(1):25–31.
11. Narayana AS, Olney LE, Loening SA, Weimar GW, Culp DA. Carcinoma of the penis: analysis of 219 cases. Cancer. 1982;49(10):2185–91.
12. Sosnowski R, Kulpa M, Kosowicz M, Wolski JK, Kuczkiewicz O, Moskal K, et al. Quality of life in penile carcinoma patients—post-total penectomy. Cent European J Urol. 2016;69(2):204–11.
13. Windahl T, Skeppner E, Andersson SO, Fugl-Meyer KS. Sexual function and satisfaction in men after laser treatment for penile carcinoma. J Urol. 2004;172(2):648–51.
14. Colecchia M, Nicolai N, Secchi P, Bandieramonte G, Paganoni AM, Sangalli LM, et al. pT1 penile squamous cell carcinoma: a clinicopathologic study of 56 cases treated by CO_2 laser therapy. Anal Quant Cytol Histol. 2009;31(3):153–60.
15. Bandieramonte G, Colecchia M, Mariani L, Lo Vullo S, Pizzocaro G, Piva L, et al. Peniscopically controlled CO_2 laser excision for conservative treatment of in situ and T1 penile carcinoma: report on 224 patients. Eur Urol. 2008;54(4):875–82.
16. Frimberger D, Hungerhuber E, Zaak D, Waidelich R, Hofstetter A, Schneede P. Penile carcinoma. Is Nd:YAG laser therapy radical enough? J Urol. 2002;168(6):2418–21.
17. Mohs FE, Snow SN, Larson PO. Mohs micrographic surgery for penile tumors. Urol Clin North Am. 1992;19(2):291–304.
18. Wells MJ, Taylor RS. Mohs micrographic surgery for penoscrotal malignancy. Urol Clin. 2010;37(3):403–9.
19. Mohs FE, Snow SN, Messing EM, Kuglitsch ME. Microscopically controlled surgery in the treatment of carcinoma of the penis. J Urol. 1985;133(6):961–6.
20. Machan M, Brodland D, Zitelli J. Penile squamous cell carcinoma: penis-preserving treatment with Mohs micrographic surgery. Dermatol Surg. 2016;42(8):936–44.
21. Ayres BE, Lam W, Al-Najjar HM, Corbishley CM, Perry MJA, Watkin NA. 1106 glans resurfacing—a new penile preserving option for superficially invasive penile cancer. Eur Urol Suppl. 2011;10(2):340.
22. Agrawal A, Pai D, Ananthakrishnan N, Smile SR, Ratnakar C. The histological extent of the local spread of carcinoma of the penis and its therapeutic implications. BJU Int. 2000;85(3):299–301.
23. Philippou P, Shabbir M, Malone P, Nigam R, Muneer A, Ralph DJ, et al. Conservative surgery for squamous cell carcinoma of the penis: resection margins and long-term oncological control. J Urol. 2012;188(3):803–8.
24. Brown CT, Minhas S, Ralph DJ. Conservative surgery for penile cancer: subtotal glans excision without grafting. BJU Int. 2005;96(6):911–2.
25. Ubrig B, Waldner M, Fallahi M, Roth S. Preputial flap for primary closure after excision of tumors on the glans penis. Urology. 2001;58(2):274–6.
26. Davis JW, Schellhammer PF, Schlossberg SM. Conservative surgical therapy for penile and urethral carcinoma. Urology. 1999;53(2):386–92.
27. Parkash S, Ananthakrishnan N, Roy P. Refashioning of phallus stumps and phalloplasty in the treatment of carcinoma of the penis. Br J Surg. 1986;73(11):902–5.
28. Piva L, Nicolai N, Di Palo A, Milani A, Merson M, Salvioni R, et al. Therapeutic alternatives in the treatment of class T1N0 squamous cell carcinoma of the penis: indications and limitations. Arch Ital Urol Androl. 1996;68(3):157–61.
29. Lümmen G, Sperling H, Pietsch M, Otto T, Rübben H. Treatment and follow-up of patients with squamous epithelial carcinoma of the penis. Urologe A. 1997;36(2):157–61.
30. Korets R, Koppie TM, Snyder ME, Russo P. Partial penectomy for patients with squamous cell carcinoma of the penis: the memorial Sloan-Kettering experience. Ann Surg Oncol. 2007;14(12):3614–9.
31. Greenberg RE. Surgical management of carcinoma of the penis. Urol Clin. 2010;37(3):369–78.
32. Djajadiningrat RS, van Werkhoven E, Meinhardt W, van Rhijn BWG, Bex A, van der Poel HG, et al. Penile sparing surgery for penile cancer-does it affect survival? J Urol. 2014;192(1):120–5.
33. Leijte JAP, Kirrander P, Antonini N, Windahl T, Horenblas S. Recurrence patterns of squamous cell carcinoma of the penis: recommendations for follow-up based on a two-centre analysis of 700 patients. Eur Urol. 2008;54(1):161–8.
34. Horenblas S, Newling DW. Local recurrent tumour after penis-conserving therapy. A plea for long-term follow-up. Br J Urol. 1993;72(6):976.
35. Ornellas AA, Kinchin EW, Nóbrega BLB, Wisnescky A, Koifman N, Quirino R. Surgical treatment of invasive squamous cell carcinoma of the penis: Brazilian National Cancer Institute long-term experience. J Surg Oncol. 2008;97(6):487–95.
36. Hegarty PK, Kayes O, Freeman A, Christopher N, Ralph DJ, Minhas S. A prospective study of 100 cases of penile cancer managed according to European Association of Urology guidelines. BJU Int. 2006;98(3):526–31.
37. Slaton JW, Morgenstern N, Levy DA, Santos MW, Tamboli P, Ro JY, et al. Tumor stage, vascular invasion and the percentage of poorly differentiated cancer: independent prognosticators for inguinal lymph node metastasis in penile squamous cancer. J Urol. 2001;165(4):1138–42.
38. Leijte JAP, Valdés Olmos RA, Nieweg OE, Horenblas S. Anatomical mapping of lymphatic drainage in penile carcinoma with SPECT-CT: implications for the extent of inguinal lymph node dissection. Eur Urol. 2008;54(4):885–90.
39. Srinivas V, Morse MJ, Herr HW, Sogani PC, Whitmore WF. Penile cancer: relation of extent of nodal metastasis to survival. J Urol. 1987;137(5):880–2.
40. Margulis V, Sagalowsky AI. Penile cancer: management of regional lymphatic drainage. Urol Clin North Am. 2010;37(3):411–9.

41. Ravi R. Morbidity following groin dissection for penile carcinoma. Br J Urol. 1993;72(6):941–5.
42. Ravi R. Prophylactic lymphadenectomy vs. observation vs. inguinal biopsy in node-negative patients with invasive carcinoma of the penis. Jpn J Clin Oncol. 1993;23(1):53–8.
43. Svatek RS, Munsell M, Kincaid JM, Hegarty P, Slaton JW, Busby JE, et al. Association between lymph node density and disease specific survival in patients with penile cancer. J Urol. 2009;182(6):2721–7.
44. Kroon BK, Horenblas S, Lont AP, Tanis PJ, Gallee MPW, Nieweg OE. Patients with penile carcinoma benefit from immediate resection of clinically occult lymph node metastases. J Urol. 2005;173(3):816–9.
45. Ficarra V, Zattoni F, Artibani W, Fandella A, Martignoni G, Novara G, et al. Nomogram predictive of pathological inguinal lymph node involvement in patients with squamous cell carcinoma of the penis. J Urol. 2006;175(5):1700–4; discussion 1704–1705.
46. Cabanas RM. Application of the sentinel node concept in urogenital cancer. In: Schlag PM, Veronesi U, editors. Lymphatic metastasis and sentinel lymphonodectomy. Berlin: Springer; 2000. p. 141–9.
47. Leijte JAP, Kroon BK, Valdés Olmos RA, Nieweg OE, Horenblas S. Reliability and safety of current dynamic sentinel node biopsy for penile carcinoma. Eur Urol. 2007;52(1):170–7.
48. Kroon BK, Horenblas S, Estourgie SH, Lont AP, Valdés Olmos RA, Nieweg OE. How to avoid false-negative dynamic sentinel node procedures in penile carcinoma. J Urol. 2004;171(6 Pt 1):2191–4.
49. Zou ZJ, Liu ZH, Tang LY, Wang YJ, Liang JY, Zhang RC, et al. Radiocolloid-based dynamic sentinel lymph node biopsy in penile cancer with clinically negative inguinal lymph node: an updated systematic review and meta-analysis. Int Urol Nephrol. 2016;48(12):2001–13.
50. Leijte JAP, Hughes B, Graafland NM, Kroon BK, Olmos RAV, Nieweg OE, et al. Two-center evaluation of dynamic sentinel node biopsy for squamous cell carcinoma of the penis. J Clin Oncol. 2009;27(20):3325–9.
51. Pettaway CA, Pisters LL, Dinney CP, Jularbal F, Swanson DA, von Eschenbach AC, et al. Sentinel lymph node dissection for penile carcinoma: the M. D. Anderson Cancer center experience. J Urol. 1995;154(6):1999–2003.
52. Spiess PE, Izawa JI, Bassett R, Kedar D, Busby JE, Wong F, et al. Preoperative lymphoscintigraphy and dynamic sentinel node biopsy for staging penile cancer: results with pathological correlation. J Urol. 2007;177(6):2157–61.
53. Catalona WJ. Modified inguinal lymphadenectomy for carcinoma of the penis with preservation of saphenous veins: technique and preliminary results. J Urol. 1988;140(2):306–10.
54. Kroon BK, Horenblas S, Deurloo EE, Nieweg OE, Teertstra HJ. Ultrasonography-guided fine-needle aspiration cytology before sentinel node biopsy in patients with penile carcinoma. BJU Int. 2005;95(4):517–21.
55. Saisorn I, Lawrentschuk N, Leewansangtong S, Bolton DM. Fine-needle aspiration cytology predicts inguinal lymph node metastasis without antibiotic pretreatment in penile carcinoma. BJU Int. 2006;97(6):1225–8.
56. Ekstrom T, Edsmyr F. Cancer of the penis; a clinical study of 229 cases. Acta Chir Scand. 1958;115(1–2):25–45.
57. Daseler EH, Anson BJ, Reimann AF. Radical excision of the inguinal and iliac lymph glands; a study based upon 450 anatomical dissections and upon supportive clinical observations. Surg Gynecol Obstet. 1948;87(6):679–94.
58. Cabanas RM. An approach for the treatment of penile carcinoma. Cancer. 1977;39(2):456–66.
59. Horenblas S, van Tinteren H, Delemarre JF, Moonen LM, Lustig V, van Waardenburg EW. Squamous cell carcinoma of the penis. III. Treatment of regional lymph nodes. J Urol. 1993;149(3):492–7.
60. Stuiver MM, Djajadiningrat RS, Graafland NM, Vincent AD, Lucas C, Horenblas S. Early wound complications after inguinal lymphadenectomy in penile cancer: a historical cohort study and risk-factor analysis. Eur Urol. 2013;64(3):486–92.
61. Koifman L, Hampl D, Koifman N, Vides AJ, Ornellas AA. Radical open inguinal lymphadenectomy for penile carcinoma: surgical technique, early complications and late outcomes. J Urol. 2013;190(6):2086–92.
62. Yao K, Tu H, Li YH, Qin ZK, Liu ZW, Zhou FJ, et al. Modified technique of radical inguinal lymphadenectomy for penile carcinoma: morbidity and outcome. J Urol. 2010;184(2):546–52.
63. Protzel C, Alcaraz A, Horenblas S, Pizzocaro G, Zlotta A, Hakenberg OW. Lymphadenectomy in the surgical management of penile cancer. Eur Urol. 2009;55(5):1075–88.
64. Thuret R, Sun M, Lughezzani G, Budaus L, Liberman D, Abdollah F, et al. A contemporary population-based assessment of the rate of lymph node dissection for penile carcinoma. Ann Surg Oncol. 2011;18(2):439–46.
65. La-Touche S, Ayres B, Lam W, Alnajjar H, Perry M, Watkin N. Trial of ligation versus coagulation of lymphatics in dynamic inguinal sentinel lymph node biopsy for staging of squamous cell carcinoma of the penis. Ann R Coll Surg Engl. 2012;94(5):344–6.
66. Culkin DJ, Beer TM. Advanced penile carcinoma. J Urol. 2003;170(2 Pt 1):359–65.
67. Lughezzani G, Catanzaro M, Torelli T, Piva L, Biasoni D, Stagni S, et al. The relationship between characteristics of inguinal lymph nodes and pelvic lymph node involvement in penile squamous cell carcinoma: a single institution experience. J Urol. 2014;191(4):977–82.
68. Graafland NM, van Boven HH, van Werkhoven E, Moonen LMF, Horenblas S. Prognostic significance of extranodal extension in patients with

pathological node positive penile carcinoma. J Urol. 2010;184(4):1347–53.
69. Kumar V, Sethia KK. Prospective study comparing video-endoscopic radical inguinal lymph node dissection (VEILND) with open radical ILND (OILND) for penile cancer over an 8-year period. BJU Int. 2017;119(4):530–4.
70. Tobias-Machado M, Tavares A, Ornellas AA, Molina WR, Juliano RV, Wroclawski ER. Video endoscopic inguinal lymphadenectomy: a new minimally invasive procedure for radical management of inguinal nodes in patients with penile squamous cell carcinoma. J Urol. 2007;177(3):953–7; discussion 958.
71. Pizzocaro G, Piva L. Adjuvant and neoadjuvant vincristine, bleomycin, and methotrexate for inguinal metastases from squamous cell carcinoma of the penis. Acta Oncol. 1988;27(6b):823–4.
72. Leijte JAP, Kerst JM, Bais E, Antonini N, Horenblas S. Neoadjuvant chemotherapy in advanced penile carcinoma. Eur Urol. 2007;52(2):488–94.
73. Bermejo C, Busby JE, Spiess PE, Heller L, Pagliaro LC, Pettaway CA. Neoadjuvant chemotherapy followed by aggressive surgical consolidation for metastatic penile squamous cell carcinoma. J Urol. 2007;177(4):1335–8.
74. Pagliaro LC, Crook J. Multimodality therapy in penile cancer: when and which treatments? World J Urol. 2009;27(2):221–5.
75. Pagliaro LC, Williams DL, Daliani D, Williams MB, Osai W, Kincaid M, et al. Neoadjuvant paclitaxel, ifosfamide, and cisplatin chemotherapy for metastatic penile cancer: a phase II study. J Clin Oncol. 2010;28(24):3851–7.
76. Giannatempo P, Paganoni A, Sangalli L, Colecchia M, Piva L, Catanzaro M, et al. Survival analyses of adjuvant or neoadjuvant combination of a taxane plus cisplatin and 5-fluorouracil (T-PF) in patients with bulky nodal metastases from squamous cell carcinoma of the penis (PSCC): results of a single high-volume center. J Clin Oncol. 2014;32(4_Suppl):377.
77. Haas GP, Blumenstein BA, Gagliano RG, Russell CA, Rivkin SE, Culkin DJ, et al. Cisplatin, methotrexate and bleomycin for the treatment of carcinoma of the penis: a southwest oncology group study. J Urol. 1999;161(6):1823–5.
78. Theodore C, Skoneczna I, Bodrogi I, Leahy M, Kerst JM, Collette L, et al. A phase II multicentre study of irinotecan (CPT 11) in combination with cisplatin (CDDP) in metastatic or locally advanced penile carcinoma (EORTC PROTOCOL 30992). Ann Oncol. 2008;19(7):1304–7.
79. Nicholson S, Hall E, Harland SJ, Chester JD, Pickering L, Barber J, et al. Phase II trial of docetaxel, cisplatin and 5FU chemotherapy in locally advanced and metastatic penis cancer (CRUK/09/001). Br J Cancer. 2013;109(10):2554–9.

Adjuvant Treatment and Follow Up 22

Kevin Arulraj, Sridhar Panaiyadiyan,
Prashant Gupta, Prabhjot Singh,
and Brusabhanu Nayak

22.1 Introduction

22.1.1 Evolution of Chemotherapy

22.1.1.1 Single-Agent Chemotherapy

Advanced carcinoma penis diagnosed with unresectable nodes or distant metastasis has a poor prognosis. Cure is seldom achieved with either surgery or radiotherapy as standalone modalities. The usage of single- or multi-agent chemotherapy in patients with advanced penile cancer is not extensively studied. Nevertheless, a myriad of single as well as multi-agent chemotherapeutic agents have shown reasonable results. Single-agent drugs such as cisplatin, bleomycin and methotrexate have been studied with modest response rates in the 1960s–1980s. Gagliano et al. from SWOG (Southwest Oncology Group) and Ahmed et al. from MSKCC (Memorial Sloan Kettering Cancer Center) used cisplatin (50–120 mg/m^2) in advanced penile cancer and observed responses in 15% and 25% of patients treated, respectively [1, 2]. Single-agent bleomycin (10–30 mg/m^2), despite having favourable response rates, was fraught with severe toxicity. Reported response rates were between 21% and 50% with one patient dying due to bleomycin-induced pulmonary toxicity [2, 3]. Single-agent methotrexate (30–3000 mg/m^2) showed responses in 8 out of 13 patients (61%) with 1 patient showing compete response and 1 patient succumbing to treatment-related sepsis [2].

22.1.1.2 Combination Chemotherapy

Following responses in single-agent chemotherapy, a three-drug study with bleomycin, methotrexate and cisplatin (BMP) was introduced. Hass et al. from SWOG used BEP (bleomycin, etoposide and cisplatin) chemotherapy for locally advanced and metastatic PSCC (primary squamous cell carcinoma). Among the 40 patients who received BMP chemotherapy, five had complete response and eight had partial response with an overall response rate (ORR) of 32.5%. However, this response was not superior to the previously reported cisplatin standalone therapy. Five patients succumbed to treatment-related adverse events among which four of them were due to bleomycin-induced pulmonary toxicity [4]. Bleomycin was then omitted, and future trials included cisplatin with other agents such as irinotecan, paclitaxel, docetaxel, ifosfamide and fluorouracil. Theodore et al. [5] reported an EORTC (European Organization for Research Treatment for Cancer) study where 28 patients were treated with double-agent chemotherapy (cisplatin and irinotecan) in patients with locally advanced and metastatic disease. Patients received either four cycles of neoadjuvant (T3, N1–N2) or eight cycles in T4/N3/M1 disease

K. Arulraj · S. Panaiyadiyan · P. Gupta · P. Singh · B. Nayak (✉)
Department of Urology, All India Institute of Medical Sciences, New Delhi, India

P. Singh et al. (eds.), *A Guide to Management of Urological Cancers*,
https://doi.org/10.1007/978-981-99-2341-0_22

with acceptable toxicity. The objective response rate was 30.8% with three patients showing no evidence of residual disease in final histopathology [5].

Pagliaro et al. used neoadjuvant paclitaxel, ifosfamide and cisplatin (TIP) in patients with bulky or fixed nodes. The regimen included four cycles of TIP followed by bilateral inguinal and bilateral or unilateral pelvic lymph node dissection in addition to control of the primary. They demonstrated an ORR of 50% and a pathologic complete response rate (pCR) of 10% with acceptable toxicity. Out of the 30 eligible patients, 22 underwent surgery. Nine patients were disease-free and alive at 34 months. This data proved the superiority of TIP regimen compared to single-agent cisplatin without any severe complications as seen with bleomycin or methotrexate [6].

Following improved response rates with TIP, the addition of docetaxel and 5-FU to cisplatin was explored. Nicholson et al. [7] evaluated the combination of docetaxel, cisplatin and 5-FU (TPF) in locally advanced and metastatic PSCC. Among the 26 patients who received TPF chemotherapy, the response rate was 38%. However, significant toxicity (grade 3 or 4) was seen in 65% of the patients. The authors concluded that addition of docetaxel was shown to increase the toxicity, and similar response rates can be achieved with cisplatin and 5-FU [7, 8]. Results from the above-mentioned studies suggest that a cisplatin-based combination chemotherapy benefits in patients with advanced and metastatic penile carcinoma. In addition, patients with bulky nodal disease were observed to benefit from neoadjuvant chemotherapy followed by lymphadenectomy.

22.1.2 Neoadjuvant Chemotherapy

The survival in cases with bulky fixed nodal metastasis is dependent upon complete control of the disease. This is seldom achieved by surgery or chemotherapy as a standalone management option [9]. Corral et al. [10] suggested that a multidisciplinary approach in patients with N3 disease helps in achieving a disease-free status and may prolong survival [10]. N3 disease carries a poor prognosis and multimodal therapy is recommended in these patients [11–13]. Neoadjuvant chemotherapy followed by consolidation surgery has shown benefit in advanced penile carcinoma. Studies have shown up to 60% response rates with chemotherapy and up to 20% showing complete response in patients undergoing consolidative ilioinguinal lymph node dissection [12–14]. Both the EAU (European Association of Urology) and the NCCN (National Comprehensive Cancer Network) guidelines have recommended neoadjuvant chemotherapy (NACT) as the preferred modality for patients with fixed, bulky or bilateral inguinal lymphadenopathy [15, 16]. Benefits of NACT include timely delivery of systemic therapy, volume reduction of lymph nodes, prognostication and enabling complete surgical consolidation. Factors to be considered when selecting an appropriate regimen include ORR, tolerability of chemotherapy, percentage of patients who receive subsequent surgical consolidation and pathological complete response (pCR). Currently, the only strong predictor for survival after NACT is the ability to attain a pCR post consolidative surgery [6].

The first study to evaluate NACT was a prospective phase 2 nonrandomized trial by Pagliaro et al. [6] from the MD Anderson Cancer Center. Their goal was to determine response rate, time to progression (TTP) and overall survival (OS). They used neoadjuvant paclitaxel, ifosfamide and cisplatin (TIP) in cases with N2–N3 disease. The regimen included four cycles of TIP followed by bilateral inguinal and either bilateral or unilateral pelvic lymph node dissection along with surgery for the primary tumour (paclitaxel, 175 mg/m^2 on day 1; ifosfamide, 1200 mg/m^2 on days 1–3; and cisplatin, 25 mg/m^2 on days 1–3, cycle repeated every 3 weeks). Among the 30 patients who received chemotherapy, 23 completed all 4 cycles (76.7%). Fifteen (50%) patients had an objective response, with 3 patients with complete response and 12 patients with a partial response. Among patients who received chemotherapy, 73% (22 patients) underwent consolidation surgery. Three patients (10%) were found to have pCR, and 9 patients (30%) had a median recurrence-free survival of 34 months. The TTP was 8 months with an OS of 17 months. The role of multimodal therapy in advanced penile cancer was first established in this prospective study, and Pagliaro et al. demonstrated that neoadjuvant chemotherapy with TIP followed by consolidation surgery is the preferred treatment option for patients with bulky lymphadenopathy [6]. Neoadjuvant TIP chemotherapy given for four cycles resulted in an ORR of 50% with 30% pCR. TIP regimen was better tolerated and had an improved response rate compared to single-agent cisplatin chemotherapy [6]. Thus, a four-cycle course of platinum- and taxane-based triple-combination regimen is currently recommended [6, 17].

Joshi et al. analysed the National Cancer Database and found that among 1123 men diagnosed with locally advanced PSCC, 727 patients underwent LND, highlighting the escalating use of chemotherapy from 38% to 48% between 2004 and 2014. Among the 338 patients with N1 disease, 31% received chemotherapy. Similarly, 40% of the 450 patients with N2 disease and 53% of the 335 patients with N3 disease underwent chemotherapy. Despite having limitations, this study emphasized the importance of lymphadenectomy in improving the overall survival on multivariate analysis [18].

The International Penile Advanced Cancer Trial (InPACT) is the first randomized trial aiming to evaluate treatment options in penile cancer. It is a multi-institutional trial which is currently underway in the UK, USA, Canada and Columbia. The study sets to answer two important questions via two independent randomizations. First is the role of NACT prior to standard surgical therapy. Patients are being randomized into three arms (chemotherapy, chemoradiotherapy and no NACT). Second is the role of prophylactic pelvic lymphadenectomy in patients who receive inguinal lymphadenectomy with high-risk pathologic factors [19]. The results of this RCT will throw light in the sequence of multimodal therapy in PSCC.

22.1.3 Adjuvant Chemotherapy

Patients with node-positive penile cancers have a high relapse rate and significant cancer-associated mortality and morbidity. Ravi et al. observed that the 5-year survival drops from 95% in node-negative disease to 76% in patients with positive inguinal nodes. The 5 year survival of pelvic node-positive cases was dismal [20]. The Milan group studied patients who were treated with adjuvant vincristine, bleomycin and methotrexate (VBM) from 1979 to 1990 and thereafter with cisplatin and 5-FU. Among the 56 node-positive patients, 25 patients received adjuvant VBM and 31 patients were treated with surgery alone. The 5-year survival in patients treated with adjuvant therapy and surgery-alone group was 82% and 37%, respectively. The group found that there is improved long-term survival in patients receiving any adjuvant therapy and a lower toxicity rate in the adjuvant 5-FU and cisplatin group. The disease-free survival in patients undergoing adjuvant chemotherapy was reported to be 84% compared to 39% in patients who do not receive any adjuvant therapy [11]. Sharma et al. in a retrospective study spanning more than 3 decades studied 84 patients from multiple centres who had pelvic nodal metastasis. Patients either did or did not receive adjuvant chemotherapy with VBM, BMP, TIP or TPF regimens. A total of 36 patients received adjuvant chemotherapy while 48 patients were managed with surgery as a standalone modality. Adjuvant chemotherapy resulted in an 11.6-month survival advantage and was associated with reduced all-cause mortality [21]. Better toxicity profile and outcomes were found with 3–4 cycles of a cisplatin, 5-FU and taxane (paclitaxel or docetaxel) regimen (TPF). Following TPF chemotherapy, 52% were disease free at 42 months [17]. It is evident from the above-mentioned studies that patients with pN2/pN3 disease benefit from adjuvant chemotherapy following lymphadenectomy. For patients with pN1 disease, no data exists concerning adjuvant therapy and is therefore not routinely considered.

22.1.4 Chemotherapy in Advanced and Relapsed Penile Cancer

The presence of visceral metastases and an ECOG (Eastern Cooperative Oncology Group) score of greater than one are considered independent poor prognostic factors for advanced penile cancer. It is still unclear as to which regimens benefit patients who do not respond to first-line chemotherapy. Nevertheless, outcomes are bleak for metastatic disease either at presentation or during the course of disease [22]. Participation in clinical trials is an option because of minimal response to available systemic chemotherapeutic regimens. Combination chemotherapy is preferred over singe-agent therapy in patients who have a good performance status to achieve a good clinical response. Factors which influence treatment decisions include type of previous chemotherapy received, disease burden and tolerability for proposed treatment and its side effects. Best supportive care is ideal for patients who are too frail to receive any further chemotherapy.

Cisplatin, as a single-agent therapy, has been shown to have some benefit in disease palliation. Gagliano et al. demonstrated a 15% overall response among 26 patients who received cisplatin with a median overall survival of close to 5 months [1]. Paclitaxel has been demonstrated to have response rates of up to 30% without major adverse events. Vinflunine, a third-generation vinca alkaloid, has been shown to have reasonable clinical outcomes with an overall response rate of 27%. This response was reported to be comparable to combination chemotherapy in other trials for advanced penile carcinoma. However, the progression-free survival was only 2.9 months with an overall survival of 8.4 months. Adverse events occurred in 10% among which the most common were constipation (64%) and neutropenia (32%) [23].

22.1.5 Role of Targeted Therapy

Both primary and metastatic penile cancer cells strongly exhibit epidermal growth factor receptor (EGFR). Despite the expectation that EGFR targeting will have good response, multiple studies have showed only a limited response with anti-EGFR therapy [24]. In addition, the HER/PTEN/Akt pathway is being explored for possible targeted therapy. Dacomitinib, a second-generation pan-HER tyrosine kinase inhibitor, which was approved for patients of non-small cell lung cancer with EGFR alterations, has been reported to show modest response in penile cancer. Necchi et al. used dacomitinib in 28 patients who had advanced or metastatic penile cancer. The overall response rate was 32% with a progression-free survival of 4.1 months and an overall survival of 13.7 months [25]. Multiple genomic studies have identified aberrancies in TP54, CDKN2A, NOTCH1 and PIK3CA, and it is estimated that about 40% of patients with metastatic disease are eligible for targeted therapy. Molecular studies have showed that up to 62% of patients with penile cancer express programmed cell death ligand 1 (PD-L1). Various studies which include single-agent (pembrolizumab, avelumab) and combination (nivolumab plus ipilimumab) immune checkpoint inhibitors are ongoing to explore this new therapeutic avenue. HPV (human papilloma virus) proteins E6 and E7 have been implicated in the development of penile cancer. Hence, targeted therapy for E6 and E7 is also being studied as a treatment option as a standalone or in combination with PD-L1 inhibition [23].

22.2 Role of Radiotherapy in Penile Cancer

22.2.1 Introduction

Squamous cell carcinomas are radiosensitive and most penile cancers are squamous cell carcinomas. Better outcomes and good response rates to chemoradiation are observed in human papilloma virus (HPV)-associated penile cancers [26]. The incidence of penile cancer, especially advanced disease, is significantly lower in developed countries compared to the rest of the world. Hence, there is a lacunae of good quality data regarding the efficacy of radiotherapy or chemoradiation in penile cancer [27]. Radiotherapy is useful as a primary modality or in the adjuvant/neoadjuvant setting. The different types of radiotherapy delivery include external beam, interstitial brachytherapy and surface mould brachytherapy.

22.2.2 Radiotherapy for Carcinoma In Situ (CIS) and Invasive PSCC

Penile preservation is feasible with radiotherapy up to T2 tumours. Men have better quality of life and sexual function with penile preservation. EBRT and mould plesiotherapy are options for management of CIS. EBRT has been employed with a local control rate of 100% in CIS [28]. With respect to invasive PSCC, curative radiotherapy can be either EBRT or brachytherapy (interstitial or mould). The 5-year organ preservation rate in patients who undergo primary EBRT for invasive penile cancer ranges between 50 to 66% [29]. Local control rate and organ preservation rate for patients treated with brachytherapy are 85% at 5 years and 70% at 10 years, respectively [30].

22.2.3 External Beam Radiotherapy

EBRT is employed in T1 and T2 disease. A circumcision is performed prior to delivery of radiation to expose the tumour, to prevent infective complications and to prevent oedema of the prepuce or phimosis. It involves in having the source of radiation away from the lesion. Adequate penile support and positioning are essential for optimal delivery of radiation and for isolation of adjacent structures from the effects of radiation. This can be achieved by placing the penis in a split-block made of wax or poly(methylmethacrylate) with a central chamber to accommodate the penis. Different sizes are required to adjust for radiotherapy-induced changes in penile size. Care is taken to eliminate air gaps for effective delivery of radiation. The clinical target volume (CTV) includes a 1 cm margin from the tumour while the planned target volume has a margin of 2 cm from the tumour to account for variations in delivery. The acceptable dose is from 66 to 70 Gy over 6.5–7 weeks. Local failure rate is increased in patients who received a dose lesser than 60 Gy, fraction size lesser than 2 Gy and treatment duration longer than 45 days [31]. The organ preservation rate and local control rate in 5 years range from 41% to 70% (average of 60%) [32]. Post EBRT changes include erythema, oedema and desquamation which take up to 4 weeks to heal.

22.2.4 Brachytherapy

22.2.4.1 Low-Dose Rate Brachytherapy

Low-dose rate brachytherapy delivers the required dose to target without excessive radiation to the penile shaft or need for a daily setup. The patient is admitted for the course of treatment (4–6 days). Under anaesthesia, interstitial needles are placed after catheterization. Ideal spacing between needles range from 12 to 18 mm. The needles are placed in two planes with or without an additional plesiotherapy plane over the side of cancer. To ensure equidistance between needles, a guide template is used. Radiation delivery can be either continuous or pulse dose. The dosage of classic LDR brachytherapy is 50–60 cGy/h. The total recommended dose is 60–65 Gy during the course of 5 days [33, 34]. The 10-year local control and penile preservation rates for LDR brachytherapy are 70–80% and 70%, respectively. Up to 20% of local failures occur 10 years after therapy and can be salvaged with surgery [29, 30, 35].

22.2.4.2 High-Dose Rate Brachytherapy

HDR brachytherapy for penile cancer is in evolution and the optimal parameters for treatment are yet to be set. The procedure is largely similar to LDR with some distinct adjustments. Ideal needle spacing is 9–12 mm, lesser than that of LDR, and spacing needs not be always equidistant. Using a universal template (with holes every 3 mm) is preferable as it is convenient to adjust spacing. Homogenous delivery of radiation is vital in HDR. An effective total dose of 45–51 Gy given as 3 Gy twice daily at 6 h intervals over 7–8 days is considered optimal [36, 37]. Penile preservation rates with HDR are between 80% and 100%. Kellas et al. reported a local failure rate of 22% with penile preservation in 80% [38].

22.2.5 Surface Mould Plesiotherapy

Surface mould plesiotherapy involves in placing a mould which contains iridium wires for a set period everyday to deliver the desired dose. Initially considered to deliver suboptimal dose (lesser than LDR), the usage of surface moulds has been re-evaluated with HDR. A dose of 40 Gy given as 4 Gy twice daily for 5 days is considered optimal. The source is positioned at 5 mm from the skin, thereby achieving 100% dose delivery at a depth of 10 mm while simultaneously limiting the exposure to skin surface. Swelling and dermatitis are expected following treatment which is maximum at 3 weeks. Complete healing is expected at 10 weeks. Surface mould plesiotherapy is still being studied and long-term data are expected [39, 40].

22.2.6 Patient Selection for Radiotherapy

Prior to treatment, a circumcision is essential. It enables complete exposure and prevents post treatment phimosis and fibrosis of the unexcised foreskin. Tumours of size 4 cm or less, confined to the glans or minimally extending beyond the coronal sulcus, are appropriate for radiotherapy. Tumour size for eligibility for interstitial brachytherapy is variable as larger tumours also respond to treatment, but a higher local failure is expected in such cases [30, 35, 41]. Tumour grade does not correlate with local control rates in brachytherapy. Nonetheless, high-grade lesions have a higher rate of nodal metastasis. Plesiotherapy is best suited for superficial tumours (up to T1b) and is not suitable for tumours with depth more than 5 mm.

22.2.7 Post Radiation Changes and Adverse Effects

Moist desquamation is seen post radiation irrespective of the mode of delivery. It heals at 10 weeks after mould therapy and takes a longer duration of about 3 months after brachytherapy. Tumour eradication results in an ulcer crater proportional to tumour depth. Local hygiene with lukewarm water is essential, and ointments such as zinc, polymyxin B or sulfadiazine can be used. Long-term effects include meatal stenosis and tissue ulceration. Meatal stenosis can occur in up to 45% of patients and is commoner when a higher dose is delivered and when the needles are closer to the meatus. Most cases are managed by meatal dilatation and regular self-calibration by patients. The need for meatoplasty and reconstruction is rare. Soft tissue ulcers occur in up to 26% of patients following brachytherapy. Higher rates of ulceration are seen in patients who receive greater than 60 Gy and have deeper tumours and when more than three planes of needles are used. Healing occurs in 3–6 months with good hygiene and topical antibiotics. Hyperbaric oxygen is an option of deeper lesions [29, 30, 35, 41].

22.2.8 Adjuvant Radiotherapy

Lymph node status is the most important prognostic factor in the management of the carcinoma penis. Surgical staging of inguinal nodes is the recommended approach as it determines further management of pelvic nodes. Radiation therapy prior to surgery is not recommended for this reason. Following surgical nodal staging, adjuvant radiotherapy is beneficial in patients who have multiple positive nodes (two or more) and extracapsular or extranodal disease and in patients with a positive margin [42]. The appropriate dose is 45 Gy in 25 fractions over 5 weeks [43]. In addition to the inguinal region, if the pelvic nodal status is unknown or if the primary disease is high risk, the pelvis is also included in the radiated area. A boost of up to 63 Gy is considered in high-risk disease (positive margins or extranodal disease).

22.2.9 Chemoradiation

Chemoradiotherapy is beneficial in squamous cell carcinoma of the head and neck, anal canal, cervical and vulva. Due to the similar pathology, nodal spread and association with HPV, vulval SCC is very often compared to penile SCC. The current recommendation for advanced nodal disease in vulvar SCC is neoadjuvant chemoradiotherapy or definitive chemoradiotherapy (1.8 Gy daily fractions to a dose of 57.6 Gy, combined with weekly cisplatin at 40 mg/m^2). In view of similar disease pattern, chemoradiotherapy for penile cancer would be an appropriate strategy in the neoadjuvant or as a definitive therapy for inoperable nodal disease. Case reports have shown the efficacy of chemoradiation in inoperable nodal disease in patients with advanced penile cancer [44, 45]. The results of IMPACT (Improving Plasma Collection Clinical Trial) trial which is underway will fill the lacunae of evidence in this topic and define the role of neoadjuvant chemoradiotherapy.

22.2.10 Palliative Radiotherapy

Palliative radiation may be considered in patients with painful bone metastases or in spinal cord compression. Short-course radiotherapy of five or ten fractions are given in these scenarios. However, this dose is not very much effective for high-volume groin disease. A consideration for combined platinum-based chemotherapy along with radiotherapy may be considered if renal function is adequate.

References

1. Gagliano RG, Blumenstein BA, Crawford ED, Stephens RL, Coltman CA, Costanzi JJ. Cis-diamminedichloroplatinum in the treatment of advanced epidermoid carcinoma of the penis: a southwest oncology group study. J Urol. 1989;141(1):66–7.
2. Ahmed T, Sklaroff R, Yagoda A. Sequential trials of methotrexate, cisplatin and bleomycin for penile cancer. J Urol. 1984;132(3):465–8.
3. Ichikawa T, Nakano I, Hirokawa I. Bleomycin treatment of the tumors of penis and scrotum. J Urol. 1969;102(6):699–707.
4. Haas GP, Blumenstein BA, Gagliano RG, Russell CA, Rivkin SE, Culkin DJ, et al. Cisplatin, methotrexate and bleomycin for the treatment of carcinoma of the penis: a southwest oncology group study. J Urol. 1999;161(6):1823–5.
5. Theodore C, Skoneczna I, Bodrogi I, Leahy M, Kerst JM, Collette L, et al. A phase II multicentre study of irinotecan (CPT 11) in combination with cisplatin (CDDP) in metastatic or locally advanced penile carcinoma (EORTC PROTOCOL 30992). Ann Oncol. 2008;19(7):1304–7.
6. Pagliaro LC, Williams DL, Daliani D, Williams MB, Osai W, Kincaid M, et al. Neoadjuvant paclitaxel, ifosfamide, and cisplatin chemotherapy for metastatic penile cancer: a phase II study. J Clin Oncol. 2010;28(24):3851–7.
7. Nicholson S, Hall E, Harland SJ, Chester JD, Pickering L, Barber J, et al. Phase II trial of docetaxel, cisplatin and 5FU chemotherapy in locally advanced and metastatic penis cancer (CRUK/09/001). Br J Cancer. 2013;109(10):2554–9.
8. Di Lorenzo G, Buonerba C, Federico P, Perdonà S, Aieta M, Rescigno P, et al. Cisplatin and 5-fluorouracil in inoperable, stage IV squamous cell carcinoma of the penis. BJU Int. 2012;110(11 Pt B):E661–6.
9. Culkin DJ, Beer TM. Advanced penile carcinoma. J Urol. 2003;170(2 Pt 1):359–65.
10. Corral DA, Sella A, Pettaway CA, Amato RJ, Jones DM, Ellerhorst J. Combination chemotherapy for metastatic or locally advanced genitourinary squamous cell carcinoma: a phase II study of methotrexate, cisplatin and bleomycin. J Urol. 1998;160(5):1770–4.
11. Pizzocaro G, Piva L. Adjuvant and neoadjuvant vincristine, bleomycin, and methotrexate for inguinal metastases from squamous cell carcinoma of the penis. Acta Oncol. 1988;27(6b):823–4.
12. Leijte JAP, Kerst JM, Bais E, Antonini N, Horenblas S. Neoadjuvant chemotherapy in advanced penile carcinoma. Eur Urol. 2007;52(2):488–94.
13. Bermejo C, Busby JE, Spiess PE, Heller L, Pagliaro LC, Pettaway CA. Neoadjuvant chemotherapy followed by aggressive surgical consolidation for metastatic penile squamous cell carcinoma. J Urol. 2007;177(4):1335–8.

14. Pagliaro LC, Crook J. Multimodality therapy in penile cancer: when and which treatments? World J Urol. 2009;27(2):221–5.
15. Hakenberg OW, Compérat EM, Minhas S, Necchi A, Protzel C, Watkin N. EAU guidelines on penile cancer: 2014 update. Eur Urol. 2015;67(1):142–50.
16. Clark PE, Spiess PE, Agarwal N, Biagioli MC, Eisenberger MA, Greenberg RE, et al. Penile cancer. J Natl Compr Cancer Netw. 2013;11(5):594–615.
17. Giannatempo P, Paganoni A, Sangalli L, Colecchia M, Piva L, Catanzaro M, et al. Survival analyses of adjuvant or neoadjuvant combination of a taxane plus cisplatin and 5-fluorouracil (T-PF) in patients with bulky nodal metastases from squamous cell carcinoma of the penis (PSCC): results of a single high-volume center. J Clin Oncol. 2014;32(4_Suppl):377.
18. Joshi SS, Handorf E, Strauss D, Correa AF, Kutikov A, Chen DYT, et al. Treatment trends and outcomes for patients with lymph node-positive cancer of the penis. JAMA Oncol. 2018;4(5):643–9.
19. Canter DJ, Nicholson S, Watkin N, Hall E, Pettaway C. InPACT executive committee. The international penile advanced cancer trial (InPACT): rationale and current status. Eur Urol Focus. 2019;5(5):706–9.
20. Ravi R. Correlation between the extent of nodal involvement and survival following groin dissection for carcinoma of the penis. Br J Urol. 1993;72(5 Pt 2):817–9.
21. Sharma P, Djajadiningrat R, Zargar-Shoshtari K, Catanzaro M, Zhu Y, Nicolai N, et al. Adjuvant chemotherapy is associated with improved overall survival in pelvic node-positive penile cancer after lymph node dissection: a multi-institutional study. Urol Oncol. 2015;33(11):496.e17–23.
22. Wang J, Pettaway CA, Pagliaro LC. Treatment for metastatic penile cancer after first-line chemotherapy failure: analysis of response and survival outcomes. Urology. 2015;85(5):1104–10.
23. Chahoud J, Kohli M, Spiess PE. Management of advanced penile cancer. Mayo Clin Proc. 2021;96(3):720–32.
24. Gu W, Zhu Y, Ye D. Beyond chemotherapy for advanced disease-the role of EGFR and PD-1 inhibitors. Transl Androl Urol. 2017;6(5):848–54.
25. Necchi A, Lo Vullo S, Perrone F, Raggi D, Giannatempo P, Calareso G, et al. First-line therapy with dacomitinib, an orally available pan-HER tyrosine kinase inhibitor, for locally advanced or metastatic penile squamous cell carcinoma: results of an open-label, single-arm, single-Centre, phase 2 study. BJU Int. 2018;121(3):348–56.
26. Djajadiningrat RS, Jordanova ES, Kroon BK, van Werkhoven E, de Jong J, Pronk DTM, et al. Human papillomavirus prevalence in invasive penile cancer and association with clinical outcome. J Urol. 2015;193(2):526–31.
27. Hernandez BY, Barnholtz-Sloan J, German RR, Giuliano A, Goodman MT, King JB, et al. Burden of invasive squamous cell carcinoma of the penis in the United States, 1998–2003. Cancer. 2008;113(S10):2883–91.
28. Mclean M, Akl AM, Wards P, Bissett R, Panzarella T, Gospodarowicz M. The results of primary radiation therapy in the management of squamous cell carcinoma of the penis. Int J Radiat Oncol Biol Phys. 1993;25(4):623–8.
29. Crook J, Ma C, Grimard L. Radiation therapy in the management of the primary penile tumor: an update. World J Urol. 2009;27(2):189–96.
30. de Crevoisier R, Slimane K, Sanfilippo N, Bossi A, Albano M, Dumas I, et al. Long-term results of brachytherapy for carcinoma of the penis confined to the glans (N- or NX). Int J Radiat Oncol Biol Phys. 2009;74(4):1150–6.
31. Sarin R, Norman AR, Steel GG, Horwich A. Treatment results and prognostic factors in 101 men treated for squamous carcinoma of the penis. Int J Radiat Oncol Biol Phys. 1997;38(4):713–22.
32. Crook J. Contemporary role of radiotherapy in the Management of Primary Penile Tumors and Metastatic Disease. Urol Clin N Am. 2016;43(4):435–48.
33. Crook J, Jezioranski J, Cygler JE. Penile brachytherapy: technical aspects and postimplant issues. Brachytherapy. 2010;9(2):151–8.
34. Kamsu-Kom L, Bidault F, Mazeron R, Baratiny C, Martin V, Maroun P, et al. Clinical experience with pulse dose rate brachytherapy for conservative treatment of penile carcinoma and comparison with historical data of low dose rate brachytherapy. Clin Oncol. 2015;27(7):387–93.
35. Mazeron JJ, Langlois D, Lobo PA, Huart JA, Calitchi E, Lusinchi A, et al. Interstitial radiation therapy for carcinoma of the penis using iridium 192 wires: the Henri Mondor experience (1970–1979). Int J Radiat Oncol Biol Phys. 1984;10(10):1891–5.
36. Sharma DN, Joshi NP, Gandhi AK, Haresh KP, Gupta S, Julka PK, et al. High-dose-rate interstitial brachytherapy for T1-T2-stage penile carcinoma: short-term results. Brachytherapy. 2014;13(5):481–7.
37. Pohanková D, Sirak I, Kasaova L, Grepl J, Paluska P, Louda M, et al. High-dose rate brachytherapy in the treatment of early stages of penile carcinoma. Klin Onkol. 2019;15:32.
38. Kellas-Sleczka S, Bialas B, Fijalkowski M, Wojcieszek P, Szlag M, Cholewka A, et al. Interstitial HDR brachytherapy for penile cancer: a thirteen-year follow up of 55 patients. Brachytherapy. 2015;14:S33.
39. Matys R, Kubicka-Mendak I, Łyczek J, Pawłowski P, Stawiarska I, Miedzinska J, et al. Pictorial essay penile cancer brachytherapy HDR mould technique used at the Holycross cancer center. J Contemp Brachytherapy. 2011;3(4):224–9.
40. Helou J, Morton G, Easton H, Jurincic L, D'Alimonte L, Ravi A. Customized penile plesiobrachytherapy using latest stereolithography techniques. Brachytherapy. 2015;14:S99–100.
41. Kiltie AE, Elwell C, Close HJ, Ash DV. Iridium-192 implantation for node-negative carcinoma of the

penis: the Cookridge hospital experience. Clin Oncol (R Coll Radiol). 2000;12(1):25–31.
42. Tang DH, Djajadiningrat R, Diorio G, Chipollini J, Ma Z, Schaible BJ, et al. Adjuvant pelvic radiation is associated with improved survival and decreased disease recurrence in pelvic node-positive penile cancer after lymph node dissection: a multi-institutional study. Urol Oncol. 2017;35(10):605.e17–23.
43. Hyde SE, Valmadre S, Hacker NF, Schilthuis MS, Grant PT, van der Velden J. Squamous cell carcinoma of the vulva with bulky positive groin nodes-nodal debulking versus full groin dissection prior to radiation therapy. Int J Gynecol Cancer. 2007;17(1):154–8.
44. Chhabra A, Schwartz D, Leaf A, Karanikolas N, Weiss JP, Schreiber D. Neoadjuvant concurrent chemoradiation for curative treatment of penile squamous cell carcinoma. Case Rep Oncol Med. 2014;2014:479376.
45. Lapierre A, Riou O, Fléchon A, Mottet N, Azria D. Advanced penile cancer with iliac lymph node involvement treated with radiation and concurrent gemcitabine. Cancer Radiother. 2017;21(2):134–7.

Part VI

Testicular Cancer

23 Diagnosis and Clinical Staging

Ravi Teja Sepuri and Gagan Prakash

23.1 Introduction

Testicular germ cell tumors are one of the few cancers with an outstanding 5-year survival rate even in advanced disease when treated with the right modality and sequence in high-volume centers.

23.2 Clinical Symptoms

Most common presenting feature of testicular cancer is painless testicular swelling. Testicular pain can occur in rare instance where rapid growth of tumor causing infarction or hemorrhage [1]. Pain is more common in NSGCT (non-seminomatous germ cell tumor) than seminomas because NSGCT are more vascular and have more rapid growth [2].Testicular trauma per se does not cause testicular tumor but makes the patient aware of the mass.

History of undescended testis and orchidopexy should be documented elaborately. Scrotal violation by means of scrotal biopsy or scrotal orchidectomy should be documented, and if systemic therapy is not required, the treatment includes revision of scar with cord by inguinal incision in case of NSGCT. If radiation therapy is planned for seminoma, the region can be included in field [3].

In around 66% of NSGCT and 15% seminomas, initial presentation will be either regional or distant metastasis, and symptoms will be present in 15% of patients. Retroperitoneal mass obstructing ureter leads to flank pain. Mass involving or infiltrating the psoas muscle or nerve roots may cause back pain, and mass causing inferior vena cava compression may cause bilateral lower limb edema [4]. Dyspnea, cough, hemoptysis, and chest pain may occur in case of pulmonary metastasis. It can also metastasize to left supraclavicular node. Gynecomastia may be present in around 2% men, and it may be due to elevated HCG levels and is most commonly seen in Leydig cell tumors [5]. In two-thirds of the men with GCT, there is an associated diminished fertility [6].

23.3 Physical Examination

Examination should be done in standing as well as supine position; comment should be made on size of the mass, consistency – hard or firm – tenderness, local rise of temperature, loss of testicular sensation, para-testicular lesions, and epididymal lesions. Loss of testicular sensation is due to pressure atrophy of neuronal endings between growing mass and tunica albuginea [7].

R. T. Sepuri · G. Prakash (✉)
Urologic Oncology Unit, Department of Surgical Oncology, Homi Bhabha National Institute, Tata Memorial Centre, Tata Memorial Hospital, Mumbai, India

P. Singh et al. (eds.), *A Guide to Management of Urological Cancers*,
https://doi.org/10.1007/978-981-99-2341-0_23

Any hard-to-firm consistency over the testis should be evaluated for neoplasm [8]. In case of hydrocele, post trauma, or complete inguinal hernia, it may be difficult to palpate mass. In such conditions, scrotal ultrasound should be used as adjunct to clinical examination.

Scrotal violation marks should be noted. Palpable inguinal lymph nodes in case of scrotal violation and orchidopexy can be appreciated [9]. In patients with undescended testis, mass in the right or left iliac fossa should be taken as testicular tumor unless proved otherwise as well as supraclavicular lymphadenopathy and mass per abdomen in case of metastasis.

23.4 Spread of the Disease

With exception of choriocarcinoma, lymphatic spread is the most common route of GCT spread. Choriocarcinoma spreads through hematogenous route [10]. In 70–80% of testicular tumors, first site of metastatic spread is retroperitoneum [11].

The draining lymph nodal stations differ for both right and left testes. Right testicular tumors drain into interaortocaval (IAC) nodes inferior to the renal vessels first and then followed by the para-aortic (PA) and para-caval nodes [12]. In case of left testicular tumors, the first landing zone is para-aortic lymph nodes and then to interaortocaval nodes. The drainage of retroperitoneal lymph is from the right to left side [13]. In this way, contralateral spread over from the definitive landing zone is common with right-sided tumors but is rarely seen with left-sided tumors [12].

Lymphatic drainage from retroperitoneum is via cisterna chyli which is located behind the right renal artery and right crus of the diaphragm [14]:

lymphatics from cisterna chyli → retrocrural LN → thoracic duct → posterior mediastinum → left supraclavicular fossa

In case of prior inguinal or pelvic surgeries, there may be retrograde spread to iliac and inguinal lymph nodes [15].

The TNM (tumor, node, and metastasis) staging of testicular cancer is described in Table 23.1.

Stage grouping				
Stage 0	pTis	N0	M0	S0
Stage I	pT1–T4	N0	M0	SX
Stage IA	pT1	N0	M0	S0
Stage IB	pT2–pT4	N0	M0	S0
Stage IS	Any pT/TX	N0	M0	S1-3
Stage II	Any pT/TX	N1-N3	M0	SX
Stage IIA	Any pT/TX	N1	M0	S0
	Any pT/TX	N1	M0	S1
Stage IIB	Any pT/TX	N2	M0	S0
	Any pT/TX	N2	M0	S1
Stage IIC	Any pT/TX	N3	M0	S0
	Any pT/TX	N3	M0	S1
Stage III	Any pT/TX	Any N	M1	SX
Stage IIIA	Any pT/TX	Any N	M1a	S0
	Any pT/TX	Any N	M1a	S1
Stage IIIB	Any pT/TX	N1-N3	M0	S2
	Any pT/TX	Any N	M1a	S2
Stage IIIC	Any pT/TX	N1-N3	M0	S3
	Any pT/TX	Any N	M1a	S3
	Any pT/TX	Any N	M1b	Any S

Table 23.1 TNM staging of testicular cancer

Pathological T staging (pT)	
pTX	Primary tumor cannot be assessed
pT0	No evidence of primary tumor
pTis	Germ cell neoplasia in situ
pT1	Tumor limited to the testis (including rete testis invasion) without lymph vascular invasion
pT1a[a]	Tumor smaller than 3 cm in size
pT1b[a]	Tumor 3 cm or larger in size
pT2	Tumor limited to the testis (including rete testis invasion) with lymph vascular invasion
	OR
	Tumor invading hilar soft tissue or epididymis or penetrating visceral mesothelial layer covering the external surface of the tunica albuginea with or without lymph vascular invasion
pT3	Tumor invades spermatic cord with or without lymph vascular invasion
pT4	Tumor invades the scrotum with or without lymph vascular invasion

Clinical nodal status (cN)	
cNX	Regional lymph nodes cannot be assessed
cN0	No regional lymph node metastasis
cN1	Metastases with a lymph node mass 2 cm or smaller in greatest dimension
	OR
	Multiple lymph nodes, not larger than 2 cm in greatest dimension

(continued)

Table 23.1 (continued)

Clinical nodal status (cN)	
cN2	Metastasis with a lymph node mass larger than 2 cm but not larger than 5 cm in greatest dimension
	OR
	Multiple lymph nodes, any one mass larger than 2 cm but not larger than 5 cm in greatest dimension
cN3	Metastasis with a lymph node mass larger than 5 cm in greatest dimension

Distant metastasis (M)	
M0	No distant metastases
M1	Distant metastases
M1a	Non-retroperitoneal nodal or pulmonary metastases
M1b	Non-pulmonary visceral metastases

Serum tumor markers (S) (pre-chemotherapy)			
SX	Serum marker studies not available or not performed		
S0	Serum marker study levels within normal limits		
	LDH (U/l)	hCG (mIU/mL)	AFP (ng/mL)
S1	<1.5 × N	<5000	<1000
S2	1.5–10 × N	5000–50,000	1000–10,000
S3	>10 × N	>50,000	>10,000

LDH lactate dehydrogenase, *hCG* human chorionic gonadotrophin, *AFP* alpha fetoprotein
[a] Subclassification of pT1 applies only to pure seminoma

T1 is divided into T1a and T1b based on the tumor size cutoff 3 cm in case of pure seminoma. Regarding spermatic cord invasion, if it is continuous involvement, it is considered T3 whereas discontinuous involvement by lymphovascular invasion is considered M1 disease. The presence of only an intravascular tumor in spermatic cord in the absence of parenchymal invasion is considered pT2.

Clinical staging:

CS I = Disease clinically confined to the testis

CS II = Regional (retroperitoneal) lymph node metastasis

CS IIA = Less than 2 cm nodal mass

CS IIB = 2–5 cm nodal mass

CS IIC = More than 5 cm nodal mass

CS III = Non-regional lymph node and/or visceral metastasis

The International Germ Cell Cancer Collaborative Group (IGCCCG) defined a prognostic factor-based staging system for advanced GCT based on identification of clinically independent adverse factors.

Good-prognosis group	
Non-seminoma (56% of cases)	*All of the following criteria:*
5-year PFS 89%	• Testis/retro-peritoneal primary
5-year survival 92%	• No non-pulmonary visceral metastases
	• AFP <1000 ng/mL
	• hCG <5000 IU/L (1000 ng/mL)
	• LDH <1.5 × ULN
Seminoma (90% of cases)	*All of the following criteria:*
5-year PFS 82%	• Any primary site
5-year survival 86%	• No non-pulmonary visceral metastases
	• Normal AFP
	• Any hCG
	• Any LDH
Intermediate-prognosis group	
Non-seminoma (28% of cases)	*Any of the following criteria:*
5-year PFS 75%	• Testis/retro-peritoneal primary
5-year survival 80%	• No non-pulmonary visceral metastases
	• AFP 1000–10,000 ng/mL or
	• hCG 5000–50,000 IU/L or
	• LDH 1.5–10 × ULN
Seminoma (10% of cases)	*All of the following criteria:*
5-year PFS 67%	• Any primary site
5-year survival 72%	• Non-pulmonary visceral metastases
	• Normal AFP
	• Any hCG
	• Any LDH
Poor-prognosis group	
Non-seminoma (16% of cases)	*Any of the following criteria:*
5-year PFS 41%	• Mediastinal primary
5-year survival 48%	• Non-pulmonary visceral metastases
	• AFP >10,000 ng/mL or
	• hCG >50,000 IU/L (10,000 ng/mL) or
	• LDH >10 × ULN
Seminoma	No patients classified as poor prognosis

The original IGCCCG risk stratification was published in 1997 and was based on patients treated from 1975 to 1990. New data was analyzed from patients between 1990 and 2013 (2451 in seminoma, 9728 in NSGCT), and results were published in 2021. This update aimed to offer a more contemporary assessment of the PFS and OS, in an era where cisplatin- and etoposide-based chemotherapy is standard.

In advanced seminoma, a 5-year overall survival rate increased from 86% to 95% in good prognostic group and from 72% in old data and 88% in intermediate prognostic group.

In advanced seminoma, a 5-year progression-free survival increased from 82% to 89% in good prognostic group and from 67% to 79% in intermediate prognostic group.

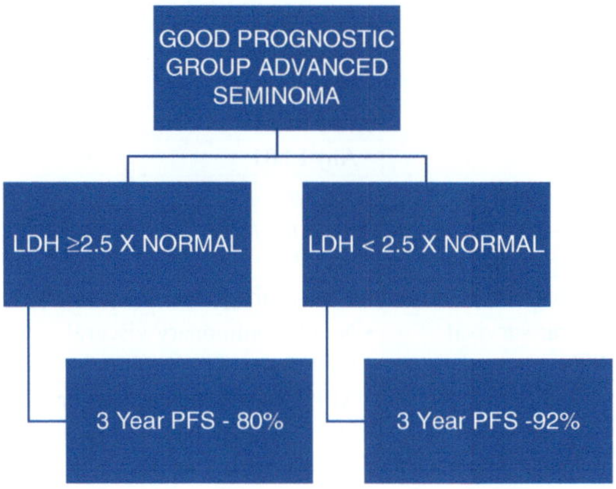

In advanced NSGCT group, for good and intermediate prognostic groups, a 5-year PFS is similar, but a 5-year OS has improved from 91% to 96% in good group and 79–89% for intermediate group. For poor risk, cancer-free survival drastically improved with the cisplatin and etoposide regimen which increased a 5-year PFS from 41% to 54% and a 5-year OS from 48% to 67%.

LDH was found to be an important prognostic factor improving the PFS, in both seminoma and advanced NSGCT. In addition, increasing age and presence of pulmonary metastases were found to be adverse prognostic factors in advanced NSGCT.

23.5 Tumor Markers

Tumor markers play an important role in diagnosis as well as management and follow-up of testicular cancer [16]. Serum tumor markers should be done at the time of diagnosis; after high inguinal orchidectomy after at least four half-lives of markers, to assess response with chemotherapy; and in the follow-up [17].

23.5.1 Alpha Fetoprotein (AFP)

AFP will be increased in around 50–60% of localized and regional nodal (CS I till CS IIB) NSGCT and 70–80% of advanced (CS IIC and III) NSGCT at the time of diagnosis [17]. Embryonal carcinoma and yolk sac tumors secrete AFP. Normal value of AFP is less than 10 ng/mL. Half-life is around 5–7 days. AFP will not be elevated in choriocarcinoma and seminomas. AFP can be elevated in other malignancies such as hepatocellular carcinoma, gastric carcinoma, pancreatic, biliary tract, and lung cancers. It will be elevated in benign conditions such as hepatitis, pancreatitis, drug induced, and hereditary tyrosinemia [17].

23.5.2 Beta Human Chorionoic Gonadotropin (β-HCG)

β-HCG will be elevated in choriocarcinoma and embryonal carcinoma. It will be elevated in 20% of CS I till IIB NSGCT and 40–50% of advanced (CS IIC and III) NSGCT and 15% seminomas [17]. Half-life is around 24–36 h. It is elevated in seminoma, choriocarcinoma, and embryonal carcinoma. It may be increased in other malignancies as well as benign conditions. Immunoassays of β-HCG has cross reactivity with LH and FSH. It can also be elevated in cases of primary hypogonadism, where values will be normalized after replacing testosterone [18].

23.5.3 Lactate Dehydrogenase (LDH)

This correlates with the tumor burden. Isochrome 12p copy numbers are directly related to LDH levels [18]. Half-life of LDH is 24 h. It does not have a role in diagnosis but has a role in prognosis of GCT. False positive can be seen in hemolysis, myocardial infarction, and rhabdomyolysis.

Post high inguinal orchidectomy after four half-lives, tumor markers are taken into consideration for staging and can decide the further management. If the tumor markers are elevated or similar compared to pre-orchidectomy, there is more likely chance of metastatic disease. If the tumor markers have normalized after orchidectomy, it is a favorable indicator, but it does not mean there is no metastatic disease. It also defines the requirement of chemotherapy or definitive primary retroperitoneal lymph node dissection. If tumor markers are elevated in CS II A and B NSGCT, then chemotherapy is given first and then RPLND (retroperitoneal lymph node dissection) is performed. If tumor markers are normal in the above situation, primary RPLND can be performed. Tumor marker values are to be with in 1 week when planned for RPLND.

For patients with advanced disease who require urgent initiation of chemotherapy, substantially the increase in AFP and/or B-hCG may be sufficient for diagnosis of GCT, without waiting for tissue diagnosis.

23.5.4 MicroRNAs (miRNAs)

These are potentially new biomarkers for GCT; initial clinical trials showed that miRNAs have more accuracy in diagnosis and treatment monitoring and for predicting recurrence of GCT particularly 371–373 (chromosomal locus 19q13.41) and miR-302/367 (4q25) [19]. Biologically they are highly stable, short, nonprotein coding RNAs. Chromosome-19-microRNA-cluster (C19MC or miR-515 ~ 526) levels are elevated in embryonal carcinoma. C19MC is expressed physiologically during pregnancy and pathologically in cases of gestational trophoblastic neoplasia and eclampsia. Complete miRNA profile will identify entire free miRNA activity which will be helpful in evaluation of underlying choriocarcinoma component in a case of NSGCT.

23.6 Imaging

23.6.1 Ultrasonography (USG) Scrotum

Ultrasonography of the scrotum with high-frequency curvilinear transducer probes (5–10 MHz) is almost 100% sensitive to pick up a lesion in the testis, but it is 100% specific enough to differentiate between benign and malignant lesions [20]. There are certain differences between seminoma and NSGCT on ultrasonography. A typical GCT looks hypoechoic. USG helps in differentiating seminoma from NSGCT, whereas the echotexture will be homogenous in the former and heterogenous in the latter [20]. On Doppler if the arterial flow increases to the testis, it is suggestive of malignancy, whereas the absence of flow does not rule out GCT [21].

In cases of advanced GCT and no mass palpable clinically, ultrasonography will be helpful to look for small scar or calcification which indicates burned out primary testis tumor. In patients with seminoma, there is chance of spontaneous regression, but GCNIS with high-risk features on ultrasound such as discrete nodule, coarse calcification, or stellate scar should be offered radical high inguinal orchidectomy as GCNIS and residual teratoma are seen frequently. Ultrasonography will be helpful in differentiating testicular from paratesticular tumors like sarcomas.

In cases of small lesions with normal STM or no metastasis, confirmation may be difficult. In such cases, size of lesion will be helpful to risk stratify. Risk of malignancy depends on size of the lesion, 50% for lesions less than 1 cm to more than 80% for more than 1–2 cm in size [22]. In such small lesions with normal STM, inguinal exploration with frozen section of the suspected lesion can be done. If there is no lesion in the testis on ultrasound, suspect primary extragonadal GCT.

Testicular microlithiasis (TML) in the contralateral testis needs to be ruled as it is associated with GCT. It is defined as innumerable tiny bright echoes diffusely and uniformly scattered throughout the substance of testes using high-frequency transducer (10 MHz). However, it is significant in the history of prior GCT or family history of GCT, history of orchidopexy, and testicular atrophy (<12 cc), and these patients need to be kept on surveillance USG [23]. <2% develop GCT within 5 years. It has been linked to common developmental defect in the seminiferous tubule formation and part of testicular dysgenesis syndrome.

1. ≥5 calcification/field
2. Diffuse
3. <2 mm size

Grading of microlithiasis: Microliths count as seen in any single view [24]

1. Minimial/mild/grade I—5–10 microliths
2. Moderate/grade II—10–20 microliths
3. Severe/grade III—>20 microliths

Indications of biopsy of TML:

Open inguinal testicular biopsy should be done if it is followed by treatment of GCNIS [24]:

1. Ipsilateral GCT and contralateral TML
2. Testicular dysgenesis syndrome
3. Cryptorchidism
4. Testicular atrophy (<12 cc)
5. Focal, clumped, and unilateral TML without clinically palpable mass
6. Severe TML
7. Grade IV or V pattern if testicular texture in USG

23.7 Testicular Nonpalpable Incidentaloma

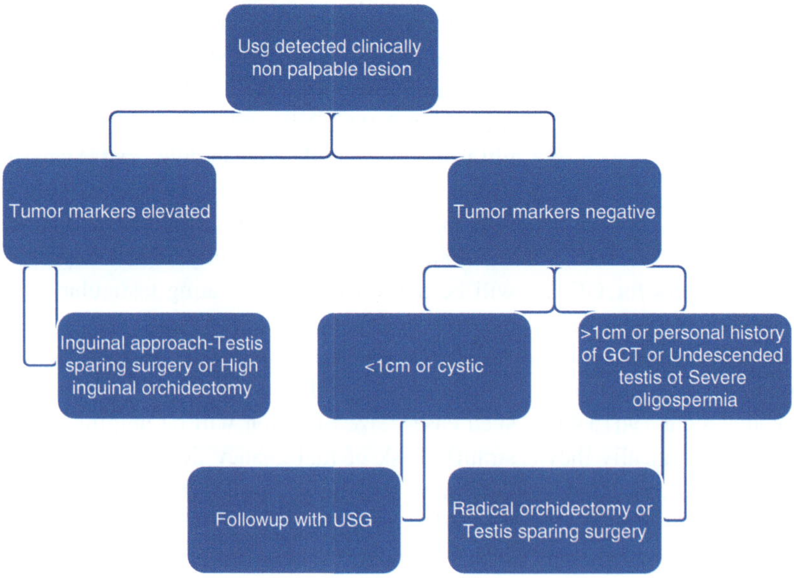

23.8 Staging Investigations

23.8.1 CECT Abdomen and Pelvis

Computed tomography of the abdomen and pelvis with intravenous and oral contrast is the most sensitive and specific noninvasive investigation useful for staging of GCT. If there is abnormality in the retroperitoneum, then CT thorax can be advised [24].

Along with retroperitoneal lymphnodal spread, it will provide information about renal vasculature, abnormal vessels, and ureteral anatomy. CT abdomen has sensitivity around 67% (range 37–100%) with specificity of around 92% (range 58–100%) [25]. In around 20% of seminomas and 70% of NSGCT, significant retroperitoneal lymphadenopathy is noticed. Definition for significant retroperitoneal lymph node is any lymph node of size more than or equal to 10 mm in the primary landing zone; it should be considered suspicious if the size is between 5 and 9 mm in the landing zone and anterior to the aorta or inferior vena cava [26]. Lymph nodes will be in infra hilar level. Hounsfield unit (HU) of seminoma is more than 30, whereas teratoma or mixed GCT is less than 30 HU [27].

Primary landing zones for right and left GCT are different. Right GCT spreads first to interaortocaval lymph node and then followed by para-caval and para-aortic. Left GCT spreads first to para-aortic lymph node and then followed by interaortocaval lymph node [27].

23.8.2 CT Thorax

All patients with testicular cancer should get chest imaging before and after chemotherapy if bleomycin is used. Lung metastasis without retroperitoneal disease is unlikely. For chest CT, sensitivity is around 100% (range 95–100%) and specificity around 93% (range is 89–97%) [25], as a routine chest x-ray has to be done in all cases as initial metastatic workup. CT thorax is recommended in cases of post-orchiectomy elevated STM, retroperitoneal lymph node enlargement CS II and III, and abnormal or suspicious chest x-ray imaging [18].

In cases of CS I NSGCT with high-risk histological features like lymphovascular invasion and predominance of embryonal carcinoma, CT thorax should be done as there is increased risk of hematogenous spread to the lung without retroperitoneal lymph node involvement. If there is mediastinal or hilar lymphadenopathy without retroperitoneal disease, there should be a high suspicion for non-GCT such as sarcoidosis or lymphoma.

23.8.3 CT Brain

CT brain is indicated in cases of highly elevated hCG (>10,000 mU/mL) where choriocarcinoma is suspected; in extensive lung metastases in symptomatic patients, CT brain is to be as initial imaging tool as there is more chance of brain metastases [19].

23.8.4 MRI in GCT

MRI of the scrotum is helpful when it is clinically indistinguishable between intra- and extra-testicular mass clinically and by USG. MRI brain is more sensitive for detecting cerebral metastases to CECT and should be preferred whenever available. However, there is no indication for routine usage for staging evaluation at present.

23.8.5 FDG PET CT

It is not routinely used in GCT except in the case of seminoma post-chemotherapy residual tumor more than 3 cm. This needs to be done at least after 6 weeks after last dose of chemotherapy.

23.9 Future Directives

Differentiating viable tumor from teratoma and tumor necrosis post-chemotherapy by miRNA and radiological features using machine learning automated integration is being evaluated as tools that could be used will prevent morbidity related to RPLND.

References

1. Smith ZL, Werntz RP, Eggener SE. Testicular cancer: epidemiology, diagnosis, and management. Med Clin North Am. 2018;102(2):251–64.
2. Cheriyan SK, Nicholson M, Aydin AM, Azizi M, Peyton CC, Sexton WJ, Gilbert SM. Current management and management controversies in early- and intermediate-stage of nonseminoma germ cell tumors. Transl Androl Urol. 2020;9(Suppl 1):S45–55.
3. Borni M, Kolsi F, Kammoun B, Kallel R, Souissi G, Boudawara MZ. Testicular non-seminomatous germ cell tumors (NSGCT) and brain metastases: about a rare location of the posterior fossa. Urol Case Rep. 2018;21:61–3.
4. Goldberg H, Klaassen Z, Chandrasekar T, Fleshner N, Hamilton RJ, Jewett MAS. Germ cell testicular tumors-contemporary diagnosis, staging and management of localized and advanced disease. Urology. 2019;125:8–19.
5. Cheng L, Albers P, Berney DM, Feldman DR, Daugaard G, Gilligan T, Looijenga LHJ. Testicular cancer. Nat Rev Dis Primers. 2018;4(1):29.
6. Jørgensen N, Rajpert-De Meyts E, Main KM, Skakkebaek NE. Testicular dysgenesis syndrome comprises some but not all cases of hypospadias and impaired spermatogenesis. Int J Androl. 2010;33(2):298–303.
7. Einhorn LH. Treatment of testicular cancer: a new and improved model. J Clin Oncol. 1990;8(11):1777–81.
8. Del Risco KR, Ruud E, Haugnes HS, Cannon-Albright LA, Thoresen M, Nafstad P, Vlatkovic L, Blaasaas KG, Næss Ø, Claussen B. Family history of cancer and risk of paediatric and young adult's testicular cancer: a Norwegian cohort study. Br J Cancer. 2019;120(10):1007–14.
9. Hanna NH, Einhorn LH. Testicular cancer—discoveries and updates. N Engl J Med. 2014;371(21):2005–16.
10. Djaladat H, Burner E, Parikh PM, Beroukhim Kay D, Hays K. The association between testis cancer and semen abnormalities before orchiectomy: a systematic review. J Adolesc Young Adult Oncol. 2014;3(4):153–9.
11. Stephenson A, Eggener SE, Bass EB, Chelnick DM, Daneshmand S, Feldman D, Gilligan T, Karam JA, Leibovich B, Liauw SL, Masterson TA, Meeks JJ, Pierorazio PM, Sharma R, Sheinfeld J. Diagnosis and treatment of early stage testicular cancer: AUA guideline. J Urol. 2019;202(2):272–81.
12. Donohue JP, Zachary JM, Maynard BR. Distribution of nodal metastases in nonseminomatous testis cancer. J Urol. 1982;128(2):315–20.
13. Dieckmann KP, Pichlmeier U. Clinical epidemiology of testicular germ cell tumors. World J Urol. 2004;22:2–14.
14. Gholam D, Fizazi K, Terrier-Lacombe MJ, et al. Advanced seminoma—treatment results and prognostic factors for survival after first-line, cisplatin-based chemotherapy and for patients with recurrent disease: a single-institution experience in 145 patients. Cancer. 2003;98:745–52.
15. Holmes L Jr, Escalante C, Garrison O, et al. Testicular cancer incidence trends in the USA (1975–2004): plateau or shifting racial paradigm? Public Health. 2008;122:862–72.
16. Karellas ME, Damjanov I, Holzbeierlein JM. ITGCN of the testis, contralateral testicular biopsy and bilateral testicular cancer. Urol Clin North Am. 2007;34:119–25.
17. Looijenga LH, Gillis AJ, Stoop H, et al. Dissecting the molecular pathways of (testicular) germ cell tumour pathogenesis: from initiation to treatment resistance. Int J Androl. 2011;34:e234–51.
18. Lackner JE, Koller A, Schatzl G, et al. Androgen deficiency symptoms in testicular cancer survivors are associated with sexual problems but not with serum testosterone or therapy. Urology. 2009;74:825–9.
19. McGlynn KA, Devesa SS, Sigurdson AJ, et al. Trends in the incidence of testicular germ cell tumors in the United States. Cancer. 2003;97:63–70.
20. Motzer RJ, Bolger GB, Boston B, et al. Testicular cancer. Clinical practice guidelines in oncology. J Natl Compr Cancer Netw. 2006;4:1038–58.
21. Raina V, Singh SP, Kamble N, et al. Brain metastasis as the site of relapse in germ cell tumor of testis. Cancer. 1993;72:2182–5.
22. Hotakainen K, Ljungberg B, Paju A, Rasmuson T, Alfthan H, Stenman UH. The free beta-subunit of human chorionic gonadotropin as a prognostic factor in renal cell carcinoma. Br J Cancer. 2002;86(2):185–9.
23. von Eyben FE. Laboratory markers and germ cell tumors. Crit Rev Clin Lab Sci. 2003;40(4):377–427.
24. Carmignani L, Morabito A, Gadda F, et al. Prognostic parameters in adult impalpable ultrasonographic lesions of the testicle. J Urol. 2005;174:1035–8.
25. De Santis M, Becherer A, Bokemeyer C, et al. (2–18) Fluoro-deoxy-D-glucose positron emission tomography is a reliable predictor for viable tumor in

postchemotherapy seminoma: an update of the prospective multicentric SEMPET trial. J Clin Oncol. 2004;22:1034–9.
26. Kreydin EI, Barrisford GW, Feldman AS, Preston MA. Testicular cancer: what the radiologist needs to know. AJR Am J Roentgenol. 2013;200(6):1215–25.
27. Tan IB, Ang KK, Ching BC, Mohan C, Toh CK, Tan MH. Testicular microlithiasis predicts concurrent testicular germ cell tumors and intratubular germ cell neoplasia of unclassified type in adults: a meta-analysis and systematic review. Cancer. 2010;116(19):4520–32.

24 Pathology and Staging

Pavithra Ayyanar and Suvendu Purkait

24.1 Introduction

Testicular tumors have diverse tumor morphology and pathogenesis as they arise from various types of cells. The 2016 World Health Organization classification of tumors of the testis radically revised the classification system and was based on the pathogenesis of tumors irrespective of the morphologic features [1]. The major changes in the germ cell tumor classification are the introduction of the term "germ cell neoplasia in situ (GCNIS)." The germ cell tumors were classified broadly into GCNIS-derived (postpubertal type) and non-GCNIS-derived (prepubertal type). The recent 2022 classification adapted the basic structure and principal nomenclature of the previous classification system [2]. Although there is a tremendous increase in the understanding of the pathobiology of the testicular tumor, the updated classification is rooted in the histological parameters. However, there are certain changes in the nomenclatures. The comparison of WHO 2016 and 2022 testicular tumor classification is mentioned in Table 24.1.

Table 24.1 2022 WHO fifth edition classification of tumors of the testis in comparison to the previous (2016) classification

2016 WHO classification	2022 WHO classification
Germ cell tumors	**Germ cell tumors**
Germ cell tumors derived from GCNIS	*Germ cell tumors derived from GCNIS*
Noninvasive GCNIS	*Noninvasive germ cell neoplasia*
	GCNIS
	Specific form of intratubular GCN
Tumors of single histologic type	Gonadoblastoma[a]
	Germinoma family of tumors[a]
	Seminoma
Non-seminomatous germ cell tumors of >1 histologic type	Seminoma with syncytiotrophoblasts
	Non-seminomatous germ cell tumors
	Postpubertal-type teratoma
	Embryonic neuroectodermal tumor[a]
	Mixed germ cell tumors of testis
Germ cell tumors of unknown type	Mixed germ cell tumors
	Polyembryoma

(continued)

P. Ayyanar · S. Purkait (✉)
Department of Pathology and Lab Medicine, AIIMS, Bhubaneswar, India
e-mail: pathol_suvendu@aiimsbhubaneswar.edu.in

P. Singh et al. (eds.), *A Guide to Management of Urological Cancers*,
https://doi.org/10.1007/978-981-99-2341-0_24

Table 24.1 (continued)

2016 WHO classification	2022 WHO classification
Germ cell tumors unrelated to GCNIS	Diffuse embryoma
	Germ cell tumors of unknown type
	Germ cell tumors unrelated to GCNIS
	Prepubertal-type teratoma
	Prepubertal-type testicular neuroendocrine tumor[a]
Sex cord-stromal tumors	**Sex cord-stromal tumors**
Pure tumors	Leydig cell tumor
Mixed and unclassified sex cord-stromal tumors	Sertoli cell tumors
Emerging entity—myoid gonadal stromal tumor	Granulosa cell tumors
	Fibroma thecoma family of tumors
	Mixed and unclassified sex cord-stromal tumors
	Signet ring stromal tumor[a]
	Myoid gonadal stromal tumor[a]
Tumors containing both germ cell and sex cord-stromal elements	–
Miscellaneous tumors of the testis	**Miscellaneous tumors of the testis**
Ovarian epithelial-type tumors	*Ovarian epithelial type tumors*
Juvenile xanthogranuloma	*Juvenile xanthogranuloma*
Hemangioma	*Hemangioma*
Hematolymphoid tumors	**Hematolymphoid tumors**
Tumors of the collecting duct and rete testis	**Tumors of the collecting duct and rete testis**
Tumors of paratesticular structures	**Tumors of paratesticular structures**
Adenomatoid tumor	Adenomatoid tumor
Mesothelioma	Mesothelioma
Well-differentiated papillary mesothelioma	Well-differentiated papillary mesothelial tumor[a]
Mesenchymal tumors of the spermatic cord and testicular adnexa	**Mesenchymal tumors of the spermatic cord and testicular adnexa**
Metastatic tumors	**Metastatic tumors**

GCNIS germ cell neoplasia in situ
[a] Changes in WHO 2022 classification

24.2 Germ cell tumors

The germ cell tumors are classified into two broad categories, based on their association with GCNIS including (i) germ cell tumors derived from GCNIS and (ii) germ cell tumors unrelated to GCNIS (Fig. 24.1). These subcategories also had distinct molecular backgrounds [3–6].

24.2.1 Germ Cell Tumors Derived from Germ Cell Neoplasia In Situ

24.2.1.1 Noninvasive Germ Cell Neoplasia

Germ Cell Neoplasia In Situ (GCNIS)

Germ cell neoplasia in situ (GCNIS) is considered a precursor lesion of invasive germ cell tumors like seminoma and other non-seminomatous tumors. It is commonly associated with testicular dysgenesis, poorly developed tubules, undifferentiated Sertoli cells, and intratubular microliths than in the normal testis.

Histopathology: There is variable involvement of the seminiferous tubules from occasional tubules with basally located atypical germ cells to complete involvement toward the luminal aspect (Fig. 24.2a, b). The neoplastic cells are usually located along the spermatogonial niche, close to the basement membrane. They have abundant clear cytoplasm, coarse chromatin, and prominent nucleoli (Fig. 24.2c, d). The Sertoli cells are relatively preserved at the abluminal side. The tumor cells can spread in a pagetoid manner and may occupy the entire seminiferous tubule.

Immunohistochemistry: The neoplastic cells express markers such as OCT3/OCT 4, NANONG, placental alkaline phosphatase (PLAP), LIN28, etc. [4–6]. These markers help to differentiate GCNIS from the maturation arrest of the gonadal cells.

Specific Forms of Intratubular Germ Cell Neoplasia

These include intratubular seminoma and intratubular non-seminoma. It is often originated from

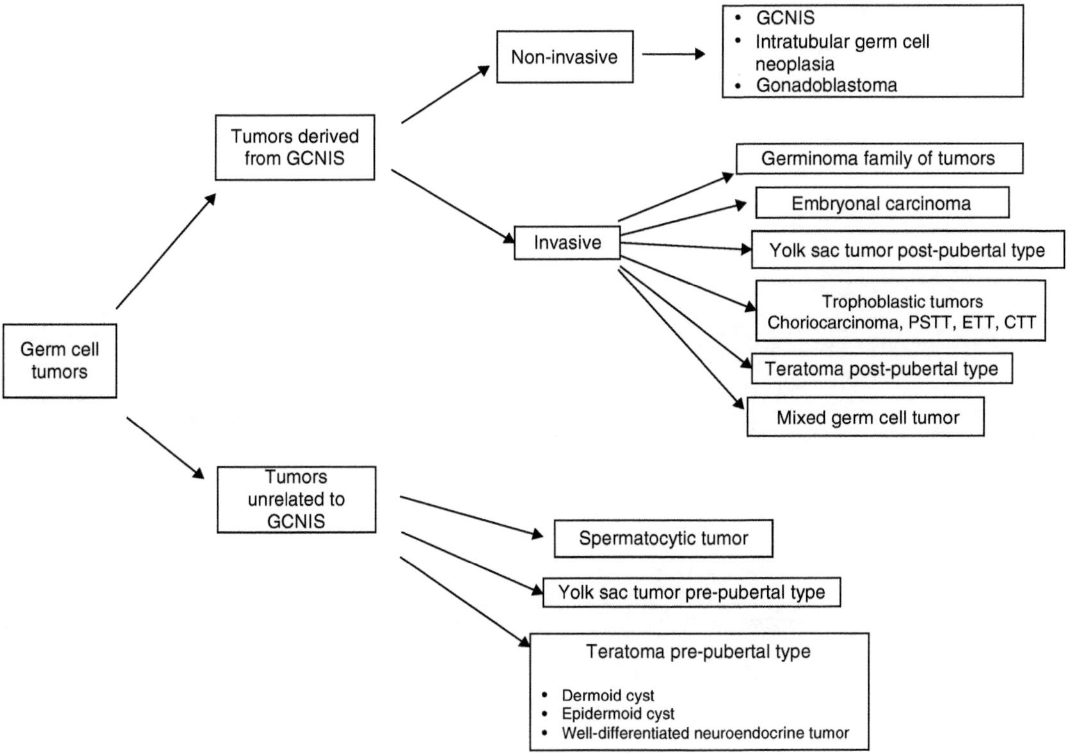

Fig. 24.1 The classification of germ cell tumors with their sub-categories

the progression of GCNIS and characterized by the complete replacement of seminiferous tubules by the neoplastic germ cells. It can show associated GCNIS and invasive malignancy foci in the surrounding part of the tumor [7].

Intratubular Seminoma

The morphology of the neoplastic cells is similar to the GCNIS and seminoma. The entire seminiferous tubule shows neoplastic germ cells. The other normal cell component such as Sertoli cells is usually absent. Immunophenotype and molecular alterations are similar to the GCNIS and seminoma.

Intratubular Non-seminoma

This category of tumors is intratubular embryonal carcinoma, intratubular trophoblast, intratubular yolk sac tumor, and intratubular teratoma. Each subtype of these tumors will have similar histomorphology and immunophenotypic features of their pure invasive malignancy counterpart as they acquire features of differentiation.

Gonadoblastoma

The 2022 WHO classification has added gonadoblastoma under noninvasive germ cell neoplasia for the first time. It was previously considered a tumor of both germ cell and sex cord-stromal tumor till the 2016 WHO classification. Most of these tumors show associated germinoma less commonly embryonal carcinoma and yolk sac tumor [8].

Histopathology: There is a biphasic cell population comprising germ cells and sex cord cells. The germ cell component usually mimics GCNIS, although heterogenous morphologic patterns ranging from cord, nests, solid/diffuse lobules to expansile patterns, etc. have been documented. The proportion of sex cord components is often similar to the immature granulosa cells, which are often highlighted by immunomarkers [9].

Immunohistochemistry: The germ cell component expresses markers similar to the GCNIS. The sex cord component is immunoreactive for α-inhibin and calretinin.

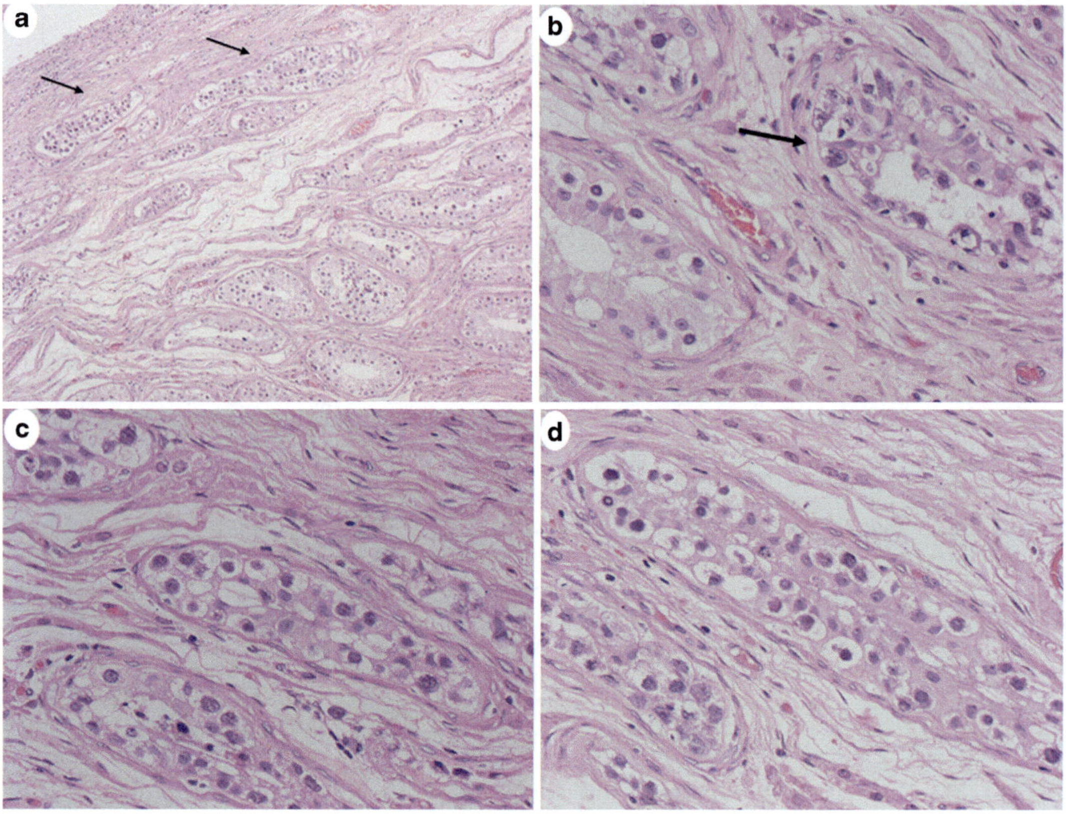

Fig. 24.2 (**a**) Germ cell neoplasia in situ (GCNIS) involving few seminiferous tubule basal aspect (black arrows) (H&E, 40X); (**b**) these atypical germ cells show clear cytoplasm, large round nucleus with coarse chromatin, and prominent nucleoli (arrow) (H&E, 400X); (**c, d**) GCNIS occupying the entire surface of the seminiferous tubules (H&E, 400X)

24.2.1.2 Germinoma Family of Tumors

It is the most common germ cell tumor in the adult age group. The WHO 2022 classification has changed the terminology of seminoma into the germinoma family of tumors, for the uniformity of tumors of a similar entity in our body [7]. It is a malignant tumor of primordial germ cell origin and develops from its precursor lesions, that is, GCNIS and intratubular seminoma.

Gross pathology: Grossly the specimen shows a solid lobulated gray-white homogenous mass with a bulging cut surface from the adjacent normal parenchyma. There may be few foci of hemorrhage and necrosis.

Microscopy: On microscopy, the tumor cells are arranged in a diffuse pattern with intervening thin fibrovascular septae, which show lymphocytic infiltration (Fig. 24.3a–c). Neoplastic cells are polygonal and have round nuclei with finely granular chromatin and prominent nucleoli. The cytoplasm is usually abundant and clear due to the presence of glycogen (Fig. 24.3c, d). A substantial proportion of cases show a granulomatous reaction in the surrounding stroma.

Immunohistochemistry: The tumor cells are positive for spalt-like, sal-like (SALL4), PLAP, c-KIT (CD117), OCT3/OCT4, and SOX 17. The expression of Pan-CK is variable. The immunostaining for CD30, EMA, and AFP is always negative [2, 8].

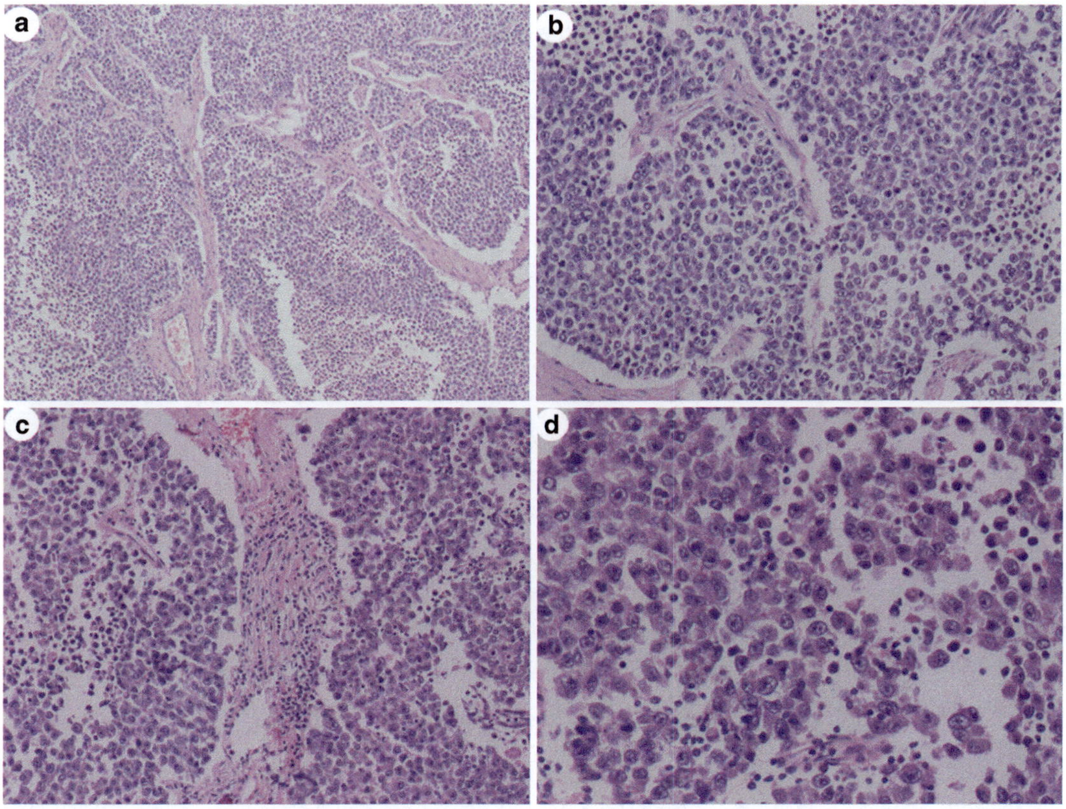

Fig. 24.3 (**a**) Sheets and lobules of tumor cell separated by fibrous septae (H&E, 20X); (**b**) sheets of monomorphic large tumor cells (H&E, 200X); (**c**) the fibrous septae shows lymphocytic infiltration (H&E, 200X); (**d**) large tumor cells with a moderate amount of eosinophilic cytoplasm, vesicular nuclear chromatin, and prominent nucleolus (H&E, 400X)

24.2.1.3 Non-seminomatous Germ Cell Tumors

Embryonal Carcinoma

It is the second most common germ cell tumor after the seminoma occurs in young adults. It has aggressive behavior with common lymphovascular invasion into the regional lymph node and other organs, commonly the liver and lung.

Gross pathology: Macroscopically, the tumor is solid with a variegated cut surface containing a variable degree of necrosis, hemorrhage, and cystic changes.

Microscopy: Several growth patterns have been documented, with the most common being solid, tubular, and papillary. Other patterns include nested, micropapillary, and blastocyst-like patterns (Fig. 24.4a, b). The neoplastic cells are large with eosinophilic cytoplasm. The nuclei are markedly pleomorphic with vesicular chromatin and multiple prominent nucleoli (Fig. 24.4c). Brisk mitosis, marked areas of necrosis, and hemorrhage are common (Fig. 24.4a).

Immunohistochemistry: The tumor cells are positive for CD30 (Fig. 24.4d), OCT3/OCT4, SOX2, and PanCK while negative for SOX17, c-KIT, EMA, glypican 3, and podoplanin [10].

Yolk Sac Tumor: Postpubertal Type

The tumor resembles the yolk sac or vitelline structures. It mostly presents as one of the main components of mixed germ cell tumors. Pure yolk sac tumor is uncommon.

Gross pathology: The gross examination of the tumor shows a solid cystic mass with focal

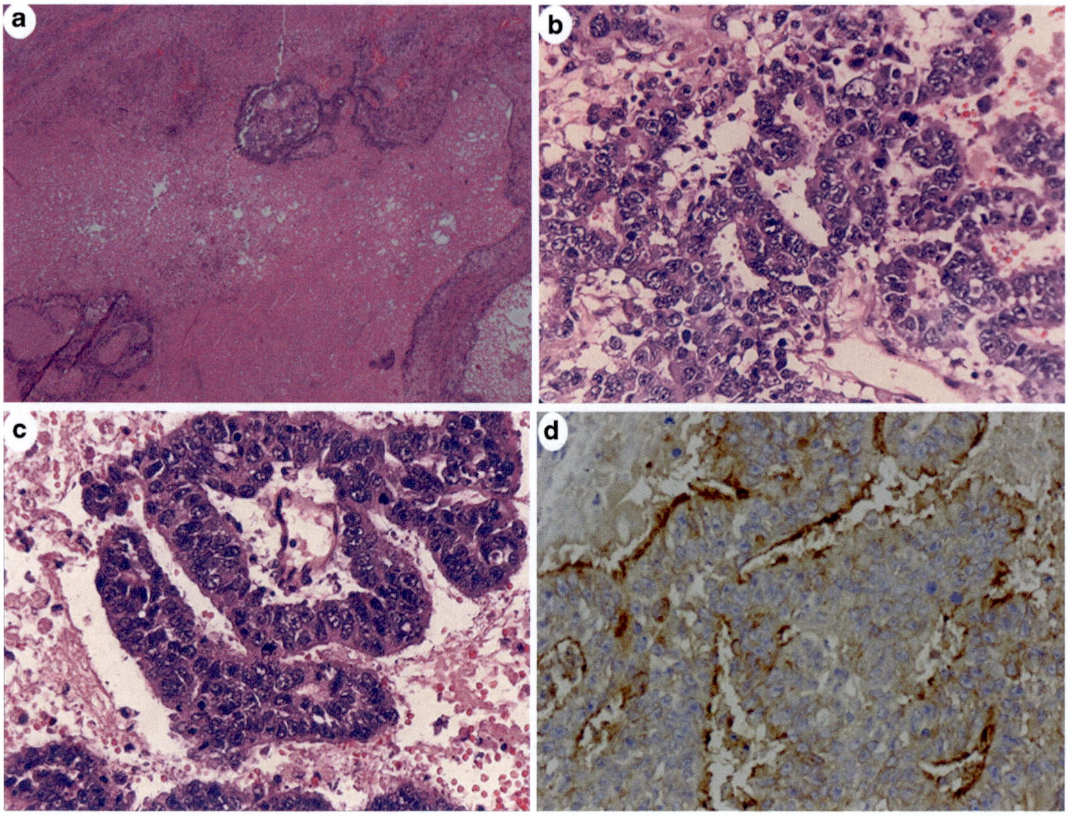

Fig. 24.4 (**a**) Extensive necrosis with few foci of tumor cells (H&E, 20X); (**b, c**) tumor cells arranged in a papillary and glandular pattern and papillae lined by many layers of large pleomorphic tumor cells with prominent nucleoli (H&E, 400X); (**d**) tumor cells show CD30 positivity (IHC, 400X)

areas of myxoid change, hemorrhage, and necrosis.

Microscopy: Similar to embryonal carcinoma, a number of histological patterns exist, including micro- or macrocytic, solid, glandular, endodermal sinus, hepatoid, papillary (Fig. 24.5a), sarcomatoid, polyvesicular vitelline, etc. [10]. Intracellular and extracellular hyaline globules (Fig. 24.5b) and basement membrane material deposits are one of the prominent features. Some of the tumors show a characteristic perivascular, glomerulus-like organization of tumor cells, also known as the Schiller-Duval body.

Immunohistochemistry: The tumor cells are positive for AFP, glypican 3, and c-KIT while negative for OCT3/OCT4 and CD30. Recently hepatocyte nuclear factor 1-beta (HNF-1β) is reported as a sensitive and specific marker for yolk sac tumors [11].

Trophoblastic Tumors

This tumor group shows trophoblastic differentiation, cytotrophoblasts, syncytiotrophoblasts, and intermediate trophoblasts. The tumor types included are choriocarcinoma, placental site trophoblastic tumor (PSTT), epithelioid trophoblastic tumor (ETT), and cystic trophoblastic tumor (CTT). The last three tumor types are often clubbed together as non-choriocarcinomatous trophoblastic tumors.

Choriocarcinoma

It is a rare, aggressive germ cell tumor that usually presents as a metastatic disease involving the liver and lung. This tumor is seen as a component of mixed germ cell tumors.

Gross pathology: The tumor is friable with marked areas of hemorrhage and congestion in the central area with focal gray-white solid areas.

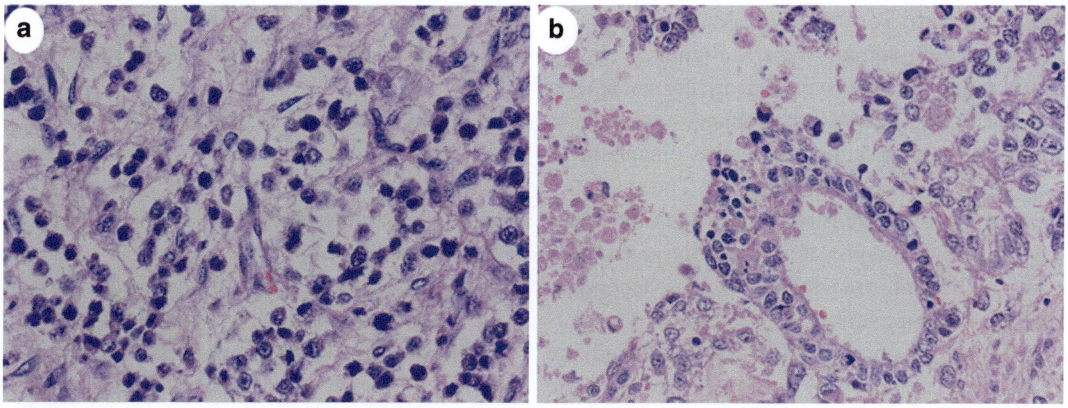

Fig. 24.5 (**a**) Tumor cells arranged in microcystic pattern and sheets (H&E, 400X); (**b**) tumor cells in papillary pattern and the presence of eosinophilic globular material predominantly in the extracellular areas and occasional cells with intracytoplasmic hyaline globules (H&E, 400X)

Microscopy: The tumor cell population comprises mono-nucleated cytotrophoblasts and intermediate-type trophoblasts, which are admixed with a variable proportion of multinucleated syncytiotrophoblastic cells. Prominent central necrosis, hemorrhage, and lymphovascular invasion are often present.

Immunohistochemistry: The tumor cells are positive β-hCG. Depending upon the composition of various trophoblastic cells, positivity for human placental lactogen, p63, and GATA3 is also noted [2, 12].

Placental Site Trophoblastic Tumor, Epithelioid Trophoblastic Tumor, and Cystic Trophoblastic Tumor (Non-choriocarcinomatous Trophoblastic Tumors)

These tumors are extremely rare in the testis; hence, they are not discussed in detail. Morphologically, trophoblastic differentiation with some tumor-specific histological features include infiltrating single cells in PSTT, nest- and cord-like arrangement in ETT, and cystic change in CTT. The immunohistochemical profile depends upon the proportion of the trophoblastic cells [12, 13].

Teratoma Postpubertal Type

These tumors are considered to arise as a result of transdifferentiation of GCNIS or seminoma. They show tumor differentiation into more than one germ cell layer. The postpubertal-type teratoma mostly presents a component of mixed germ cell tumor.

Gross pathology: Gross appearance depends upon the tumor components. The cut surface is usually a solid cystic mass with the bone, cartilage, and mucinous or pultaceous material depending upon the present different germ cell layers.

Microscopy: It contains derivatives of one or more germ cell derivatives with variable proportions, including the skin, bronchial epithelium, components of the gastrointestinal tract, urogenital tract, neuroepithelial/glial tissue, bone, cartilage, adipose tissue, etc. Cellular atypia is relatively common. Immature components of mesenchymal and neuroectodermal structures can be identified.

Immunohistochemistry: It is of limited value except in cases of mixed germ cell tumors [14].

Teratoma with Somatic-Type Malignancy

Teratoma with somatic-type malignancy can be either carcinoma or sarcoma arising in a teratoma. The presence of a malignant component in at least more than 5 mm diameter is diagnostic as per the 2022 WHO classification. The measurement of the field size is recommended rather than a 4× objective low-power field. The term somatic-type malignant transformation or secondary malignant component is not preferred.

The most common sarcomas identified are rhabdomyosarcoma and leiomyosarcoma, while most carcinomas are adenocarcinoma. Further, there is a change in nomenclature from "testicular carcinoid" to "testicular neuroendocrine tumor" and "primitive neuroectodermal tumor" to "embryonic-type neuroectodermal tumor" [2, 15, 16].

24.2.1.4 Mixed Germ Cell Tumors of the Testis

These tumors contain more than one germ cell tumor component. Even if seminoma is present as one of the components in a mixed germ cell tumor, the tumor is considered non-seminomatous.

Grossly the tumor usually has a variegated appearance. The histological features and immunohistochemical features correspond to the specific tumor subtypes [2, 8] (Fig. 24.6a–f; case of mixed germ cell tumor containing seminoma, embryonal carcinoma, and mature and immature teratoma components).

24.2.1.5 Germ Cell Tumors of Unknown Type: Regressed Germ Cell Tumors

These are the germ cell tumors which are undergone spontaneous regression and are replaced by fibrotic nodules. The clinical presentation of this entity is metastatic disease. Microscopic features are fibrosis, calcification, chronic inflammation, and infarcted tubules [8].

24.2.2 Germ Cell Tumors Unrelated to Germ Cell Neoplasia In Situ

24.2.2.1 Spermatocytic Tumor

It is a rare testicular tumor. There is no associated GCNIS lesion or disorders of the testis and arises from the postpubertal type of germ cells.

Gross pathology: The tumor has a lobular appearance with a fleshy to the myxoid cut surface. Foci of hemorrhage may be seen.

Microscopy: There is a nodular to diffuse pattern of arrangement of tumor cells with three types of cells, including small lymphocyte-like cells, medium-sized cells with filamentous chromatin, and large giant tumor cells. Unlike seminoma, this tumor rarely shows lymphocytic infiltration or granulomatous inflammation.

Immunohistochemistry: Immunostaining for OCT3/OCT4, PLAP, CD30, AFP, and beta-HCG is negative. Staining for SALL-4, c-KIT, MAGEA4, and OCT-2 is usually positive [17].

24.2.2.2 Teratoma: Prepubertal Type

This tumor lacks association with GCNIS. Components from one or more germ cell layers may be seen. In contrast to its postpubertal counterpart, this tumor shows more organoid architecture and lesser cytological atypia. The benign testicular teratomas like dermoid and epidermoid cysts are largely included in this group [2, 8].

24.2.2.3 Other Prepubertal-Type Tumors: Yolk Sac Tumor, Prepubertal Type; and Mixed Teratoma and Yolk Sac Tumor, Prepubertal Type: and Testicular Neuroendocrine Tumor, Prepubertal Type

These tumors lack GCNIS, otherwise morphologically similar to the postpubertal type.

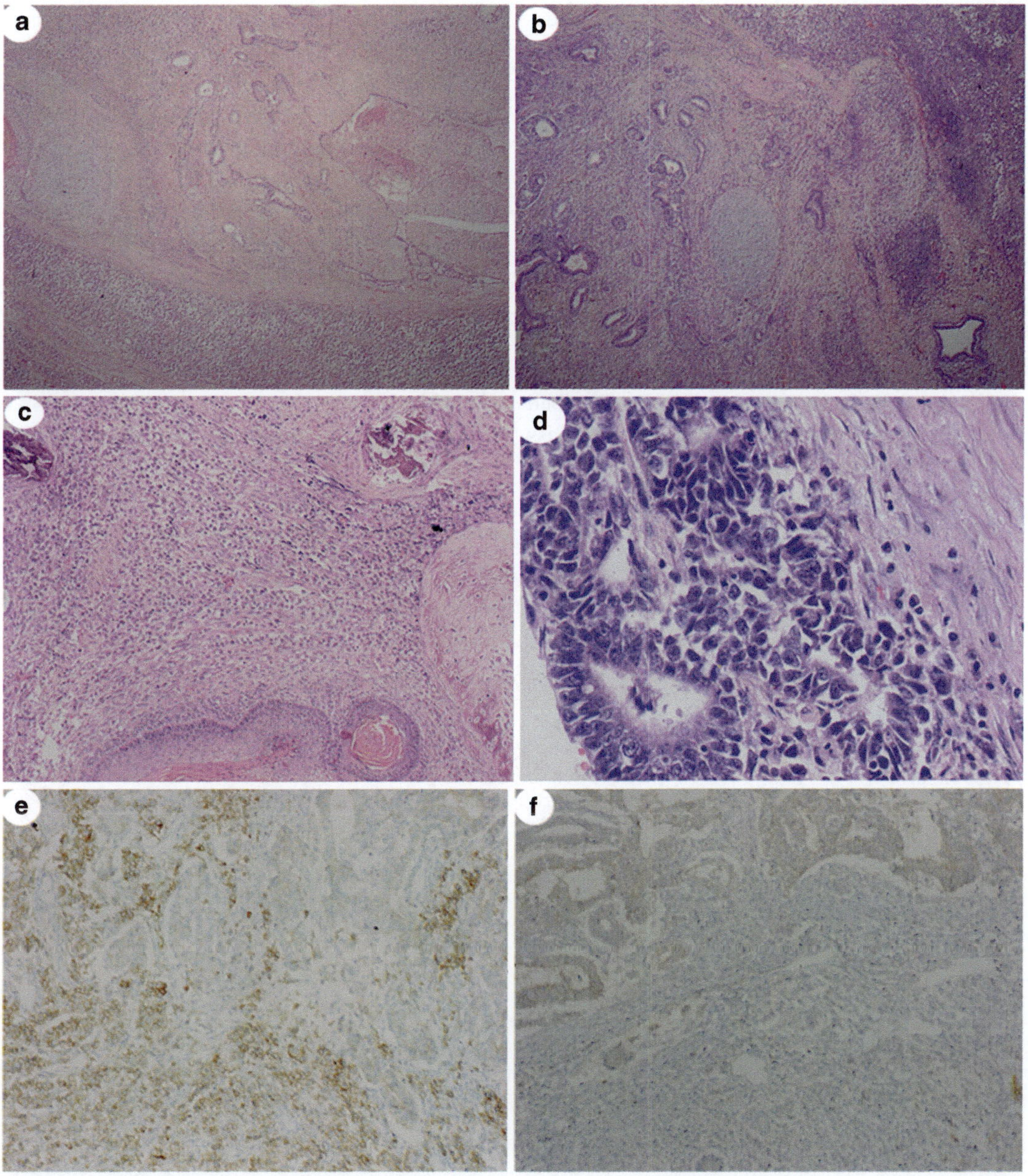

Fig. 24.6 (**a, b**) Mixed germ cell tumor composed of seminoma and mature teratoma components, hyaline cartilage, and stratified squamous epithelium with keratin (H&E, 40X and 100X); (**c**) seminoma tumor cells with hyaline cartilage and ossification (H&E, 100X); (**d**) immature component—primitive neuroepithelial cells (H&E, 400X); (**e**) seminoma cells show CD117 positivity (IHC, 100X); (**f**) embryonal carcinoma cells show CD30 positivity (weak and membranous)

24.3 Sex Cord-Stromal Tumors

Sex cord-stromal tumors account for 4% of testicular tumors and are common in pediatric age groups. It includes tumors arising from Leydig cells, Sertoli cells, granulosa cells, theca cells, and fibroblasts. It can be a pure type or mixed type of sex cord-stromal component. Most of the tumors are nonfunctional and benign. The classification of sex cord-stromal tumors is depicted in Table 24.1.

24.3.1 Leydig Cell Tumors

These are the most common sex cord-stromal tumors and are characterized by the tumor morphology resemblance to normal Leydig cells of the testis.

Gross pathology: The macroscopic features are predominantly unilateral well-circumscribed solid homogenous yellow to gray-brown mass with a soft consistency. Focal areas of hemorrhage and necrosis can be seen.

Microscopy: The tumor cells are arranged in nodules, nests, and sheets containing monomorphic cells separated by collagenous tissue (Fig. 24.7a, b). The other uncommon patterns are trabecular, ribbon-like, sarcomatoid, and microcystic. The individual tumor cells have abundant eosinophilic cytoplasm, which may contain Reinke crystals and lipofuscin pigment and centrally placed round nucleus, and prominent nucleoli and has no atypia (Fig. 24.7b) [18]. The criteria for malignancy (≥2 features required) are size >50 mm, infiltrative borders, cytological atypia, mitotic figures ≥3/10 high-power fields, vascular involvement, and necrosis [19].

Immunohistochemistry: The tumor cells are positive for inhibin (Fig. 24.7c), calretinin (Fig. 24.7d), SF1, melan A, and CD99 and negative for beta-catenin (nuclear stain).

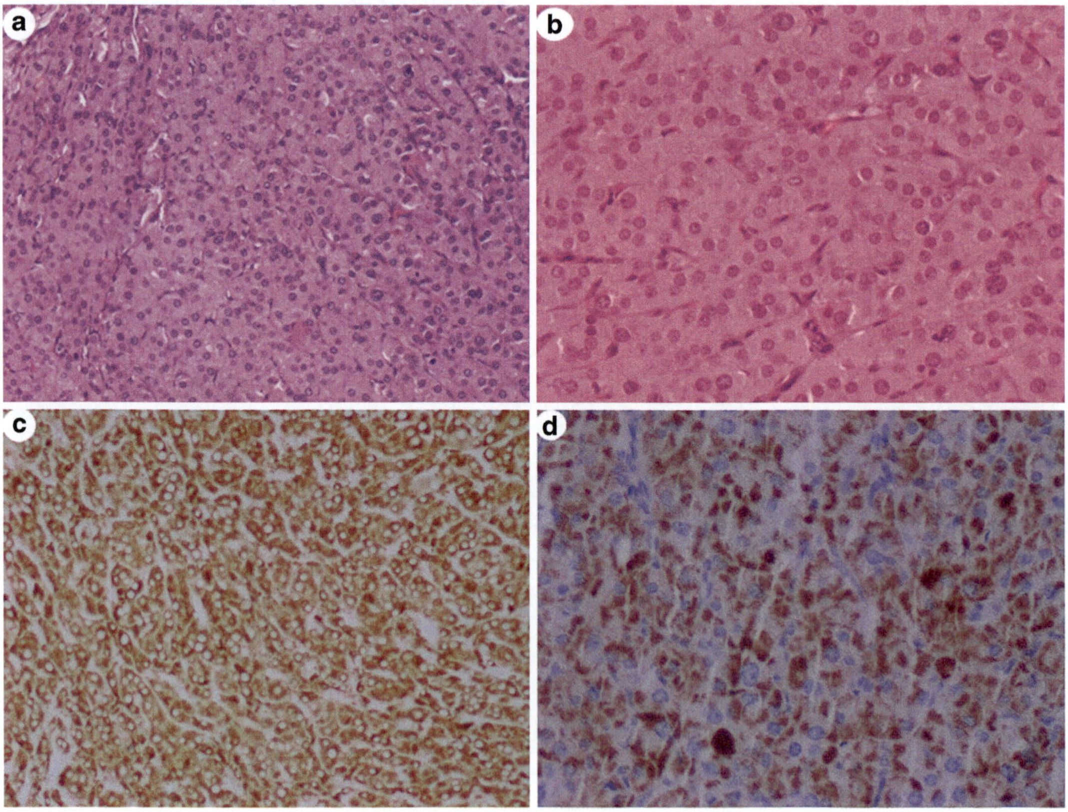

Fig. 24.7 (**a**) Nests and cords of tumor cells (H&E, 100X); (**b**) tumor cells are monomorphic and contain abundant eosinophilic cytoplasm, centrally placed round nucleus, and fine chromatin and inconspicuous nucleolus (H&E, 200X); (**c**) these cells are diffuse and strongly immunopositive for inhibin (IHC, 200X); (**d**) tumor cells are positive for calretinin (IHC, 200X)

24.3.2 Sertoli Cell Tumors

Sertoli cell tumors commonly occur in adult age groups. The molecular abnormality includes mutation involving the CTNNB1 gene [20].

Gross pathology: The gross features are similar to the Leydig cell tumor except that this tumor will show soft to a firm consistency.

Microscopy: The microscopic features include nodular, tubular, cords, nests, or diffuse growth patterns with less collagenous stroma. Tumor cells have moderate eosinophilic cytoplasm and may show abundant, lipid-rich vacuolated appearance without cytological atypia. The features of malignancy are similar to those mentioned in the Leydig cell tumor [21].

Immunohistochemistry: On IHC, the tumor cells are positive for inhibin, calretinin, SF1, WT1, melan A, CD99, and beta-catenin (nuclear staining).

24.3.2.1 Large Cell Calcifying Sertoli Cell Tumor

It is characterized by Sertoli cells with marked areas of calcification. It occurs as a bilateral multifocal tumor in the case of the Carney complex [22]. Tumor cells are positive for inhibin, S 100, and SF1 and negative for beta-catenin (nuclear staining). The genetic mutation involves the PRKAR1A gene [23].

24.3.2.2 Intratubular Large Cell Hyalinizing Sertoli Cell Neoplasms

They are characterized by intratubular proliferation of Sertoli cells with basement membrane deposits. It is commonly associated with Peutz-Jeghers syndrome with STK11 gene mutation [24].

24.3.3 Granulosa Cell Tumors

This category of tumors includes adult and juvenile types with similar morphology to that seen in their ovarian counterparts. Adult-type granulosa cell tumors account for <5% of all testicular tumors [25].

Gross pathology: Grossly it is a well-circumscribed solid lobulated mass.

Microscopy: The histopathological features are nodules, diffuse, microfollicle, trabeculae, cords, nest (Fig. 24.8a, b), and rarely sarcomatoid pattern of tumor cells with a characteristic small oval nucleus with grooving, inconspicuous nucleoli (Fig. 24.8c). Juvenile-type granulosa cell tumors will show a solid and macrofollicular pattern, conspicuous nucleoli, and presence of mitotic figures without any nuclear groove [26, 27].

Immunohistochemistry: The tumor cells are positive for inhibin (Fig. 24.8d), FOXL2, calretinin, melan A, and CD99 and negative for beta-catenin (nuclear stain) and EMA [25].

24.3.4 Tumors in the Fibroma Thecoma Group

These are very rare and benign tumors that are derived from gonadal stroma or tunica albuginea.

Gross pathology: The gross features are solid, white, and firm mass.

Microscopy: It shows a fascicular and storiform pattern (Fig. 24.9a) of spindle cells without nuclear atypia (Fig. 24.9b).

Immunohistochemistry: IHC shows positive for inhibin, calretinin, melan A, PanCK, S100, Desmin, CD34, and BCL2 [1, 28].

24.3.5 Mixed and Unclassified Sex Cord-Stromal Tumors

These tumors show more than two types of sex cord-stromal elements and unclassified indicated the lack of differentiation of tumor cells [1].

24.3.6 Myoid Gonadal Stromal Tumor

This was an emerging entity in the 2016 WHO classification. 2022 WHO classification includes this new entity in the sex cord-stromal tumors. The clin-

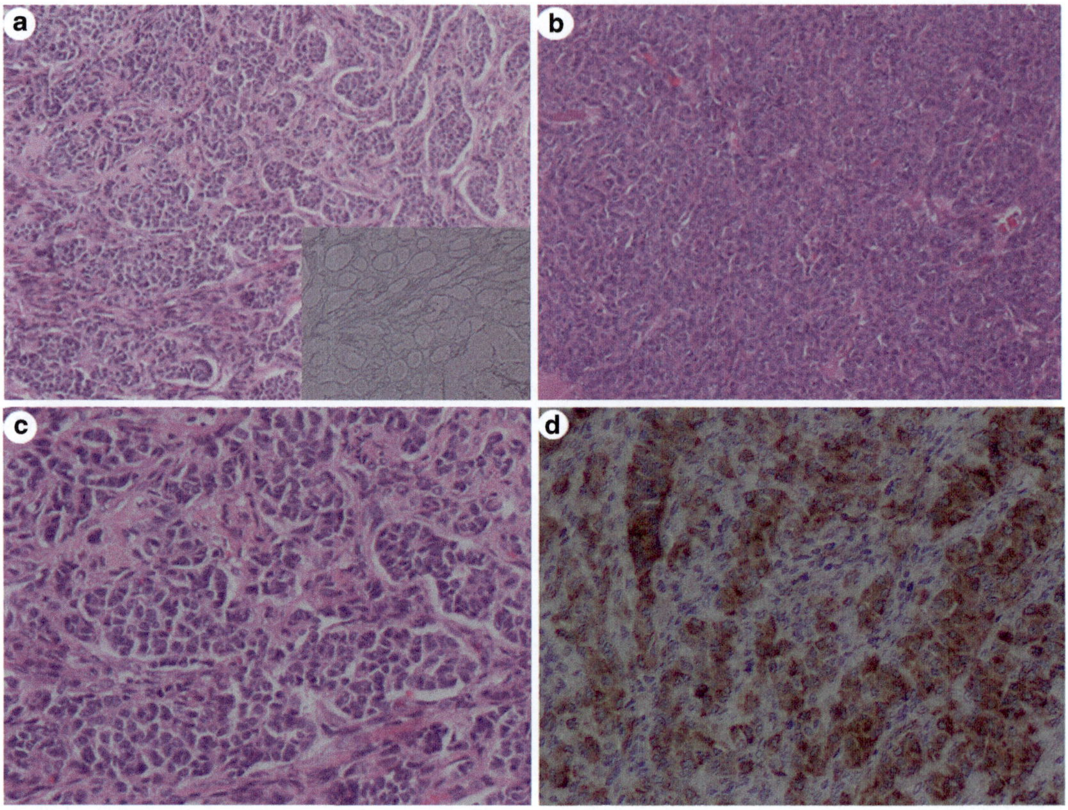

Fig. 24.8 (**a**) Nests and cords of tumor cells (H&E, 100X). Inset—Reticulin stain highlights the reticulin-rich areas around these nests (Reticulin, 100x); (**b**) diffuse pattern of tumor cells (H&E, 100X); (**c**) these tumor cells are monomorphic with an oval nucleus and nuclear grooves and inconspicuous nucleolus ((H&E, 200X); (**d**) tumor cells are positive for inhibin (IHC, 200X)

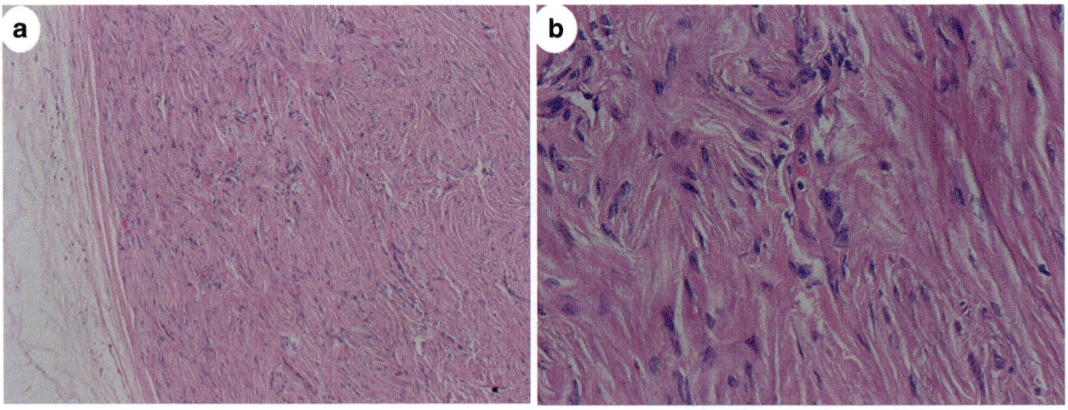

Fig. 24.9 (**a**) Encapsulated storiform pattern of spindle cells (H&E, 100X); (**b**) these spindle cells have oval to elongated nucleus with fine nuclear chromatin and inconspicuous nucleoli and embedded in the collagenous stroma (H&E, 400X)

ical and morphologic features may overlap with fibroma thecoma group tumors or leiomyoma.

Gross pathology: The gross features are similar to the fibroma group of tumors.

Microscopy: The microscopic features include a nodular and short fascicular pattern of spindle cells in a collagenous stroma. The individual tumor cell shows moderate eosinophilic cytoplasm, a fusiform nucleus with tapered ends, and can show mitotic figures.

Immunohistochemistry: These cells are positive for SF-1, SMA, smooth muscle myosin, S100, and FOXL2 and focal weak positive for inhibin [2, 29].

24.3.7 Signet-Ring Stromal Tumor

These are benign tumors similar to their ovarian counterpart. This entity is also added new in the sex cord-stromal tumors in WHO 2022 classification. It can show mutations involving the CTNNB1 gene [30].

Histopathology: Microscopically they show solid nodules separated by fibrous tissue and edematous stroma. The tumor shows cytoplasmic vacuoles and eccentrically placed nuclei.

Immunohistochemistry: The tumor cells are immunopositive for vimentin, β-catenin (nuclear positivity), cyclin D1, synaptophysin, NSE, CD10, and S100, while negative for inhibin, calretinin, desmin, and melan A.

24.4 Miscellaneous Tumors of the Testis

This group includes ovarian surface epithelial-type tumors, juvenile xanthogranuloma, and hemangioma. These tumors are rare.

24.4.1 Ovarian Surface Epithelial-Type Tumors

This category of tumors accounts for <1% of testicular tumors and is the same entity as its ovarian counterparts. It includes serous, mucinous, endometrioid, clear cell, and Brenner cell morphology of benign, borderline, and malignant tumors. Among these benign serous followed by mucinous types are the common tumors [31].

24.4.2 Juvenile Xanthogranuloma

This tumor is common in the infant age group. Histomorphology shows sheets of foamy macrophages admixed with Touton-type giant cells.

24.4.3 Hemangioma

The benign vascular tumor can be cavernous, capillary, and epithelioid morphology.

24.5 Hematolymphoid Tumors

Primary non-Hodgkin lymphoma accounts for 9% of testicular neoplasms. Diffuse large B cell lymphoma (DLBCL) is the common type. The other tumors include T and B-lymphoblastic lymphoma, Burkitt lymphoma, extranodal NK/T cell lymphoma, follicular lymphoma, plasmacytoma, and myeloid sarcoma [32]. The clinical features including age, other lymph nodal and bone marrow involvements, peripheral blood smear findings, and histomorphology of small, intermediate, and large atypical lymphoid cells with the immunohistochemistry will help to arrive at a correct diagnosis.

24.6 Tumors of Collecting the Duct and Rete Testis

These include adenoma and adenocarcinoma of the rete testis. These tumors are rare in occurrence. Microscopic features are glandular, tubular, and papillary patterns with minimal cytological atypia in benign tumors. Adenocarcinoma features are complex tubulocystic and spindle cell morphology with infiltrative border, desmoplasia, necrosis, and cytological atypia.

24.7 Tumors of Paratesticular Structures

Tumors under this category include tumors of paratesticular mesothelial origin (adenomatoid tumor and mesothelioma), epididymis (papillary cystadenoma, adenocarcinoma, squamous cell carcinoma, melanotic neuroectodermal tumors), and others (nephroblastoma and paraganglioma).

24.7.1 Adenomatoid Tumors

This is a benign tumor of mesothelial cells commonly seen in adults. Histopathological features are glandular and interconnected vascular-like patterns of tumor cells having scant cytoplasm in a fibrocollagenous stroma. Tumor cells are positive for PanCK, WT1, and calretinin and negative for CK5/CK6, BerEP4, and CD31.

24.7.2 Mesothelioma

These are the malignant mesothelial tumors arising from the tunica vaginalis. It includes mesothelioma (epithelioid, sarcomatoid, and biphasic type) and well-differentiated papillary mesothelial tumor. The term well-differentiated papillary mesothelioma is not recommended as per the recent WHO classification [24].

The histological features are similar to other serous body cavity mesotheliomas.

Tumor cells show positivity for calretinin, EMA, CK5/CK6, and p53 and are negative for CEA.

24.8 Mesenchymal Tumors of the Spermatic Cord and Testicular Adnexa

These are the tumors of the adipocytic, smooth muscle, skeletal muscle, fibroblastic and myofibroblastic, nerve sheath, origin, and others (desmoplastic small round cell tumor).

24.9 Metastatic Tumors

These are the secondary tumors that involve the testicular parenchyma. The most common primary tumors are the prostate, kidney, gastrointestinal tract, and lung. The detailed clinical history and histomorphology along with immunohistochemistry for the primary origin of the tumor will help to diagnose these tumors.

24.10 Staging of Testicular Tumors

The American Joint Committee on Cancer (AJCC), eighth edition, is being followed now for the pathological staging (pTNM) of testicular tumors and has been discussed in previous chapter [33].

24.10.1 Pathological T-Stage

The parameters which are important for pathological staging include tumor size, extension through the tunica albuginea, rete testis invasion, hilar soft tissue invasion, spermatic cord invasion, epididymal invasion, and lymphovascular invasion. The T1 sub-staging for pure seminoma based on the tumor size is recommended [30] (Fig. 24.10).

24.10.2 Pathological N-Stage

This denotes the regional nodal involvement status. It is important to note that the size of the largest involved lymph node rather than the size of the metastatic deposit is considered for the staging. Obviously, the number of the involved lymph node is another important criterion.

24.10.3 M-Stage

Involvement of non-retroperitoneal lymph node, lung, or other visceral organs is included in the M1 sub-staging. The changes made in the pM staging are the discontinuous involvement of the spermatic cord by the lymphovascular invasion.

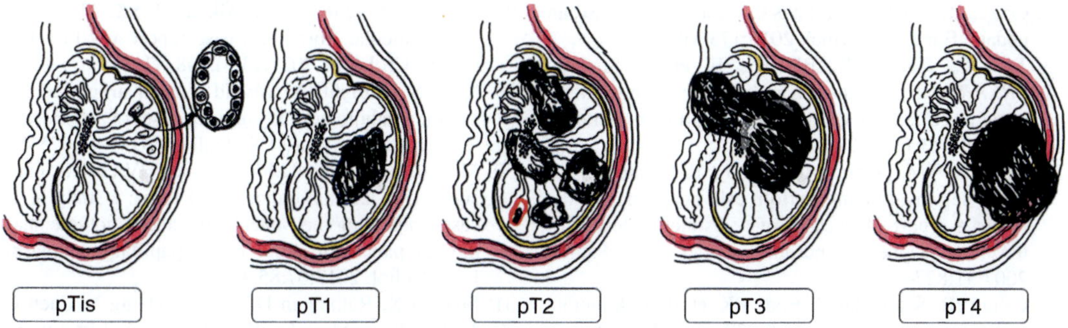

Fig. 24.10 Schematic diagram of the testicular tumor AJCC pathological T-staging

References

1. Moch H, Humphrey PA, Ulbright TM, Reuter V. WHO classification of Tumours of the urinary system and male genital organs. Lyon: International Agency for Research on Cancer; 2016.
2. WHO. Classification of tumors of the urinary system and male genital organs. 5th ed. Lyon: International Agency for Research on Cancer; 2022.
3. Mostert M, Rosenberg C, Stoop H, et al. Comparative genomic and in situ hybridization of germ cell tumors of the infantile testis. Lab Investig. 2000;80:1055–64.
4. Sheikine Y, Genega E, Melamed J, et al. Molecular genetics of testicular germ cell tumors. Am J Cancer Res. 2012;2:153–67.
5. Boublikova L, Buchler T, Stary J, et al. Molecular biology of testicular germ cell tumors: unique features awaiting clinical application. Crit Rev Oncol Hematol. 2014;89:366–85.
6. Looijenga LH, Gillis AJ, Stoop HJ, et al. Chromosomes and expression in human testicular germ-cell tumors: insight into their cell of origin and pathogenesis. Ann N Y Acad Sci. 2007;1120:187–214.
7. Berney DM, Stoneham S, Arora R, Shamash J, Lockley M. Ovarian germ cell tumor classification: views from the testis. Histopathology. 2020;76:25–36.
8. Al-Obaidy KI, Idrees MT. Testicular tumors: a contemporary update on morphologic, Immunohistochemical and molecular features. Adv Anat Pathol. 2021;28(4):258–75.
9. Kao CS, Idrees MT, Young RH, Ulbright TM. "Dissecting gonadoblastoma" of scully: a morphologic variant that often mimics germinoma. Am J Surg Pathol. 2016;40:1417–23.
10. Kao CS, Ulbright TM, Young RH, et al. Testicular embryonal carcinoma: a morphologic study of 180 cases highlighting unusual and unemphasized aspects. Am J Surg Pathol. 2014;38:689–97.
11. Gallo A, Fankhauser C, Hermanns T, et al. Hnf1beta is a sensitive and specific novel marker for yolk sac tumor: a tissue microarray analysis of 601 testicular germ cell tumors. Mod Pathol. 2020;33:2354–60.
12. Idrees MT, Kao CS, Epstein JI, Ulbright TM. Nonchoriocarcinomatous trophoblastic tumors of the testis: the widening spectrum of trophoblastic neoplasia. Am J Surg Pathol. 2015;39(11):1468–78.
13. Allan RW, Algood CB, Shih IM. Metastatic epithelioid trophoblastic tumor in a male patient with a mixed germ-cell tumor of the testis. Am J Surg Pathol. 2009;33(12):1902–5.
14. Zhang C, Berney DM, Hirsch MS, et al. Evidence supporting the existence of benign teratomas of the postpubertal testis: a clinical, histopathologic, and molecular genetic analysis of 25 cases. Am J Surg Pathol. 2013;37:827–35.
15. Ulbright TM, Hattab EM, Zhang S, et al. Primitive neuroectodermal tumors in patients with testicular germ cell tumors usually resemble pediatric-type central nervous system embryonal neoplasms and lack chromosome 22 rearrangements. Mod Pathol. 2010;23:972–80.
16. Looijenga LH, Stoop H, Biermann K. Testicular cancer: biology and biomarkers. Virchows Arch. 2014;464:301–13.
17. Hu R, Ulbright TM, Young RH. Spermatocytic seminoma: a report of 85 cases emphasizing its morphologic spectrum including some aspects not widely known. Am J Surg Pathol. 2019;43:1–11.
18. Ulbright TM, Srigley JR, Hatzianastassiou DK, et al. Leydig cell tumors of the testis with unusual features. Adipose differentiation, calcification with ossification, and spindle-shaped tumor cells. Am J Surg Pathol. 2002;26:1424–33.
19. Kim I, Young RH, Scully RE. Leydig cell tumors of the testis. A clinicopathological analysis of 40 cases and review of the literature. Am J Surg Pathol. 1985;9:177–19.
20. Kao CS, Kum JB, Idrees MT, et al. Sclerosing sertoli cell tumor of the testis: a clinicopathologic study of 20 cases. Am J Surg Pathol. 2014;38:510–7.
21. Young RH, Koelliker DD, Scully RE. Sertoli cell tumors of the testis, not otherwise specified: a clinicopathologic analysis of 60 cases. Am J Surg Pathol. 1998;22:709–21.

22. Correa R, Salpea P, Stratakis CA. Carney complex: an update. Eur J Endocrinol. 2015;173:M85–97.
23. Tatsi C, Faucz FR, Blavakis E, et al. Somatic *PRKAR1A* gene mutation in a nonsyndromic metastatic large cell calcifying sertoli cell tumor. J Endocr Soc. 2019;3:1375–82.
24. Ulbright TM, Amin MB, Young RH. Intratubular large cell hyalinizing sertoli cell neoplasia of the testis: a report of 8 cases of a distinctive lesion of the Peutz-Jeghers syndrome. Am J Surg Pathol. 2007;31:827–35.
25. Grogg JB, Schneider K, Bode PK, et al. Risk factors and treatment outcomes of 239 patients with testicular granulosa cell tumors: a systematic review of published case series data. J Cancer Res Clin Oncol. 2020;146:2829–41.
26. Hes O, Vanecek T, Petersson F, et al. Mutational analysis (c.402c>g) of the foxl2 gene and immunohistochemical expression of the foxl2 protein in testicular adult type granulosa cell tumors and incompletely differentiated sex cord-stromal tumors. Appl Immunohistochem Mol Morphol. 2011;19:347–51.
27. Kao CS, Cornejo KM, Ulbright TM, et al. Juvenile granulosa cell tumors of the testis: a clinicopathologic study of 70 cases with emphasis on its wide morphologic spectrum. Am J Surg Pathol. 2015;39:1159–69.
28. Algarni AM, Junejo NN, Alkhateeb SS, Al-Hussain TO. Testicular fibroma: a case report and literature review. Urol Ann. 2021;13(3):308–11.
29. Kao CS, Ulbright TM. Myoid gonadal stromal tumor: a clinicopathologic study of three cases of a distinctive testicular tumor. Am J Clin Pathol. 2014;142:675–82.
30. Michalova K, Michal M Jr, Kazakov DV, et al. Primary signet ring stromal tumor of the testis: a study of 13 cases indicating their phenotypic and genotypic analogy to pancreatic solid pseudopapillary neoplasm. Hum Pathol. 2017;67:85–93.
31. Shadhu K, Ramlagun D, Zhu K, Zhang Y, Chen C, Xi D, Zhu J, Miao C, Wang Y, Qin C. Testis tumor of ovarian epithelial type: a rare case. Urology. 2018;115:e9–e10.
32. Gundrum JD, Mathiason MA, Moore DB, et al. Primary testicular diffuse large B-cell lymphoma: a population-based study on the incidence, natural history, and survival comparison with primary nodal counterpart before and after the introduction of rituximab. J Clin Oncol. 2009;27:5227–32.
33. Amin MB, Greene FL, Edge SB, et al. The eighth edition AJCC cancer staging manual: continuing to build a bridge from a population based to a more "personalized" approach to cancer staging. CA Cancer J Clin. 2017;67:93–9.

25 Management

Praful Pandey and Ranjit Kumar Sahoo

25.1 Introduction

As per the GLOBOCAN database, testicular germ cell tumors amounted to 74,458 cases (cumulative lifetime risk: 0.14) and 9334 deaths (cumulative lifetime risk: 0.02) globally in 2020. Cumulative lifetime risk of TGCT is higher in high-income countries, but the lifetime risk of dying from TGCT does not vary with the income status highlighting the higher proportional mortality in lower-middle income countries (LMIC) [1]. The rarity of testicular cancer is indicated by the fact that it occurs in less than <1 man/100,000 population. The reported incidence of testicular cancer in India is 0.5/100,000, much lower than the global incidence [2]. Increasing incidence in western countries [3] but gradual reduction in LMIC [4] showcases a similar disparity in temporal trends as well. The western rise of TGCT incidence is driven more by seminomas than NSGCTs (non-seminomatous germ cell tumors) [5]. The reason for this temporal shift is unknown, and in utero exposure to diethylstilbestrol, early exposure to viruses, environmental influences, and testicular trauma are postulated causes [6]. Although uncommon overall [7], it is the second most common malignancy (after thyroid cancer) in patients aged 20–29 years [8]. Peak incidence for non-seminoma and mixed GCT is in the third decade versus in the fourth decade for pure seminomas [9].

Patients in western countries typically have limited disease at presentation. As per one study, 79.1% seminomas and 47.6% NSGCT patients have stage 1 disease at presentation. Only 7% had metastasis at presentation, 80% with good prognosis as per International Germ Cell Cancer Collaborative Group (IGCCCG) [10]. Patients in the LMIC typically present with more advanced disease [11, 12], as shown by an Indian study reporting that 35% patients have metastasis at presentation (only 48% good risk as per IGCCCG) [11]. Approximately 2% patients have bilateral disease at presentation [10]. Analysis of histological subtypes showcases a similar dichotomy with Western literature reporting a preponderance of seminomas [10] (60%) as compared to LMIC literature reporting NSGCT as being more common [11, 12]. Amongst NSGCT cases, teratoma component is found in slightly less than half of all cases [10].

Independent from socioeconomic influences, race also impacts TGCT incidence and natural history. African-American men have a four times lesser age-matched incidence of TGCT. However, they typically present with more advanced stage reflecting differential health-seeking behavior [13].

P. Pandey · R. K. Sahoo (✉)
Department of Medical Oncology,
DR. B.R.A.I.R.C.H, All India Institute of Medical Sciences (AIIMS), New Delhi, India

P. Singh et al. (eds.), *A Guide to Management of Urological Cancers*,
https://doi.org/10.1007/978-981-99-2341-0_25

25.2 Risk Factors

There are a number of known risk factors for testicular neoplasia which predispose to the development of carcinoma in situ (CIS) and invasive testicular cancer:

1. Cryptorchidism—Increased risk of testicular cancer is well documented, and prophylactic orchiectomy is prudent, especially in cases of the intra-abdominal testis (as compared to inguinal cryptorchidism) [14].
2. Hypospadias—A health registry study from Denmark (n = 5541) reported a significant increase in the incidence of TGCT (relative risk 2.13, 95% CI 1.26–3.61) [15].
3. Contralateral testicular cancer—In an epidemiological study (n = 29,515), 175 (0.6%) had a synchronous contralateral cancer [16]. Multiple studies report around 2% 15-year cumulative risk of a contralateral (metachronous) testicular cancer [17, 18].
4. Extragonadal Germ cell tumor—Retroperitoneal extragonadal GCT portends higher risk than mediastinal disease. Non-seminomatous histology has higher risk than seminomas [19].
5. Family History—About 1–3% of patients have a positive family history (more than expected by chance) [20, 21]. Many familial cases are associated with isochromosome 12p [22]. TGCT are enriched with reciprocal loss-of-heterozygosity (double-strand DNA break signature) [23], and certain patients may have germline predisposition via CHEK2 mutations [24].
6. HIV infection—HIV-infected men have modestly increased incidence of TGCT (mostly seminomas), with one study reporting a standardized incidence ratio of 0.7:1.8 [25].
7. Androgen insensitivity syndromes and mixed gonadal dysgenesis—Intersex individuals (androgen insensitivity syndrome/mixed gonadal dysgenesis) have a high risk of GCNIS and germinal and nongerminal neoplasms [26].
8. Klinefelter syndrome and Down syndrome: Klinefelter and Down syndrome are associated with mediastinal and testicular GCT, respectively [27–29].

25.3 The Impact of Delays in Diagnosis on Clinical Outcomes

Multiple single-center studies report a 6-month delay between symptom onset and diagnosis [30]. Overreliance on the emblematic "painless testicular lump" and failure to examine the external genitalia in the appropriate patient are probable causes. Delay in TC diagnosis relates to more advanced disease requiring intensive chemotherapy treatment with increased morbidity and decreased survival [31–33].

25.4 The Symptoms Suggestive of Metastasis from Testicular Germ Cell Tumors

Around 10% (range: 5–19%) of TGCT cases have symptoms from distant disease alone highlighting the importance of testicular examination in the appropriate patient. The most common symptoms are back pain (from infiltration into lumbar venous plexus or the psoas muscle), epigastric swelling or lump, palpable supraclavicular adenopathy, and weight loss [30]. An uncommon patient may have the following:

1. Cough or shortness of breath alone from pulmonary metastasis
2. Retro duodenal lymphadenopathy causing gastric outlet obstruction and GI bleeding
3. Bony pains
4. Symptoms of direct nervous system involvement
5. Pedal edema (unilateral/bilateral) because of iliac/caval obstruction or thrombosis [34]

25.5 The Paraneoplastic Syndromes Associated with Testicular Germ Cell Tumors

25.5.1 Gynecomastia in Testicular Germ Cell Tumors

Testicular tumors cause only 1% of all cases of gynecomastia [35] with Leydig cell tumors having a higher penetrance (25–30%) [36] compared to TGCT (7–11% via clinical assessment) [30]. Patients at high risk of paraneoplastic gynecomastia (recent onset, painful/tender, or more than 4 cm) may show elevated estradiol and suppressed luteinizing hormone (LH) levels prompting a testicular ultrasound to look for site of peripheral aberrant estrogen production [37]. Leydig cell tumors directly secrete estradiol, while TGCT causes gynecomastia via β-hCG elevation and resultant inhibition of cytochrome P450c17 and activation of Leydig cell aromatase [38]. Accordingly, β-hCG levels are typically normal in Leydig cell tumors and elevated in TGCT (although a sizeable minority may have normal levels) [37].

hCG is secreted typically by choriocarcinoma, embryonal cell carcinoma, or trophoblastic cell component. Gynecomastia in TGCT is predominantly β-hCG driven (although a sizeable minority may have normal levels), a surrogate marker of disease burden with prognostic impact [39]. Along these lines, studies exploring prognostic utility of quantitative assessment of gynecomastia in the initial staging CT have provided valuable insights as follows [39, 40]. First, subclinical gynecomastia is found in one-fourth of all patients (23.4%) [40]. Second, β-hCG levels account for half of the inter-patient variability in mean glandular breast diameter [40]. Third, although more common in NSGCT given higher β-hCG levels (30%), up to 16.7% patients with pure seminomas also have a mean breast diameter > 25 mm [40]. Lastly, CT-based assessment of gynecomastia may or may not predict prognosis or presence of metastasis with current evidence showing contradictory results [39, 40].

Timing of onset of gynecomastia in TGCT is of particular importance. Up to 15% patients have new-onset gynecomastia after successful treatment which typically goes within a year of onset. Compensatory rise in LH levels stemming from testicular epithelial damage is the postulated cause [41].

To summarize, while clinical gynecomastia at presentation may prompt the diagnosis of a testicular neoplasm, neither clinical nor radiological gynecomastia can suggest probable histology, likelihood of metastasis, outcomes, or relapse.

25.5.2 Paraneoplastic Hyperthyroidism

The β-subunit of hCG is a weak agonist at the TSH receptor but may cause clinical disease at high levels seen in some TGCT patients [42]. A prospective study assessing thyroid function tests in cases of disseminated NSGCT recorded a prevalence of 3.5% and 2% for clinical (elevated thyroxin, suppressed TSH) and subclinical hyperthyroidism (suppressed TSH alone), respectively. Almost all patients with clinical hyperthyroidism were symptomatic, although weight loss (the most common recorded symptom) was equally prevalent in the euthyroid group as well. Notably, clinical hyperthyroidism was noted exclusively in patients with β-hCG levels >50,000 IU/mL (mean levels: 1, 325, and 147 IU/mL). Thyroxin levels normalized by day 26 in all patients treated with BEP chemotherapy [43].

As such, assessing for hyperthyroidism in cases of disseminated NSGCT with markedly elevated β-hCG levels may allow initiation of symptomatic therapy (beta-blockers), allowing better tolerance of initial chemotherapy.

25.5.3 Paraneoplastic Encephalitis

Rarely patients present with paraneoplastic encephalitis with severe neurological manifestations with KLH11 autoantibodies especially due to seminoma (both gonadal and extra-gonadal).

25.6 The Utility and Shortcomings of Scrotal Ultrasonography

Scrotal ultrasound with a high-frequency (7–10 MHz) linear array probe has 100% sensitivity for detecting testicular masses [44] and should be done in all patients with suspected TGCT regardless of the presence or absence of a clinically palpable mass [30]. As explained in the following sections, scrotal ultrasound is yet to supplant high inguinal orchidectomy (HIO) given its inadequacy at confirmation of malignant nature, histological subtyping, or T-staging [45, 46] and exists currently as a crucial preliminary test only.

25.7 Can Scrotal Ultrasound Predict Histology?

While certain ultrasonographic features cluster by histology, none (alone or in combination) provide clinically relevant discrimination (seminoma vs. NSGCT) [9]. For instance, while seminomas are more commonly well-defined lesions without cystic areas as compared to the irregular, heterogenous (cystic and calcified areas) appearance of NSGCT, radiopathological correlation is only 70% accurate [45]. The concordance remains mostly unchanged despite addition of scrotal MRI [47].

Difficult visualization of tunica albuginea leads to inaccurate T-staging, which is further impaired by the ill-defined margins typically seen in NSGCT lesions. Consequently, radiopathological concordance for T-staging as assessed by scrotal ultrasound was 8% in NSGCT and 44% in seminomas in one study [45].

25.8 Incidental Lesions on Ultrasound-Clinical Approach

In patients presenting with a palpable testicular lump or symptomatic distant disease, TGCT is the most likely diagnosis prompting a radical inguinal orchidectomy [9]. However, the same cannot be said for small nonpalpable lesions incidentally detected on scrotal ultrasonography typically done as a part of evaluating male infertility. A study reported 46 cases of incidental asymptomatic testicular lesions smaller than 1 cm amongst 4418 men undergoing scrotal ultrasound for infertility evaluation. Only three of the eight patients undergoing surgery had a neoplasm (two with Leydig cell tumors and one with seminoma) [48]. Similarly, a prospective study reported that only half of all incidentally detected subcentimetric lesions were malignant in nature, while Leydig cell tumors were the most common amongst benign lesions [49].

Given the higher proportion of benign lesions and the underlying infertility being evaluated, ruling out malignancy noninvasively is of paramount importance [50]. Localization of the testicular lump may help since intratesticular masses are typically malignant while para-testicular masses are typically benign, although exceptions exist [51]. A prospective study evaluating utility of quantitative contrast-enhanced ultrasonography reported contrast enhancement as a diagnostic feature of neoplastic lesions (benign or malignant). Furthermore, rapid washin and delayed washout patterns were suggestive of malignant (77%, $p < 0.001$) and benign lesions (93%, $p < 0.001$), respectively. Combination of unenhanced and quantitative contrast-enhanced scrotal ultrasonography was 82% sensitive and 91% specific in the differential diagnosis of benign versus malignant lesions. However, the following caveats compromise the external validity of these results. First, only patients of infertility with incidentally detected lesions (nonpalpable, most <1.5 cm) were enrolled. Second, contrast washout pattern was observer dependent [49].

25.9 Management of Stage 1 Seminomas (CS1S)

25.9.1 Overview

The diagnosis of stage 1 seminoma relies on comprehensive HPE evaluation of the primary specimen, no AFP elevation, post HIO normalization of tumor markers, and a normal staging abdominal CT scan with thoracic radiograph/CT [9]. Accounting for almost 80% of all seminoma cases [10], stage 1 seminomas have nearly 100% disease-specific survival with either of the modalities: active surveillance [52], single-dose carboplatin [53], and para-aortic radiotherapy [54].

25.9.2 Active Surveillance

Roughly 15% patients with stage 1 seminoma have occult retroperitoneal disease which manifests clinically at a later time-point. Vast majority relapse in the retroperitoneum with near universal chemotherapy sensitivity and a disease-specific overall survival nearing 100%. Notably, these percentages are based on studies monitoring patients with a CT scan every 3–4 moths for the first 3–5 years [52, 53, 55]. Although justified in patients with NSGCT, such active surveillance protocols might be overkilled in seminomas. Along these lines, a recent randomized trial assessing rates of relapse with advanced disease (stage IIA or higher) with a factorial design (CT vs. MRI, follow-up schedules of three scans in 3 years vs. seven scans in 5 years) reported the following outcomes: MRI was noninferior to CT (0.6% vs. 2.6%), more frequent scanning detected more relapses, but non-inferiority margin met (2.8% vs. 0.3%). Notably, almost all relapses were picked up at protocol assessments possibly highlighting the modest symptom burden. Also, the difference in rate of relapse detection had no impact on outcomes [56]. Thus, less intensive follow-up standards may be standard in the future.

25.9.3 Para-aortic Radiotherapy

Relapse rates after para-aortic radiotherapy are 1–3% [54, 57, 58], owing to the radiosensitivity of seminomas. Given the impressive efficacy, studies have instead focused on adverse effect reduction via de-escalation. Because of the physiological nodal drainage of the testis, irradiation of the pelvic nodes may not be needed. A study reported similar relapse rates with better quality of life when pelvic nodal irradiation was omitted, making para-aortic strip irradiation the standard of care. Notably, at least moderately severe GI toxicity was seen in 60% and 5% in the acute and chronic phase, respectively [54]. A subsequent study demonstrated non-inferiority of 20 Gy versus 30 Gy with lesser fatigue at 4 weeks (5% vs. 20%), making 20 Gy the standard dose. Thus, para-aortic strip radiotherapy at a dose of 20 Gy is a current standard of care option in cases of stage 1 seminomas [9].

Risk of second malignant neoplasms (SMN), cardiovascular diseases (CVD), and gonadal damage makes radiotherapy a less preferred option versus its counterparts [59]. A study evaluating contralateral gonadal toxicity with scattered radiation reported thermoluminescent dosimetry (TLD) readings of 3.89 cGY versus 1.48 cGY without and with scrotal shielding, respectively, showcasing that gonadal toxicity cannot be completely negated [60]. A retrospective study of 2629 patients of stage 1 seminoma treated with para-aortic strip RT reported an SIR of 1.61 for SMN compared to observation alone. Notably, most SMN were in the RT field [61]. However, whether adjuvant chemotherapy is any better in terms of long-term toxicity is doubtful (discussed subsequently).

Thus, para-aortic strip RT at a dose of 20 Gy consistently reports relapse rates less than 5% with long-term morbidity which may not be significantly greater compared to adjuvant chemotherapy.

25.9.4 Adjuvant Carboplatin

Given the potential hazards of SMN and CVD from para-aortic radiotherapy, carboplatin adjuvant therapy was evaluated in stage 1 seminomas. In 2005, the results of the MRC TE19/EORTC 80982 non-inferiority trial were published, reporting a 2-year relapse rate of 5.1% and 4.1% in patients receiving carboplatin and para-aortic radiotherapy, respectively, with lesser acute adverse events and a better QoL (after day 3) in the carboplatin arm. This difference of −1.0%

(90% CI: −2.5 to −0.5) was within the prespecified non-inferiority margin of 3%, and adjuvant chemotherapy was deemed non-inferior to adjuvant para-aortic radiotherapy with added advantages of lesser SMN, CAD, and contralateral TGCT rates [62]. However, longer follow-up (median: 6.5 years) revealed a breach in the non-inferiority margin (difference in relapse-free rates −1.3%, 90% CI: −3.5 to 0.7), with most of the relapses being in the retroperitoneum necessitating ongoing serial CT scan-based assessment. Although no differences were evident in rates of SMN and CVD, longer follow-up is prudent for meaningful inference [63]. In this regard, a prospective single-arm study with a longer follow-up (median: 9 years) reported statistically nonsignificant but numerically higher rates of ischemic heart disease as well as cerebrovascular disease. Additionally, no difference in rates of contralateral TGCT was evident [64]. Another retrospective study reported similar incidence rates of SMN and CVD with chemotherapy and radiotherapy compared to active surveillance [65].

Aforementioned studies have enrolled unselected patients with stage 1 seminomas, a cohort where approximately 80% patients may not need any adjuvant therapy whatsoever, necessitating delineation of high-risk subsets [52]. A pooled analysis of four surveillance studies elucidated the following risk factors for relapse: primary size >4 cm and invasion of rete testis invasion. Five-year relapse rates were 12%, 16%, and 32% in patients none, one, or two risk factors, respectively [66]. Notably, while two pivotal nonrandomized studies administered adjuvant chemotherapy based on these criteria [53, 67, 68], other studies failed to validate these risk factors [53, 69]. The SWENOTECA study administered one cycle of adjuvant carboplatin to patients with either or both risk factors and reported a modest reduction in relapse rates (absolute, 6.5%; relative, 50%). Thus, carboplatin therapy reduced the number of patients relapsing from 1 in 10 to 1 in 7. Additionally, since most patients relapsed in the retroperitoneum (90%), obviation of serial CT scans was also not achieved. Contrasting with these results, a retrospective study of patients with primary size >6 cm reported a 90% reduction in relapse rates with adjuvant dogleg RT (24–26 Gy), with most relapses being outside the radiotherapy portal [68]. Non-inferiority of adjuvant chemotherapy has been demonstrated in an unselected population where a vast majority of patients needed no therapy whatsoever, which may have caused a regression to mean [62]. The same does not seem to hold true when higher-risk patients are assessed specifically. However, neither does dose reduction to 20 Gy or omission of pelvic radiotherapy [54, 57].

Two instead of one dose of adjuvant carboplatin is a possible answer. A pooled analysis of Spanish trials reported relapse rates as low as 1.4% (range: 1.4–6%) in patients with both risk factors [67]. The following need to be considered while analyzing these percentages: First, limitations of cross-study comparisons apply. Second, relapse rates of patients with none/one/two risk factors overlap defeating the purpose of risk stratification. Third, median follow-up is only 3 years while as many as 15% relapses happen after 3 years [63]. In this regard, a recent retrospective study of 159 patients receiving two cycles of adjuvant carboplatin with a longer follow-up (median: 106 months) has reported the following outcomes: 15-year RFS of 99.4%, SMN rate of 7.6%, and contralateral TGCT rate of 3.85%. Notably, this study enrolled an unselected population, and neither primary size nor rete testis invasion was associated with a higher relapse rate [70]. Thus, while evidence is limited, longer follow-up seems to reveal a steeper price for the benefits of more carboplatin cycles.

A few important points about administration of carboplatin warrants discussion should this modality be chosen. Regarding dose calculation, Cr^{51}-labelled EDTA clearance-based estimation of GFR is the recommended standard in two of the largest prospective studies [53, 62]. While 24 h urinary creatine level-based creatine clearance was also used, a 15% dose reduction was done as a part of the protocol given the overestimation of GFR typically seen. Additionally, while a small subset of patients received doses calculated based on cystatin C clearance or serum creatinine-based estimated GFR, these patients were more likely to be underdosed. However, this underdosing did not have an impact on release rates [53]. Therapy is typically instituted within 8 weeks of orchidectomy. Up to 5% patients experience grade 3/grade 4 thrombocytopenia after carboplatin therapy [53].

25.10 Management of Persistently Elevated Tumor Markers Post-orchiectomy

Post-orchidectomy tumor marker levels are integral for staging [71]. Expected normalization of serum tumor markers (STM) post high inguinal orchidectomy is 4–6 days for lactate dehydrogenase (LDH) and hCG as compared to 20–28 days for alpha fetoprotein (AFP) [72]. While a multitude of cases explain mild persistent elevation post-orchidectomy, markedly elevated levels/rising levels indicate (and are treated as) metastatic disease regardless of the findings on cross-sectional imaging [73]. Although implications of LDH elevations in patients with seminomas are less clear, normal post-orchidectomy levels are needed for considering active surveillance or carboplatin chemotherapy (although para-aortic strip radiotherapy may still be considered) [74].

In patients with persistent elevation/serial rise of STM post-orchidectomy, ultrasonographic assessment of the contralateral testis along with cross-sectional imaging of all possible metastatic sites is to be done [75]. Lack of visualized disease on imaging along with normal contralateral testis implies a clinical stage of IS with management and prognosis identical to IGCCCG good prognosis metastatic NSGCT. One retrospective review of 114 cases of stage IS TGCT reported that 94% cases were good risk by the IGCCCG prognostic classification. Five-year DFS and 10-year DFS were 87% and 85%, respectively. Embryonal cell carcinoma component in the primary tumor was independently predictive of requirement of further therapy [76].

25.11 Evidence-Based Management of Good Risk Seminomas (Stage 2/Stage 3)

A prospective trial demonstrated equivalent efficacy and lesser toxicity with three cycles of BEP compared to four cycles in good risk TGCT [77]. Another option, four cycles of EP chemotherapy, is endorsed by the plethora of evidence documenting long-term survival more than 90% [53, 78–81]. Thus, three cycles of BEP and four cycles of EP chemotherapy are the current standards of care [9].

While no trials have compared EP and BEP chemotherapy in good risk seminomas, retrospective studies consistently report long-term survival rates of more than 90% with EP chemotherapy [53, 78, 80, 81]. A prospective study reported a 3-year PFS and OS of 93% and 99%, respectively, when treating good risk seminomas with four cycles of standard dose EP [82]. Given the cumulative dose-dependent risks of therapy-related AML (tAML) with etoposide therapy in TGCT patients [83], a prospective study evaluated an attenuated EP chemotherapy schedule in good risk seminomas (400 mg/m^2 etoposide per cycle) and reported CR rates, 3y PFS, and 3y OS of 69%, 89%, and 97%, respectively [84]. However, given the low magnitude of risk (1.3% tAML cases in patients with cumulative dose of etoposide >2 g/m^2) [83], potential drop in efficacy is not justified.

Carboplatin is another potential route for therapy de-escalation in these patients. Multiple phase two studies reported a 3-year OS nearing 90% with single-agent carboplatin [85–87]. Building on this, two phase three trials evaluating carboplatin monotherapy with cisplatin-based combinations reported inferior PFS with monotherapy without an impact on overall survival. Since the trials were not powered adequately to detect a survival difference, carboplatin monotherapy is not currently used. However, efficacy of carboplatin-based combinations currently remains unknown [88].

To summarize, both EP (four cycles) and BEP (three cycles) are acceptable options with no prospectively proven superior. Decision-making may be based on patient wishes, impact of therapy duration, and risks of bleomycin-induced pulmonary toxicity [81]. Carboplatin monotherapy is suboptimal and its combinations are largely unexplored.

25.12 Management of Intermediate-Risk Seminomas

No randomized trials specifically focus on this uncommon subgroup of patients. Acceptable options for management are four cycles of BEP or VIP chemotherapy based on risk of bleomycin-induced lung injury [9]. A prospective study treating intermediate-risk seminomas with VIP chemotherapy reported 87% long-term survival, but no comparator arm limits the external validity of these results [82].

25.13 Evidence-Based Management of Good Risk NSGCT

Given the thresholds used for classification in the IGCCCG initiative, these patients by definition have long-term survival rates of more than 90% [9]. Thus, the bulk of research has been dedicated to minimization of therapy-related toxicity. The current options for management are four cycles of EP chemotherapy or three cycles of BEP chemotherapy [9].

25.14 Four Cycles of EP Versus Three Cycles of BEP

The optimal choice between BEP and EP chemotherapy in patients of good risk NSGCT remains a topic of active debate. Multiple phase three trials have assessed the impact of bleomycin omission, but heterogeneity in chemotherapy backbone and definition of "good risk" obviates simple interpretation.

While initial phase three trials suggested adverse impact of bleomycin omission, a closer look challenges the external validity of these findings. The initial trial by R de Wit et al. used a chemotherapy backbone having suboptimal doses (etoposide dose per cycle: 360 mg/m^2) [89]. The trial by Levi et al. assessed a vinblastine-based backbone which is no longer standard [90]. Similarly, the trial by Loehrer et al. evaluated three cycles of EP instead of the standard, four cycles [91]. Furthermore, neither of these three trials is recruited by the IGCCCG risk classification (since they predated it).

A retrospective analysis of two pooled trials comparing four cycles of standard-dose EP reported outcomes at par with most prior BEP datasets. However, lack of randomized nature and recruitment by a center-specific algorithm defining "good risk" as CR probability >0.5 limits its external validity. To troubleshoot this, a subsequent analysis reclassifying these patients by IGCCCG classification reported similar impressive outcomes in the good risk NSGCT group [92]. These results primed four cycles of EP as a potential standard of care.

A subsequent trial by R de Wit et al. aimed at finding out the optimal dose and duration of BEP chemotherapy. Findings were notable for equivalence of three and four cycles in terms of efficacy. Furthermore, a 3-day BEP regime was found to be more GI and neurotoxic although adverse effect rates reached significance in the a four-cycle subset only [93]. This study established three cycles of conventional 5-day BEP as the optimal bleomycin containing standard of care, and a randomized trial comparing three cycles of BEP (etoposide 500 mg/m^2 per cycle) with four cycles of EP was needed. On these lines, the GETUG T93BP trial evaluated three cycles of BEP with four cycles of EP and reported nonsignificant trend toward better PFS and OS with BEP. The trial however recruited by the Gustave Roussy prognostic model and a subsequent mature analysis specific to the IGCCCG good risk group reported higher 4-year EFS in the BEP arm (93% vs. 86%, $p = 0.052$) [81]. However, the definition of an "event" here needs clarification. Any viable tumor in the residual mass was an event, as was any subsequent teratoma resection. When these outcomes are taken in the true clinical sense (CR with chemotherapy and surgery), the distribution of events is identical across groups. Apart from the obvious negation of pulmonary toxicity, several other factors may impact decision-making. Neurological toxicity, skin rash, and Raynaud's phenomenon were more common in the BEP arm. On the other hand, residual masses in BEP-treated patients were less likely to have viable cancer (1% vs. 6%).

25.15 Other Routes to De-intensification of BEP

Carboplatin-based combinations have been tried upfront given the lower propensity for nephrotoxicity, neurotoxicity, and emesis. A trial comparing cisplatin (20 mg/m²/day × 5 days) or carboplatin (500 mg/m² on day 1) addition to etoposide (100 mg/m²/day × 5 days) reported inferior outcomes with carboplatin-based therapy [94]. Another trial reported inferior outcomes with carboplatin substitution in the BEP regime. However, inadequate doses of etoposide (360 mg/m²/cycle) and bleomycin (30 U single dose per cycle) hinder generalizability. Notably, the BEP arm reported CR rates, 1-year FFS, and 2-year OS of 86%, 91%, and 97%, respectively [95]. Building on this, a randomized trial evaluated efficacy of a BEP regime with reduced doses and reported inferior outcomes with four cycles of $B_{30}E_{360}P$ compared to three cycles of $B_{90}E_{500}P$ [96]. Prolonged bleomycin infusions have been tried to reduce pulmonary toxicity based on preclinical and retrospective data. However, a randomized trial failed to confirm this hypothesis, and bleomycin boluses remain the standard of care [97].

Capping of bleomycin dose and periodic pulmonary function testing (DLCO) are also helpful in prudent de-escalation. A retrospective study of TGCT patients receiving 30 IU bleomycin/week reported symptomatic and fatal pneumonitis in 5–16% and 0–3% cases, respectively. On the other hand, a prospective study administering 15 IU/m² bleomycin weekly and stopping therapy in cases showing more than 25% decline of DLCO reported the following: asymptomatic pneumonitis in 10%, symptomatic (clinical/radiological) pneumonitis in 2%, and fatal pneumonitis in 0.2%. Notably, patients with lesser median cumulative bleomycin doses (100 IU/m²) did not have compromised oncological outcomes compared to patients receiving higher doses (median: 140 IU/m²) [98]. Thus, periodic DLCO monitoring may reduce symptomatic cases of bleomycin toxicity without impact on oncological outcomes. Furthermore, capping the dose at 150 IU/m² and using adjusted doses of 15 IU/m² weekly are additional risk-reducing measures.

To summarize the available evidence, optimizing de-escalation of chemotherapy in good risk NSGCT is an interplay of bleomycin versus chemotherapy backbone. While bleomycin is probably dispensable in the face of optimal doses and cycles of EP, its addition does not negate suboptimal doses, cycles, or carboplatin substitution highlighting the reliance on etoposide and cisplatin for efficacy in this patient population. However, capping the dose at 150 IU/m², monitoring via periodic DLCO, and using BSA adjusted doses are prudent risk-reducing steps with no compromise of oncological outcomes. Whether lesser bleomycin per cycle is permissible with a $E_{500}P$ backbone is currently unknown. Infusional bleomycin offers no advantages in lieu of its logistic challenges.

25.16 Evidence-Based Management of Intermediate-Risk NSGCT

Four cycles of BEP chemotherapy remain the time-tested standard. Randomized trials evaluating four cycles of VIP chemotherapy [98] and T-BEP chemotherapy [99] failed to show improved outcomes along with poorer tolerability. However, temporal increment in survival is evident with the same chemotherapy backbone with more recent studies reporting 5-year OS near 90% as compared to the initial ICGGGC classifier of 80% [100, 101].

25.17 The Current Evidence-Based Standard for High-Risk NSGCT

25.17.1 Current Standard of Therapy: Four Cycles of BEP

Most guidelines and prospective studies recommend/use four cycles of BEP chemotherapy followed by resection of residual masses as the treatment of choice [9]. However, outcomes are modest for this subset of patients with most estimates of 2-year EFS nearing 50% and 2-year OS nearing 70% [102–105]. Given that a multitude of approaches have failed to consistently improve outcomes in this setting (detailed below), adhering to evidence-based management is crucial. A retrospective study reported as many as half of relapsed TGCT patients receiving inappropriate first-line therapy with most common errors being unjustified reduction in intensity, inappropriate delay in chemotherapy cycles, and delayed/omitted resection of residual masses. These findings reinforce the value of managing these cases at an experienced high-volume center [106].

25.17.2 Intensification of Frontline Therapy

Given the encouraging data for ifosfamide in relapsed/refractory settings, a randomized trial comparing VIP (etoposide, ifosfamide, cisplatin) versus BEP chemotherapy reported equivalent efficacy but higher hematological toxicity [102]. However, VIP chemotherapy may be used in patients at high risk of/with features of bleomycin-induced lung injury. The TIP regime (paclitaxel, ifosfamide, cisplatin) is another option in such settings where etoposide omission is needed as well [107]. A more promising approach is based on tailoring intensification on rate of STM decline. A randomized trial evaluating a dose-dense protocol incorporating upfront oxaliplatin, paclitaxel, and infusional bleomycin in patients with poor marker decline reported improvement in 3-year PFS by 34%. However, given the higher toxicity rates and lack of impact on overall survival, it is seldom used in clinical practice although a discussion of pros and cons is warranted with the patient [105].

25.17.3 High-Dose Chemotherapy and Autologous Stem Cell Transplantation

The following rationale makes autologous stem cell transplantation a viable option for TGCT management: first, multiple agents with synergistic action and no demonstrated plateau in the dose-response curve; second, rarity of bone marrow metastasis; and third, young patients with lesser comorbidities [108]. Chemotherapy agents with the aforementioned properties include carboplatin, etoposide, and cyclophosphamide. Carboplatin (and not cisplatin) is used in this setting given a lack of neurotoxicity, ototoxicity, and nephrotoxicity seen with this agent along with reports of safety of carboplatin monotherapy up to doses of 1600 mg/m^2 except for myelotoxicity [109]. For etoposide, no dose-response curve is known till doses as high as 2400 mg/m^2 [110]. Synergy with cyclophosphamide at such high doses is an added benefit of etoposide [111].

Given the plethora of evidence in relapsed settings, multiple phase 1/phase 2 studies evaluated HDT-ASCT in frontline settings. A French study failed to demonstrate any benefit [112]. A subsequent retrospective analysis from MSKCC (Memorial Sloan Kettering Cancer Center) reported that frontline ASCT was better tolerated versus subsequent line ASCT and achieved outcomes superior to historic first-line cohorts [113]. A German phase 1/phase 2 study reported 80% long-term survival with upfront HDT-ASCT (potential 20% gain vs. historic cohorts) [114]. A subsequent multivariate matched-pair analysis reported better 2-year PFS (75% vs. 59%, p = 0.0056) and 2-year OS (82% vs. 71%, p = 0.0184) [115]. This body of evidence prompted phase 3 trials to evaluate role of frontline HDT-ASCT in poor risk NSGCT.

An initial phase 3 trial failed to show benefit from HDT-ASCT, but the therapy given as active control (vinblastine, etoposide, and cisplatin) limits generalizability [116]. Two subsequent phase 3 trials have evaluated HDT-ASCT versus BEP chemotherapy [103, 104]. While neither showed improved survival, the trial by Daugaard showed numerically higher 2-year FFS (58.2% vs. 44.8%, $p = 0.06$). Compliance with therapy and included patient subsets may explain this difference. The study by Daugaard et al. administered ASCT to 95.4% cases with about 75% cases completing all four cycles [103], as compared to only 77% receiving ASCT in the study by Motzer et al. [104]. Additionally, while Daugaard et al. included only poor risk NSGCT [103], Motzer et al. included seminomas (2% of all cases) and IGCCCG intermediate risk as well (21% of all cases) [104]. Thus, while frontline ASCT has no role in the current scenario, studies with more better patient selection and tolerable regimes may change this in the future.

25.18 Can We Give Initial Low-Intensity Chemotherapy in High-Burden Disease?

Subsets with target organ damage may be better treated with initial abbreviated chemotherapy to tide over the crisis without compromising long-term outcomes. Patients with extensive pulmonary metastasis along with dyspnea at rest/room air $PaO_2 < 80$ mmHg/both are at a high risk of alveolar hemorrhage from necrosis (and superadded neutropenic infections) with full-dose chemotherapy. A single-arm study of 25 patients reported significant reduction in acute respiratory distress syndrome (87% vs. 30%) and better survival (27% vs. 40%, $p = 0.01$) with initial 3-day EP and bleomycin omission with subsequent therapy on day 15 [117].

A similar study evaluating the baby-BOP (bBOP) regime (cisplatin 50 mg/m^2, vincristine 2 mg, and bleomycin 30 U on day 1 only) in patients with complicated disease (organ failure, vena cava obstruction, poor performance status from overwhelming disease) showed better initial tolerability without impact on overall long-term survival. Conventional chemotherapy may be initiated 7 days after bBOP at the physician's discretion [118].

25.19 Management of Testicular GCT with CNS Metastasis

Incidence of CNS metastasis in TGCT ranges from 1% to 3% at baseline [119–121] to as high as 40% in autopsy studies with around 10% patients having CNS metastasis at some point of time of their disease antemortem [122]. Seen almost exclusively in patients with NSGCT [123], this is an especially poor prognostic subset given that the 5-year survival of GCT patients with CNS, bony, and hepatic metastasis is 33%, 35%, and 50%, respectively [119]. This adverse prognostic impact combined with relative paucity of cases impels decisions not based on prospective randomized evidence [75]. Based on clinical features, outcomes, and prognostic impact of various therapeutic modalities, GCT patients with CNS involvement can be categorized as follows: (1) patients with CNS metastasis at baseline, (2) patients with early isolated CNS relapse, and (3) patients with CNS as well as systemic relapse on/after platinum-based chemotherapy [123 125].

25.20 CNS Metastasis at Baseline

Compared to patients with CNS disease at relapse, these patients have significantly higher β-hCG values (more than half with values >100,000 IU/L), multiple CNS lesions (67% vs. 56%, $p < 0.05$), widespread systemic disease (99% vs. 72%), hepatic/bone metastasis (46% vs. 25%), and pulmonary metastasis (94% vs. 62%) [123]. These findings may partly be explained by the inclusion of isolated CNS relapses in the other cohort. Notably, around half of all patients with CNS metastasis are asymptomatic [123], necessitating CNS-directed imaging in case of high baseline β-hCG levels [75].

Risk-adapted, platinum-based, multi-agent chemotherapy is the backbone of management. Components of the BEP regime are known to cross the blood-brain barrier in patients with CNS involvement [126], with around two-thirds of treated patients achieving CR [125]. Utility of CNS-directed therapy is controversial in these settings. The largest retrospective dataset published reported the impact of CNS-directed therapy on outcomes. All patients received chemotherapy and 55% patients received some form of CNS-directed therapy (neurosurgical resection/radiotherapy) [123]. In contrast, the following are reasons for supporting CNS-directed therapy: first, most CNS relapses happen within 3–6 months [123, 125] of therapy completion with some having CNS only relapses, pointing at the possibility of CNS as a sanctuary site [120].

References

1. 28-testis-fact-sheet. https://gco.iarc.fr/today/data/factsheets/cancers/28-Testis-fact-sheet.pdf.
2. Shanmugalingam T, Soultati A, Chowdhury S, Rudman S, Van Hemelrijck M. Global incidence and outcome of testicular cancer. Clin Epidemiol. 2013;5:417–27.
3. Nigam M, Aschebrook-Kilfoy B, Shikanov S, Eggener S. Increasing incidence of testicular cancer in the United States and Europe between 1992 and 2009. World J Urol. 2015;33(5):623–31.
4. Cancer over time. https://gco.iarc.fr/overtime.
5. McGlynn KA, Devesa SS, Sigurdson AJ, Brown LM, Tsao L, Tarone RE. Trends in the incidence of testicular germ cell tumors in the United States. Cancer. 2003;97(1):63–70.
6. Zheng T, Holford TR, Ma Z, Ward BA, Flannery J, Boyle P. Continuing increase in incidence of germ-cell testis cancer in young adults: experience from Connecticut, USA, 1935–1992. Int J Cancer. 1996;65(6):723–9.
7. Cancer today. http://gco.iarc.fr/today/home.
8. Miller KD, Fidler-Benaoudia M, Keegan TH, Hipp HS, Jemal A, Siegel RL. Cancer statistics for adolescents and young adults, 2020. CA Cancer J Clin. 2020;70(6):443–59.
9. Laguna MP, Pizzocaro G, Klepp O, Algaba F, Kisbenedek L, Leiva O. EAU guidelines on testicular cancer. Eur Urol. 2001;40(2):102–10.
10. Dieckmann KP, Richter-Simonsen H, Kulejewski M, Ikogho R, Zecha H, Anheuser P, et al. Testicular germ-cell Tumours: a descriptive analysis of clinical characteristics at first presentation. Urol Int. 2018;100(4):409–19.
11. Nair LM, Krishna KJ, Kumar A, Mathews S, Joseph J, James FV. Prognostic factors and outcomes of nonseminomatous germ cell tumours of testis—experience from a tertiary cancer centre in India. 2020. http://ecancer.org/en/journal/article/1145-prognostic-factors-and-outcomes-of-nonseminomatous-germ-cell-tumours-of-testis-experience-from-a-tertiary-cancer-centre-in-india.
12. Joshi A, Zanwar S, Shetty N, Patil V, Noronha V, Bakshi G, et al. Epidemiology of male seminomatous and nonseminomatous germ cell tumors and response to first-line chemotherapy from a tertiary cancer center in India. Indian J Cancer. 2016;53(2):313.
13. Gajendran VK, Nguyen M, Ellison LM. Testicular cancer patterns in African-American men. Urology. 2005;66(3):602–5.
14. Batata MA, Chu FC, Hilaris BS, Whitmore WF, Golbey RB. Testicular cancer in cryptorchids. Cancer. 1982;49(5):1023–30.
15. Schnack TH, Poulsen G, Myrup C, Wohlfahrt J, Melbye M. Familial coaggregation of cryptorchidism, hypospadias, and testicular germ cell cancer: a nationwide cohort study. J Natl Cancer Inst. 2010;102(3):187–92.
16. Fosså SD, Chen J, Schonfeld SJ, McGlynn KA, McMaster ML, Gail MH, et al. Risk of contralateral testicular cancer: a population-based study of 29,515 U.S. men. J Natl Cancer Inst. 2005;97(14):1056–66.
17. Blok JM, Groot HJ, Huele EH, de Wit R, Horenblas S, Nuver J, et al. Dose-dependent effect of platinum-based chemotherapy on the risk of Metachronous contralateral testicular cancer. J Clin Oncol. 2021;39(4):319–27.
18. Kier MGG, Lauritsen J, Almstrup K, Mortensen MS, Toft BG, Rajpert-De Meyts E, et al. Screening for carcinoma in situ in the contralateral testicle in patients with testicular cancer: a population-based study. Ann Oncol. 2015;26(4):737–42.
19. Stang A, Trabert B, Wentzensen N, Cook MB, Rusner C, Oosterhuis JW, et al. Gonadal and extragonadal germ cell tumors in the United States, 1973–2007. Int J Androl. 2012;35(4):616–25.
20. Harland SJ. Conundrum of the hereditary component of testicular cancer. Lancet. 2000;356(9240):1455–6.
21. Forman D, Oliver RT, Brett AR, Marsh SG, Moses JH, Bodmer JG, et al. Familial testicular cancer: a report of the UK family register, estimation of risk and an HLA class 1 sib-pair analysis. Br J Cancer. 1992;65(2):255–62.
22. Bosl GJ, Ilson DH, Rodriguez E, Motzer RJ, Reuter VE, Chaganti RS. Clinical relevance of the i(12p) marker chromosome in germ cell tumors. J Natl Cancer Inst. 1994;86(5):349–55.
23. Taylor-Weiner A, Zack T, O'Donnell E, Guerriero JL, Bernard B, Reddy A, et al. Genomic evolution and chemoresistance in germ-cell tumours. Nature. 2016;540(7631):114–8.

24. AlDubayan SH, Pyle LC, Gamulin M, Kulis T, Moore ND, Taylor-Weiner A, et al. Association of Inherited Pathogenic Variants in checkpoint kinase 2 (CHEK2) with susceptibility to testicular germ cell tumors. JAMA Oncol. 2019;5(4):514–22.
25. Grulich AE, van Leeuwen MT, Falster MO, Vajdic CM. Incidence of cancers in people with HIV/AIDS compared with immunosuppressed transplant recipients: a meta-analysis. Lancet. 2007;370(9581):59–67.
26. Gourlay WA, Johnson HW, Pantzar JT, McGillivray B, Crawford R, Nielsen WR. Gonadal tumors in disorders of sexual differentiation. Urology. 1994;43(4):537–40.
27. Hasle H, Mellemgaard A, Nielsen J, Hansen J. Cancer incidence in men with Klinefelter syndrome. Br J Cancer. 1995;71(2):416–20.
28. Hasle H, Jacobsen BB, Asschenfeldt P, Andersen K. Mediastinal germ cell tumour associated with Klinefelter syndrome. A report of case and review of the literature. Eur J Pediatr. 1992;151(10):735–9.
29. Dexeus FH, Logothetis CJ, Chong C, Sella A, Ogden S. Genetic abnormalities in men with germ cell tumors. J Urol. 1988;140(1):80–4.
30. Moul JW. Timely diagnosis of testicular cancer. Urol Clin North Am. 2007;34(2):109–17; abstract vii.
31. Bosl GJ, Goldman A, Lange PH, Vogelzang NJ, Fraley EE, Levitt SH, et al. Impact of delay in diagnosis on clinical stage of testicular cancer. Lancet. 1981;318(8253):970–3.
32. Öztürk Ç, Fleer J, Hoekstra HJ, Hoekstra-Weebers JEHM. Delay in diagnosis of testicular cancer; a need for awareness programs. PLoS One. 2015;10(11):e0141244.
33. Vasudev NS, Joffe JK, Cooke C, Richards F, Jones WG. Delay in the diagnosis of testicular tumours—changes over the past 18 years. Br J Gen Pract. 2004;54(505):595–7.
34. Bosl GJ, Motzer RJ. Testicular germ-cell cancer. N Engl J Med. 1997;337(4):242–54.
35. Mieritz MG, Christiansen P, Jensen MB, Joensen UN, Nordkap L, Olesen IA, et al. Gynaecomastia in 786 adult men: clinical and biochemical findings. Eur J Endocrinol. 2017;176(5):555–66.
36. Gabrilove JL, Nicolis GL, Mitty HA, Sohval AR. Feminizing interstitial cell tumor of the testis: personal observations and a review of the literature. Cancer. 1975;35(4):1184–202.
37. Clinical features, diagnosis, and evaluation of gynecomastia in adults—UpToDate. https://www.uptodate.com/contents/clinical-features-diagnosis-and-evaluation-of-gynecomastia-in-adults?sectionName=Further%20evaluation%20to%20rule%20out%20breast%20cancer&topicRef=7466&anchor=H409071425&source=see_link#H409071425.
38. Forest MG, Lecoq A, Saez JM. Kinetics of human chorionic gonadotropin-induced Steroidogenic response of the human testis. II. Plasma 17α-Hydroxyprogesterone, Δ4-Androstenedione, Estrone, and 17β-estradiol: evidence for the action of human chorionic gonadotropin on intermediate enzymes implicated in steroid biosynthesis*. J Clin Endocrinol Metabol. 1979;49(2):284–91.
39. Polat AV, Öztürk M, Çamlıdağ İ, Akyüz B. Is gynecomastia related to the disease characteristics and prognosis in testicular germ cell tumor patients? Diagn Interv Radiol. 2019;25(3):189–94.
40. Klang E, Rozendorn N, Raskin S, Portnoy O, Sklair M, Marom EM, et al. CT measurement of breast glandular tissue and its association with testicular cancer. Eur Radiol. 2017;27(2):536–42.
41. Turner AR, Morrish DW, Berry J, MacDonald RN. Gynecomastia after cytotoxic therapy for metastatic testicular cancer. Arch Intern Med. 1982;142(5):896–7.
42. Yoshimura M, Hershman JM. Thyrotropic action of human chorionic gonadotropin. Thyroid. 1995;5(5):425–34.
43. Oosting SF, de Haas EC, Links TP, de Bruin D, Sluiter WJ, de Jong IJ, et al. Prevalence of paraneoplastic hyperthyroidism in patients with metastatic non-seminomatous germ-cell tumors. Ann Oncol. 2010;21(1):104–8.
44. Rifkin MD, Kurtz AB, Pasto ME, Goldberg BB. Diagnostic capabilities of high-resolution scrotal ultrasonography: prospective evaluation. J Ultrasound Med. 1985;4(1):13–9.
45. Marth D, Scheidegger J, Studer UE. Ultrasonography of testicular tumors. Urol Int. 1990;45(4):237–40.
46. Benson CB. The role of ultrasound in diagnosis and staging of testicular cancer. Semin Urol. 1988;6(3):189–202.
47. Schultz-Lampel D, Bogaert G, Thüroff JW, Schlegel E, Cramer B. MRI for evaluation of scrotal pathology. Urol Res. 1991;19(5):289–92.
48. Toren PJ, Roberts M, Lecker I, Grober ED, Jarvi K, Lo KC. Small incidentally discovered testicular masses in infertile men—is active surveillance the new standard of care? J Urol. 2010;183(4):1373–7.
49. Isidori AM, Pozza C, Gianfrilli D, Giannetta E, Lemma A, Pofi R, et al. Differential diagnosis of nonpalpable testicular lesions: qualitative and quantitative contrast-enhanced US of benign and malignant testicular tumors. Radiology. 2014;273(2):606–18.
50. Rocher L, Criton A, Gennisson JL, Creze M, Albiges L, Ferlicot S, et al. Characterization of testicular masses in adults: performance of combined quantitative shear wave elastography and conventional ultrasound. Ultrasound Med Biol. 2019;45(3):720–31.
51. McDonald MW, Reed AB, Tran PT, Evans LA. Testicular tumor ultrasound characteristics and association with histopathology. Urol Int. 2012;89(2):196–202.
52. Mortensen MS, Lauritsen J, Gundgaard MG, Agerbæk M, Holm NV, Christensen IJ, et al. A nationwide cohort study of stage I seminoma patients followed on a surveillance program. Eur Urol. 2014;66(6):1172–8.

53. Tandstad T, Ståhl O, Dahl O, Haugnes HS, Håkansson U, Karlsdottir Å, et al. Treatment of stage I seminoma, with one course of adjuvant carboplatin or surveillance, risk-adapted recommendations implementing patient autonomy: a report from the Swedish and Norwegian Testicular Cancer Group (SWENOTECA). Ann Oncol. 2016;27(7):1299–304.
54. Fosså SD, Horwich A, Russell JM, Roberts JT, Cullen MH, Hodson NJ, et al. Optimal planning target volume for stage I testicular seminoma: a Medical Research Council randomized trial. Medical Research Council Testicular Tumor Working Group. J Clin Oncol. 1999;17(4):1146.
55. Kollmannsberger C, Tandstad T, Bedard PL, Cohn-Cedermark G, Chung PW, Jewett MA, et al. Patterns of relapse in patients with clinical stage I testicular cancer managed with active surveillance. J Clin Oncol. 2015;33(1):51–7.
56. Joffe JK, Cafferty FH, Murphy L, Rustin GJS, Sohaib SA, Swift S, et al. Imaging modality and frequency in surveillance of stage I seminoma testicular cancer: results from a randomized, phase III, factorial trial (TRISST). J Clin Oncol. 2021;39(6_Suppl):374.
57. Jones WG, Fossa SD, Mead GM, Roberts JT, Sokal M, Horwich A, et al. Randomized trial of 30 versus 20 Gy in the adjuvant treatment of stage I testicular seminoma: a report on Medical Research Council trial TE18, European Organisation for the research and treatment of cancer trial 30942 (ISRCTN18525328). J Clin Oncol. 2005;23(6):1200–8.
58. Melchior D, Hammer P, Fimmers R, Schüller H, Albers P. Long term results and morbidity of para-aortic compared with paraaortic and iliac adjuvant radiation in clinical stage I seminoma. Anticancer Res. 2001;21(4B):2989–93.
59. Patel HD, Srivastava A, Alam R, Joice GA, Schwen ZR, Semerjian A, et al. Radiotherapy for stage I and II testicular seminomas: secondary malignancies and survival. Urol Oncol. 2017;35(10):606.e1–7.
60. Bieri S, Rouzaud M, Miralbell R. Seminoma of the testis: is scrotal shielding necessary when radiotherapy is limited to the Para-aortic nodes? Radiother Oncol. 1999;50(3):349–53.
61. Horwich A, Fossa SD, Huddart R, Dearnaley DP, Stenning S, Aresu M, et al. Second cancer risk and mortality in men treated with radiotherapy for stage I seminoma. Br J Cancer. 2014;110(1):256–63.
62. Oliver RTD, Mason MD, Mead GM, von der Maase H, Rustin GJS, Joffe JK, et al. Radiotherapy versus single-dose carboplatin in adjuvant treatment of stage I seminoma: a randomised trial. Lancet. 2005;366(9482):293–300.
63. Oliver RTD, Mead GM, Rustin GJS, Joffe JK, Aass N, Coleman R, et al. Randomized trial of carboplatin versus radiotherapy for stage I seminoma: mature results on relapse and contralateral testis cancer rates in MRC TE19/EORTC 30982 study (ISRCTN27163214). J Clin Oncol. 2011;29(8):957–62.
64. Powles T, Robinson D, Shamash J, Moller H, Tranter N, Oliver T. The long-term risks of adjuvant carboplatin treatment for stage I seminoma of the testis. Ann Oncol. 2008;19(3):443–7.
65. van den Belt-Dusebout AW, de Wit R, Gietema JA, Horenblas S, Louwman MWJ, Ribot JG, et al. Treatment-specific risks of second malignancies and cardiovascular disease in 5-year survivors of testicular cancer. J Clin Oncol. 2007;25(28):4370–8.
66. Warde P, Specht L, Horwich A, Oliver T, Panzarella T, Gospodarowicz M, et al. Prognostic factors for relapse in stage I seminoma managed by surveillance: a pooled analysis. J Clin Oncol. 2002;20(22):4448–52.
67. Aparicio J, Germà JR, del Muro XG, Maroto P, Arranz JA, Sáenz A, et al. Risk-adapted management for patients with clinical stage I seminoma: the second Spanish Germ Cell Cancer Cooperative Group Study. J Clin Oncol. 2005;23(34):8717–23.
68. Mortensen MS, Bandak M, Kier MGG, Lauritsen J, Agerbæk M, Holm NV, et al. Surveillance versus adjuvant radiotherapy for patients with high-risk stage I seminoma. Cancer. 2017;123(7):1212–8.
69. Chung P, Daugaard G, Tyldesley S, Atenafu EG, Panzarella T, Kollmannsberger C, et al. Evaluation of a prognostic model for risk of relapse in stage I seminoma surveillance. Cancer Med. 2015;4(1):155–60.
70. Chandran EA, Chindewere A, North R, Jameson MB. Two cycles of adjuvant carboplatin for clinical stage 1 testicular seminoma in New Zealand centres: a retrospective analysis of efficacy and long-term events. Cancer Rep (Hoboken). 2020;4(2):e1310.
71. Amin MB, Greene FL, Edge SB, Compton CC, Gershenwald JE, Brookland RK, et al. The eighth edition AJCC cancer staging manual: continuing to build a bridge from a population-based to a more "personalized" approach to cancer staging. CA Cancer J Clin. 2017;67(2):93–9.
72. Milose JC, Filson CP, Weizer AZ, Hafez KS, Montgomery JS. Role of biochemical markers in testicular cancer: diagnosis, staging, and surveillance. Open Access J Urol. 2011;4:1–8.
73. Gilligan TD, Hayes DF, Seidenfeld J, Temin S. ASCO clinical practice guideline on uses of serum tumor markers in adult males with germ cell tumors. JOP. 2010;6(4):199–202.
74. Salem M, Gilligan T. Serum tumor markers and their utilization in the management of germ-cell tumors in adult males. Expert Rev Anticancer Ther. 2011;11(1):1–4.
75. Krege S, Beyer J, Souchon R, Albers P, Albrecht W, Algaba F, et al. European consensus conference on diagnosis and treatment of germ cell cancer: a report of the second meeting of the European Germ Cell Cancer Consensus Group (EGCCCG): part I. Eur Urol. 2008;53(3):478–96.
76. Aparicio J, Sánchez MA, Ochenduszko S, Gumà J, Fernández AA, Garcíadel MX, et al. Treatment and outcome of patients with stage IS testicular cancer:

a retrospective study from the Spanish Germ Cell Cancer Group. J Urol. 2019;202(4):742–7.
77. Einhorn LH, Williams SD, Loehrer PJ, Birch R, Drasga R, Omura G, et al. Evaluation of optimal duration of chemotherapy in favorable-prognosis disseminated germ cell tumors: a southeastern cancer study group protocol. J Clin Oncol. 1989;7(3):387–91.
78. Mencel PJ, Motzer RJ, Mazumdar M, Vlamis V, Bajorin DF, Bosl GJ. Advanced seminoma: treatment results, survival, and prognostic factors in 142 patients. J Clin Oncol. 1994;12(1):120–6.
79. Culine S, Abs L, Terrier-Lacombe MJ, Théodore C, Wibault P, Droz JP. Cisplatin-based chemotherapy in advanced seminoma: the Institut Gustave Roussy Experience. Eur J Cancer. 1998;34(3):353–8.
80. Gholam D, Fizazi K, Terrier-Lacombe MJ, Jan P, Culine S, Theodore C. Advanced seminoma—treatment results and prognostic factors for survival after first-line, cisplatin-based chemotherapy and for patients with recurrent disease: a single-institution experience in 145 patients. Cancer. 2003;98(4):745–52.
81. Culine S, Kerbrat P, Kramar A, Théodore C, Chevreau C, Geoffrois L, et al. Refining the optimal chemotherapy regimen for good-risk metastatic nonseminomatous germ-cell tumors: a randomized trial of the Genito-Urinary Group of the French Federation of Cancer Centers (GETUG T93BP). Ann Oncol. 2007;18(5):917–24.
82. Fizazi K, Delva R, Caty A, Chevreau C, Kerbrat P, Rolland F, et al. A risk-adapted study of cisplatin and etoposide, with or without ifosfamide, in patients with metastatic seminoma: results of the GETUG S99 multicenter prospective study. Eur Urol. 2014;65(2):381–6.
83. Kollmannsberger C, Beyer J, Droz JP, Harstrick A, Hartmann JT, Biron P, et al. Secondary leukemia following high cumulative doses of etoposide in patients treated for advanced germ cell tumors. J Clin Oncol. 1998;16(10):3386–91.
84. Arranz Arija JA, García del Muro X, Gumà J, Aparicio J, Salazar R, Saenz A, et al. E400P in advanced seminoma of good prognosis according to the international germ cell cancer collaborative group (IGCCCG) classification: the Spanish germ cell cancer group experience. Ann Oncol. 2001;12(4):487–91.
85. Horwich A, Dearnaley DP, A'Hern R, Mason M, Thomas G, Jay G, et al. The activity of single-agent carboplatin in advanced seminoma. Eur J Cancer. 1992;28A(8–9):1307–10.
86. Schmoll HJ, Harstrick A, Bokemeyer C, Dieckmann KP, Clemm C, Berdel WE, et al. Single-agent carboplatinum for advanced seminoma. A phase II study. Cancer. 1993;72(1):237–43.
87. Oliver RT, Lore S, Ong J. Alternatives to radiotherapy in the management of seminoma. Br J Urol. 1990;65(1):61–7.
88. Bokemeyer C, Kollmannsberger C, Stenning S, Hartmann JT, Horwich A, Clemm C, et al. Metastatic seminoma treated with either single agent carboplatin or cisplatin-based combination chemotherapy: a pooled analysis of two randomised trials. Br J Cancer. 2004;91(4):683–7.
89. de Wit R, Stoter G, Kaye SB, Sleijfer DT, Jones WG, ten Bokkel Huinink WW, et al. Importance of bleomycin in combination chemotherapy for good-prognosis testicular nonseminoma: a randomized study of the European Organization for Research and Treatment of Cancer Genitourinary Tract Cancer Cooperative Group. J Clin Oncol. 1997;15(5):1837–43.
90. Levi JA, Raghavan D, Harvey V, Thompson D, Sandeman T, Gill G, et al. The importance of bleomycin in combination chemotherapy for good-prognosis germ cell carcinoma. Australasian germ cell trial group. J Clin Oncol. 1993;11(7):1300–5.
91. Loehrer PJ, Johnson D, Elson P, Einhorn LH, Trump D. Importance of bleomycin in favorable-prognosis disseminated germ cell tumors: an eastern cooperative oncology group trial. J Clin Oncol. 1995;13(2):470–6.
92. Kondagunta GV, Bacik J, Bajorin D, Dobrzynski D, Sheinfeld J, Motzer RJ, Bosl GJ. Etoposide and cisplatin chemotherapy for metastatic good-risk germ cell tumors. J Clin Oncol. 2005;23(36):9290–4.
93. de Wit R, Roberts JT, Wilkinson PM, de Mulder PH, Mead GM, Fosså SD, et al. Equivalence of three or four cycles of bleomycin, etoposide, and cisplatin chemotherapy and of a 3- or 5-day schedule in good-prognosis germ cell cancer: a randomized study of the European Organization for Research and Treatment of Cancer Genitourinary Tract Cancer Cooperative Group and the Medical Research Council. J Clin Oncol. 2001;19(6):1629–40.
94. Bajorin DF, Sarosdy MF, Pfister DG, Mazumdar M, Motzer RJ, Scher HI, et al. Randomized trial of etoposide and cisplatin versus etoposide and carboplatin in patients with good-risk germ cell tumors: a multiinstitutional study. J Clin Oncol. 1993;11(4):598–606.
95. Horwich A, Sleijfer DT, Fosså SD, Kaye SB, Oliver RT, Cullen MH, et al. Randomized trial of bleomycin, etoposide, and cisplatin compared with bleomycin, etoposide, and carboplatin in good-prognosis metastatic nonseminomatous germ cell cancer: a multiinstitutional Medical Research Council/European Organization for Research and Treatment of cancer trial. J Clin Oncol. 1997;15(5):1844–52.
96. Grimison PS, Stockler MR, Thomson DB, Olver IN, Harvey VJ, Gebski VJ, et al. Comparison of two standard chemotherapy regimens for good-prognosis germ cell tumors: updated analysis of a randomized trial. J Natl Cancer Inst. 2010;102(16):1253–62.
97. Shamash J, Sarker SJ, Huddart R, Harland S, Joffe JK, Mazhar D, et al. A randomized phase III study of 72 h infusional versus bolus bleomycin in BEP (bleomycin, etoposide and cisplatin) chemotherapy to treat IGCCCG good prognosis metastatic germ cell tumours (TE-3). Ann Oncol. 2017;28(6):1333–8.

98. Lauritsen J, Kier MGG, Bandak M, Mortensen MS, Thomsen FB, Mortensen J, et al. Pulmonary function in patients with germ cell cancer treated with bleomycin, etoposide, and cisplatin. J Clin Oncol. 2016;34(13):1492–9.
99. de Wit R, Stoter G, Sleijfer DT, Neijt JP, ten Bokkel Huinink WW, de Prijck L, et al. Four cycles of BEP vs. four cycles of VIP in patients with intermediate-prognosis metastatic testicular non-seminoma: a randomized study of the EORTC genitourinary tract cancer cooperative group. European Organization for Research and Treatment of Cancer. Br J Cancer. 1998;78(6):828–32.
100. de Wit R, Skoneczna I, Daugaard G, De Santis M, Garin A, Aass N, et al. Randomized phase III study comparing paclitaxel-bleomycin, etoposide, and cisplatin (BEP) to standard BEP in intermediate-prognosis germ-cell cancer: intergroup study EORTC 30983. J Clin Oncol. 2012;30(8):792–9.
101. Seidel C, Daugaard G, Tryakin A, Necchi A, Cohn Cedermark G, Ståhl O, et al. Intermediate prognosis in metastatic germ cell tumours-outcome and prognostic factors. Eur J Cancer. 2018;94:16–25.
102. Olofsson SE, Tandstad T, Jerkeman M, Dahl O, Ståhl O, Klepp O, et al. Population-based study of treatment guided by tumor marker decline in patients with metastatic nonseminomatous germ cell tumor: a report from the Swedish-Norwegian testicular cancer group. J Clin Oncol. 2011;29(15):2032–9.
103. Nichols CR, Catalano PJ, Crawford ED, Vogelzang NJ, Einhorn LH, Loehrer PJ. Randomized comparison of cisplatin and etoposide and either bleomycin or ifosfamide in treatment of advanced disseminated germ cell tumors: an eastern cooperative oncology group, southwest oncology group, and cancer and leukemia group B study. J Clin Oncol. 1998;16(4):1287–93.
104. Daugaard G, Skoneczna I, Aass N, De Wit R, De Santis M, Dumez H, et al. A randomized phase III study comparing standard dose BEP with sequential high-dose cisplatin, etoposide, and ifosfamide (VIP) plus stem-cell support in males with poor-prognosis germ-cell cancer. An intergroup study of EORTC, GTCSG, and Grupo germinal (EORTC 30974). Ann Oncol. 2011;22(5):1054–61.
105. Motzer RJ, Nichols CJ, Margolin KA, Bacik J, Richardson PG, Vogelzang NJ, et al. Phase III randomized trial of conventional-dose chemotherapy with or without high-dose chemotherapy and autologous hematopoietic stem-cell rescue as first-line treatment for patients with poor-prognosis metastatic germ cell tumors. J Clin Oncol. 2007;25(3):247–56.
106. Fizazi K, Pagliaro L, Laplanche A, Fléchon A, Mardiak J, Geoffrois L, et al. Personalised chemotherapy based on tumour marker decline in poor prognosis germ-cell tumours (GETUG 13): a phase 3, multicentre, randomised trial. Lancet Oncol. 2014;15(13):1442–50.
107. Thibault C, Fizazi K, Barrios D, Massard C, Albiges L, Baumert H, et al. Compliance with guidelines and correlation with outcome in patients with advanced germ-cell tumours. Eur J Cancer. 2014;50(7):1284–90.
108. Feldman DR, Hu J, Srinivas S, Stadler WM, Costello BA, Appleman LJ, et al. Multicenter randomized phase 2 trial of paclitaxel, ifosfamide, and cisplatin (TIP) versus bleomycin, etoposide, and cisplatin (BEP) for first-line treatment of patients (pts) with intermediate- or poor-risk germ cell tumors (GCT). J Clin Oncol. 2018;36(15_Suppl):4508.
109. Voss MH, Feldman DR, Motzer RJ. High-dose chemotherapy and stem cell transplantation for advanced testicular cancer. Expert Rev Anticancer Ther. 2011;11(7):1091–103.
110. Shea TC, Flaherty M, Elias A, Eder JP, Antman K, Begg C, et al. A phase I clinical and pharmacokinetic study of carboplatin and autologous bone marrow support. J Clin Oncol. 1989;7(5):651–61.
111. Wolff SN, Johnson DH, Hainsworth JD, Greco FA. High-dose VP-16-213 monotherapy for refractory germinal malignancies: a phase II study. J Clin Oncol. 1984;2(4):271–4.
112. Buckner CD, Clift RA, Fefer A, Funk DD, Glucksberg H, Neiman PE, et al. High-dose cyclophosphamide (NSC-26271) for the treatment of metastatic testicular neoplasms. Cancer Chemother Rep. 1974;58(5 Pt 1):709–14.
113. Chevreau C, Droz JP, Pico JL, Biron P, Kerbrat P, Cure H, et al. Early intensified chemotherapy with autologous bone marrow transplantation in first line treatment of poor risk non-seminomatous germ cell tumours. Preliminary results of a French randomized trial. Eur Urol. 1993;23(1):213–7. discussion 218
114. Motzer RJ, Mazumdar M, Bajorin DF, Bosl GJ, Lyn P, Vlamis V. High-dose carboplatin, etoposide, and cyclophosphamide with autologous bone marrow transplantation in first-line therapy for patients with poor-risk germ cell tumors. J Clin Oncol. 1997;15(7):2546–52.
115. Bokemeyer C, Harstrick A, Beyer J, Metzner B, Rüther U, Hartmann JT, et al. The use of dose-intensified chemotherapy in the treatment of metastatic nonseminomatous testicular germ cell tumors. German testicular cancer study group. Semin Oncol. 1998;25(2 Suppl 4):24–32; discussion 45–48.
116. Bokemeyer C, Kollmannsberger C, Meisner C, Harstrick A, Beyer J, Metzner B, et al. First-line high-dose chemotherapy compared with standard-dose PEB/VIP chemotherapy in patients with advanced germ cell tumors: a multivariate and matched-pair analysis. J Clin Oncol. 1999;17(11):3450–6.
117. Droz JP, Kramar A, Biron P, Pico JL, Kerbrat P, Pény J, et al. Failure of high-dose cyclophosphamide and etoposide combined with double-dose cisplatin and bone marrow support in patients with high-volume metastatic nonseminomatous germ-cell tumours: mature results of a randomised trial. Eur Urol. 2007;51(3):739–46; discussion 747–748.
118. Massard C, Plantade A, Gross-Goupil M, Loriot Y, Besse B, Raynard B, et al. Poor prognosis

nonseminomatous germ-cell tumours (NSGCTs): should chemotherapy doses be reduced at first cycle to prevent acute respiratory distress syndrome in patients with multiple lung metastases? Ann Oncol. 2010;21(8):1585–8.
119. Gillessen S, Powles T, Lim L, Wilson P, Shamash J. Low-dose induction chemotherapy with baby-BOP in patients with metastatic germ-cell tumours does not compromise outcome: a single-Centre experience. Ann Oncol. 2010;21(8):1589–93.
120. International Germ Cell Consensus Classification: a prognostic factor-based staging system for metastatic germ cell cancers. International germ cell cancer collaborative group. J Clin Oncol. 1997;15(2):594–603.
121. Gerl A, Clemm C, Kohl P, Schalhorn A, Wilmanns W. Central nervous system as sanctuary site of relapse in patients treated with chemotherapy for metastatic testicular cancer. Clin Exp Metastasis. 1994;12(3):226–30.
122. Bower M, Newlands ES, Holden L, Rustin GJ, Begent RH. Treatment of men with metastatic non-seminomatous germ cell tumours with cyclical POMB/ACE chemotherapy. Ann Oncol. 1997;8(5):477–83.
123. Williams SD, Einhorn LH. Brain metastases in disseminated germinal neoplasms: incidence and clinical course. Cancer. 1979;44(4):1514–6.
124. Feldman DR, Lorch A, Kramar A, Albany C, Einhorn LH, Giannatempo P, et al. Brain metastases in patients with germ cell tumors: prognostic factors and treatment options—an analysis from the global germ cell cancer group. J Clin Oncol. 2016;34(4):345–51.
125. Bokemeyer C, Nowak P, Haupt A, Metzner B, Köhne H, Hartmann JT, et al. Treatment of brain metastases in patients with testicular cancer. J Clin Oncol. 1997;15(4):1449–54.
126. Fosså SD, Bokemeyer C, Gerl A, Culine S, Jones WG, Mead GM, et al. Treatment outcome of patients with brain metastases from malignant germ cell tumors. Cancer. 1999;85(4):988–97.

Retroperitoneal Lymph Node Dissection

26

Ajit Gujela and Gagan Prakash

26.1 Lymphatic Drainage and Templates

The lymphatic route of dissemination to the retroperitoneal nodes is the most common pathway of spread for testicular GCT with the exception of choriocarcinoma which has a propensity for hematogenous spread.

The lymphatic drainage of the testis follows predictable and preferential pathways [1]. For right testis tumours (primary right side) [2], the inter aortocaval zone is the most common site of tumour deposition followed by paracaval zone. The preaortic and left paraaortic areas are the most common sites of left testis tumour nodal spread (primary left side) [1]. The pattern of lymphatic drainage is right to left in the retroperitoneum.

Historically, systematic bilateral retroperitoneal lymph node dissection—extending to the renal pedicles superiorly, to the bifurcation of the aorta inferiorly and to the ureters—laterally was performed [3]. Additionally resection of interiliac tissue up to the level of bifurcation of common iliac arteries often along with suprahilar tissue (above renal vessels up to the diaphragm) bilaterally was conducted for complete removal of disease [1, 3].

However, management of GCT and RPLND has undergone revolutionary changes on account of the advent of highly effective cisplatin-based chemotherapy, information about primary landing zones of right versus left primary disease and the need to preserve the post-sympathetic ganglionic fibres for the preservation of ejaculatory function. The findings of Ray and associates [3] put forth the idea of the feasibility of limiting retroperitoneal lymph node dissection for clinical stage I disease to those areas in which solitary metastases occur. Thus modified RPLND templates were introduced and supported later by scientific literature [1].

As a result, several modified templates have been presented, all of which follow four basic principles as follows:

(a) Include ipsilateral lymph node areas between the levels of the renal hilum and the bifurcation of common iliac vessels as a minimum template.
(b) For right-sided primary tumours, the interaortocaval lymph nodes are to be included.
(c) Avoid dissection in the contralateral sympathetic trunk region.
(d) To avoid harm to the sympathetic postganglionic fibres and hypogastric plexus, avoid contralateral dissection below IMA [4] (Fig. 26.1).

A. Gujela · G. Prakash (✉)
Department of Surgical Oncology (Uro Oncology Unit), Homi Bhabha National Institute, Tata Memorial Centre, Tata Memorial Hospital, Mumbai, India

P. Singh et al. (eds.), *A Guide to Management of Urological Cancers*,
https://doi.org/10.1007/978-981-99-2341-0_26

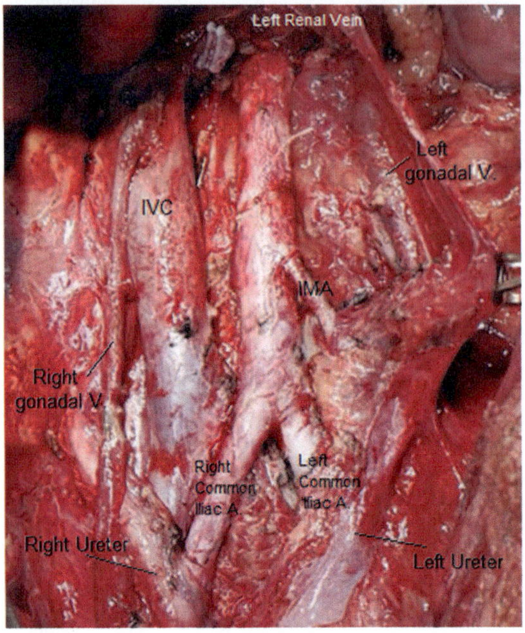

Fig. 26.1 RPLND template

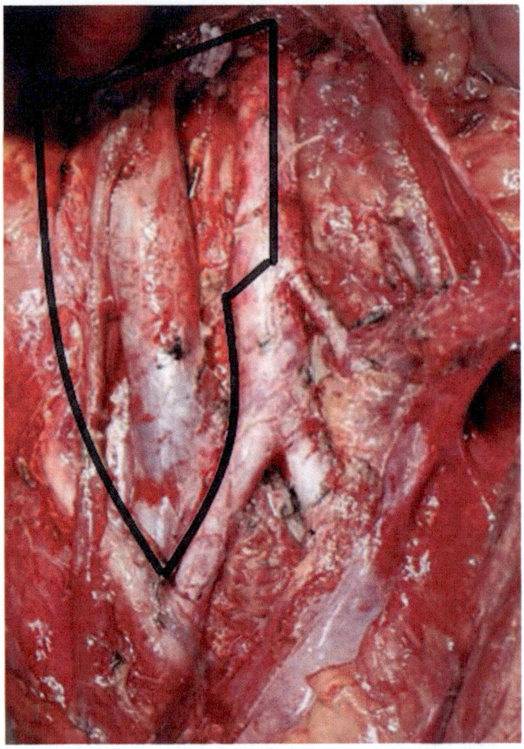

Fig. 26.2 Right modified template

26.1.1 Modified Template Resection of the Right Side

Boundary of resection—laterally, right ureter; cranially, right renal vessels; and caudally, right ureter crossing the right common iliac vessels and medially including the interaortocaval lymph nodes up to the inferior mesenteric artery. Thus the lymph node packet includes the precaval, caval, paracaval, retrocaval and inter-aortocaval regions, as well as the region lateral to the common iliac vessels with sparing of the left sympathetic nerves [5] (Fig. 26.2).

26.1.2 Modified Template Resection of the Left Side

Boundary of resection—laterally, left ureter; cranially, left renal vessels; and caudally, left ureter crossing the left common iliac vessels and medially including the superficial interaortocaval and preaortal lymph nodes up to the inferior mesenteric artery. Thus the lymph node packets include the preaortic, retro-aortic and paraaortic lymph nodes with sparing of the right sympathetic nerves [5] (Fig. 26.3).

Avoiding suprahilar dissection reduced the risk of chylous ascites, renal injury and pancreatic and/or duodenal injuries. Preservation of antegrade ejaculatory function in the majority of men was possible by avoiding the interiliac and contralateral retroperitoneum.

Many worldwide facilities continue to employ modified surgical templates that minimise contralateral dissection to increase rates of antegrade ejaculation postoperatively [4, 6]. However, studies have recently cast doubt on their utility based on viable extra-template disease in at least 7–32% of patients in the postchemotherapy scenario [7, 8] depending on the template utilised. As attempt to spare ejaculation at the risk of incomplete cancer removal is never a good idea, a complete bilateral infrahilar template bounded laterally by ureters, cranially by renal vessels and caudally by aortic

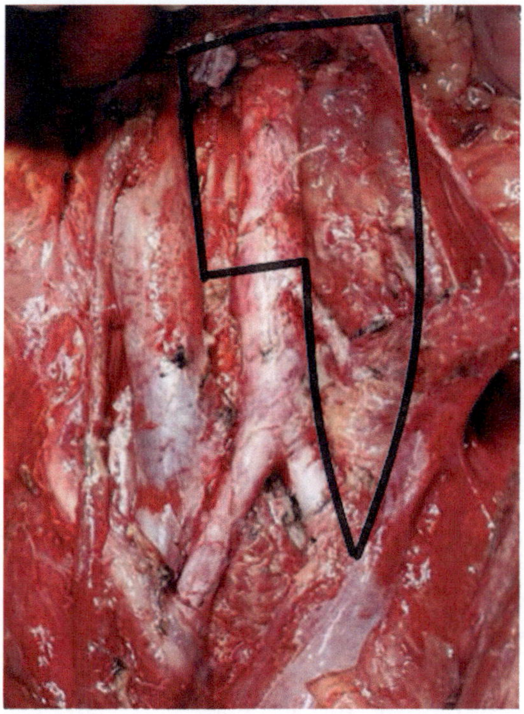

Fig. 26.3 Left modified template

bifurcation is the most judicious option oncologically, and nerve-sparing procedures should be used only when absolutely necessary [9].

26.2 Types of RPLND

- Primary RPLND—Upfront RPLND performed after orchidectomy with serum tumour markers in normal range in CSI high-risk NSGCT or CSII low-volume (N1) NSGCT [10].
- Postchemotherapy RPLND (PC-RPLND)—After induction chemotherapy for residual retroperitoneal masses ≥1 cm with serum tumour markers in normal range. Residual or growing masses after chemotherapy are the results of either teratoma or viable GCT [10].
- Salvage postchemotherapy RPLND—After both induction and salvage chemotherapy with serum tumour markers in normal range with residual radiographic disease. After salvage chemotherapy, RPLND has to be performed independent of the residual tumour diameter [11].
- Desperation RPLND—After at least two lines of chemotherapy with elevated serum tumour markers. Elevated serum tumour markers are associated with both a lower OS and higher risks of finding active cancer [12].
- Redo or reoperative RPLND—After a previous RPLND for any residual masses. Risk factors—tumour biology, that is, teratoma and inadequate surgical clearance—are left para-aortic and left renal hilar regions are the most common sites of retroperitoneal failure [13, 14].
- RPLND for late relapse—For relapse >24 months after complete response due to primary therapy (which may or may not have included RPLND).

26.3 Approaches for RPLND

Three approaches of RPLND include the following:

- Open (O-RPLND)
- Laparoscopic (L-RPLND)
- Robotic (RA RPLND)

26.3.1 O-RPLND

Open RPLND traditionally has been done using the midline transperitoneal approach. It has been described later in this chapter. Another approach is the midline extraperitoneal approach. Studies from a few centres have shown that this approach can be performed safely in selected patients without compromising the completeness of the resection even in the postchemotherapy setting and is associated with rapid return of bowel function, minimal rates of ileus and short hospital stay [15, 16].

26.3.2 L-RPLND

L-RPLND is a technically challenging operation with a steep learning curve that should only be attempted by experienced surgeons who are comfortable and skilled with advanced techniques. Although some surgeons employ an extraperitoneal technique, most prefer a transperitoneal approach since the working anatomical space is larger and more familiar and also facilitates bilateral dissection when needed. Generally, supine position is preferred; however, some surgeons favour slightly elevating the ipsilateral flank when performing a unilateral template dissection.

Four 10 mm trocars are implanted in the midline, uniformly spaced from the xyphoid process to the public symphysis, for L-RPLND. An additional 5 mm port may be placed laterally to assist with the spermatic cord (SC) dissection [17, 18].

Surgical technique and templates are similar to that of O-RPLND beginning with bowel mobilisation to expose the retroperitoneum followed by defining the template for lymphadenectomy. L-RPLND allows for a faster recovery with a shorter hospital stay, as well as issues similar to O-RPLND. L-RPLND is a viable and effective method that offers the advantages of minimally invasive surgery [17, 18].

26.3.3 RA-RPLND

Similar to L-RPLND, RA-RPLND is a technically demanding surgery requiring high level of skills and experience in robotic as well as open retroperitoneal surgeries. RA-RPLND could be performed in modified flank position with ipsilateral side up or the more accepted technique of patient in supine with Trendelenburg position allowing access to bilateral retroperitoneum. All ports are placed infra-umbilically (Fig. 26.4).

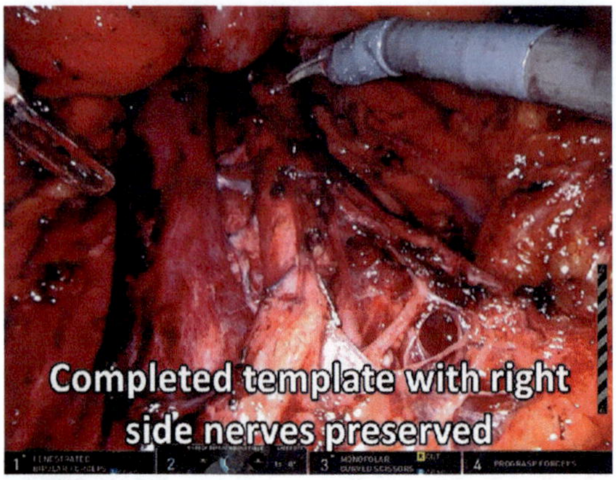

Fig. 26.4 Robotic RPLND with right lumbar sympathetic nerves preserved

Access to the retroperitoneum is achieved by incising the posterior peritoneum immediately medial to the cecum and extending to the Treitz ligament. Suturing both cut ends of the parietal peritoneum to the anterior abdominal wall 'raises a curtain' exposing the retroperitoneum. Technique of RPLND in supine approach was same as in open RPLND. Some concerns about an unusual pattern of recurrence have been raised recently. Bleeding is the commonest cause for conversion to open surgery, and vascular injury is the most common intraoperative complication.

26.4 Surgical Technique

26.4.1 Presurgical Planning

Basic preoperative assessment should include the following:

- CECT abdomen and pelvis scan within 4–6 weeks of surgery. It helps in planning surgery by understanding patient anatomy and disease extent better and plan for intraoperative consultation.
- No preoperative bowel preparation required.
- Preoperative sperm banking should be offered and recommended to all patients who desire future paternity.
- Assessment for pulmonary toxicity due to preoperative chemotherapy regimen (bleomycin-based) and discussion with anaesthesia team for the same.

26.4.2 Open RPLND

Position—supine position with the arms extended slightly below a 90-degree angle. A midline incision is carried from the level of the xyphoid to just few centimetres above pubic symphysis, and the peritoneal cavity is entered sharply and the falciform towards the superior IVC is released to avoid hepatic injury from retraction. For some patients, an extraperitoneal approach has been promoted since it gives a shorter length of stay [19] and a faster recovery of bowel function.

26.4.3 Exposure of the Retroperitoneum

From the tip of the cecum to the medial aspect of the inferior mesenteric vein, an incision is made. The peritoneal reflection (white line of Toldt) is incised up the ascending colon to the level of the foramen of Winslow–Cattell Braasch manoeuvre if complete bowel mobilisation is needed, followed by placement of the intestines on the chest. The inferior mesenteric vein can be sacrificed to help in the exposure of the left retroperitoneum in situations of big left-sided malignancies.

The peritoneal reflection (white line of Toldt) of the descending colon is incised if a modified left-sided approach is used—Mattox procedure. A plane is formed between the mesentery and the retroperitoneal fat. Identifying the gonadal vein and ureter and keeping anterior to these structures may make it easier to find the plane. The pancreas' inferior surface and the duodenum are released from the surface of the renal vessels, IVC and aorta. Liberal use of clips in this area helps reduce the chance of a postoperative chylous leak.

26.4.4 Split-and-Roll Technique

Fascia and tissue over the great vessels is spilt—beginning with the IVC or aorta in cranial-caudal or caudal-to-cranial approach depending upon the surgeon's preference and the template planned. The ability to locate the superior hypogastric plexus using the postganglionic sympathetic nerves originating from the right side may be one advantage of starting on the aorta. The objective is to locate this plexus and protect it from harm if a nerve-sparing procedure is planned.

26.4.5 Anatomy of Sympathetic Nerves

Four post ganglionic efferent sympathetic fibres (L1, L2, L3, L4) are responsible for antegrade ejaculation in men. Some of these fibres fuse to form three efferent fibres which exit the right sympathetic chain beneath the IVC travel in the interaortocaval space and join the three paraaortic fibres which exit the left parasympathetic chain, to generate the hypogastric plexus over the aortic surface.

26.4.6 Paracaval Node Dissection

While separating the paracaval nodal tissue from Gerota's fascia, care must be made to dissect and preserve the right ureter. The right gonadal vein may be ligated; thus nodal tissue may be easily detached from the caval adventitia, which is free of sympathetic tissue. A varied number of lumbar veins (typically 2–3) may appear when the IVC is rolled to the left. The plane between the paracaval nodal tissue and the fascia overlaying the psoas major muscle can be split with a right-sided approach to reveal the sympathetic chain. These may be mistaken for lymphatic tissue or vessels but should be preserved, particularly in a nerve-sparing RPLND [9].

26.4.7 Interaortocaval Node Dissection

The plane between the interaortocaval nodal tissue and the caval adventitia can be separated without encountering sympathetic nerves using the split-and-roll method on the IVC. The left lumbar veins (variable) can be identified by following this plane, which are often seen draining centrally. After the lumber veins have been ligated, complete control of the veins should be accomplished, and the IVC can be fully mobilised. To locate the lumbar sympathetic nerves, thorough dissection of the right sympathetic chain should be performed anteriorly.

Normally, two lumbar sympathetic nerves connect the infrarenal region of the aortic plexus, separated about one vertebral level apart; however, auxiliary lumbar sympathetic nerves of equivalent size, coursing alongside and in parallel with the LSN proper, are a regular occurrence. For reference, vessel loops should be put around the LSNs. The right chord of the aortic plexus can be seen by following the right lumbar sympathetic nerves anteriorly. The infrarenal abdominal aorta has a longitudinal nerve that runs along the antero-medial side which contributes to the formation of the superior hypogastric plexus [9] (Fig. 26.5).

The preaortic nodes can be divided with care to maintain any preaortic nerves that may link with the contralateral cord of the aortic plexus once the right-sided nerves have been preserved. Following that, dissection might progress down the aortic adventitia to determine the lumbar arteries. Typically, three pairs of lumbar arteries run along the infrarenal abdominal aorta, with the origin of the IMA used to approximate the site of the middle pair (third lumbar arteries). The anterior and lateral attachments of the lymph node packet are totally freed at this stage. To avoid a postoperative chylous leak, the lymphatics should be ligated at the cephalad level at this stage.

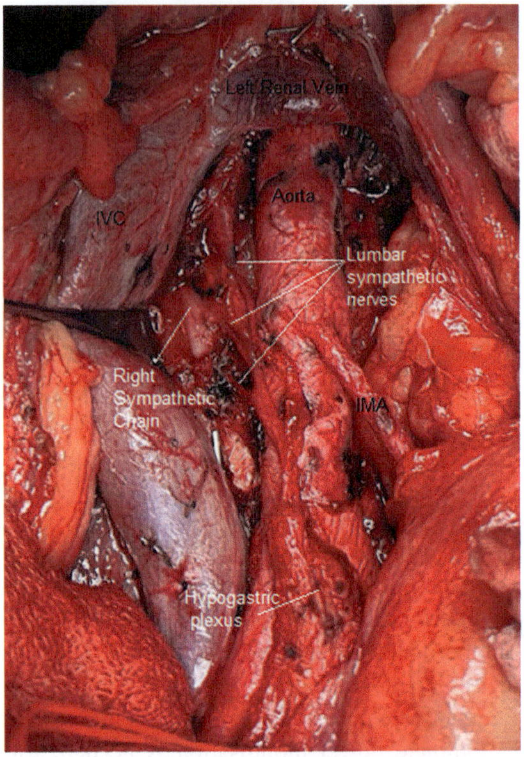

Fig. 26.5 Right lumbar sympathetic nerves preserved

26.4.8 Paraaortic Node Dissection

The paraaortic dissection is frequently difficult, especially at the superior border, which might be a cause of in-field recurrence. The anterior split along the aorta and iliac vessels continues caudally until the ureter crossing, which will encompass about a portion of the left common iliac artery while preserving the inferior mesenteric artery. Accessing the inferior paraaortic nodal tissue can be achieved by incising the white line of Toldt to mobilise the descending colon, facilitating medial reflection of the distal bowels and their mesentery. The left lumbar arteries can be identified and ligated by dissecting along the plane of the aortic adventitia. Studies have shown that there is a significant propensity for the lumbar arteries to be located at comparable levels; the position of the right lumbar arteries can aid in identifying left lumbar arteries.

While the aortic plexus is frequently bilaterally symmetric in its organisation, it is important to note that it seldom shows a bilateral symmetric location. As a result, the location of the right LSNs cannot be utilised to identify the position of the left LSNs. Near the IMA's beginning and near the intersection of the second infrared LSN, the inferior mesenteric ganglion and the left chord of the aortic plexus may be detected [9] (Fig. 26.6).

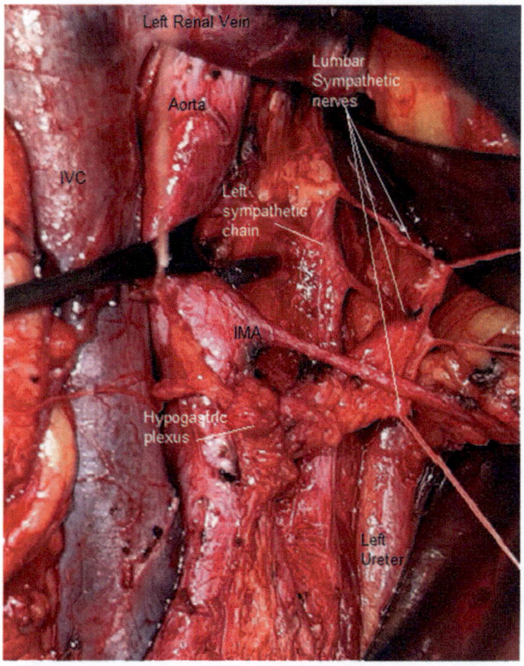

Fig. 26.6 Left sympathetic nerves preserved

26.5 Adjuvant/Additional Surgical Procedures

Adjuvant/additional surgical procedures are typically required in PC-RPLND setting with incidence rate of up to 30% [20–22]. A detailed study of preoperative imaging helps in identification of patients at increased risk. Most common adjuvant procedure is nephrectomy followed by vascular reconstruction.

26.5.1 Nephrectomy

- Incidence up to 30% [21, 23, 24]
- High-risk settings—post-salvage chemotherapy, desperation RPLND, late relapse, reoperative RPLND and bulky disease >10 cm [21].
- Renal replacement therapy or substitution for cisplatin due to compromised renal function in case of relapse is not required due to young age of patient and good renal reserve [23].

26.5.2 Vascular Reconstructions

- Incidence up to 15% [25, 26].
- High-risk settings—multiple cytotoxic regimens, presence of cisplatin refractory germ cell tumours ,residual masses encasing vessel by more than 50%, residual tumour size ≥5 cm and intermediate or poor risk germ cell tumours [26, 27].
- Incidence of intraluminal thrombus at PC RPLND is 5.8%. Active cancer or teratoma is identified in 44.9% of thrombi. Most common site—right primary tumour, IVC followed by right renal vein and iliac vein for left, and primary tumour, left renal vein. Thrombus in the aorta is very rare [28].
- IVC reconstructions—primary repair, lateral venography, patch venoplasty, interposition bypass replacement and vena cava resection.
- Aortic reconstructions—Mostly required in cases of subadventitial dissection in densely adherent masses requiring polytetrafluoroethylene [29] or Dacron graft.

26.5.3 Liver Resections

- About 30–40% of individuals with NSGCT will develop extra-retroperitoneal metastases, with the liver being affected in 2–15% of instances [30–32].
- Despite the fact that PC-RPLND histology predicts extra-retroperitoneal histology better than other clinical factors in various studies, it cannot overcome the significant histologic discordance between different locations of residual disease [32–35].
- Because the histology of PC-RPLND cannot properly predict the histology of other locations, it should not be used to determine whether or not to resect remaining hepatic masses, as unresected residual disease puts patients at risk for late relapse [29, 35].
- Management options—individualised—biopsy and observation, microwave ablation and surgical resection.

Other adjuvant procedures include bowel and pelvic resections.

26.6 RPLND Outcomes

26.6.1 Primary RPLND

As no prospective randomised control trial exists for primary RPLND for clinical stage I or IIA disease resolve the debate between modified/unilateral template and full bilateral template dissections for primary RPLND remains unresolved. Even though the seminal work of Ray et al. [3] further supported by Donohue et al. 1982 and Weissbach et al. [1, 2] support the use of modified unilateral templates with its advantages, the study by Eggener et al. puts forth the risk of leaving disease behind in 3–23% of patients by using the modified unilateral templates [8]. It is obvious from the data described here that with proper patient selection, excellent surgical skill and the judicious use of adjuvant chemotherapy, better outcomes can be predicted in the vast majority of patients. Whether either a complete bilateral template or a modified/unilateral template should be required to be used to accomplish such outcomes is still unknown. Post primary RPLND–pN0 patients are to be observed with no adjuvant therapy. However, for pN1 or pN2 disease, controversies regarding further management in form of observation versus adjuvant chemotherapy exist except in cases of Teratoma wherein only observation is warranted.

26.6.2 PC-RPLND

In the postchemotherapy setting, the standard of care is a resection of the residual mass and a full bilateral infrahilar RPLND because it provided excellent control of the retroperitoneum, albeit at the cost of significant potential morbidity and frequent ejaculatory dysfunction in patients for whom a nerve-saving approach was not possible. Like in case of primary RPLND, there have been no prospective randomised control trials of full bilateral versus modified unilateral template approaches to PC-RPLND. Pathological outcomes of PC-RPLND—relative frequencies of teratoma, fibrosis and viable germ cell malignancy—are generally around 45%, 40% and 15%, respectively [36–39]. Presence of viable germ cell malignancy represents the resistance to chemotherapy regimen and warrants individualised treatment in form of systemic chemotherapy. No additional treatment is recommended for either fibrosis/necrosis or teratoma on final pathology after PC-RPLND [5-year about 50%].

26.6.3 Salvage RPLND

In salvage setting, that is, after primary and second-line/third-line chemotherapy regimens with residual retroperitoneal masses with normal serum tumour markers—the incidence of viable germ cell malignancy is two to three times of that in PC-RPLND with worse overall survival [5-year about 70%] [11, 40, 41].

26.6.4 Desperation RPLND

Desperation RPLND done in the setting of persistently elevated serum tumour markers despite chemotherapy has worse outcomes [5-year about 50%] due to higher relapses and progression, higher incidence of viable germ cell malignancy and malignancy outside retroperitoneum [40, 42, 43]. The favourable prognostic factors include elevation of α-fetoprotein alone, complete resection of residual disease, histological finding of differentiated teratoma in the resected tissues and normalisation of tumour markers after desperation—RPLND [44].

26.6.5 Reoperative RPLND

Lack of volume and experience in performing RPLND results in technical failure of the first operation leaving behind residual disease at primary staging RPLND or PC-RPLND. Risk factors include teratoma and inadequate surgical clearance mostly involving the left renal hilar and paraaortic regions [13, 14]. Re-do RPLND is associated with higher incidences of surgical complications and poorer oncological outcomes.

26.7 Late Relapse

Late relapse is seen in only 2–4% of patients mostly in retroperitoneum [45]. As the disease is resistant to chemotherapy, resectable disease should be subjected to RPLND [46]. No previous treatment, asymptomatic presentation and a single site of recurrence are all factors that indicate increased survival at the time of late relapse. During RPLND for late relapse, complete resection is related to considerably better survival [35].

26.8 Complications of RPLND

Overall complication rates for PC-RPLND—3.7% to 32% [47–49] with risk of peri-operative mortality –0.26% [49] and the incidence of intraoperative as well as postoperative complications is higher for bilateral PC-RPLND than for unilateral PC-RPLND [50]. Overall complication rates for primary RPLND—1.3–24% [19, 48, 51] with risk of mortality generally be zero [19, 48, 52].

26.8.1 Complications

Intra-operative: Ureteric injury and vascular injuries with resultant haemorrhage are most common intraoperative complications [50].

26.8.2 Lymphatic

Lymphocele—Localised accumulation of lymphatic fluid in surgical bed symptomatic/asymptomatic in nature. Meticulous ligation/clipping of lymphatic channels helps in prevention of lymphatic leak. Management options include observation and aspiration/drainage.

26.8.3 Chylous Ascites

Chylous ascites is the collection of chylomicron-containing lymphatic fluid in the retroperitoneal and peritoneal compartments. It has been reported that it occurs in 0.2–2.1% of patients in the primary setting, with greater incidence of 2–7% in postchemotherapy populations [2, 5, 8]. It commonly occurs in the second or third week after surgery, with symptoms including abdominal distention, anorexia, nausea, vomiting and difficulty in breathing.

The physical examination reveals the typical symptoms of an abdominal fluid thrill, with imaging demonstrating the diffuse presence of fluid throughout the abdominal cavity. The diagnosis is based on paracentesis, which reveals milky fluid. The fluid will be found to be an alkaline, triglyceride-rich fluid that stains positive for Sudan black. Dissections that include the suprahilar region as well as disruption of the cisterna chyli and its tributaries are more likely to result in this complication.

Management options take a step-by-step approach, beginning with paracentesis and assessing symptom remission. The implementation of a low-fat/medium-chain triglyceride diet and surveillance is beneficial, and many patients will not require any additional therapy. However, in the case of rapid reaccumulation and the development of recurring symptoms, an indwelling tunnelled drain is inserted, and complete parenteral nourishment is initiated, with oral intake restricted.

In the case of refractory or chronic large-volume ascites, a peritoneovenous (LeVeen) shunt and surgical exploration with attempted lymphatic leak closure are the final resorts [53].

26.8.4 Neurologic

Temporary neuropraxia in the thigh normally resolves after 4 weeks, although it might last for months. Symptomatic relief with opioids and nerve pain medicines such as gabapentin and nonsteroidal anti-inflammatories is only marginally beneficial. One of the most devastating neurologic complications that can occur with extensive residual masses, combined retroperitoneal and mediastinal dissection with division of lumbar and intercostal arteries and previous abdominal irradiation is spinal cord ischaemia with subsequent lower extremity paralysis [53].

26.8.5 Gastrointestinal

Following RPLND, postoperative paralytic ileus is a common complication. The use of an extraperitoneal technique may reduce this probability significantly. The majority of patients do not need regular postoperative nasogastric tubes. Small intestinal blockage needing surgical intervention is known to occur in less than 1% of cases. This has been observed to happen within 30 days of RPLND as well as years later.

26.8.6 Pulmonary

Pulmonary problems are uncommon; however they do occur more frequently after chemotherapy because of bleomycin-associated pulmonary damage. PE, pneumonia and acute respiratory distress syndrome with mechanical ventilation are examples of these consequences. The need of an expert anaesthesiologist in dealing with intraoperative and postoperative pulmonary problems cannot be overstated. Intraoperative fluid resuscitation is kept to a minimum and is not influenced by intraoperative urine output.

26.8.7 Venous Thromboembolism

RPLND, like all major abdominal procedures, has the risk of venous thromboembolism (VTE). However, because of the young patient group, the incidence of VTE consequences is less than 1%. The use of sequential compression devices, early mobilisation and ambulation and pharmacologic thromboprophylaxis when needed all contribute to a reduction in thromboembolic events.

26.9 Future Directions

For individuals with node-positive seminoma, the current standard of care is radiation or chemotherapy, which are linked with severe long-term morbidity, including secondary cancers, cardiovascular disease, metabolic syndrome and pulmonary toxicity. The PRIMETEST and SEMS trials support the use of RPLND in patients with clinical stage II A/B seminoma [54, 55].

The potential use of miR-371a-3p as a reliable predictor of PC-RPLND histopathology in residual masses has been studied. As a considerable fraction of patients have necrosis/fibrosis exclusively, miRNA may aid in patient selection for PC-RPLND and avoid a potentially morbid surgery [56, 57].

CT radiomics is an intriguing new method for better predicting the existence of malignant histology in retroperitoneal LN metastases from NSTGCTs, with the goal of decreasing overtreatment in this young patient population, and is being explored [58, 59].

References

1. Donohue JP, Zachary JM, Maynard BR. Distribution of nodal metastases in nonseminomatous testis cancer. J Urol. 1982;128(2):315–20.
2. Weissbach L, Boedefeld EA. Localization of solitary and multiple metastases in stage II nonseminomatous testis tumor as basis for a modified staging lymph node dissection in stage I. J Urol. 1987;138(1):77–82.
3. Ray B, Hajdu SI, Whitmore WF Jr. Distribution of retroperitoneal lymph node metastases in testicular germinal tumors. Cancer. 1974;33(2):340–8.
4. Katz MH, Eggener SE. The evolution, controversies, and potential pitfalls of modified retroperitoneal lymph node dissection templates. World J Urol. 2009;27(4):477–83.
5. Hiester A, Nini A, Fingerhut A, Große Siemer R, Winter C, Albers P, et al. Preservation of ejaculatory function after postchemotherapy retroperitoneal lymph node dissection (PC-RPLND) in patients with testicular cancer: template vs. bilateral resection. Front Surg. 2019;5:80.
6. Doerr A, Skinner EC, Skinner DG. Preservation of ejaculation through a modified retroperitoneal lymph node dissection in low stage testis cancer. J Urol. 1993;149(6):1472–4.
7. Carver BS, Shayegan B, Eggener S, Stasi J, Motzer RJ, Bosl GJ, et al. Incidence of metastatic nonsemi-

nomatous germ cell tumor outside the boundaries of a modified postchemotherapy retroperitoneal lymph node dissection. J Clin Oncol. 2007;25(28):4365–9.
8. Eggener SE, Carver BS, Sharp DS, Motzer RJ, Bosl GJ, Sheinfeld JJ. Incidence of disease outside modified retroperitoneal lymph node dissection templates in clinical stage I or IIA nonseminomatous germ cell testicular cancer. J Urol. 2007;177(3):937–43.
9. Beveridge TS, Allman BL, Johnson M, Power A, Sheinfeld J, Power NE. Retroperitoneal lymph node dissection: anatomical and technical considerations from a cadaveric study. J Urol. 2016;196(6):1764–71.
10. Speir RW, Cary C, Masterson TA. Surgical salvage in patients with advanced testicular cancer: indications, risks and outcomes. Transl Androl Urol. 2020;9(Suppl 1):S83.
11. Albers P, Nini A, Hiester A, Winter C, Lusch A, Lorch A. Postchemotherapy retroperitoneal lymph node dissection (PC-RPLND) in patients with testis cancer in the salvage setting. Eur Urol. 2019;37(7_Suppl):524.
12. Coogan CL, Foster RS, Rowland RG, Bihrle R, Smith ER Jr, Einhorn LH, et al. Postchemotherapy retroperitoneal lymph node dissection is effective therapy in selected patients with elevated tumor markers after primary chemotherapy alone. Urology. 1997;50(6):957–62.
13. Pedrosa JA, Masterson TA, Rice KR, Bihrle R, Beck SD, Foster RS. Reoperative retroperitoneal lymph node dissection for metastatic germ cell tumors: analysis of local recurrence and predictors of survival. J Urol. 2014;191(6):1777–82.
14. Murphy AM, McKiernan JM. Reoperative retroperitoneal lymph-node dissection for testicular germ cell tumor. World J Urol. 2009;27(4):501–6.
15. Syan-Bhanvadia S, Bazargani ST, Clifford TG, Cai J, Miranda G, Daneshmand S. Midline extraperitoneal approach to retroperitoneal lymph node dissection in testicular cancer: minimizing surgical morbidity. Eur Urol. 2017;72(5):814–20.
16. Kim P, Syan-Bhanvadia S, Djaladat H, Faber K, Tadros NN, Nichols C, et al. Midline extraperitoneal approach for retroperitoneal lymph node dissection for testicular germ cell tumor. Urology. 2012;80(4):941–5.
17. Hillelsohn JH, Duty BD, Okhunov Z, Kavoussi LR. Laparoscopic retroperitoneal lymph node dissection for testicular cancer. Arab J Urol. 2012;10(1):66–73.
18. Shishido T, Okegawa T, Hayashi K, Masuda K, Taguchi S, Nakamura Y, et al. Laparoscopic retroperitoneal lymph node dissection versus open retroperitoneal lymph node dissection for testicular cancer: a comparison of clinical and perioperative outcomes. Asian J Urol. 2022;9(2):119–24.
19. Heidenreich A, Albers P, Hartmann M, Kliesch S, KÖHrmann K-U, Krege S, et al. Complications of primary nerve sparing retroperitoneal lymph node dissection for clinical stage I Nonseminomatous germ cell tumors of the testis: experience of the German testicular cancer study group. J Urol. 2003;169(5):1710–4.
20. Heidenreich A, Paffenholz P, Nestler T, Pfister DJ. Primary and postchemotherapy retroperitoneal lymphadenectomy for testicular cancer. Oncol Res Treat. 2018;41(6):370–8.
21. Cary KC, Beck SD, Bihrle R, Foster RS. Clinical and pathological features predictive of nephrectomy at post-chemotherapy retroperitoneal lymph node dissection. J Urol. 2013;189(3):812–7.
22. Blok JM, Meijer RP, van der Poel HG, Bex A, van Vooren J, van Urk JJ, et al. Additional surgical procedures and perioperative morbidity in post-chemotherapy retroperitoneal lymph node dissection for metastatic testicular cancer in two intermediate volume hospitals. World J Urol. 2021;39(3):839–46.
23. Stephenson AJ, Tal R, Sheinfeld JJ. Adjunctive nephrectomy at post-chemotherapy retroperitoneal lymph node dissection for nonseminomatous germ cell testicular cancer. J Urol. 2006;176(5):1996–9.
24. Macleod LC, Rajanahally S, Nayak JG, Parent BA, Ramos JD, Schade GR, et al. Characterizing the morbidity of postchemotherapy retroperitoneal lymph node dissection for testis cancer in a national cohort of privately insured patients. Urology. 2016;91:70–6.
25. Djaladat H, Nichols C, Daneshmand SJ. Adjuvant surgery in testicular cancer patients undergoing post-chemotherapy retroperitoneal lymph node dissection. Ann Surg Oncol. 2012;19(7):2388–93.
26. Heidenreich A, Haidl F, Paffenholz P, Pape C, Neumann U, Pfister DJ. Surgical management of complex residual masses following systemic chemotherapy for metastatic testicular germ cell tumours. Ann Oncol. 2017;28(2):362–7.
27. Winter C, Pfister D, Busch J, Bingöl C, Ranft U, Schrader M, et al. Residual tumor size and IGCCCG risk classification predict additional vascular procedures in patients with germ cell tumors and residual tumor resection: a multicenter analysis of the German Testicular Cancer Study Group. Eur Urol. 2012;61(2):403–9.
28. Johnston P, Beck SD, Cheng L, Masterson TA, Bihrle R, Kesler K, et al. Incidence, histology and management of intraluminal thrombus at post-chemotherapy retroperitoneal lymph node dissection. J Urol. 2013;190(3):874–7.
29. Sheinfeld JJ. Risks of the uncontrolled retroperitoneum. Ann Surg Oncol. 2003;10(2):100.
30. Hartmann J, Candelaria M, Kuczyk M, Schmoll H-J, Bokemeyer CJ. Comparison of histological results from the resection of residual masses at different sites after chemotherapy for metastatic non-seminomatous germ cell tumours. Eur J Cancer. 1997;33(6):843–7.
31. Fizazi K, Tjulandin S, Salvioni R, Germà-Lluch JR, Bouzy J, Ragan D, et al. Viable malignant cells after primary chemotherapy for disseminated nonseminomatous germ cell tumors: prognostic factors and role of postsurgery chemotherapy—results from an international study group. J Clin Oncol. 2001;19(10):2647–57.

32. Carver BS, Sheinfeld JJ. Management of post-chemotherapy extra-retroperitoneal residual masses. World J Urol. 2009;27(4):489–92.
33. Masterson TA, Shayegan B, Carver BS, Bajorin DF, Feldman DR, Motzer RJ, et al. Clinical impact of residual extraretroperitoneal masses in patients with advanced nonseminomatous germ cell testicular cancer. Urology. 2012;79(1):156–9.
34. Jacobsen N-EB, Beck SD, Jacobson LE, Bihrle R, Einhorn LH, Foster RS. Is retroperitoneal histology predictive of liver histology at concurrent post-chemotherapy retroperitoneal lymph node dissection and hepatic resection? J Urol. 2010;184(3):949–53.
35. Sharp DS, Carver BS, Eggener SE, Kondagunta GV, Motzer RJ, Bosl GJ, et al. Clinical outcome and predictors of survival in late relapse of germ cell tumor. J Clin Oncol. 2008;26(34):5524.
36. Hendry WF, Norman AR, Dearnaley DP, Fisher C, Nicholls J, Huddart RA, et al. Metastatic nonseminomatous germ cell tumors of the testis: results of elective and salvage surgery for patients with residual retroperitoneal masses. Cancer. 2002;94(6):1668–76.
37. Spiess PE, Tannir NM, Tu SM, Brown GA, Liu P, Kamat AM, et al. Viable germ cell tumor at post-chemotherapy retroperitoneal lymph node dissection: can we predict patients at risk of disease progression? Cancer. 2007;110(12):2700–8.
38. Carver BS, Bianco FJ Jr, Shayegan B, Vickers A, Motzer RJ, Bosl GJ, et al. Predicting teratoma in the retroperitoneum in men undergoing post-chemotherapy retroperitoneal lymph node dissection. J Urol. 2006;176(1):100–4.
39. Albers P, Weissbach L, Krege S, Kliesch S, Hartmann M, Heidenreich A, et al. Prediction of necrosis after chemotherapy of advanced germ cell tumors: results of a prospective multicenter trial of the German Testicular Cancer Study Group. J Urol. 2004;171(5):1835–8.
40. Donohue J, Leviovitch I, Foster R, Baniel J, Tognoni P. Integration of surgery and systemic therapy: results and principles of integration. Semin Urol Oncol. 1998;16(2):65–71.
41. Eggener SE, Carver BS, Loeb S, Kondagunta GV, Bosl GJ, Sheinfeld JJ. Pathologic findings and clinical outcome of patients undergoing retroperitoneal lymph node dissection after multiple chemotherapy regimens for metastatic testicular germ cell tumors. Cancer. 2007;109(3):528–35.
42. Albers P, Ganz A, Hannig E, Miersch WD, Müller SC. Salvage surgery of chemorefractory germ cell tumors with elevated tumor markers. J Urol. 2000;164(2):381–4.
43. Beck SD, Foster RS, Bihrle R, Einhorn LH, Donohue JP. Outcome analysis for patients with elevated serum tumor markers at postchemotherapy retroperitoneal lymph node dissection. J Clin Oncol. 2005;23(25):6149–56.
44. Ong TA, Winkler MH, Savage PM, Seckl MJ, Christmas T. Retroperitoneal lymph node dissection after chemotherapy in patients with elevated tumour markers: indications, histopathology and outcome. BJU Int. 2008;102(2):198–202.
45. Baniel J, Foster R, Rowland R, Bihrle R, Donohue JJ. Testis cancer: complications of post-chemotherapy retroperitoneal lymph node dissection. J Urol. 1995;153(3S):976–80.
46. Michael H, Lucia J, Foster RS, Ulbright TM. The pathology of late recurrence of testicular germ cell tumors. Am J Surg Pathol. 2000;24(2):257–73.
47. Mosharafa AA, Foster RS, Koch MO, Bihrle R, Donohue JP. Complications of post-chemotherapy retroperitoneal lymph node dissection for testis cancer. J Urol. 2004;171(5):1839–41.
48. Subramanian VS, Nguyen CT, Stephenson AJ, Klein EA. Complications of open primary and post-chemotherapy retroperitoneal lymph node dissection for testicular cancer. Urol Oncol. 2010;28(5):504–9.
49. Cary C, Masterson TA, Bihrle R, Foster RS. Contemporary trends in postchemotherapy retroperitoneal lymph node dissection: additional procedures and perioperative complications. Urol Oncol. 2015;33(9):389.e15–21.
50. Gerdtsson A, Håkansson U, Törnblom M, Jancke G, Negaard HF, Glimelius I, et al. Surgical complications in postchemotherapy retroperitoneal lymph node dissection for nonseminoma germ cell tumour: a population-based study from the Swedish Norwegian Testicular Cancer Group. Eur Urol Oncol. 2020;3(3):382–9.
51. Beck SDW, Peterson MD, Bihrle R, Donohue JP, Foster RS. Short-term morbidity of primary retroperitoneal lymph node dissection in a contemporary Group of Patients. J Urol. 2007;178(2):504–6.
52. Donohue JP, Thornhill JA, Foster RS, Rowland RG, Bihrle R. Retroperitoneal lymphadenectomy for clinical stage a testis cancer (1965 to 1989): modifications of technique and impact on ejaculation. J Urol. 1993;149(2):237–43.
53. Cary C, Foster RS, Masterson TA. Complications of retroperitoneal lymph node dissection. Urol Clin North Am. 2019;46(3):429–37.
54. Albers P, Lusch A, Che Y, Arsov C, Niegisch G, Hiester A. The PRIMETEST trial: Prospective phase II trial of primary retroperitoneal lymph node dissection (RPLND) in stage II A/B patients with seminoma. Eur Urol. 2022;40(6_Suppl):420.
55. Daneshmand S, Cary C, Masterson TA, Einhorn L, Boorjian SA, Kollmannsberger CK, et al. SEMS trial: result of a prospective, multi-institutional phase II clinical trial of surgery in early metastatic seminoma. Am Soc Clin Oncol. 2021;39:375.
56. Leão R, van Agthoven T, Figueiredo A, Jewett MA, Fadaak K, Sweet J, et al. Serum miRNA predicts viable disease after chemotherapy in patients with testicular nonseminoma germ cell tumor. J Urol. 2018;200(1):126–35.
57. Kremer L, von Brandenstein M, Wittersheim M, Koeditz B, Paffenholz P, Hellmich M, et al. The combination of microRNA-371a-3p and 375-5p can distinguish viable germ cell tumor and teratoma from

necrosis in postchemotherapy retroperitoneal lymph node dissection specimens. Transl Androl Urol. 2021;10(4):1647–55.

58. Baessler B, Nestler T, Pinto dos Santos D, Paffenholz P, Zeuch V, Pfister D, et al. Radiomics allows for detection of benign and malignant histopathology in patients with metastatic testicular germ cell tumors prior to post-chemotherapy retroperitoneal lymph node dissection. Eur Radiol. 2020;30(4):2334–45.
59. Nestler T, Baeßler B, Santos DPD, Pfister DJKP, Maintz D, Heidenreich A. Predicting vital retroperitoneal residual tumors of metastatic testicular tumor patients after chemotherapy using radiomics. J Clin Oncol. 2019;37(7_Suppl):527.

GPSR Compliance

The European Union's (EU) General Product Safety Regulation (GPSR) is a set of rules that requires consumer products to be safe and our obligations to ensure this.

If you have any concerns about our products, you can contact us on ProductSafety@springernature.com

In case Publisher is established outside the EU, the EU authorized representative is:

Springer Nature Customer Service Center GmbH
Europaplatz 3
69115 Heidelberg, Germany

Batch number: 10732799

Printed by Printforce, the Netherlands